PEDIATRICS, CHILD AND ADOLESCENT HEALTH

CHRONIC DISEASE AND DISABILITY

THE PEDIATRIC HEART

SECOND EDITION

Pediatrics, Child and Adolescent Health

Joav Merrick - Series Editor

National Institute of Child Health and Human Development,
Ministry of Social Affairs, Jerusalem

Chronic Disease and Disability: The Pediatric Heart, Second Edition
Donald E. Greydanus, Premchand Anne, John D. Rowlett and Joav Merrick (Editors)
2020. ISBN: 978-1-53617-656-8 (Hardcover)
2020. ISBN: 978-1-53617-657-5 (ebook)

Adolescence: Behavioural Risk Factors of Non-Communicable Diseases
Supa Pengpid, Karl Peltzer and Joav Merrick (Editors)
2020. ISBN: 978-1-53617-704-6 (Hardcover)
2020. ISBN: 978-1-53617-705-3 (e-book)

Adolescence in Curaçao
Soraya Verstraeten, Supa Pengpid, Karl Peltzer and Joav Merrick (Editors)
2020. ISBN: 978-1-53617-522-6 (softcover)
2020. ISBN: 978-1-53617-523-3 (e-book)

Building Youth for the Future: Suicide Prevention Aspects
Hatim A. Omar *and Joav Merrick (Editors)*
2019. ISBN: 978-1-53615-799-4 (Hardcover)
2019. ISBN: 978-1-53616-565-4 (e-book)

Vaccine: Measles and Rubella Vaccination Experience in Zambia
Mazyanga L. Mazaba-Liwewe, Seter Siziya and Joav Merrick (Editors)
2019. ISBN: 978-1-53615-799-4 (Hardcover)
2019. ISBN: 978-1-53615-800-7 (e-book)

The Boko Haram Terror: Adversary to the Wellbeing of Nigerian Kids
Miracle A. Adesina, Kehinde K. Kanmodi and Joav Merrick (Editors)
2019. ISBN: 978-1-53615-443-6 (Softcover)
2019. ISBN: 978-1-53615-444-3 (e-book)

Chronic Disease and Disability: Pediatric Obesity Perspectives
Marisha Agana, Donald E. Greydanus, Manmohan K. Kamboj and Joav Merrick (Editors)
2019. ISBN: 978-1-53615-240-1 (Hardcover)
2019. ISBN: 978-1-53615-241-8 (e-book)

Substance Use Disorders in Adolescents and Young Adults: A Manual for Pediatric and Primary Care Clinicians. Second Edition
Donald E. Greydanus, Gabriel Kaplan, Dilip R. Patel and Joav Merrick (Editors)
2019. ISBN: 978-1-53615-359-0 (Hardcover)
2019. ISBN: 978-1-53615-360-6 (e-book)

Building Youth for the Future: A Path towards Suicide Prevention
Hatim A. Omar and Joav Merrick (Editors)
2018. ISBN: 978-1-53613-768-2 (Hardcover)
2018. ISBN: 978-1-53613-769-9 (e-book)

Soft Skills and Aspirations in Chinese Children and Youth
Daniel T.L. Shek, Janet TY Leung and Joav Merrick (Editors)
2018. ISBN: 978-1-53614-092-7 (Hardcover)
2018. ISBN: 978-1-53614-093-4 (e-book)

Childhood and Adolescence: Tribute to Emanuel Chigier, 1928-2017
Joav Merrick (Editor)
2018. ISBN: 978-1-53613-574-9 (Hardcover)
2018. ISBN: 978-1-53613-574-9 (e-book)

Child Health and Human Development Yearbook 2017
Joav Merrick (Editor)
2018. ISBN: 978-1-53613-628-9 (Hardcover)
2018. ISBN: 978-1-53613-629-6 (e-book)

Child and Adolescent Health Yearbook 2017
Joav Merrick (Editor)
2018. ISBN: 978-1-53613-594-7 (Hardcover)
2018. ISBN: 978-1-53613-595-4 (e-book)

Chronic Disease and Disability: The Pediatric Gastrointestinal Tract
Donald E Greydanus, Orhan Atay, and Joav Merrick (Editors)
2018. ISBN: 978-1-53612-948-9 (Hardcover)
2018. ISBN: 978-1-53612-949-6 (e-book)

Multiple Sclerosis in Children and Adolescents
Hatim Omar and Joshua Chalkley (Editors)
2018. ISBN: 978-1-53612-979-3 (Hardcover)
2018. ISBN: 978-1-53612-980-9 (e-book)

Childhood and Adolescence: Tribute to Emanuel Chigier, 1928-2017
Joav Merrick (Editor)
2018. ISBN: 978-1-53613-574-9 (Softcover)
2018. ISBN: 978-1-53613-575-6 (e-book)

Chronic Disease and Disability: The Pediatric Lung
Donald E Greydanus, Myrtha M Gregoire-Bottex, Kevin W Cates and Joav Merrick (Editors)
2018. ISBN: 978-1-53613-577-0 (Hardcover)
2018. ISBN: 978-1-53613-578-7 (e-book)

Bicycles: Helmet Use of Adolescents at Independent Schools
Ronald Chow, Michael Borean, Drew Hollenberg, Jaclyn Viehweger, Tharani Anpalagan and Anna Rzepka (Editors)
2017. ISBN: 978-1-53612-458-3 (Hardcover)
2017. ISBN: 978-1-53612-459-0 (e-book)

Positive Youth Development: Long Term Effects in a Chinese Program
Daniel TL Shek, Cecilia MS Ma, Janet TY Leung and Joav Merrick (Editors)
2017. ISBN: 978-1-53612-539-9 (Hardcover)
2017. ISBN: 978-1-53612-540-5 (e-book)

Adolescence: Bicycle and Helmet Use of Adolescents and Young Adults
Ronald Chow and Joav Merrick (Editors)
2017. ISBN: 978-1-53612-039-4 (Hardcover)
2017. ISBN: 978-1-53612-060-8 (e-book)

Suicide: A Global View on Suicidal Ideation among Adolescents
Mazyanga L. Mazaba, Seter Siziya and Joav Merrick (Editors)
2017. ISBN: 978-1-53611-788-2 (Hardcover)
2017. ISBN: 978-1-53611-799-8 (e-book)

Children and Youth: Post-Traumatic Stress Disorder and Motor Vehicle Crashes
Donald E. Greydanus, Roger W. Apple, Kathryn White, and Joav Merrick (Editors)
2017. ISBN: 978-1-53611-102-6 (Hardcover)
2017. ISBN: 978-1-53611-255-9 (e-book)

Child and Adolescent Health Yearbook 2016
Joav Merrick (Editor)
2017. ISBN: 978-1-53610-948-1 (Hardcover)
2017. ISBN: 978-1-53610-957-3 (e-book)

Child Health and Human Development Yearbook 2016
Joav Merrick (Editor)
2017. ISBN: 978-1-53610-946-7 (Hardcover)
2017. ISBN: 978-1-53610-958-0 (e-book)

Chronic Disease and Disability: The Pediatric Kidney
Donald E Greydanus, Vimal Master Sankar Raj, and Joav Merrick (Editors)
2016. ISBN: 978-1-63483-793-4 (Hardcover)
2015. ISBN: 978-1-63483-809-2 (e-book)

Child and Adolescent Health Yearbook 2015
Joav Merrick (Editor)
2016. ISBN: 978-1-63484-512-0 (Hardcover)
2016. ISBN: 978-1-63484-543-4 (e-book)

Child Health and Human Development Yearbook 2015
Joav Merrick (Editor)
2016. ISBN: 978-1-63484-513-7 (Hardcover)
2016. ISBN: 978-1-63484-544-1 (e-book)

Pain Management Yearbook 2015
Joav Merrick (Editor)
2016. ISBN: 978-1-63484-515-1 (Hardcover)
2016. ISBN: 978-1-63484-545-8 (e-book)

Children and Childhood:
Some International Aspects
Joav Merrick (Editor)
2016. ISBN: 978-1-63484-587-8
(Hardcover)
2016. ISBN: 978-1-63484-594-6
(e-book)

Children and Adolescents:
Future Challenges
Daniel TL Shek, Tak Yan Lee,
and Joav Merrick (Editors)
2016. ISBN: 978-1-63484-616-5
(Hardcover)
2016. ISBN: 978-1-63484-627-1
(e-book)

Adolescence: Positive Youth
Development Programs
in Chinese Communities
Daniel TL Shek, Florence KY Wu,
Janet TY Leung, and Joav Merrick
(Editors)
2016. ISBN: 978-1-63484-044-6
(Hardcover)
2016. ISBN: 978-1-63484-677-6
(e-book)

Growing Up in the Middle East:
The Daily Lives and Well-Being
of Israeli and Palestinian Youth
Yossi Harel-Fisch, Ziad Abdeen
and Miriam Navot
2016. ISBN: 978-1-63484-746-9
(Hardcover)
2016. ISBN: 978-1-63484-765-0
(e-book)

Sexuality:
Some International Aspects
Joav Merrick
and Donald E Greydanus (Editors)
2016. ISBN: 978-1-63484-707-0
(Hardcover)
2016. ISBN: 978-1-63484-719-3
(e-book)

Chronic Disease and Disability:
The Pediatric Heart
Donald E Greydanus,
Devika Malhotra
and Joav Merrick (Editors)
2016. ISBN: 978-1-63484-828-2
(Hardcover)
2016. ISBN: 978-1-63484-842-8
(e-book)

Diabetes Mellitus:
Childhood and Adolescence
Manmohan K Kamboj,
Donald E Greydanus
and Joav Merrick (Editors)
2016. ISBN: 978-1-53610-095-2
(Hardcover)
2016. ISBN: 978-1-53610-104-1
(e-book)

Chronic Disease and Disability:
Abuse and Neglect in Childhood
and Adolescence
Donald E Greydanus,
Vincent J Palusci
and Joav Merrick (Editors)
2016. ISBN: 978-1-53610-129-4
(Hardcover)
2016. ISBN: 978-1-53610-142-3
(e-book)

Clinical Aspects of Psychopharmacology in Childhood and Adolescence, Second Edition
Donald E Greydanus, Joseph L Calles, Jr, Dilip R Patel, Ahsan Nazeer and Joav Merrick (Editors)
2016. ISBN: 978-1-53610-241-3 (Hardcover)
2016. ISBN: 978-1-53610-253-6 (e-book)

Chronic Disease and Disability: The Pediatric Pancreas
Donald E Greydanus, Manmohan K Kamboj and Joav Merrick (Editors)
2016. ISBN: 978-1-53610-055-6 (Hardcover)
2016. ISBN: 978-1-53610-065-5 (e-book)

A Pediatric Resident Pocket Guide: Making the Most of Morning Reports
Arthur N Feinberg
2015. ISBN: 978-1-63482-141-4 (Softcover)
2015. ISBN: 978-1-63482-186-5 (e-book)

Child and Adolescent Health Yearbook 2014
Joav Merrick (Editor)
2015. ISBN: 978-1-63482-162-9 (Hardcover)
2015. ISBN: 978-1-63482-206-0 (e-book)

Tropical Pediatrics: A Public Health Concern of International Proportions Second Edition
Richard R Roach, Donald E Greydanus, Dilip R Patel and Joav Merrick (Editors)
2015. ISBN: 978-1-63463-381-9 (Hardcover)
2015. ISBN: 978-1-63463-404-5 (e-book)

Child and Adolescent Health Issues (A Tribute to the Pediatrician Donald E Greydanus)
Joav Merrick (Editor)
2015. ISBN: 978-1-63463-574-5 (Hardcover)
2015. ISBN: 978-1-63463-576-9 (e-book)

Child Health and Human Development Yearbook 2014
Joav Merrick (Editor)
2015. ISBN: 978-1-63482-163-6 (Hardcover)
2015. ISBN: 978-1-63482-207-7 (e-book)

Behavioral Pediatrics, 4th Edition
Donald E Greydanus, Dilip R Patel, Helen D Pratt, Joseph L Calles Jr, Ahsan Nazeer and Joav Merrick (Editors)
2015. ISBN: 978-1-63483-027-0 (Hardcover)
2015. ISBN: 978-1-63483-052-2 (e-book)

Disability, Chronic Disease and Human Development
Joav Merrick
2015. ISBN: 978-1-63483-029-4 (Hardcover)
2015. ISBN: 978-1-63483-057-7 (e-book)

Caribbean Adolescents: Some Public Health Concerns
Cecilia Hegamin-Younge and Joav Merrick (Editors)
2015. ISBN: 978-1-63483-341-7 (Hardcover)
2015. ISBN: 978-1-63483-343-1 (e-book)

Adolescence and Health: Some International Perspectives
Joav Merrick (Editor)
2015. ISBN: 978-1-63483-791-0 (Hardcover)
2015. ISBN: 978-1-63483-808-5 (e-book)

Youth Suicide Prevention: Everybody's Business
Hatim A Omar (Editor)
2015. ISBN: 978-1-63483-786-6 (Softcover)
2015. ISBN: 978-1-63483-820-7 (e-book)

Human Developmental Research: Experience from Research in Hong Kong
Daniel TL Shek, Cecilia Ma, Yu Lu and Joav Merrick (Editors)
2014. ISBN: 978-1-62808-166-4 (Hardcover)
2013. ISBN: 978-1-62808-167-1 (e-book)

School, Adolescence and Health Issues
Joav Merrick, Ariel Tenenbaum and Hatim A Omar (Editors)
2014. ISBN: 978-1-62948-702-1 (Hardcover)
2014. ISBN: 978-1-62948-707-6 (e-book)

Adolescence and Sexuality: International Perspectives
Joav Merrick, Ariel Tenenbaum and Hatim A Omar (Editors)
2014. ISBN: 978-1-62948-711-3 (Hardcover)
2014. ISBN: 978-1-62948-724-3 (e-book)

Child and Adolescent Health Yearbook 2013
Joav Merrick (Editor)
2014. ISBN: 978-1-63117-658-6 (Hardcover)
2014. ISBN: 978-1-63117-668-5 (e-book)

Adoption: The Search for a New Parenthood
Gary Diamond and Eva Arbel
2014. ISBN: 978-1-63117-710-1 (Hardcover)
2014. ISBN: 978-1-63117-713-2 (e-book)

Adolescence: Places and Spaces
Myra F Taylor, Julie Ann Pooley and Joav Merrick (Editors)
2014. ISBN: 978-1-63117-847-4 (Hardcover)
2014. ISBN: 978-1-63117-850-4 (e-book)

Child Health and Human Development Yearbook 2013
Joav Merrick (Editor)
2014. ISBN: 978-1-63117-939-6 (Hardcover)
2013. ISBN: 978-1-63117-958-7 (e-book)

Born into this World: Health Issues
Donald E Greydanus, Arthur N Feinberg, and Joav Merrick (Editors)
2014. ISBN: 978-1-63321-667-9 (Hardcover)
2014. ISBN: 978-1-63321-669-3 (e-book)

Caring for the Newborn: A Comprehensive Guide for the Clinician
Donald E Greydanus, Arthur N Feinberg and Joav Merrick (Editors)
2014. ISBN: 978-1-63321-760-7 (Hardcover)
2014. ISBN: 978-1-63321-781-2 (e-book)

Environment and Hope: Impoving Health, Reducing AIDS and Promoting Food Security in the World
Leslie Rubin and Joav Merrick (Editors)
2014. ISBN: 978-1-63321-772-0 (Hardcover)
2014. ISBN: 978-1-63321-782-9 (e-book)

Pain Management Yearbook 2013
Joav Merrick (Editor)
2014. ISBN: 978-1-63117-944-0 (Hardcover)
2014. ISBN: 978-1-63117-959-4 (e-book)

Pediatric and Adolescent Dermatology: Some Current Issues
Donald E Greydanus, Arthur N Feinberg and Joav Merrick (Editors)
2014. ISBN: 978-1-63321-853-6 (Hardcover)
2014. ISBN: 978-1-63321-863-5 (e-book)

Adolescence and Behavior Issues in a Chinese Context
Daniel TL Shek, Rachel CF Sun, and Joav Merrick (Editors)
2013. ISBN: 978-1-62618-614-9 (Hardcover)
2013. ISBN: 978-1-62618-692-7 (e-book)

Advances in Preterm Infant Research
Jing Sun, Nicholas Buys and Joav Merrick
2013. ISBN: 978-1-62618-696-5 (Hardcover)
2013. ISBN: 978-1-62618-775-7 (e-book)

Child Health and Human Development: Social, Economic and Environmental Factors
Leslie Rubin and Joav Merrick (Editors)
2013. ISBN: 978-1-62948-166-1 (Hardcover)
2013. ISBN: 978-1-62948-169-2 (e-book)

Children, Violence and Bullying: International Perspectives
Joav Merrick, Isack Kandel and Hatim A Omar (Editors)
2013. ISBN: 978-1-62948-342-9 (Hardcover)
2013. ISBN: 978-1-62948-345-0 (e-book)

Chinese Adolescent Development: Economic Disadvantages, Parents and Intrapersonal Development
Daniel TL Shek, Rachel CF Sun and Joav Merrick (Editors)
2013. ISBN: 978-1-62618-622-4 (Hardcover)
2013. ISBN: 978-1-62618-694-1 (e-book)

Chronic Disease and Disability in Childhood
Joav Merrick
2013. ISBN: 978-1-62808-865-6 (Hardcover)
2013. ISBN: 978-1-62808-868-7 (e-book)

Environmental Health Disparities in Children: Asthma, Obesity and Food
Leslie Rubin and Joav Merrick (Editors)
2013. ISBN: 978-1-62948-122-7 (Hardcover)
2013. ISBN: 978-1-62948-135-7 (e-book)

Environmental Health: Home, School and Community
Leslie Rubin and Joav Merrick (Editors)
2013. ISBN: 978-1-62948-155-5 (Hardcover)
2013. ISBN: 978-1-62948-158-6 (e-book)

Guidelines for the Healthy Integration of the Ill Child in the Educational System: Experience from Israel
Yosefa Isenberg
2013. ISBN: 978-1-62808-350-7 (Hardcover)
2013. ISBN: 978-1-62808-353-8 (e-book)

Internet Addiction: A Public Health Concern in Adolescence
Artemis Tsitsika, Mari Janikian, Donald E Greydanus, Hatim A Omar and Joav Merrick (Editors)
2013. ISBN: 978-1-62618-925-6 (Hardcover)
2013. ISBN: 978-1-62618-959-1 (e-book)

Playing with Fire: Children, Adolescents and Firesetting
Hatim A. Omar, Carrie Howell Bowling and Joav Merrick (Editors)
2013. ISBN: 978-1-62948-471-6 (Softcover)
2013. ISBN: 978-1-62948-474-7 (e-book)

Promotion of Holistic Development of Young People in Hong Kong
Daniel TL Shek, Tak Yan Lee and Joav Merrick (Editors)
2013. ISBN: 978-1-62808-019-3 (Hardcover)
2013. ISBN: 978-1-62808-040-7 (e-book)

University and College Students: Health and Development Issues for the Leaders of Tomorrow
Daniel TL Shek, Rachel CF and Joav Merrick (Editors)
2013. ISBN: 978-1-62618-586-9 (Hardcover)
2013. ISBN: 978-1-62618-612-5 (e-book)

Break the Cycle of Environmental Health Disparities: Maternal and Child Health Aspects
Leslie Rubin and Joav Merrick (Editors)
2013. ISBN: 978-1-62948-107-4 (Hardcover)
2013. ISBN: 978-1-62948-133-3 (e-book)

Child and Adolescent Health Yearbook 2012
Joav Merrick (Editor)
2012. ISBN: 978-1-61942-788-4 (Hardcover)
2012. ISBN: 978-1-61942-789-1 (e-book)

Child Health and Human Development Yearbook 2011
Joav Merrick (Editor)
2012. ISBN: 978-1-61942-969-7 (Hardcover)
2012. ISBN: 978-1-61942-970-3 (e-book)

Child and Adolescent Health Yearbook 2011
Joav Merrick (Editor)
2012. ISBN: 978-1-61942-782-2 (Hardcover)
2012. ISBN: 978-1-61942-783-9 (e-book)

Tropical Pediatrics: A Public Health Concern of International Proportions
Richard R Roach, Donald E Greydanus, Dilip R Patel, Douglas N Homnick and Joav Merrick (Editors)
2012. ISBN: 978-1-61942-831-7 (Hardcover)
2012. ISBN: 978-1-61942-840-9 (e-book)

Child Health and Human Development Yearbook 2012
Joav Merrick (Editor)
2012. ISBN: 978-1-61942-978-9 (Hardcover)
2012. ISBN: 978-1-61942-979-6 (e-book)

Developmental Issues in Chinese Adolescents
Daniel TL Shek, Rachel CF Sun and Joav Merrick (Editors)
2012. ISBN: 978-1-62081-262-4 (Hardcover)
2012. ISBN: 978-1-62081-270-9 (e-book)

Positive Youth Development: Theory, Research and Application
Daniel TL Shek, Rachel CF Sun and Joav Merrick (Editors)
2012. ISBN: 978-1-62081-305-8 (Hardcover)
2012. ISBN: 978-1-62081-347-8 (e-book)

Understanding Autism Spectrum Disorder: Current Research Aspects
Ditza A Zachor and Joav Merrick (Editors)
2012. ISBN: 978-1-62081-353-9 (Hardcover)
2012. ISBN: 978-1-62081-390-4 (e-book)

Positive Youth Development: A New School Curriculum to Tackle Adolescent Developmental Issues
Hing Keung Ma, Daniel TL Shek and Joav Merrick (Editors)
2012. ISBN: 978-1-62081-384-3 (Hardcover)
2012. ISBN: 978-1-62081-385-0 (e-book)

Transition from Pediatric to Adult Medical Care
David Wood, John G Reiss, Maria E Ferris, Linda R Edwards and Joav Merrick (Editors)
2012. ISBN: 978-1-62081-409-3 (Hardcover)
2012. ISBN: 978-1-62081-412-3 (e-book)

PEDIATRICS, CHILD AND ADOLESCENT HEALTH

CHRONIC DISEASE AND DISABILITY

THE PEDIATRIC HEART

SECOND EDITION

DONALD E. GREYDANUS, MD, DrHC (Athens)
PREMCHAND ANNE, MD
JOHN D. ROWLETT, MD
AND
JOAV MERRICK, MD, MMedSci, DMSc
EDITORS

Medicine & Health
New York

Library of Congress Cataloging-in-Publication Data

Names: Greydanus, Donald E., editor.
Title: Chronic disease and disability: the pediatric heart / Donald E.
Greydanus, Premchand Anne, John D. Rowlett, Joav Merrick, editors.
Other titles: Pediatric heart
Identifiers: LCCN 2020010692 (print) | LCCN 2020010693 (ebook) |
ISBN 9781536176568 (hardcover) | ISBN 9781536176575 (adobe pdf)
Subjects: LCSH: Pediatric cardiology. | Chronic diseases in children. |
Heart--Growth. | Heart--Physiology.
Classification: LCC RJ421 .C49 2020 (print) | LCC RJ421 (ebook) | DDC 618.92/12--dc23
LC record available at https://lccn.loc.gov/2020010692
LC ebook record available at https://lccn.loc.gov/2020010693

Published by Nova Science Publishers, Inc. † New York

DEDICATION

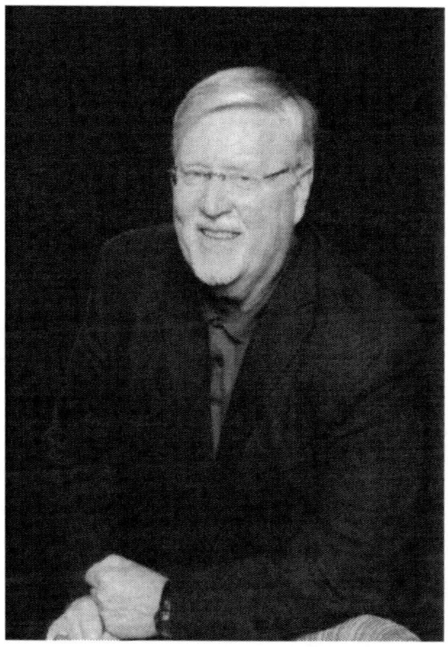

Eugene F Luckstead Sr, MD (1938-2013)

This book *"Chronic disease and disability: The pediatric heart, Second edition"* is dedicated to Eugene F Luckstead Sr, MD, a man who poured his own heart and soul into caring for the hearts of pediatric and adolescent patients.

Eugene was born and raised in Iowa where he excelled in both academics and athletics. He pursued higher education at the University of Iowa, where he graduated in 1959 with a degree in biology and in 1963 with a medical doctorate degree. He completed a residency in pediatrics, while serving in the Navy as Lieutenant Commander in Oakland, California. He continued his naval service while stationed in Long Beach, California, until 1968. He then completed a fellowship in pediatric cardiology at the University of Kansas.

Throughout his professional life, Eugene served as medical faculty at the University of Kansas, the University of Oklahoma, and the University of Iowa while he served as Chairman of the Department of Pediatrics at Blank Children's Hospital in Des Moines, Iowa. He also served as Medical Director of Cook Fort Worth Children's Hospital (Texas) and as Executive

Medical Director at Kings Daughters Children's Hospital in Norfolk, Virginia, where he also served as Professor of Pediatrics at Eastern Virginia Medical School. Finally, he served as Professor of Pediatrics at Texas Tech University Health Sciences center, while continuing to practice as a pediatric cardiologist until his death in 2013.

Selflessly serving others was the hallmark of Eugene's life. He cherished people and took great joy in helping his patients. Additionally, he was passionate about teaching and loved mentoring medical students, residents, and young physicians. He was an extensively published author of articles and texts on the topics of pediatric cardiology and pediatric and adolescent sports medicine as well as being a worldwide guest speaker on topics concerning sports medicine. Although Gene left a rich legacy as a skilled clinician, teacher, author, and speaker, his patients and those closest to him fondly reflect on his living out the philosophy that "every heart matters."

Eugene F Luckstead Jr, MD
Lubbock, Texas, United States of America
Email: eluckstead@suddenlink.net

Contents

INTRODUCTION

"Chronic disease and disability: The pediatric heart, Second edition" is written for health care professionals to help update knowledge of pediatric cardiology from the Aristotelean heart era and particularly from the past several decades. The current and future shortage of pediatric cardiologists necessitates steady, rejuvenated information on the Aristotelean heart for primary care clinicians as they care for the child as well as adolescent/young adult with cardiovascular dilemmas and disorders (1,2). In view of this shortage and the rapidly increasing knowledge in pediatric cardiology as well as understanding indications for referral to pediatric cardiologists in the 21st century, au courant assiduous information aimed at primary care clinicians in these areas becomes increasingly important (3-12).

Chapters in this book cover cardiologic problems in different pediatric ages from newborns to young adults. We begin with a history of medical knowledge regarding the heart starting when writing began in ancient Mesopotamia and progress to ancient Egypt, ancient Greece (Hippocrates, Aristotle) and beyond. Modern scientific knowledge of the human heart gradually emerged from what Aristotle taught (i.e., The Aristotelean heart) to our current understanding that is subject to further change with ongoing insight and research from current as well as future scholars.

As noted by some of the ancient polymaths, the heart does not exist in isolation but is involved in other aspects of the body---thus, we include discussions on hypertension that may involve renal pathophysiology and hyperlipidemia as well as obesity that involves various organ systems (13,14). Indeed, the interplay of the heart with the kidney and other bodily systems is a key aspect of modern research as well as clinical practice (13-23). Sleep health and sleep disorders are included to remind all clinicians of its critical importance for all pediatric persons—those with and without chronic illnesses such as cardiovascular disorders (24-31). We also look at issues of cardiac death in pediatric patients from various viewpoints (27,28,30,32-38).

Behavioral/psychiatric aspects of chronic diseases, including cardiac disorders, are also considered because of the importance that cardiac (and chronic) diseases have on all human beings including the newborn, child, adolescent and young adult. The interplay of physiology and psychology (including neurodevelopmental outcomes) in human health as well as disease is complex and often enigmatically Delphic (39-50). Thus, this book provides various aspects of both as 21st century research seeks further clarity on this often misunderstood and ignored interplay.

It is easy for a non-cardiologist to become lost in the complexities of cardiac physiology, diagnosis, and treatment—i.e., to miss the forest for the trees. It is not unusual for one to "fall" into the circulatory system and not return after being weighed down by a seemingly skimble-skamble litany of cardiac sagacities! We include some overlap in various discussions to help in this regard. Thus, one can ask: "what is the role ("the forest") of the primary care clinician in the diagnosis and management of pediatric cardiac disorders ("the trees")?"

The editors of this book thank our erudite experts for this Promethean perlustration as we plan our next edited enchiridion. The editors dedicate this work to a pediatric cardiologist and sports expert of sophisticated skills—a larger than life person, Eugene F Luckstead Sr, MD—who touched so many in his life as beautifully outlined by his son, Eugene Luckstead Jr, MD in his dedication. I (DEG) had the privilege of knowing Gene and worked with him on various projects that we shared (51,52). He particularly appreciated the interplay of pediatric cardiology and sports medicine as well as the blend of past with current medical knowledge (53-55).

Gene would have agreed with the premise of this book—helping all primary care clinicians in pediatric cardiology knowledge and improving the quality of life for those with cardiovascular disease (56). That was Gene Luckstead's legacy to the many fortunate enough to know him. Aristotle would have enjoyed knowing Gene and would be amazed by the knowledge about his Aristotelean heart that has been accumulated in the past two and half millennia as well as how concepts of cardiac complexity continue to be unraveled as the 21st century unfolds (55,57-60)!

"Mine is the first step and therefore a small one, though worked out with much thought and hard labor. You, my readers or hearers of my lectures, if you think I have done as much as can fairly be expected of an initial start. . . will acknowledge what I have achieved and will pardon what I have left for others to accomplish"

Aristotle (385 BC-322 BC)

References

[1] Jewett EA, Anderson MR, Gilchrist GS. The pediatric subspecialty workforce: public policy and forces for change. Pediatrics 2005;116(5):1192-202.

[2] Marelli AJ, Gurvitz M. From numbers to guidelines. Prog Cardiovasc Dis 2011;53(4):239-46.

[3] Hansen LK, Birkebaek NH, Oxhøj H. Initial evaluation of children with heart murmurs by non-specialized paediatrician. Eur J Pediatr 1995;154(1):15-7.

[4] Abdurrahman L, Bockoven JR, Pickoff AS, Ralston MA, Ross JE. Pediatric cardiology update: Office-based practice of pediatric cardiology for the primary care provider. Curr Probl Pediatr Adolesc Health Care 2003;33(10):318-47.

[5] Benun J, Fisher SD, Oray EJ, Schwartz ML, Exil V, Messere C, et al. Cardiac management by pediatricians versus pediatric cardiologists in an inpatient academic center. Am Heart J 2003;145(3):424-9.

[6] Geggel RL. Conditions leading to pediatric cardiology consultation in a tertiary academic hospital. Pediatrics 2004;114(4):e409-17.

[7] Lantin-Hermoso MR. Pediatric cardiology for the primary care pediatrician. Indian J Pediatr 2005;72(6):513-8.

[8] Washington R. Sports cardiology in the adolescent athlete: concerns for the pediatrician. Pediatr Ann 2007;36(11):698-702.

[9] Khushu A, Kelsall AW, Usher-Smith JA. Outcome of children [corrected] with heart murmurs referred from general practice to a paediatrician with expertise in cardiology. Cardiol Young 2015;25(1):123-7.

[10] Greydanus DE. The cardiovascular system. In: Hofman AD, ed. Adolescent medicine. Menlo Park, CA: Addison-Wesley, 1983:68-85.

[11] Greydanus DE, Hofmann AD. The cardiovascular system. In: Hofmann AD, Greydanus DE, eds. Adolescent medicine, 2nd edition. Norwalk, CT: Appleton Lange, 1989:99-122.

[12] Rowlett JD, Greydanus DE. The cardiovascular system. In: Hofmann AD, Greydanus DE, eds. Adolescent medicine, 3rd edition. Norwalk, CT: Appleton Lange, 1997:147-76.

[13] Margineau CO, Melit LE, Hutanu A, Ghiga DV, Sasaran MO. The adipokines and the inflammatory status in the era of pediatric obesity. Cytokine 2019;126:154925. doi: 10.1016/j.cyto.2019.154925.

[14] Andonian C, Langer F, Beckmann J, Bischoff G, Ewert P, Freilinger S, et al. Overweight and obesity: an emerging program in patients with congenital heart disease. Cardiovasc Diagn Ther 2019;9(Suppl 2):S360-8.

[15] Hames DL, Ferguson MA, Kaza AK, Rajagopal S Thiagarajan RR, Teele SA, et al. Renal replacement therapy in the pediatric cardiac intensive care unit. J Thorac Cardiovasc Surg 2019;158(5):1446-55.

[16] Fuhrman DY, Nguyen L, Hindes M, Kellum JA. Baseline tubular biomarkers in young adults with congenital heart disease as compared to healthy young adults: Detecting subclinical kidney injury. Congenit Heart Dis 2019 Dec 2. doi: 10.1111/chd.12862.

[17] Liem RI, Lanzkron S, D Coates T, DeCastro L, Desai AA, Ataga KI, et al. American Society of Hematology 2019 guidelines for sickle cell disease: cardiopulmonary and kidney disease. Blood Adv 2019;3(23):3867-97.

[18] Ezekian JE, Hill KD. Management of pulmonary arterial hypertension in the pediatric patient. Curr Cardiol Rep 2019;21(12):162. doi: 10.1007/s11886-019-1229-2.

[19] Nagdyman N, Mebus S, Kügel J, Zachoval R, Clevert DA, Braun SL, et al. Non-invasive assessment of liver alternations in Senning and Mustard patients. Cardiovasc Diagn Ther 2019;9(Suppl 2):S198-S208.

[20] Leerink JM, Feijen ELAM, van der Pal HJH, Kok WEM, Mavinkurve-Groothuis AMC, Kapusta L, et al. Diagnostic tools for early detection of cardiac dysfunction in childhood cancer survivors: Methodological aspects of the Dutch late effects after childhood cancer (LATER) cardiology study. Am Heart J 2019;219:89-98.

[21] Mandawat A, Eberly L, Border W. A cardio-oncology data commons: Lessons from pediatric oncology. Curr Cardiol Rep 2019;21(10):128. doi: 10.1007/s11886-019-1212-y.

[22] Abdelmohsen G, Mohamed H, Mohsen M, Abdelaziz O, Ahmed D, Abdelsamal M, et al. Evaluation of cardiac function in pediatric patients with mild to moderate bronchial asthma in the era of cardiac strain imaging. Pediatric Pulmonol 2019;54(12):1905-13.

[23] Lerner RK, Gruber N, Pollak U. Congenital heart disease and thyroid dysfunction: Combination, association, and implication. World J Pediatr Congenit Heart Surg 2019;10(5):605-615.

[24] Hoevenaar-Blom MP, Spijkerman AM, Kromhout D, van den Berg JF, Verschuren WM. Sleep duration and sleep quality in relation to 12-year cardiovascular disease incidence: The MORGEN study. Sleep 2011;34(11):1487-92.

[25] Cappuccio FP, Cooper D, D'Elia L, Strazzullo P, Miller MA. Sleep duration predicts cardiovascular outcomes: a systematic review and meta-analysis of prospective studies. Eur Heart J 2011;32(11):1484-92.

[26] Gianfagna F, Veronesi G, Bertù L, Cesana G, Grassi G, Stranges S, et al. Influence of sleep disturbances on age at onset and long-term incidence of major cardiovascular events: the MONICA-Brianza and PAMELA cohort studies. Sleep Med 2016;21:126-32.

[27] Hulsegge G, Looman M, Smit HA, Daviglus ML, van der Schouw YT, Verschuren WM. Lifestyle changes in young adulthood and middle age and risk of cardiovascular disease and all-cause mortality: The Doetinchem Cohort Study. J Am Heart Assoc 2016;5(1). pii: e002432. doi: 10.1161/JAHA.115.002432.

[28] Yin J, Jin X, Shan Z, Li S, Huang H, Li P, et al. Relationship of sleep duration with all-cause mortality and cardiovascular events: A systematic review and dose-response meta-analysis of prospective cohort studies. J Am Heart Assoc 2017;6(9). pii: e005947. doi: 10.1161/JAHA.117.005947.

[29] Yunus FM, Khan S, Mitra DK, Mistry SK, Afsana K, Rahman M. Relationship of sleep pattern and snoring with chronic disease: Findings from a nationwide population-based survey. Sleep Health 2018;4(1):40-8.

[30] Kwok CS, Kontopantelis E, Kuligowski G, Gray M, Muhyaldeen A, Gale CP, et al. Self-reported sleep duration and quality and cardiovascular disease and mortality: A dose-response meta-analysis. J Am Heart Assoc 2018;7(15):e008552. doi: 10.1161/JAHA.118.008552.

[31] Petrovic D, Haba-Rubio J, de Mestral Vargas C, Kelly-Irving M, Vineis P, Kivimäki M, et al. The contribution of sleep to social inequalities in cardiovascular disorders: a multi-cohort study. Cardiovasc Res 2019 Nov 22. pii: cvz267. doi: 10.1093/cvr/cvz267.

[32] Burstein R, Henry NJ, Collison ML, Marczak LB, Sligar A, Watson S, et al. Mapping 123 million neonatal, infant and child deaths between 2000 and 2017. Nature 2019;574(7778):353-8.

[33] Gray B, Ackerman MJ, Semsarian C, Behar ER. Evaluation after sudden death in the young. Circ Arrhythm Electrophysiol 2019;12(8):e007453. doi: 10.1161/CIRCEP.119.007453.

[34] Norrish G, Ding T, Field E, Ziólkowska L, Olivoto I, Limongelli G, et al. Development of a novel risk prediction model for sudden cardiac death in childhood hypertrophic cardiomyopathy (HCM Risk-Kids). JAMA Cardiol 2019 Aug 14. doi: 10.1001/jamacardio.2019.2861.

[35] Ackerman MJ, Giudicessi JR. Findings of uncertain significance and a family history of sudden death: Worth the FUSs? J Am Coll Cardiol 2019;74(6):771-3.

[36] Webster G, Olson R, Schoppen ZJ, Giancola N, Balmert LC, Cherny S, et al. Cardiac evaluation of children with a family history of sudden death. J Am Coll Cardiol 2019;74(6):759-70.

[37] Moynihan KM, Snaman JM, Kaye EC, Morrison WE, DeWitt AG, Sacks LD, et al. Integration of pediatric palliative care into cardiac intensive care: A champion-based model. Pediatrics 2019;144(2). pii: e20190160. doi: 10.1542/peds.2019-0160.

[38] Kaufman BD, Cohen HJ. Palliative care in pediatric heart failure and transplantation. Curr Opin Pediatr 2019;31(5):611-6.

[39] Kasparian NA, Kan JM, Sood E, Wray J, Pincus HA, Newburger JW. Mental health care for parents of babies with congenital heart disease during intensive care unit admission: Systematic review and statement of best practice. Early Hum Dev 2019;139:104837. doi: 10.1016/j.earlhumdev.2019.104837.

[40] Khairandish Z, Jamali L, Haghbin S. Role of anxiety and depression in adolescents with chest pain referred to a cardiology clinic. Cardiol Young 2017;27(1):125-30.

[41] Kenar A, Örun UA, Yoldas T, Kayali S, Bodur S, Karademir S. Anxiety, depression, and behavioural rating scales in children with non-cardiac chest pain. Cardiol Young 2019;29(10):1268-71.

[42] White BR, Rogers LS, Kirschen MP. Understanding advances in our understanding of neurodevelopmental outcomes in congenital heart disease. Curr Opin Pediatr 2019;31(6):783-8.

[43] Fifer CG, Cohen MS, Peng DM. A noncompliant teen needs a second heart transplant. Ann Thorac Surg 2019;108(5):1282-4.

[44] Gakenheimer-Smith L, Glotzbach K, Ou Z, Presson AP, Puchalski M, Jones C, et al. The impact of neurobehavior on feeding outcomes in neonates with congenital heart disease. J Pediatr 2019;214:71-78.e2.

[45] Goldberg CS, Hu C, Brosig C, Gaynor JW, Mahle WT, Miller T, et al. Behavioral and quality of life at 6 years for children with hypoplastic left heart syndrome. Pediatrics 2019;144(5). pii: e20191010. doi: 10.1542/peds.2019-1010.

[46] Sigmon ER, Kelleman M, Susi A, Nylund CM, Oster ME. Congenital heart disease and autism: A case-control study. Pediatrics 2019;144(5). pii: e20184114. doi: 10.1542/peds.2018-4114.

[47] Cutitta K, Lantin-Hermoso MR. Evaluating quality of life in young school-aged children with hypoplastic left heart syndrome. Pediatrics 2019;144(5). pii: e20191664. doi: 10.1542/peds.2019-1664.

[48] Nielsen C, Ratiu I, Esfandiarei M, Chen A, Selamet Tierney ES. A review of psychosocial factors in Marfan syndrome: Adolescents, adults, families, and providers. J Pediatr Genet 2019;8(3):109-22.

[49] van der Mheen M, Meentken MG, van Beynum IM, van der Ende J, van Galen E, Zirar A, et al. CHIP-Family intervention to improve the psychosocial well-being of young children with congenital heart disease and their families: results of a randomised controlled trial. Cardiol Young 2019;29(9):1172-82.

[50] Komulainen K, Mittleman MA, Ruohonen S, Laitinen TT, Pahkala K, Elovainio M, et al. Childhood psychosocial environment and adult cardiac health: A causal mediation approach. Am J Prev Med 2019;57(6):e195-e202.

[51] Luckstead EF, Greydanus DE. Medical care of the adolescent athlete. Los Angeles, CA: Practice Management Information Corporation, 1993.

[52] Luckstead Sr EF, Noubani H. Cardiovascular disorders in the adolescent. In: Greydanus DE, Patel DR, Pratt HD, eds. Essential adolescent medicine. New York: McGraw-Hill Medical, 2006:129-56.

[53] Molossi S, Grenier M. The management of athletes with congenital heart disease. Clin Sports Med 2015;34(3):551-70.

[54] Pagourelias ED, Kouidi E, Vassilikos VP. Recommendations for participation in competitive sports in athletes with hypertrophic cardiomyopathy: opening the sacks of Aeolus. Eur Heart J 2019;40(36):3064. doi: 10.1093/eurheartj/ehz475.

[55] Iftikhar PM, Uddin MF, Ali F, Arastu AH, Khan J, Munawar M, et al. The top most-cited and influential published articles in atrial fibrillation from 1900 to 2019. Am J Cardiol 2019 Nov 9. pii: S0002-9149(19)31240-8. doi: 10.1016/j.amjcard.2019.10.053.

[56] Schrøder M, Boisen KA, Reimers J, Teilmann G, Brok J. Quality of life in adolescents and young adults with CHD is not reduced: A systematic review and metal-analysis. Cardiol Young 2015;12:1-11.

[57] Brown AE, Bradbrook KE, Casey FE. A survey of adult and pediatric cardiology fellows on training received in family planning counseling. J Women's Health (Larchmt) 2019 Jan 25. doi: 10.1089/jwh.2018.7186.

[58] Abrignani MG, Lucá F, Favilli S, Benvenuto M, Rao CM, Di Fusco SA, et al. Lifestyles and cardiovascular prevention in childhood and adolescence. Pediatr Cardiol 2019;40(6):1113-25.

[59] Soler-Botija C, Gálvez-Montón C, Bayés-Genis A. Epigenetic biomarkers in cardiovascular diseases. Front Genet 2019;10:950. doi: 10.3389/fgene.2019.00950.

[60] Cohen M. Editorial: A contemporary look at pediatric cardiology in 2020. Curr Opin Cardiol 2020;35(1):35-6.

Donald E Greydanus, MD, DrHC (Athens), FAAP
Premchand Anne, MD, MBA, MPH, FACC, FAAP, FACP
John D Rowlett, MD, FAAP, FACP
Joav Merrick, MD, MMedSci, DMSc

SECTION 1: MEDICAL ISSUES OF THE PEDIATRIC HEART

In: Chronic Disease and Disability
Editors: DE Greydanus, P Anne, JD Rowlett et al.
ISBN: 978-1-53617-656-8

Chapter 1

PROMETHEAN PROGRESS IN UNDERSTANDING THE PEDIATRIC HEART: FROM THE ANCIENT EGYPTIAN HEART AND THE ARISTOTELIAN HEART TO THE 20TH CENTURY HEART WITH THE BLALOCK-TAUSSIG SHUNT: STANDING ON THE SHOULDERS OF GIANTS

Donald E Greydanus[1,*], MD, DrHC (Athens) and Joav Merrick[2-5], MD, MMedSc, DMSc

[1]Department of Pediatric and Adolescent Medicine, Western Michigan University Homer Stryker MD School of Medicine, Kalamazoo, Michigan, United States of America
[2]National Institute of Child Health and Human Development, Jerusalem
[3]Division of Pediatrics, Hadassah Hebrew University Medical Center, Mt Scopus Campus, Jerusalem, Israel
[4]Kentucky Children's Hospital, University of Kentucky College of Medicine, Lexington, Kentucky, United States of America
[5]Center for Healthy Development, School of Public Health, Georgia State University, Atlanta, Georgia, United States of America

ABSTRACT

The first book in English on cardiology by Allan Burns of Glasgow in 1809 was on observations of the most frequent and important diseases of the heart. This included a section on malformations or congenital heart defects—the beginning of pediatric cardiology. The first great school of cardiology was in Paris in 1806 with French physician Jean-Nicolas Corvisart (1755-1821), who also was the personal physician to Napoléon Bonaparte (1769-1821). A further stimulation for the birth of pediatric cardiology was

* Correspondence: Donald E Greydanus, MD, DrHC (Athens), Professor of Pediatrics and Founding Chair, Department of Pediatric and Adolescent Medicine, Western Michigan University, Homer Stryker MD School of Medicine, 1000 Oakland Drive D48G, Kalamazoo, MI 49008-1284, United States. Email: Donald.Greydanus@med.wmich.edu.

struggles to deal with the ravages of rheumatic fever that was first identified by the English physician Thomas Sydenham (1624-1689). It was the link of heart disease to rheumatic fever and the identification of heart malformations (congenital heart disease) that led to the development of pediatric cardiology in the 20th century. The acknowledged founder of pediatric cardiology in the minds of many experts is Helen Brooke Taussig (1898-1986). Surviving tuberculosis (that, when she was nine years of age, killed her mother), prejudice in school, and adult-onset deafness, she became one of the prime movers in pediatric cardiology in the 20th century. Her work in pediatric cardiology began in 1930 in caring for children with rheumatic heart disease based on the work of previous giants.

> If I have seen further than others, it is by standing upon the shoulders of giants
> Sir Isaac Newton (1642-1727)

INTRODUCTION

The study of life began with the emergence of Homo sapiens over 200,000 years ago (1-6). Prior to the emergence of writing by the Sumerians in 3500 BCE on clay tablets that emerged from earlier Neolithic writing, we can only guess at what ancient humans thought of the this muscular organ located in the chest's center that we call the heart (cor, Herz, hart, hjerte, καρδιά, сердце, cœur, corazón).

Rudimentary knowledge of this organ is traced to Mesopotamia (3100 BCE to 332 BCE) that included Sumer and the Akkadian, Babylonian, and Assyrian empires in modern-day Iraq. The word, Mesopotamia, is Greek for "land between rivers" and indeed was between the Tigris and Euphrates rivers—major waterways of antiquity. Sumerian scholars, as now, thought of the heart in philosophical terms as seen by this poem from Sumer:

> It is not the heart which leads to enmity; It is the tongue which leads to enmity..... A hating heart destroys the home.... (3)

ANCIENT EGYPTIAN MEDICINE

> My heart, my mother; my heart, my mother! My heart whereby I came into being!
> (The Prayer of Ani, Book of the Death) (7)

Perhaps the most famous reference to the heart in ancient history is that regarding the weighing of the heart in the afterlife from the 'Book of the dead," which was an Egyptian funerary book used from 1550 BCE to 50 BCE (7). In the process of mummification, the heart which ancient Egyptians believed to be the person's center of thought (as well as memory and emotion), was preserved along with added jeweled heart scarabs to serve as a heart replacement if needed. The deceased heart was weighed on the scale of Maat against what was called the "feather of truth" by the jackal-headed Anubis and the result was recorded by the scribe of the gods (the ibis-headed Thoth) (7). The dead person was allowed to go into the afterlife with his heart returned if the weight of the heart was the same as the feather; however, it was not, then the person was eaten by the Ammit—a creature with the triad body of a hippopotamus, lion, and crocodile.

Knowledge of ancient Egyptian medicine is known from such work reflected in the 1875 discovery by the German Egyptologist Georg Ebers (1837-1898) of what is called the Ebers Papyrus that dates to the reign of Amenophis I (second King of the 18th Dynasty) in 1536 BCE (7, 8). This document was over 20 meters in length and had 108 columns of text with a series of prescriptions organized by different diseases (7). The oldest known surgical document or text is the Edwin Smith Papyrus which was discovered in 1862 near Luxor, Egypt (8). Edwin Smith (1822-1906) was an American dealer and collector whose name was given to this papyrus.

Ancient Egyptian physicians were pioneers in a detailed cardiovascular examination which involved brilliant insights into cardiovascular anatomy and physiology influencing medicine for 30 centuries from 3500 BCE (9). These trailblazing clinicians of ancient Egypt wrote the first book of cardiology called "treaty of the heart" that identified the importance of the pulse as it related to heart contractions (10, 11). Ancient Egyptian physicians concluded that various channels or tubes were connected to the heart that allowed passage of blood, air, urine, and the soul. Early concepts of heart failure are attributed by some scholars to the work of these ancient physicians who used such terms as "weakness of the heart and cardiac dysfunction (11, 12)." Translations of the Ebers Papyrus noted such words as: "his heart is bored, the heart weakens, debility has risen in the heart, his heart is flooded," and "his heart of over flooded (12)."

Ancient Hebrews who learned much from the ancient Egyptians also paid much attention to the heart (as well as the kidneys [reins] as a way of judging the worth of a human being (13).

> ...Examine me, O Lord, and prove me; try my reins and my heart
> (Psalms 26:2—1000 BCE).
> ...I, the Lord, search the heart, I try the reins, even to give every man according to his ways, and according to the fruit of his doings
> (Jeremiah [Yirmeyahu] 17:10—600 BCE

Ancient Greek physicians

The first known Greek medical school was in Cnidus in 700 BCE and one of its early medical scholars was Alcmaeon of Croton (born around 510 BCE) who helped to establish the principle of observing patients to understand disease (14). Alcmaeon noted that arteries and veins were not the same based on his dissection of animals. He was a student of the famous Ionian Greek philosopher and mathematician, Pythagoras (570-490 BCE). Though certainly influenced by ancient Egyptian medicine, the Greek physicians sought to move the knowledge of medicine further and indeed they did as they established the basis for modern Western medicine.

One of the earlier movers in this direction was the Greek historian and political philosopher, Thucydides (460-400 BCE) of Athens who wrote the famous incunabulum, History of the Peloponnesian War, that detailed the 5th century BC war between the ancient enemies, Athens and Sparta. Thucydides is called the father of scientific history whose writings were based on verifiable data that did not include the effects of the Greek gods in the lives of human beings and rejected theories based on apotropaism. He noted that prayers were not effective in the treatment of medical disorders such as the plague. The age of scientific discovery was now born though based on the classic theory of humorism or the balance of the four classic humours (i.e., black bile, yellow bile, phlegm, and blood)–this Zeitgeist ancient Greece persisted well after the Renaissance period into the 16th century!

The father of modern Western medicine was Hippocrates of Kos (460-370 BCE) whose works extended conclusions of ancient Egyptian physicians and reflected in the Corpus Hippocraticum—a collection of over 60 medical works (15). These Greek physicians of Kos and ancient Greece sought to understand illnesses apart from religious theories and Hippocrates is identified with the first description of nail clubbing or clubbing of the fingers (called "Hippocrates fingers") which can reflect a number of conditions including cyanotic heart disease.

> ....He made a finer end, and went away an it had been any christom child. He parted ev'n just between twelve and one, ev'n at the turning o' th' tide; for after I saw him fumble with the sheets and play with flowers and smile upon his finger's end...... and all was as cold as any stone.
>
> (William Shakespeare, Henry V, Act II, Scene iii —1599 AD)

An early writer about the life and accomplishments of Hippocrates was the Greek physician, Soranus of Ephesus, who live at the end of the first century and the beginning of the second century AD. Hippocrates was the son of a physician (Heraclides) who learned medicine from his father and grandfather. Hippocrates trained at the Kos Asklepieion and set the stage for Western Medicine.

The classic Greek philosopher and polymath of noesis, Aristotle (384-322 BCE) founded the Peripatetic School of Philosophy in Athens. Aristotle was a student of Plato who in turn had been a student of the Socrates whose maieutic or Socratic method of teaching changed the Western world. His father was a physician who took care of King Philip of Macedon and assigned his son, Aristotle, to tutor Alexander the Great at age 13 years. Alexander the Great was so impressed with this teaching that he later gave Aristotle money to start his Peripatetic School in Athen's Lyceum.

Aristotle was also a physician who secerned that the human soul was housed in the heart and not the brain; he also noted that the heart was the seat of the senses and was a hot organ that needed the lungs and the brain to cool it (16). Aristotle sought to understand his world with a scientific approach and, based on his study of chick embryos, concluded the heart was the first organ to develop (17). He provided one of the earliest and accurate descriptions of the cardiovascular system that included anatomy of the heart and blood vessels in his classic Historia Animalium (18). He described the human heart as having three venticles (right, left, and middle) and regarded the right atrium as a venous dilatation (19).

Praxagoras (340 BCE-280 BCE) was born in Kos, Greece and was an anatomist who distinguished between arteries and veins. Arteries were identified as air tubes (as noted with the trachea and bronchi) that carried the mystic life force called "pneuma" while veins carried blood. Arteries came from the heart and veins came from the liver. Other Greeks who studied anatomy around this time include Greek physicians Herophilus (335-280 BCE) and Erasistratus (304-250 BCE) founded a school of anatomy in Alexandria, Egypt.

Herophilus of Chalcedon was the first anatomist and he described the anatomy of heart valves while Erasistratus further distinguished between veins and arteries in which one had a pulse (artery) and one (vein) did not based on vivisection work on the necks of pigs (16). Herophilus noted that arteries were thicker than veins and Erasistratus demonstrated the presence of semilunar valves. Based on the conclusions of the earlier philosophers (such as Plato and Aristotle) that the human body had no role after death, these Greek scientists at Alexandria began to dissect humans both dead and alive (i.e., vivisection).

Their work allowed physicians to conclude that the heart was not the center of sensations but was a pump to keep one alive. Erasistratus showed how blood was stopped from retrograde flow in normal conditions and that arteries were filled with air carrying "pneuma" or the "animal spirit (13)." He concluded that the blood flowed via vacuums. The removal of the anatomical location of the soul from the heart in ancient thought to the whole body and beyond was a process of many millennia that was stimulated by the knowledge of the heart as a pump (20, 21).

FIRST CENTURY AD

Only by this historical route can many problems in medicine be approached profitably
Sir William Osler, MD, 1849-1919

Roman physicians of the first century, often Greeks from Asia Minor (Anatolia, now present day Turkey), began to push the boundaries of knowledge about the heart. Pedanius Dioscorides (40-90 AD) wrote the famous De Materia Medica (Latin for "on Medical Material") in about 60 AD that became the standard encyclopedic pharmacopoeia of herbs and medicines from the mid-first century until the Renaissance period. In this five volume document this Greek physician, pharmacologist, and botanist wrote about herbs to improve heart disease such as use of the herb Hawthorn (Crataegus oxyacantha) for heart failure (22). The discovery of foxglove (Digitalis purpurea) had to wait for the 17th century as reviewed later.

Galen of Pergamos (Aelius Galenus or Claudius Galenus--AD 129– c.200/c.216), father of modern and experimental Western medicine, was a physician, surgeon, and philosopher. He was the son of a wealthy architect (Aelius Nicon) who shared a love of knowledge with his son. Galen noted that the heart was the second most important organ in the body (surpassed only by the liver), that it was the derivation of the person's heat, and in contrast to Aristotle, the heart was not the mainspring of the nerves (23). Galen described two independent networks of arteries and veins and this theory prevailed in Western medicine until William Harvey's work in the 17st century. In this Galenic view the liver produced the blood from food that is eaten and the blood was centrifugally sent to the body while air (pneuma) was absorbed into the pulmonary veins and distributed to the body by arteries.

Blood passed from veins to arteries by way of invisible holes (pores) in the peripheral areas as well as the interventricular septum which was felt by Galen to be a porous septum (24). Galen wrote that the human body has three systems: 1) the natural spirit (veins and the liver for nutrition); 2) the vital spirit (involving the heart and blood in arteries mixed with air from the lungs); and 3) the animal spirit (25). A number of arteries connected to a structure at the brain's based called "rete mirabile" and was a place for the change of vital spirits to be altered to animal spirits and then sent to the through nerves thought to be hollow tubes. His work was based on animal dissection and not human dissection and thus errors arose that would be corrected 15 centuries later (26).

Oribasius (325-403 AD) was a Greek physician living in the Oriental Roman empire (Byzantium) who, utilizing magnifying lenses, confirmed Erasistratus' concept of a connection (anastomosis which he called capillaries) between arteries and veins (26). Oribasius also identified circulation in the kidneys that including blood flow through the aorta's renal artery branch with venous return via the inferior vena cava's renal vein branch (26).

Table 1. Arab/Persian clinicians of the Golden Age of the Islamic era (27) (partial list)

Ali at-Taberi (838-870 AD)
Ar-Razi (Rhazes:865-925 AD)
Ali ibn al-Abbas al-Magusi (Haly: died around 990 AD)
ibn al-Qasim al-Zahrawi (Abulcasis: 936-1013 AD)
ibn al-Haitam (Alhazen: 965-1040 AD)
ibn Sina (Avicenna: 980-1037 AD)
ibn Abi al-Ala Zuhr (Avenzor: 1091-1131 AD)
ibn Rushd (Averroes: 1126-1198 AD)
ibn al-Baitar (1197-1248 AD)
ibn al-Nafis (1213-1288 AD)

Golden Ages of Islamic Era: 9TH to 12TH Centuries

The Fall of Rome in 476 AD led to a loss of medical knowledge in Europe though medicine was kept alive and advanced by brilliant Arab and Persian physicians in the 9th century and beyond (see Table 1). Persian-born physicians include Doctors Taberi, Magusi, and Razi. Perhaps the most influential Islamic physician/philosopher was Ibn Sina (Avicenna: 980-1037 AD) who wrote a medical encyclopedia called Cannon of Medicine and a work on cardiac drugs (26). His encyclopedic work, "The book of healing" became well-known (26). Avicenna was born in Bukhara (present-day Uzbekistan) and died in Hamadan; he was a scholar in various fields including medicine, mathematics, physics, Islamic theology, astronomy, geology, and poetry. His father was a respected scholar and installed this love of scholarship in his son.

Avicenna refined Galen's theory of pulses and provided details on a number of drugs that effected the heart. He made mention of pericardial disease and prevention of cardiac diseases including the importance of a "healthy" diet for those with heart disease. In his book on drugs for heart disease there is mention of various drug treatments that came from mineral, vegetable, and animal sources (27, 28). He was the first to use a drug that eventually was classified as a calcium channel drug (29). He described the Willis circle, capillary circulation, cardiac tamponade, hypertension, palpitation, stroke, hypersensitivity and its link with vasovagal syncope, and the connections of emotion with cardiac action (28, 30). Avicenna's work was influential for the next several centuries (31).

Ibn al-Nafis (1213-1288) was an Arab physician who challenged the Galenic theory of circulation and did not agree with the belief in a porous interventricular septum (27, 32, 33). Ibn al-Nafis described the pulmonary circulation and wrote about pores between the pulmonary artery and vein that four centuries later were called pulmonary capillaries by Marcello Malpighi (32-35). Some have incorrectly noted that the 16th century European scientists discovered the pulmonary circulation but this distinction belongs to Ibn al-Nafis in the minds of some scholars (35-38). He was a famous ophthalmologist who also described the coronary circulation (27, 37). Contributions of Inn al-Nafis sometimes are confused in the English speaking world since his and other works of physicians in the Islamic Golden Age of Medicine were published in

Persian and/or Arabic. The exact contributions with reference to the Renaissance scholars continues to be debated (27, 37, 38). In 1924 a manuscript was discovered in Europe written by Ib Nafis that notes his description of the pulmonary circulation (37).

> If I don't know that my work will not last up to ten thousand years after me, I would not write them
>
> Ibn al-Nafis (27)

MEDICAL RENAISSANCE (15TH TO 17TH CENTURIES): EXORDIUM OF MODERN CARDIOLOGY

> At one and the same time, in one and the same subject, two opposite motions cannot take place, that is, repentance and desire. Therefore, if the right upper (auricle) and lower ventricles are the one and the same, it is necessary that the whole should cause at the same time one and the same effect and not two effects arising from diametrically opposite purposes as one sees in the case of the right ventricle with the lower, for whenever the lower contracts, the upper dilates to accommodate the blood which has been driven out of the lower ventricle
>
> (Leonardo da Vinci (22))

LEONARDO DA VINCI (1452-1564)

The practice of human dissection began in Europe in the 13th and 14th centuries by a number of physician-anatomists such as the Italian Mondino de Luzzi (Mundinus: 1270-1326), the Italian Guido da Vigevano (Guido da Pavia: 1280-1349), and the French father of surgery, Henri de Mondeville (1260-1316) (39). Leonardo da Vinci (1452-1564) sketched the heart based on the Galenic model and recognized the heart as a muscle in which systole is this organ's active stage (40). His research allowed him to link heart action with the pulse, connect the auricles and pulmonary veins, explain valve functioning, and even describe effects of aging on the cardiac tissue (40). This brilliant artist, scientist, and inventor also described the sinuses of Valsalva function (nearly 2 centuries before Valsalva provided them his name) as well as presented information that was a precursor to current understanding of atherosclerosis (41, 42). His famous painting of Mona Lisa from 1507 may represent the first presentation of familial hypercholesterolemia in which there a suspicious lesion on her left upper eyelid and also on the right hand (43).

MICHAEL SERVETUS (1511-1553)

Michael Servetus (Miguel Servet, Miguel Serveto, Revés, Miguel Serveto Conesa) was a Spanish theologian and physician who is identified by history as the first European to describe the pulmonary circulation in his 1553 work, Christianismi Restitutio; he accomplished this independently---apparently not aware of the 13th century contributions of the brilliant Arab physician Ibn al-Nafis (27, 44-47). Though a true polymath who was versed in other fields as well (i.e., geography, astronomy, mathematics), he was entangled in the theological cacophony of the 16th century in Europe and was burned at the stake in Geneva in 1553 (46, 47). A major contributor to the anger at him was his boldness in challenging the theories of Hippocrates and Galen whose ideas were predominant in medical circles for 14 to 18 centuries. The courage of Michael Servetus allowed others to challenge the Hippocratic-Galenic views and eventually allow a more correct understanding of the heart and the circulatory system (48).

Andreas Vesalius (1514-1564)

Andreas Vesalius was born in Brussels, Belgium and graduated from the University of Padua in 1537 with an MD degree (49). He studied anatomy there based on his work in dissections and became Chair of Anatomy and Surgery there for six years. He left this job at age 28 years to become the court physician to Emperor Charles V and then to his son, Phillip II of Spain (49, 50). This Flemish genius published three seminal books on anatomy (49-52): Tabulae Anatomicae Sex (1538), Epitome (1543), and his towering work—De Humani Corporis Fabrica (1543). Though he initially accepted the Galenic view of a porous interventricular septum, he later rejected it because he could not find it in his dissections. Andreas Vesalius also noted that blood vessels did not come from the liver as in the Galenic view, but from the heart. His detailed anatomical descriptions of the human body changed the science of anatomy with influence to current times (53).

Vesalius taught that understanding of anatomy should be derived from direct observation via dissection and not acceptance of traditional books (49). Such a view was not well received in his era and was perceived as a challenge to established religious and academic groups (54, 55). He spoke against the Inquisition and was headed to being burned at the stake until the Spanish Court intervened that led to a forced pilgrimage to Jerusalem (51). Vesalius died on this return journey from Jerusalem on the Greek island of Zante where he was put to shore alone (51, 54). Contributions of such brilliant scholars as Servetus and Vesalius are that more remarkable considering the danger they were in when challenging their academic and religious dogma. For example, the work of Galen was held in such high esteem for so many centuries that change to more accurate science was very difficult and a high price was paid by those who dared to offer a challenge.

Realdo Colombo (1511-1559)

Realdo Colombo (Matteo Realdo Colombo) was the Italian professor who succeeded Andreas Versalius as Chair of Anatomy and Surgery at the University of Padua after having been his student. He was also a professor at the University of Pisa and the Papal University (Sapienza); in the latter position he was surgeon to Pope Julius III (56). His views validation of pulmonary circulation were published in his De re anatomica ("On Things Anatomical) in 1559 that was later acknowledged by William Harvey (26). Realdo Colombo is known as an anatomist who accurately placed the right kidney below that of the left kidney and provided an improved description of pulmonary circulation with blood moving between the two ventricles via the lungs (56). One of his famous patients was Michelangelo whom Professor Colombo unsuccessfully tried to convince in illustrating his treatise on anatomy (56). Matteo Realdo Colombo remains one of the great anatomists and professors of the Renaissance era though he is often underappreciated (57).

HIERONYMUS FABRICIUS (1537-1619)

Hieronymus Fabricius (Girolamo Fabrizio) was an Italian anatomist and surgeon who is called the father of embryology (58-60). His teacher was Gabriele Falloppio whom he succeeded as Professor of anatomy and surgery at the University of Padua. Fabricius designed the first public theater for anatomical dissections and had many students who went on to fame including William Harvey (1578-1657). Fabricius is credited with the discovery of valves ("membranous folds") in veins in his 1603 De Venarum Ostiolis, though he did not understand their role in antegrade flow of blood to the heart.

ANDREA CESALPINO (1519-1603)

Andrea Cesalpino (Andreas Cæsalpinus) was an Italian physician and botanist who was a pioneer in classification by classifying plants according to their seeds and fruits versus other methods such as an alphabetical scheme or medical characteristics (61, 62). He provided a concept of blood circulation different than what William Harvey proposed (63).

WILLIAM HARVEY (1578-1657)

William Harvey was born in Folkestone, England and was the oldest of 7 sons whose father was a farmer. William Harvey received the MD degree from the University of Padua (Università degli Studi di Padova', UNIPD), Italy in 1602. One of his advisors was Hieronymus Fabricius who undoubtedly agreed with the quote (vide supra) about Harvey doing well on his examinations and that it was a sign of his amazing potential (64, 65). He became the Court Physician to England's King James I and also Charles I. In addition to his work on the heart he also studied embryology and emphasized the primacy of the egg in contrast to primacy of sperm in procreation. In his 1651 work, Exercitationes de generatione animalum he noted the idea of "omne vivum ex ovo" (all life comes from the egg). In his work on the heart he used vivisection on animals such as deer provided to him from his King.

Using a combination of intelligence and brilliant experimentation, William Harvey provided a new view of the cardiovascular system that challenged the centuries-held views of Galen (66). He described a system with two explicit arrangements of blood vessels (i.e., arteries and veins) (23) and a heart that circulated blood by its contraction. The liver was no longer the maker of blood and the ebb-flow method of blood movement seen in Galenism was no longer valid. The heart was now the center of circulation and not the liver (67). The porous interventricular septum of Galen was also replaced and there was a view of pulmonary circulation with blood moving through the lung circulation from the right ventricle to the left atrium and to the left ventricle (67). The heart had two phases—contraction (systole) and rest (diastole).

The medical world was awaken and shaken in 1628 with Harvey's monumental publication, De Motu Cordis (Exercitatio Anatomica de Motu Cordis et Sanguinis in Animalibus[An Anatomical Dissertation Upon the Movement of the Heart and Blood in Animals]) which was a masterpiece of analysis of anatomy, physiology, volumetric circulatory flow and understanding of the continuity principle (68). Harvey's 1628 De motu cordis was published in Latin and the first English edition was in 1653 (69). The 1628 edition was 72 pages and it was released to the world at an annual book event in Frankfurt, Germany (22, 23).

He predicted the existence of capillaries linking arteries and veins but history would await the discovery of the microscope and the work of Malpighi to confirm this prediction (67). The future work of Anton van Leeuwhoek also clarified qualities of blood in different vessels of the body (67). The field of experimental cardiology was born and William Harvey was able to remove underlying theology from physiology so that science was free to explore proven ideas and change ideas as more evidence arose (70)

This work confronted the current medical thinking of its day that his views were initially rejected and it was not until after his death that the accuracy and brilliance of William Harvey's contributions were appreciated (23, 71). Many of his contemporaries worried that if one could not accept this aspect of Galenism, then perhaps all of Galen's ideas (as that of the ancient scholars) were not to be believed! However, as the Greek mythic hero, Hercules, used major effort to clean the Augean stable, so did real hero, Harvey, use major effort to clean medical minds from incorrect views (24). Harvey followed in the tradition of Aristotle as opposed to Galen (70).

One of the first scholars to accept Harvey's work was the great French philosopher, Rene Descartes (1596-1650), the father of modern philosophy and conceptualizer of Cogito ergo sum (I think, therefore I am) (22). Though the location of the soul remained controversial, it essentially became medical dogma that the heart was the center of the circulatory system and details of the anatomy as well as the physiology of the circulatory system were revealed in astonishing detail by William Harvey (21).

> ...I found the task so truly arduous...that I was almost tempted to think...that the movement of the heart was only to be comprehended by God. For I could neither rightly perceive at first when the systole and when the diastole took place by reason of the rapidity of the movement...
>
> William Harvey (72).

Robert Hooke (1635-1703)

Robert Hooke was an English architect and philosopher involved in a number of fields including using telescopes and microscopes. In 1665 he published a work called "Micrographia" that published descriptions of 60 objects (biologic and inorganic) seen with the microscope that included the first description of the microfungus Mucor and developed the term, cell (73-75). He was curator of the then newly developed Royal Society in London and also used his architectural skills to help deal with the aftermath of the Great Fire in London of 1666 (76, 77). Robert Hooke and Antony van Leeuwenhoek set the stage for microscopic discoveries in medicine and many other fields.

ANTONY VAN LEEUWENHOEK (1632-1723)

Antony van Leeuwenhoek was a draper from Delft, Netherlands and was a Delft contemporary of the great Dutch painter, Johannes Vermeer (1632-1675). He build his own microscopes that were the best of his era and with his own observations became the acknowledged father of microbiology, optic microscopy, protozoology, protistology and micromorphology (78-83). He was able to grind lens to provide the best magnification available (up to an estimated x266) and he combined this talent with the ability to provide precise observation and recording of what he saw (84, 85). Of the more than 500 single lens microscopes he made, only nine are still in existence (85).

Antony van Leeuwenhoek was a normal citizen of Delft, the Netherlands who began his observations in his 40s, but without formal scientific training, he changed the world of science by seeing and describing microbes and providing microscopic details about animals, plants, and minerals (86). Though at first ridiculed by incredulous scientists of his day, such as those at the Royal Society of London, his amazing descriptions of his "strange little animals" ("wee animalicules") including protozoa that were sent in letters to the Royal Society of London were eventually accepted and he was honored—especially well after his death by scientists in the19th and especially 20th century (79, 84, 87-89). He is the unsung hero of microscopy who was the first to see spermatozoa, red blood cells, protozoa, bacterial and other structures under his wonderful microscopes (81, 82). He was far ahead of his times with his amazing work and marvelous microscopes (90). Thucydides (460-400 BCE) of Athens would have been impressed with such detailed and verifiable work!

MARCELLO MALPHIGHI (1628-94)

The father of microscopic anatomy, Marcello Malphighi, used the then newly invented microscope for great advancements in science that included advancing the achievements of William Harvey by identifying pulmonary capillaries and alveoli (63, 91). Marcello Malphighi's magnus opus was published in 1666 and called De viscerum structura exercitatio anatomica that advanced many fields including nephrology, neurology, gastroenterology, dermatology and gynecology (92). He did not believe in Galen's hepatocentrism but endorsed Harvey's cardiocentrism (93). Marcello Malphighi provided many contributions to the field of embryology, and as with other giants of science, had to content with critics of his era who did not want to challenge "comfortable" views of the natural world (93, 94). This Italian genus of the 17th century helped moved scientists into the modern biology and life sciences era (93, 94).

CARDINAL CONCEPTS IN CARDIOLOGY: THE 18TH CENTURY

William Withering (1741-1799) was an English polymath whose skills included being a botanist and physician. Such prowess allowed him to investigate why an elderly female with "dropsy" (edema and swelling from congestive heart failure) improved after taking a local herbal remedy (95-97). This was a major observation since the recommended treatment in that era was bleeding. He was able to determine the key ingredient was from the flowering plant, Digitalis purpurea (foxglove, common foxglove, lady glove, purple foxglove) which lead to the more than two centuries use of digitalis for the treatment of heart failure (98). Based on talent and obsession to observe and record, this pioneer moved the field of cardiology into active treatment utilizing plants as therapy. He also meticulously identified features of digitalis toxicity and a prepared a plan for titrating this medical to maximize benefit and avoid digitalis toxicity. (97-100). William Withering was able to move the work of Pedanius Dioscorides (40-90 AD) on the herb Hawthorn (Crataegus oxyacantha) to another level for the benefit of Homo sapiens (22).

Withering's 1785 research was a cohort study of 163 patients with dropsy (hydropsy) who were given foxglove and he reported the results for responders (with congestive heart failure) and non-responders; the study was called "An account of the Foxglove, and some of its medical uses: with practical remarks on dropsy, and other diseases" (101). Edema (oedema) was originally called dropsy, a word first recorded in the penultimate decade of the 13th century and later connected to heart and renal disease in the 18th and 19th centuries.

Withering was among the first to look at the effects of a drug on treatment of a condition and avoiding his era'a practice of looking at response based on the four humors theory, paved the way for modern research on drug effects (99). He was a well-known member of the Lunar Society that was a dinner gathering of prominent citizens in Birmingham, England between 1765 and 1813; they would meet during the full moon (99).

William Withering's legacy in cardiology is profound and remains with us today even as other medications are replacing the use of digitalis in the 21st century in the treatment of congestive heart failure and atrial fibrillation (102). Withering taught future doctors to use a standard protocol in preparing a drug from a natural plant to avoid uneven benefit and results (100). Twenty-first century proponents of medial cannabis need to read the work of William Withering in the 18th century!

We have learned much about the cardiac glycoside digitoxin since the death of Dr. Withering. Differences in reaction to a drug can be due to changes in sensitivities of involved receptors and differences in how the drug is disposed (100). Mechanism of cardiac glycoside action involves inhibition of ATPase activity involving the sodium potassium ATPase pump.

JEAN-ANTOINE NOLLET (1700-1770)

Jean-Antoine Nollet was a French physicist and priest (Abbé Nollet) involved in work on electricity. Using a Leyden jar (named by Dutch physicist Pieter van Musschenbroek (1692-1761) after the place of its discovery) he provided a jolt of electricity through a number of Royal Guards to King Louis XV in 1746. He contributed to the use of electricity in medicine that developed over the next two centuries (103, 104).

LUIGI GALVANI (1737-1798)

Luigi Galvani was an Italian physician and physicist whose work on muscles of frogs' legs led to the concept of animal electricity that can be traced to the idea of static electricity found in the Leyden jar (105-107). His work with dissected frog legs led to contraction of these muscles inducing Luigi Galvani to conclude that the source of electricity was in the animal muscles and nerves. Alessandro Volta (1745-1927) was an Italian chemist and physicist who was the inventor of the electrical battery; by the turn of the 19th century Volta concluded that the electricity in Galvani's experiments was due to the use of two different metals with the frog body fluid serving as the conductor.

Galvani was given credit for starting research that was the beginning point of electrophysiology. The process of placing a zinc layer over steel was called galvanism and Andre Ampére (1775-1836) invented the galvanometer naming it after Luigi Galvani; later, the electrocardiogram would later be developed which is a form of a galvanometer (107). Andre Ampére was a French mathematician and physicist who is credited as one of the developers of classical electromagnetism despite differences between Galvani and Volta noted in the halls of history (107-114). The work of this great scientist set off a fury of research activity in the 19th century and beyond that led to the development of electrophysiology, electromagnetism, electrochemistry, and the electrical battery (115).

> I had dissected and prepared a frog in the usual way and while I was attending to something else I laid it on a table on which stood an electrical machine at some distance from its conductor and separated from it by a considerable space. Now when one of the persons present touched accidentally and lightly the inner crural nerves of the frog with the point of the scalpel, all the muscles of the legs seem to contract again and again as if they were affected by powerful cramps
>
> Luigi Galvani, September 20, 1786 (116)

CARDINAL CONCEPTS IN CARDIOLOGY: THE 19TH CENTURY

The 19th and 20th century brought forth scintillating scholars, who, standing on the shoulders of previous giants, advanced the field of clinical cardiology to its current level. An example of this statement is seen in the English scientist, Michael Faraday (1791-1867), who developed concepts of electrolysis, electromagnetic induction and electrolysis (117-123). Concepts bearing his name include Faradays law of induction, Faraday wave, Faraday paradox, Faraday constant, and others. This was all the more remarkable considering the fact that he had received limited education in science.

His 1832 paper on electromagnetic induction is a major work that helped to transform his world (124). His research at England's Royal Institute led to the startling concept of an electric current induced to flow through a conductor and was a harbinger of the Scottish scientist James Clerk Maxwell's (1831-1879) theory of classical electromagnetism (124). This work also led to the development of the electric dynamo and electric motor that are major structures in the 21st century (124). He and his colleagues developed terminology based on his electrochemical research and based on knowledge of Greek, coined terms that have become part of modern science; these include electrolyte, electrode, and ion (125).

Michael Faraday's work influenced many others during his time and beyond. For example, knowledge about brain electricity and epileptic electrical discharges involved the work of the great Irish neurologist Robert Bentley Todd (1809-1860) in London who was shaped by Michael Faraday's work on electromagnetism (126, 127). Michael Faraday became Professor of Chemistry at the Royal Institution of Great Britain, succeeding the famous Cornish chemist Humphrey Davy (1778-1889). In 1818 Faraday contributed to anesthesia by concluding that inhaling the vapor of ether caused the same effects on sedation as that of inhaling nitrous oxide (laughing gas)—the agent that was Professor Davy's discovery (128, 129). Michael Faraday's contributions to archeological chemistry are also well known (130). This amazing scholar who became the greatest electrical scientist was also astute in communicating his research to the world (131).

Willem Einthoven (1860-1927)

Willem Einthoven was a Dutch physician and physiologist who developed the first clinically useful, practical electrocardiogram (EKG) in 1903 (132-137). The first to record the electrical activity of the heart was the British physiologist Augustus Desiré Waller (1856-1922) who was the son of the famous British neurophysiologist, Augustus Volney Waller (1816-1870) (138-143). Waller used a mercury capillary electrometer and provided the first recording in 1987 at St. Mary's Hospital in London, England. However, it was of poor quality with minimal clinical usefulness.

Willem Einthoven demonstrated his keen ability to make insightful views on research topics. In his post-medical training life, he began with research to accurately identify and record heart sounds with a capillary electrometer. He as others during his time knew that the heart produces electricity as it beats but precisely measuring this electric activity was problematic until Willem Einthoven looked at this arena. Despite various difficulties and standing on the shoulders of giants Einthoven went on to develop his string galvanometer to provide a clinically useful electrocardiogram starting in 1901 and 1903 (144-146). The 1901 article was his first publication on this instrument and his 1903 publication provided more details of his cutting-edge contribution (147).

From 1894 to 1913 his diligent work established essential features of modern electrocardiography (148). He developed the Einthoven triangle and provided the naming of the recording with P, Q, R, S, and T based on mathematical foundations of the 17th century French mathematician and philosopher, René Descartes as well as others (147, 149, 150). Einthoven was eloquently able to combine a number of disciplines in developing a clinically useful electrocardiogram that included electromagnetism, quartz chemistry, optics, and method of recording (143).

His own version of the galvanometer contained a quartz string that was silver coated (151). Using his string galvanometer Einthoven was able to provide electrocardiographic characterizations of cardiovascular conditions (152). Though not accepted at first even by his local Dutch colleagues, his work was eventually appreciated and Willem Einthoven received the Novel Prize for Medicine and Physiology in 1924 "for the discovery of the mechanism of the electrocardiogram." (143, 147, 153-156). Indeed, Willem Einthoven is the father of electrocardiography (155, 157).

WILHELM KONRAD RÖNTGEN (1845-1923)

Wilhem Konrad Röntgen was a German physicist who developed and identified electromagnetic radiation in November of 1895 that were called X-rays or Röntgen rays in his honor for which he received the Novel Prize in 1901 (158-173). Though born in Germany (Lennep on the lower Rhine), his family moved to the Netherlands when he was three years of age because of political unrest; he lived 17 years in the Netherlands (167). He was expelled from school in his youth and was not a good student of physics (167, 173). However, later he was taught by a famous German physicist, August Adolf Eduard Eberhard Kundt (1839-1894) of the Polytechnicum in Zurich, Switzerland (173).

Details of Röntgen's discovery in Würzburg, Germany were never provided by Wilhem Röntgen and the earliest notes of his dates to November 15, 1895 which was about one week after his original experiment that some in history date to November 8, 1895 (168, 171). Röntgen sent information to several of his compatriots in January of 1896 and news was quickly spread by newspapers and colleagues in Berlin, Vienna and other places to the world including persons such as the German Emperor William II (Friedrich Wilhelm Viktor Albrecht von Preußen [1859-1941]) (169). Basic diagnostic radiologic emerged quickly in the first few decades of Wilhem Röntgen's contribution to science (170).

The term X-rays was in reference to his being unclear what this type of energy or electromagnetic radiation was in terms of its nature or meaning; this stimulated much research by various individuals with reference to study of x-rays in physics and medicine in the 20th and now 21st centuries (162-167, 171). Professor Röntgen set the stage for the later development of diagnostic and therapeutic radiology (radiotherapy, nuclear medicine and radiodiagnostics) along with the work of such luminaries as the French physicist Antoine Henri Becquerel (1852-1908) and Polish/French physicist/chemist Marie Sklodowska-Curie (1867-1934); both these French scientists received the Novel Prize in Physics in 1903 for their monumental work (163).

The impact of medical physics on medicine, including cardiology, have been far-reaching and still expanding (166, 172). The impactful discovery of x-rays would lead to the development of x-ray tube science, hot cathode Coolidge tube (invented by American physicist William David Coolidge [1873-1975] in 1913), and eventually diagnostic radiology physics (165). Physics in the 20th century took off with innovative scientists reaching for the stars based on the electromagnetic theory of the Scottish mathematical physicist James Clerk Maxwell (1831-1879), quantum physics of the German physicist Max Karl Ernst Ludwig Planck (1858-1947), and the general theory of relativity of the German-born physicist Albert Einstein (1879-1955) (162, 164).

Information obtained seven decades after this Nobel Prize was given reveal the Nobel Committee had suggested that this prize be divided between Wilhem Konrad Röntgen and another German physicist, Philipp Eduard Anton von Lenard (167). Philipp Lenard (1862-1947) was later awarded the Nobel Prize for physics in 1905 for his research on cathode rays.

SCIPIONE RIVA-ROCCI (1863-1937)

Accurate measurement of blood pressure was a task that required a number of individuals after William Harvey (1578-1657) concluded there was a limited amount of blood that circulated through the body in one direction (174). For example, the French physicist Jean Léonard Marie Poiseuille (1797-1869) revealed the mercury hydrodynometer (U-tube mercury manometer) with measurements in mm Hg units (174-176). The German physician, Karl von Vierordt (1818-1884) developed a sphygomograph in 1854 that was the precursor to the modern sphygmomanometer (174).

Samuel Siegfried Karl Ritter von Basch (1837-1905) was an Austrian-Jewish physician credited by some with the development of the sphygmomanometer or blood pressure meter (176, 177). He is perhaps better known as the physician to the Mexican emperor Ferdinand Maximilian Joseph (1832-1867). Another advancement was the contribution of "Korotkov sounds" and identification of the diastolic blood pressure by the Russian surgeon Nikolai-Sergeyevich Korotkov in 1905 (1874-1920) (175, 176, 178).

History typically credits the Italian physician Scipione Riva-Rocci (1863-1937) for the development of a clinically useful sphygmomanometer for blood pressure measurements (174-181). He initially published his method of blood pressure in 1896 and 1897 which was based on compression of the brachial artery in contrast to previous methods based on compression on the radial artery (178). His blood pressure technique was spread to the United States and Europe after he was visited by the famous American neurosurgeon Harvey Cushing (1869-1939).

Sir Thomas Lauder Brunton (1844-1916)

Thomas Lauder Brunton was a Scottish physician who is credited with use of the vasodilator, amyl nitrite, for management of angina pectoris (182-184). He was able to use his knowledge of pharmacology to conclude that a vasodilator would dilate coronary arteries and thus utilized amyl nitrite for this purpose. This was part of the effort to use medication to treat cardiac conditions, as noted in the spirit of William Withering in the 18th century. Brunton was knighted in 1900 and he also converted to Islam as noted with his new name: Jalaluddin Lauder Brunton.

Cardinal concepts in cardiology: The 20th century

It is not beyond peradventure to note that, standing on the shoulders of giants from other lands (ancient Mesopotamia, Egypt, Greece, Rome, Arab countries, Renaissance Europeans, 18th and 19th century Europeans), remarkable achievements in the understanding of cardiac physiology and cardiac disease management resulted from the remarkable achievements of a variety of scientists and clinicians in the 20th century in Europe and also in the United States. Some researchers, as already noted, lived in both centuries and ushered in remarkable achievements in cardiology in the 20th century. One example is provided by Willem Einthoven (1860-1927) whose work on the electrocardiogram began the understanding of abnormal heart rhythms (arrhythmias).

Another is that of Karel Frederick Wenckebach (1864-1940) who was a Dutch anatomist who in the penultimate year of the penultimate decade of the 19th century wrote about an abnormal heart rhythm cause by partial clogging of atrioventricular (AV) conduction leading to what has been called a second degree AV block or the Wenckebach phenomenon (or Mobitz type I) (185-187).

Sir Thomas Lewis (1881-1945)

Sir Thomas Lewis was a British cardiologist who is the father of clinical cardiac electrophysiology and corresponded with a number of experts in his era, including Willem Einthoven, to understand the complex area of cardiac disease including arrhythmias (188-192). He studied the connection with cardiac rhythm and some cases of syncope (193). In 1909 he (along with Scottish cardiologist Sir James MacKenzie [1853-1925]) started the journal, Heart: A Journal for the Study of Circulation that was called Clinical Science in 1933. He published his first book in this field in 1913 called Clinical Electrocardiography.

The legacy of Sir Thomas Lewis, Sir James MacKenzie, Karel Frederick Wenckebach, and many others was that cardiology was developing as a powerful research and clinical field in the early 20th century that would increase exponentially as this century progressed.

Frank Norman Wilson (1890-1952)

Frank Norman Wilson was an American cardiologist credited with initiating the modern era of electrocardiography (194-199). He was the son of a farmer who became a Professor of Internal Medicine at the University of Michigan (Ann Arbor, Michigan, USA) and was there from 1914 to 1952 (197). World War I brought him to England where he met Sir Thomas Lewis with whom he shared a passion for electrocardiography and also photography of birds (197). His work on electrocardiography and the ventricles made him internationally acclaimed (198). Professor Wilson, standing on the shoulders of giants, such as Willem Einthoven (1860-1927) and Sir Thomas Lewis (1881-1945), and pushed the field further into the modern era by brilliantly developing clinically useful applications of the electrocardiogram (199).

After his death, more work continued to understand the QRS origin and in the 1970s, progress in understanding cardiac cell communication occurred (199). More information regarding causes and management of cardiac arrhythmias continued as the 20th century progressed that included work on tachycardias in the 1960s and 1970s, use of external and implantable defibrillators in the 1960s and 1980s, surgery for arrhythmias in 1980s, and catheter ablation for supraventricular tachycardias in the final decade of the 20th century (200, 201).

The 20th Century and the Rise of Cardiac Catheterization

As knowledge of the heart was growing in the 20th century, progress in diagnostic methods also was seen. A German physician, Werner Theodor Otto Forßmann (1904-1979), inserted a catheter into a vein of an arm and passed the catheter into his heart, initiating the field of cardiac catheterization (202-204). A variety of researchers, such as French physician André Frédéric Cournand (1895-1988) and American physician Dickinson Woodruff Richards (1895-1973), performed right heart catheterization on a regular basis starting in the 1940s (202, 205-207). The 1956 Nobel Prize in Physiology or Medicine was awarded to Werner Theodor Otto Forßmann (1904-1979), André Frédéric Cournand (1895-1988), and Dickinson Woodruff Richards (1895-1973) - for development of the monumental 20th century procedure, cardiac catheterization (208).

These 1956 Nobel Laureates represent the 20th century triumvirate of cardiac catheterization. History is replete with triumvirates of note. For example, the First Triumvirate of ancient Rome was Julius Caesar, Pompey (Gnaeus Pompeius Magnus) and Crassus (Marcus Licinius Crassus) in 60 BC and the Second Triumvirate was Antony (Mark Antony), Lepidus (Marcus Aemilius Lepidus), and Octavian (Gaius Julius Octavius) in 43 BC.

Other giants of cardiology emerged for the betterment of human beings and angiocardiography developed in a number of countries in the 20th century between 1929 and 1959 (202). Frank Mason Sones Jr, MD (1918-1985) was an American physician who has been called the father of modern pioneering research developing cinecoronary arteriography (202, 203, 209). This field continued with the work of Andreas Gruentzig regarding cardiac catheterization interventions in 1977 with the development of balloon angioplasty (203, 204).

Andreas Roland Gruentzig (1949-1985) was a German cardiologist who opened up medicine to providing interventions directly in arteries without the need for open surgical procedures with its inherent risks of surgery under general anesthesia (210-213). He performed the first femoral angioplasty in 1975, and first procedure with his developed double-lumen catheter in 1975, and presented the results of four cases of angioplasty at the 1977 American Heart Association meeting in Miami, Florida, USA. Gruentzig died in a plane crash in 1985.

> Without the work of Mason Sones—the most important contributor to modern cardiology—all our efforts in myocardial revascularization would be fruitless René Favaloro—Argentina (209)

Emergence and Emanation of Pediatric Cardiology from Adult Cardiology in the 20th Century

Though there are many other giants who work led to current knowledge of adult cardiology, this synopsis now turns to consideration of the focus of this book—the Pediatric Heart. Indeed, countless millennia past before attention was turned to the child and the pediatric heart. History identifies Soranus of Ephesus (98 AD-138 AD) as the world's first pediatrician (214). Fifteen centuries later the first book on pediatrics in the Western world was published in 1544 AD by Thomas Phaer (1510-1560)—a truly assiduous Renaissance man of sagacity---physician, lawyer, poet, philosopher, and father of English pediatrics (215). Progress in gaining knowledge in adult cardiology has been reviewed both before and after this book was published.

The monumental work, De Motu Cardis by William Harvey in 1628 set the stage for both adult and pediatric cardiology that would slowly emerge on the shoulders of other giants (63-72). The first description of what was later to be called tetralogy of Fallot was by 17th century Danish physician and anatomist, Niels Stensen (1638-1686) (216-218). History has assigned this tetralogy eponym as the tetraology of Fallot in honor of the French physician from Marseille, Étienne-Louis Arthur Fallot (1850-1911) (219-221). One of the reasons to call this tetralogy after Fallot was the work of the great Canadian pathologist, Maude E. Abbott (1869-1940) (222).

Eighty eight year before Maude E Abbott was born, one of the great clinicians of his and any era was born---- René Théophile Hyacinthe Lënnec (1781-1826) who is credited with the invention of the stethoscope in 1816 as well as a pioneer in carefully correlating physical signs with autopsy findings (223-227). The monumental work of this great French physician "De l'Auscultation Médiate" published in 1819 is considered the beginning of pulmonary medicine (224). He is the father of clinical auscultation, wrote the first descriptions of bronchiectasis, and classified various disorders---as pneumonia, pleurisy, pneumothorax, and others (226).

Identification of heart sounds was now unleased and more auscultation discoveries were seen. The 19th century was a golden age of discoveries based on giants standing on the shoulders of other giants. The impression of clinicians since Hippocrates was that the heart was immune to disease: cor aegrotari non potest (228). Pope Clement XI (1649-1721) had asked his physician Giovanni Lancisi (1654-1720) of Rome to write about this and Lancisi responded by authoring his work, De subitaneis mortibus (On sudden death) in 1707. The work of René Théophile Hyacinthe Lënnec decades later added to the ability to learn about the diseases of the heart, an organ apparently not immune to disease despite the theory of Hippocrates.

The first book in English on cardiology was by Allan Burns of Glasgow who wrote in 1809: Observations on some of the most frequent and important diseases of the heart (228). This included a section on malformations or congenital heart defects—the beginning of pediatric cardiology. The first great school of cardiology was in Paris in 1806 with French physician Jean-Nicolas Corvisart (1755-1821). This famous physician to Napoléon Bonaparte (1769-1821) was able to combine the technique of percussion from Austrian physician Josef Leopold Auenbrugger (Leopold von Auenbrugger [Avenbrugger]: 1722-1809) with Lënnec's auscultation.

Now enter the great English cardiologist, Thomas Bevill Peacock (1812-1882) who advanced medicine in many ways (228-232). He was a Quaker physician who identified various aspects of cardiology between 1846 and 1868 that included concepts of dissecting aneurysms, valvular heart disease (such as pulmonary stenosis), and congenital heart disease (228-232). Based on lectures given to students starting in 1854 at London's St Thomas Hospital, he wrote his magnus opus in 1858 "On malformations of the human heart" that had five sections including one on malformations (congenital heart disease) (228).

> Peacock was not a specialist in the modern sense of the world. He was essentially a general physician with a particular interest in pathology. His main contributions were in cardiology to which he added knowledge by keen observation, punctilious description and illustration, and a flair for arranging his material in a neat and orderly fashion (228)

A further stimulation for the birth of pediatric cardiology was struggles to deal with the ravages of rheumatic fever that was first identified by English physician Thomas Sydenham (1624-1689) (233). Called the English Hippocrates, Syndenham's views of medicine were aligned with the Hippocratic school of medicine in which observation of the patient was key to advancement in medicine as reflected in his 1676 "Magnus Opus Observationes Medicae" (234-238). The understanding of the cardiac manifestations found in rheumatic fever would take many decades to unravel as noted by French anatomist Raymond Vieussens (1636-1715) who provided the first autopsy results of mitral valve stenosis and aortic valve insufficiency

(239-242). Other 19th century contributors in linking heart damage with rheumatic fever were the French physician, Jean-Baptiste Bouillaud (1796-1881) (243, 244) and English paediatrician Walter Butler Cheadle (1836-1910) (245-247). It was the link of heart disease to rheumatic fever and the identification of heart malformations (congenital heart disease) that led to the development of pediatric cardiology in the 20th century.

HELEN BROOKE TAUSSIG (1898-1986)

The acknowledged founder of pediatric cardiology in the minds of many experts is Helen Brooke Taussig (233, 248-252). Surviving tuberculosis (that, when she was nine years of age, killed her mother), prejudice in school, and adult-onset deafness, she became one of the prime movers in pediatric cardiology in the 20th century. Her work in pediatric cardiology began in 1930 in caring for children with rheumatic heart disease based on the work of previous giants such as Raymond Vieussens (1636-1715), Jean-Baptiste Bouillaud (1796-1881) and English pediatrician Walter Butler Cheadle (1836-1910) (233, 239-247).

As noted by Taussig herself, the development of her knowledge in congenital heart disease was traced to knowing the great McGill University pathologist Maude E Abbott (1869-1940) (222). Helen Taussig had read the famous "Abbott atlas of congential cardiac disease" of 1936 and also had a friendship with this famous Canadian pathologist who became the founder of the International Academy of Pathology. Abbott was a colleague of the legendary Canadian physician Sir William Osler (1849-1919) who encouraged Abbott in this work that provided a unique atlas of 1,000 congenital heart disease cases (222, 253). Maude E Abbott is the only Canadian and the only female found on the great mural of the history of cardiology by the famous Mexican painter and muralist Diego Rivera (1886-1957) in Mexico City, Mexico (253, 254).

The link to this Osler-Abbott-Taussig triad was solidified in 1935 when Taussig helped to have Abbott meet American adult cardiologist Paul Dudley White (1886-1973), whose 1931 book "Heart disease" contained research by Abbott (255). Indeed, one can note that the link of Osler-Abbott-White-Taussig was the link to two centuries and the foundation of congenital heart disease knowledge for the 20th and now 21st century (255).

As Helen Taussig work in cardiology continued, she was also helped with the gradual link established between rheumatic fever and streptococcal infection, the discovery of penicillin by Sir Alexander Fleming (1881-1955) in 1928, and sulfonamide by German pathologist-bacteriologist Gerhard Johannes Paul Domagk (1895-1964)in 1932 (256-262). As cardiology clinics were less frequently filled with rheumatic heart disease because of the use of these novel antibiotics, cardiologists turned their attention to understanding and managing congenital heart disease (233).

> When I woke up just after dawn on September 28, 1928, I certainly didn't plan to revolutionize all medicine by discovering the world's first antibiotic, or bacteria killer. But I suppose that was exactly what I did
>
> Sir Alexander Fleming (260).

As researchers and clinicians contemplated the management of congenital heart disease, a major event occurred in this regard when 33 year old American surgeon, Robert Edward Gross

(1905-1988) auspiciously ligated the patent ductus of a seven year old girl in Boston, Massachusetts (233, 263-265). One can conclude that this was the beginning of 20th century pediatric cardiology and/or pediatric cardiac surgery when congenital heart disease was being directly treated (263-265). Helen Taussig and Maude Abbott discussed patent ductus surgery and Helen Taussig had the brilliant idea of developing a patient ductus arteriosus shunt in blue babies with cyanotic congenital disease so that pulmonary blood flow would be improved (255).

After Robert Edward Gross was not interested in doing this surgery, Helen Taussig continued with her vision and approached American Alfred Blalock (1899-1964) who then with the technical aid of Viven Thomas performed this landmark surgery in 1944, which involved creating the first subclavian-pulmonary artery shunt for a patient with tetralogy of Fallot (266, 267). The Taussig-Blalock shunt was created and these two innovators worked together in 1944 and 1945 to management many blue babies and stimulate the field of cardiac surgery for children with cyanotic congenital heart disease (255). Helen Taussig's "Congenital malformations of the heart" was published in 1947.

From William Harvey (1578-1657), Niels Stensen (1638-1686), Étienne-Louis Arthur Fallot (1850-1911), Sir William Osler (1849-1919) and Maude E Abbott (1869-1940)—the baton was passed to Helen Taussig, who with Viven Thomas and the Alfred Blalock made an incredible feat of progress in the mid-20th century. Though they did not receive a Nobel Prize for such an accomplishment, their legacy endures and the field of pediatric cardiology exploded in the later part of the 20th and now early part of the 21st century (233, 268, 269).

University of Minnesota Chair and Professor of Surgery Owen H Wangenesteen (1898-1981): "The outstanding contribution to the advancement of surgery in the 20th century has been the development of open-heart surgery" (273).

There are many experts and giants who have come along since the work of Peter Gross and Helen Tausig to advance the field of pediatric cardiology and pediatric cardiac surgery over the last half of the 20th century and a decade and a half of the 21st century (233, 269-275). These amazing accounts have been beautifully recorded by a variety of experts for the interested reader who will learn about the work of John Heysham Gibbon Jr (designer of extracorporeal circulatory support) (1903-1973) (276), pioneer pediatric cardiologist Alexander S Nadas (1913-2000) (269, 277, 278), Floyd John Lewis (1916-1933) (279), Mayo Clinic cardiovascular surgeon John Webster Kirklin (1917-2004) (280), father of open heart surgery Clarence Walton ("Walt") Lillehei (1918-1999) (281, 282), pediatric cardiologist Williams J Rashkind (1922-1986 [Rashkind balloon atrial septostomy]) (269, 283), Italian cardiac surgeon Giancarlo Rastelli (1922-1970 [Rastelli procedure for repair of transposition of the great arteries]) (284), and so many more. The first successful open heart surgery was performed by Floyd John Lewis in 1952 (279). Owen H Wangenesteen (1898-1981), in his book "Rise of surgery," noted that "Walt Lillehei was one of the surgical immortals" (282).

CHAPTER DENOUEMENT

Determination, persistence, and stubbornness were the most important components important components of research and successful discovery Clarence Walton ("Walt") Lillehei (282)

In the spirit of Wilhelm Konrad Röntgen (1845-1923) progress in imaging has been spectacular that includes computerized tomograms (CTs), magnetic resonance imaging (MRIs), and nuclear scans (233, 285, 286). In the spirit of William Withering (1741-1799) research in pharmacology had led to management of ductus arteriosus with prostaglandins (287-290), pharmacology of tetralogy of Fallot spells (i.e., ß-blockers, midazolam, others) (291-293), and hypertension management with angiotensin-converting enzyme inhibitors, calcium channel blockers, and vasodilators (233, 291-298).

In the spirit of Andreas Vesalius (1514-1564), appreciation of anatomy in heart disease remains important for health care providers in the 21st century (299).

In the spirit of Willem Einthoven (1860-1927), Karel Frederick Wenckebach (1864-1940), Sir Thomas Lewis (1881-1945) and other giants of the past, arrhythmias continue to be clarified in the 21st century including concepts in fetal arrhythmias and channelopathies (300, 301).

In the spirit of Ibn al-Nafis (1213-1288) and Michael Servetus (1511-1553), scholars in the 21st century continue to explore the pulmonary circulation (302). In the spirit of Walter Butler Cheadle (1836-1910), Sir Alexander Fleming (1881-1955) and Gerhard Johannes Paul Domagk (1895-1964), research in the 21st century continues to explore how infection affects the heart and its valves as well as methods of management (303). In this same spirit of complex inflammatory disease involving the heart and in the case of Kawasaki disease, the heart's blood vessels (including coronary artery aneurysms)—as identified by Japanese pediatrician, Tomisaku Kawasaki (1925-) in 1961--continues to be explored in the 21st century (304, 305).

Transitional care of pediatric patients with congenital heart disease to adult care providers as these individuals mature into adulthood remains an important priority in the 21st century (306-309). The Human Genome studies have led to improved knowledge on genetic causes of heart disease. (310-316) Valve replacement is being improved with studies on bioengineered valves (317, 318). Cardiac transplantation may be replaced by research on techniques to grow myocardial cells and alter the need for patients in the future who need a heart transplantation (319-323). The history of pediatric transplantation as other aspects of pediatric cardiology is rich with principles to teach us about the past, the present, and the future (324-335).

> If a man can grow a heart, he can build one
> Willem Johan Kolff (1911-2009)

References

[1] Evolution of modern humans: Early modern Homo sapiens. URL: http://anthro.palomar.edu/homo2/mod_homo_4.htm.

[2] Magner LN. A history of the life sciences, 3rd ed. New York: Marcel Dekker, 2002.

[3] Kramer SN. The Sumerians. Chicago, IL: University of Chicago Press, 1963:225-63.

[4] Jastrow M. The liver in antiquity and the beginnings of anatomy. Philadelphia, PA: Transactions College of Physicians, 1907;XXIX:117.

[5] Roth MT. Law collections from Mesopotamia and Asia Minor. Atlanta, GA: Scholars Press, 1997.

[6] Geller MJ, Horstmanshoff HFJ, Stol M, Tilburg C, eds. West meets East: Early Greeks and Babylonian diagnosis. Magic and rationality in ancient Near Eastern and Graeco-Roman Medicine. Boston, MA: Brill, 2004.

[7] Taylor JH, ed. Ancient Egyptian book of the dead: Journey through the afterlife. London: British Museum Press, 2010;54.

[8] Hallmann-Mikolajczak A. Ebers Papyrus. The book of the medical knowledge of the 16th century BCE Egyptians. Arch Hist Filoz Med 2004;67(1):5-14. [Polish]

[9] Stiefel M, Shaner A, Schaefer SD. The Edwin Smith Papyrus: The birth of analytical thinking in medicine and otolaryngology. Laryngoscope 2006;116(2):182-8.

[10] Ziskind B. The cardiovascular examination in the light of the medical papyruses of old Egypt. Hist Sci Med 2006;40(1):61-8. [French]

[11] Ziskind B, Halioua B. Contribution of ancient Egypt to cardiovascular medicine. Arch Mal Coeur Vaiss 2004;97(4):370-4. [French]

[12] Saba MM, Ventura HO, Saleh M, Mehra MR. Ancient Egyptian medicine and the concept of heart failure. J Card Fail 2006;12(6):416-21.

[13] Bongartz LG, Cramer J, Joles JA. Origins of the cardiorenal syndrome and the cardiorenal connection. URL: http://cdn..intechopen.com/pdfs-wm/32307/pdf.

[14] Codellas PS. Alcmaeon of Croton: His life, work, and fragments. Proceed Royal Soc Med 1931;25(4):1041-6.

[15] Schiefsky MJ. Hippocrates: on ancient medicine. Leiden: Brill, 2005.

[16] Mason, Stephen F. A history of the sciences. New York: Collier Books, 1956.

[17] Dunn PM. Aristotle (384-322 BC): Philosopher and scientist of ancient Greece. Arch Dis Child Fetal Neonatal 2006;91(1):F76-7.

[18] Shoja MM, Tubbs RS, Loukas M, Ardalan MR. The Aristotelian account of "heart and veins." Int J Cardiol 2008;125(3):304-10.

[19] Van Praagh R, Van Praagh S. Aristotle's "triventricular" heart and the relevant history of the cardiovascular system. Chest 1983;84(4):462-8.

[20] Loukas M, Hanna M, AlsaieMason Stephen F. gh N, Shoja MM, Tubbs RS. Clinical anatomy as practiced by ancient Egyptians. Clin Anat 2011;24(4):409-15.

[21] Santoro G, Wood MD, Merio L, Anastasi GP, Tomasello F, Germanò A. The anatomical location of the soul from the heart, through the brain, to the whole body and beyond: a journey through Western history, science, and philosophy. Neurosurgery 2009;65(4):633-43.

[22] A history of the heart. URL: http://web.stanford.edu/class/history13/earlysciencelab/body/heartpages/heart.html.

[23] Aird WC. Discovery of the cardiovascular system: From Galen to William Harvey. J Thromb Haemost 2011;9(Suppl 10):118-29.

[24] O'Rourke Boyle M. Harvey, by Hercules! The hero of the blood's circulation. Med Hist 2013;57(1):6-27.

[25] Ancient Greek medicine. URL: https://en.wikipedia.org/wiki/Ancient_Greek_medicine.

[26] Bestetti RB, Baraldi C, Restini BA, Couto LB. Development of anatomophysiologic knowledge regarding the cardiovascular system: from Egyptians to Harvey. Arq Bras Cardiol 2014;103(6):538-545.

[27] Masic I, Dilic M, Solakovic E, Rustemepasic N, Ridjanovic Z. Why historians of medicine called Ibn al-Nafis the second Avicenna? Med Arh 2008;62(4):244-9.

[28] Chamsi-Pasha MAR, Chamsi-Pasha H. Avicenna' contribution to cardiology.l Avicenna J Med 2014;4(1):9-12.

[29] Faridi P, Zarshenas MM. Ibn Sina's book on drugs for cardiovascular diseases. Int J Cardiol 2010;145:223.

[30] Tekol Y. The medieval physician Avicenna used an herbal calcium channel blocker, Taxus baccata L. Phytother Res 2007;21:701-2.

[31] Zarshenas MM, Zargaran A. A review on the Avicenna's contribution to the field of cardiology. Int J Cardiol 2015;182:237-41.

[32] Majeed A. How Islam changed medicine. BMJ 2005;331:1486-7.

[33] West JB. Ibn al-Nafis, the pulmonary circulation, and the Islamic Golden age. J Appl Physiol 1985;105(6):1877-80.

[34] Bittar EE. A study of Ibn Nafis. Bull Hist med 1955;29:352-368.

[35] Coppola ED. The discovery of the pulmonary circulation: A new approach. Bull Hist Med 1957;31:44-77.

[36] Loukas M, Lam R, Tubbs RS, Shoja MM, Apaydin N. Ibn al-Nafis (1210-1288): The first description of the pulmonary circulation. Am Surg 2008;74(5):440-2.
[37] Masic I. On the occasion of 800th anniversary of birth of Ibn al-Nafis—Discoverer of cardiac and pulmonary circulation. Med Arh 2010;64(5):309-13.
[38] Akmal M, Zulkifle M, Ansari A. Ibn Nafis—A forgotten genius in the discovery of pulmonary blood circulation. Heart Views 2010;11(1):26-30.
[39] Gurunluoglu R, Gurunluoglu A, Williams SA, Cavdar S. The history and illustration of anatomy in the Middle Ages. J Med Biogr 2013;21(4):219-29.
[40] Shoja MM, Agutter PS, Loukas M, Benninger B, Shokouhi G, Namdar H, et al. Leonardo da Vinci's studies of the heart. Int J Cardiol 2013;167(4):1126-33.
[41] Boon B. Leondardo da Vinci on atherosclerosis and the function of the sinuses of Valsalva. Neth Heart J 2009;17(12):496-499.
[42] Jones R. Leonardo da Vinci: anatomist. Br J Gen Pract 2012;62(599):319.
[43] Ose L. The real code of Leonardo da Vinci. Curr Cardiol Rev 2008;4(1):60-2.
[44] Persaud TV. Historical development of the concept of a pulmonary circulation. Can J Cardiol 1989;5(1):12-6.
[45] Bosmia A, Watanabe K, Shoja MM, Loukas M, Tubbs RS. Michael Servetus (1511-1553): physician and heretic who described the pulmonary circulation. Int J Cardiol 2013;167(2):318-21.
[46] Pai-Dhungat JV, Parikh F. Michael Servetus—Discoverer of pulmonary circulation and a heretic. J Assoc Physicians India 2014;62(5):447-8.
[47] Gracia Guillén D. Michael Servetus: symphony in <<re-major>>. An R Acad Nac Med (Madr) 2004;121(3):453-68. [Spanish]
[48] Stefanadis C, Karamanou M, Androutsos G. Discovery of pulmonary circulation. Hellenic J Cardiol 2009;50:373-8.
[49] Benini A, Bonar SK. Andreas Vesalius 1514-1564. Spine (Phila Pa 1976) 1996;21(11):1388-93.
[50] Izumi H. Andreas Vesalius in the Spanish Court. Nihon Ishigaku Zasshi 2004;50(4):591-616. [Japanese]
[51] Lasky II. The martyrdom of Doctor Andreas Vesalius. Clin Orthop Relat Res 1990;259:304-11.
[52] Zampieri F, Basso C, Thiene G. Andreas Vesalius' Tabulae anatomicae sex (1538) and the seal of the American College of Cardiology. J Am Coll Cardiol 2014;63(7):694-5.
[53] Toledo-Pereyra LH. Medical Renaissance. J Invest Surg 2015;28(3):127-30.
[54] Ambrose CT. Andreas Vesalius (1514-1564)—An unfinished life. Acta Med Hist Adriat 2014;12(2):217-30.
[55] Mesquita ET, de Souza Júnior CV, Ferreira TR. Andreas Vesalius 500 years—A Renaissance that revolutionized cardiovascular knowledge. Rev Bras Cir Cardiovasc 2015;30(2):260-5.
[56] Eknoyan G, De Santo NG. Realdo Colombo (1516-1559): A reappraisal. Am J Nephrol 1997;17(3-4):261-8.
[57] Tubbs RS, Linganna S, Loukas M. Matteo Realdo Colombo (c.1516-1559): The anatomist and surgeon. Am Surg 2008;74(1):84-6.
[58] Rosenberg SL. Hieronymus Fabricius Ab Aquapendente: Part I. Cal West Med 1933;38(3):173-6.
[59] Rosenberg SL. Hieronymus Fabricius Ab Aquapendente: Part II. Cal West Med 1933;38(4):260-3.
[60] Rosenberg SL. Hieronymus Fabricius Ab Aquapendente: Part III. Cal West Med 1933;38(5):367-70.
[61] Buoncristiani A. Andrea Cesalpino as a pioneer in classification. Kos 2003;212:38-41.
[62] Morton AG. A letter of Andrea Cesalpino. Arch Nat Hist 1987;14(2);169-73.
[63] Khan IA, Daya SK, Gowda RM. Evolution of the theory of circulation. Int J Cardiol 2005;98(3):519-21.
[64] Power D. William Harvey: Masters of medicine. London: T Fisher Unwin 1897:26-7.
[65] McKenna M. William Harvey, 1. That incomparable invention of Dr Harvey's. Can J Surg 1987;30(2):139-41.
[66] Tsukisawa M. Reconstruction of the "conversion theory" from the primacy of the heart to the primacy of the blood—William Harvey's observation, logic and the construction of the exercitatio. Kagakushi Kenkyu 1995;34(194):118-28. [Japanese]

[67] Martins e Silva J. From the discovery of the circulation of the blood to the first steps in hemorheology: Part I. Rev Port Cardiol 2009;28(11):1245-68. [English/Portuguese]

[68] Pasipoularides A. Historical perspective: Harvey's epoch-making discovery of the circulation, its historical antecedents, and some initial consequences on medical practice. J Appl Physiol (1985) 2013;114(11):1493-503.

[69] White JS. The 1653 English edition of De motu cordis, shown to be Harvey's vernacular original and revealing crucial aspects of his pre-circulation theory and its connection to the discovery of the circulation of the blood. Hist Philos Life Sci 1999;21(1):65-91.

[70] Pasipoularides A. Greek underpinnings to his methodology in unraveling De Motu Cordis and what Harvey has to teach us still today. Int J Cardiol 2013;168(4):3173-82.

[71] de Micheli A, Izaquirre-Avila R. Evolution of knowledge on blood and its movement. 1st part. Integration of circulatory doctrine. Iatrophysics of blood. Rev Invest Clin 2004;56(6):783-92. [Spanish]

[72] Power D. William Harvey: Masters of medicine. London: T Fisher Unwin, 1897:193.

[73] Gest H. The discovery of microorganisms by Robert Hooke and Antoni van Leeuwenhoek, fellows of the Royal Society. Notes Rec R Soc Lond 2004;58(2):187-201.

[74] Gest H. The remarkable vision of Robert Hooke (1635-1703): First observer of the microbial world. Perspect Biol Med 2005;48(2):266-72.

[75] Gest H. Homage to Robert Hooke (1635-1703): New insights from the recently discovered Hooke Folio. Perspect Biol Med 2009;52(3):392-9.

[76] Rowbury R. Robert Hooke, 1635-1703. Sci Prog 2012;95(Pt 3):238-54.

[77] West JB. Robert Hooke: Early respiratory physiologist, polymath, and mechanical genius. Physiology (Bethesda) 2014;29(4):222-33.

[78] Tugui I. 250 years after the death of Antony van Leeuwenhoek, the man who first saw microbes. Microbiol Parazitol Epidemiol (Bucur). 1973;18(6):537-40. [Romanian]

[79] Corliss JO. Three centuries of protozoology: A brief tribute to its founding father: A. van Leeuwenhoek of Delft. J Protozool 1975;22(1):3-7.

[80] Corliss JO. A salute to Antony van Leeuwenhoek of Delft, most versatile 17th century founding father of protistology. Protist 2002;153(2):177-90.

[81] Karamanou M, Poulakou-Rebelakou E, Tzetis M, Androutsos G. Anton van Leeuwenhoek (1632-1723): Father of micromorphology and discoverer of spermatozoa. Rev Argent Microbiol 2010;42(4):311-4.

[82] Zwick RK, Schmidt BA. When Anton van Leeuwenhoek looked through his early microscopes in the 1600s, he realized the world was teeming with microbial organisms. Introduction, Yale J Biol Med 2014;87(1):1.

[83] Pai-Dhungat JV, Parikh F. Antony van Leeuwenhoek (1632-1723). J Assoc Physicians India 2015;63(3):34-5.

[84] Toledo-Pereyra LH. The strange little animals of Antony van Leeuwenhoek surgical revolution. J Invest Surg 2009;22(1):4-8.

[85] Van Zuylen J. The microscopes of Antony van Leeuwenhoek. J Microsc 1981;121 (Pt 3):309-28.

[86] Anderson D. Still going strong: Leeuwenhoek at eighty. Antonie van Leeuwenhoek 2014;106(1):3-26.

[87] Finlay BJ, Esteban GF. Exploring Leeuwenhoek's legacy: the abundance and diversity of protozoa. Int Microbiol 2001;4(3):125-33.

[88] Amato K. Little animals observed by Antony van Leeuwenhoek. Nihon Saikingaku Aasshi 2014;69(2):315-30. [Japanese]

[89] Lane N. The unseen world: reflections on Leeuwenhoek (1677) 'Concerning little animals'. Philos Trans R Soc Lond B Biol Sci 2015;370(1666). doi: 10.1098/rstb.2014.0344.

[90] James J. Van Leeuwenhoek's discovery of bacteria: a look too far ahead. Ned Tijdschr Geneeskd 2004;148(52):2590-4. [Dutch]

[91] West JB. Marcello Malpighi and the discovery of the pulmonary capillaries and alveoli. Am J Physiol Lung Cell Mol Physiol 2013;304(6):L383-90.

[92] Mezzogiorno A, Mezzogiorno V. Marcello Malpighi (1628-1694). Am J Nephrol 1997;17(3-4):269-73.

[93] DiDio LJ. Marcello Malpighi: The father of microscopic anatomy. Ital J Anat Embryol 1995;100(Suppl 1):3-9.
[94] Piccolino M. Marcello Malphighi and the difficult birth of modern life sciences. Endeavour 1999;23(4):175-9.
[95] Wilkinson KD. William Withering. Br Heart J 1950;12(1):1-9.
[96] Fisch C. William Withering: An account of the foxglove and some of its medical uses 1785-1985. J Am Coll Cardiol 1985;5(5 Suppl A):1A-2A.
[97] Krikler DM. The foxglove: "The old woman from Shropshire" and William Withering. J Am Coll Cardiol 1985;5(5 Suppl A):3A-9A.
[98] Wade OL. Digoxin 1785-1985. I. Two hundred years of digitalis. J Clin Hosp Pharm 1986;11(1):3-9.
[99] Buchtel L, Ventura HO. Lunar Society and the discovery of digitalis. J La State Med Soc 2006;158(1):26-30.
[100] Breckenridge A. William Withering legacy---for the good of the patient. Clin Med 2006;6(4):393-7.
[101] Pagliaro L, Colli A, Bobbio M. Individual response to treatment: from Withering to contemporary medicine. Recenti Prog Med 2015;106(7):308-15.
[102] Weisse AB. A fond farewell to the foxglove? The decline in the use of digitalis. J Card Fail 2010;16(1):45-8.
[103] Benguigui I. Nollet's theory of electricity and its application to medicine as deduced from his unpublished correspondence with Jallabert. Gesnerus 1981;38(1-2):225-35. [French]
[104] Renner C. Birth of medical electricity. Hist Sci Med 2007;41(4):353-8. [French]
[105] Wenzel E. Luigi Galvani-Alexander von Humboldt-Hans Berger—From the history of electroencephalography. Munch Med Wochenschr 1962;104:1146-50. [German]
[106] No authors listed. Aloysio Luigi Galvani (1737-1798) discoverer of animal electricity. JAMA 1967;201(8):626-7.
[107] Haas LF. Luigi Galvani (1737-98). J Neurol Neurosurg Psychiatry 1993; 56(10):1084.
[108] Bresadola M. Medicine and science in the life of Luigi Galvani (1737-1798). Brain Res Bull 1998;46(5):367-80.
[109] Piccolino M. Luigi Galvani and animal electricity: two centuries after the foundation of electrophysiology. Trends Neurosci 1997;20(10):443-8.
[110] Piccolino M. Luigi Galvani's path to animal electricity. C R Biol 2006;329(5-6):303-18.
[111] Goldensohn ES. Animal electricity from Bologna to Boston. Electroencephalogr Clin Neurophysiol 1998;106(2):94-100.
[112] De Micheli-Serra A. Remembering Luigi Galvani on the bicentennial of his death. Gac Med Mex 1999;135(3):323-8. [Spanish]
[113] Isler H. Romantic origins of electrophysiology. Schweiz Rundsch Med Prax 1992;81(49):1485-8. [German]
[114] Piccolino M. Visual images in Luigi Galvani's path to animal electricity. J Hist Neurosci 2008;17(3):335-48.
[115] Cajavilca C, Varon J, Sternbach GL. Resuscitation great. Luigi Galvani and the foundations of electrophysiology. Resuscitation 2009;80(2):159-62.
[116] ECG timeline: History of the electrocardiogram. URL: http:///www.ecglibrary.com/ecghist.html.
[117] Swann WF. Michael Faraday. Science 1931;73(1895):433-9.
[118] Cragg RH. 'Work, finish, and publish" the chemistry of Michael Faraday 1791-1867. Chem Br 1967;3(11):482-6.
[119] Williams LP. Michael Faraday and the physics of 100 years ago. Science 1967;156(3780):1335-42.
[120] Balmer H. Michael Faraday to his 100th birthday on 25 August 1967. Gesnerus 1967;24(3):152-6. [German]
[121] Rowe RC. Michael Faraday: An inspiration to all scientists. Private prescription: A thought-provoking tonic on the lighter side. Drug Discov Today 2001;6(23):1196-1197.
[122] Roth BJ. Michael Faraday and painless defibrillation. Heart Rhythm 2005;2(10):1114-5.
[123] Sera-Shriar E. The correspondence of Michael Faraday. Ann Sci 2015;72(3):401-6.
[124] Al-Khalili J. The birth of the electric machines: a commentary on Faraday (1832) 'Experimental researches in electricity." Philos Trans A Math Phys Eng Sci 2015;373(2039). pii: 20140208.

[125] Giddens WR. The origin of electrochemical nomenclature. J La State Med Soc 2001;153(9):471-5.
[126] Reynolds EH. Todd, Faraday, and the electrical basis of epilepsy. Epilepsia 2004; 45(8):985-92.
[127] Reynolds E. Todd, Faraday and the electrical basis of brain activity. Pract Neurol 2007;7(5):331-5.
[128] Bergman NA. Michael Faraday and his contribution to anesthesia. Anesthesiology 1992;77(4):812-6.
[129] Fujita T. Sir Humphrey Davy, the discoverer of anesthetic action of nitrous oxide—Davy and poets of British Romanticism and inhalation of laughing gas by his friends. Masui 1998;47(1):102-6. [Japanese]
[130] Moshenska G. Michael Faraday's contributions to archaeological chemistry. Ambix 2015;62(3):266-86.
[131] Gross AG. The continuity of scientific discovery and its communication: the example of Michael Faraday. J Biomed Discov Collab 2009;4:3.
[132] Lewis T. Willem Einthoven, MD, PhD. Br Med J 1927;2(3483):664-5.
[133] Williams HB. Willem Einthoven. Science 1928;67(1740):456-8.
[134] No authors listed. Willem Einthoven (1860-1927). JAMA 1965;191:494-5.
[135] No authors listed. Einthoven, Willem. Rev Gastroenterol 1950;17(5):397.
[136] De Waart. Einthoven commemoration. Am Heart J 1961;61:357-60.
[137] Gottlieb LS. Willem Einthoven, MD, PhD, 1860-1927. Centenary of the father of electrocardiography. Arch Intern Med 1961;107:447-9.
[138] No authors listed. Augustus Desiré Waller (1856-1922), electrocardiographer. JAMA 1967;202(2):139-40.
[139] Tenczer J. Centenary of electrocardiography. Remembering Augustus Desiré Waller. Orv Hetil 1987;128(48):2533. [Hungarian]
[140] Cope Z. Augustus Desiré Waller (1856-1922). Med Hist 1973;17(4):380-5.
[141] Acierno LJ. Augustus Desiré Waller. Clin Cardiol 2000;23(4):307-9.
[142] Lüderitz B. Augustus Desiré Waller (1856-1922)—the first to record the electrical activity of the human heart. J Interv Card Electrophysiol 2003;9(1):59-60.
[143] Shapiro E. Willem Einthoven's fortuitous invention. Am J Cardiol 1977;40(6):987-8.
[144] Bergovec M. 100 years of clinical electrocardiography. Lijec Vjesn 2003;125(11-12):329-33.
[145] de Micheli A. On the first studies of electrophysiology. Arch Cardiol Mex 2011;81(4):337-42. [Spanish]
[146] Barold SS. Willem Einthoven and the birth of clinical electrocardiography a hundred years ago. Card Electrophysiol Rev 2003;7(1):99-104.
[147] Schwartze D. Willem Einthoven. Thoughts on the occasion of his 125th anniversary. Z Gesamte Inn Med 1985;40(11):356-60. [German]
[148] Schweitzer P, Keller S. Willem Einthoven—inventor of electrocardiography. Vnitr Lek 2002;48(Suppl 1):20-3.
[149] Henson JR. Descartes and he ECG lettering series. J Hist Med Allied Sci 1971;21:181-186.
[150] Wyers PJ. The string of Einthoven's string galvanometer. Gewina 1996;19(2):80-94. [Dutch]
[151] Einthoven W. Le telecardiogramme. Arch Int de Physiol 1906;4:132-64. (Translated into English: Einthoven W. The telecardiogram. Am Heart J 1957;53:602-15).
[152] Rivera-Ruiz M, Cajavilca C, Varon J. Einthoven's String Galvanometer. Tex Heart Inst J 2008;35(2):174-178.
[153] Cajavilca C, Varon J. Resuscitation great. Willem Einthoven: The development of the human electrocardiogram. Resuscitation 2008;76(3):325-8.
[154] Wyers PJ. Adaptation of Einthoven's string galvanometer for electrocardiography in the Netherlands. Ned Tijdschr Geneeskd 2001;145(51):2465-9. [Dutch]
[155] Ershler I. Willem Einthoven—The man. The string galvanometer electrocardiograph. Arch Intern Med 1988;148(2):453-5.
[156] Einthoven W. Über die form des menschlichen electrocardiogramms. Arch f d Ges Physiol 1895;60:101-23. [German]
[157] Einthoven W. The different forms of the human electrocardiogram and their significance. Lancet 1912(1):853-861.
[158] Underwood EA. Wilhelm Conrad Röntgen (1845-1923) and the early development of radiology.Proc R Soc Med 1945;38(12):697-706.

[159] Underwood EA. Wilhelm Conrad Röntgen (1845-1923) and the early development of radiology. Can Med Assoc J 1946;54:61-7.
[160] Schindler J. Wilhelm Conrad Röntgen and Switzerland. SSO Schweiz Monatsschr Zahnheilkd 1955;65(10):954-8. [German]
[161] Cohen M, Trott NG. Wilhelm Conrad Röntgen, 1845-1923. Br J Radiol 1973;46(542):81-2.
[162] Tubiana M. Wilhelm Conrad Röntgen and the discovery of x-rays. Bull Acad Natl Med 1996;180(1):97-108. [French]
[163] Roth J. The consequences of the discovery by W.C. Röntgen for present-day medical physics and radiation protection. Experimentia 1995;51(7):640-51.
[164] Rosenow UF. Notes on the legacy of the Röntgen rays. Med Phys 1995;22(11 Pt 2):1855-67.
[165] Mould RF. The early history of x-ray diagnosis with emphasis on the contributions of physics 1895-1915. Phys Med Biol 1995;40(11):1741-87.
[166] Cohen M, Trott NG. Radiology, physical science, and the emergency of medical physics. Med Phys 1995;22(11 Pt 2):1889-97.
[167] Johansen JG. Circumstances surrounding the discovery of Röntgen rays. Tidsskr Nor Laegeforen 1995;115(30):3745-8. [Norwegian]
[168] Dörfel G. Röntgen's strange order—A contribution to the history of the discovery of Röntgen's rays. Rofo 2010;182(10):879-82. [German]
[169] Schüttmann W. The response to Wilhem Conrad Röntgen's discovery in Berlin. Sudhoffs Arch 1995;79(1):1-12. [German]
[170] Lentle B, Aldrich J. Radiological sciences, past and present. Lancet 1997;350(9073):280-5.
[171] Frankel RI. Centennial of Röntgen's discovery of x-rays. West J Med 1996;164(6):497-501.
[172] Fleming LW. The Röntgen centenary. Scott Med J 1995;40(5):153-5.
[173] Langfeldt B. Wilhelm Konrad Röntgen 1845-1923. Dan Medicinhist Årbog 1995;115-21. [Danish]
[174] Roguin A. Scipione Riva-Rocci and the men behind the mercury sphygmomanometer. Int J Clin Pract 2006;60(1):73-7.
[175] Karamanou M, Papaioannou TG, Tsoucalas G, Tousoulis D, Stefanadis C, Androutsos G. Blood pressure measurement: lessons learned from our ancestors. Curr Pharm Des 2015;21(6):700-4.
[176] Chávez Domínguez R, de Micheli A. Epistemological focus on sphygmomanometry. Rev Invest Clin 2002;54(1):84-91. [Spanish]
[177] Solo-Perez-de-Celis E. Karl Samuel Von Basch: The sphygmomanometer and the Empire. J Hypertens 2007;25(7):1507-9.
[178] van Gijn J, Gijselhart JP. Riva-Rocci and blood pressure. Ned Tijdschr Geneeskd 2013;157(3):A5536. [Dutch]
[179] Benassi E. Scipione Riva-Rocci. Mal Cardiovasc 1963;33:843-7. [Italian]
[180] Pellegrini G. The scientific work of Scipione Riva-Rocci. Minerva Med 1964;21:900-3. [Italian]
[181] Mancia G. Scipione Riva-Rocci. Clin Cardiol 1997;20(5):503-4.
[182] Fye B. T. Brunton and amyl nitrite: a Victorian vasodilator. Circulation 1986; 74(2):222-9.
[183] Fye WB. T. Lauder Brunton (1844-1916). Clin Cardiol 1989;12(11):675-6.
[184] Berry D. History of cardiology: Sir Thomas Brunton MD. Circulation 2006;116(14):f164.
[185] James TN. The connecting pathways between the sinus node and the A-V node and between the right and left atrium in the human heart. Am Heart J 1963;66(4):498-508.
[186] Cooper J, Marriott HJ. To Wenckebach: A centenary salute. Tex Heart Inst 1999;26(1):8-11.
[187] Mendoza-Davila N, Varon J. Resuscitation great. Karel Wenckebach: the story behind the block. Resuscitation (Ireland) 2008;79(2):189-92.
[188] No authors listed. Sir Thomas Lewis. Can Med Assoc J 1945;52(6):616-7.
[189] Burchell H. Sir Thomas Lewis: his impact on American cardiology. Br Heart J 1981;46(1):1-4.
[190] Krikler DM. Historical aspects of electrocardiography. Cardiol Clin 1987;5(3):349-55.
[191] Hollman A. Sir Thomas Lewis: clinical scientist and cardiologist, 1881-1945. J Med Biogr 1994;2(2):63-70.
[192] Pai-Dhungat JV, Parikh F. Sir Thomas Lewis (1881-1945). J Assoc Physicians India 2015;63(3):103.
[193] Cannom DS. History of syncope in the cardiac literature. Prog Cardiovasc Dis 2013;55(4):334-8.
[194] No authors listed. Frank Norman Wilson, MD. Med Bull (Ann Arbor). 1952;18(9):274-5.

[195] Rijlant P. Frank N. Wilson; 1890-1952. Acta Cardiol 1952;7(5):469-70.
[196] Johnston FD. Frank N. Wilson—in memoriam. J Mich State Med Soc 1953;52(1):76-7.
[197] Kahn JK, Howell JD. Frank Normal Wilson. Clin Cardiol 1987;10:616-618.
[198] Schwartze D. Frank N. Wilson and his significance for cardiology. Z Gesamte Inn Med 1991;46(5):160-3.
[199] Scher AM. Studies of the electrical activity of the ventricles and the origin of the QRS complex. Acta Cardiol 1995;50(6):429-65.
[200] Janse MJ, Rosen MR. History of arrhythmias. Handb Exp Pharmacol 2006;(171):1-39.
[201] Wellens HJ. Cardiac arrhythmias: the quest for a cure: a historical perspective. J Am Coll Cardiol 2004;44(6):1155-63.
[202] Meruane J. Historic perspective of cardiac catheterization. Rev Med Chil 1992;120(10):1184-90. [Spanish]
[203] Bourassa MG. The history of cardiac catheterization. Can J Cardiol 2005; 21(12):1011-4.
[204] Wilms G, Baert AL. The history of angiography. J Belge Radiol 1995;78(5):299-302.
[205] Riley RL. The award of the Trudeau Medal for 1971 (Andre F. Cournand). Am Rev Respir Dis 1971;104(4):615-7.
[206] Cournand A. Dickinson Woodruff Richards: October 20, 1895-February 23, 1973. Biogr Mem Natl Acad Sci 1989;58:459-87.
[207] Cournand A. Dickinson Woodruff Richards, 1895-1973. Trans Assoc Am Physicians 1973;86:22-8.
[208] Raju TN. The Nobel chronicles. 1956: Werner Forssmann (1904-1979), Frédéric Cournand (1895-1988) and Dickinson Woodruff Richards Jr. (1895-1973). Lancet 1999;353(9167):1891.
[209] Hall RJ. In memoriam. F. Mason Sones, Jr, MD. Tex Heart Inst J 1985;12(4):356-358.
[210] Hurst JW, King SB 3rd, Greene L. In memory of Andreas Roland Gruentzig and Margaret Anne Thornton Gruentzig. Am J Cardiol 1986;57(4):333-6.
[211] Hurst JW. Andreas Roland Gruentzig, MD: The teaching genius. Clin Cardiol 1986;9(1):35-7.
[212] Núñez Gn. Andreas Roland Grüntzig, 1939-1985. Rev Soc Venez Hist Med 1990;39(57):65-9. [Spanish]
[213] Jerie P. Thirty years of the balloon catheter—A Grüntzig and percutaneous balloon angioplasty. Cas Lek Cesk 2004;143(12):866-71. [Czech]
[214] Dunn PM. Soranus of Ephesus (circa AD 98-138) and perinatal care in Roman times. Arch Dis Child Fetal Neonatal Ed 1995;73(1):F51-2.
[215] Bloch H. Thomas Phaer, MD (1510-1560): Father of English pediatrics. South Med J 1990;83(6):672-4.
[216] Perrini P, Lanzino G, Parenti GF. Niels Stensen (1638-1686): Scientist, neuroanatomist, and saint. Neurosurgery 2010;67(1):3-9.
[217] Tubbs RS, Gianaris N, Shoja MM, Loukas M, Cohen Gadol AA. “The heart is simply a muscle” and first description of the tetralogy of “Fallot.” Early contributions to cardiac anatomy and pathology by bishop and anatomist Niels Stensen (1638-1686). Int J Cardiol 2012;154(3):312-5.
[218] Pai-Dhungat JV, Parikh F. Niels Stensen (1638-1686). J Assoc Physicians India 2015;63(3):35.
[219] Van Gijn J, Gijselhart JP. Fallot and his tetralogy. Ned Tijdschr Geneeskd 2010;154:A1546. [Dutch]
[220] Evans WN. “Tetralogy of Fallot” and Etienne-Louis Arthur Fallot. Pediatric Cardiol 2008;29(3):637-40.
[221] Van Praagh R. Etienne-Louis Arthur Fallot and his tetralogy: a new translation of Fallot’s summary and a modern reassessment of this anomaly. Eur J Cardiothorac Surg 1989;3(5):381-6.
[222] Waugh D. Maudie: the life and times of McGill’s Maude Abbott. Mod Pathol 1992;5(6):597-9.
[223] Thayer WS. Laennec-One hundred years after. Address in Medicine. Can Med Assoc J 1919;9(9):769-82.
[224] Sakula A. RTH Laënnec-1781-1826-his life and work: a bicentenary appreciation. Thorax 1981; 36(2):81-90.
[225] Rapoport J. Laënnec and the discovery of auscultation. Isr J Med Sci 1986;22(7-8):597-601.
[226] Roguin A. Rene Theophile Hyacinthe Lënnec (1781-1826): the man behind the stethoscope. Clin Med Res 2006;4(3):230-5.
[227] Pai-Dhungat JV. RT Laennec (1781-1826). J Assoc Physicians India 2015;63(3):44-5.

[228] Porter IH. The nineteenth-century physician and cardiologist Thomas Bevill Peacock (1812-1882). Med Hist 1962;6:240-54.

[229] No authors listed. Thomas Bevill Peacock (1812-1882)-19th century cardiologist. JAMA 1968;203(9):801.

[230] Fye WB. Thomas Bevill Peacock. Clin Cardiol 1990;13(6):447-8.

[231] Greenberg M. Thomas Bevill Peacock, pioneer occupational and environmental physician. Am J Ind Med 1992;21(3):443-7.

[232] Storey GA. Thomas Bevill Peacock: Quaker physician. J Friends Hist Soc 1999;58(3):271-76.

[233] Noonan JA. A history of pediatric specialties: the development of pediatric cardiology. Pediatr Res 2004;56:298-306.

[234] Person SA Thomas Syndenham -the founder of clinical medicine (275th anniversary of his detail). Klin Med (Mosk) 1965;43(11):139-44. [Russian]

[235] Taylor FK. Sydenham's disease entities. Psychol Med 1982;12(2):243-50.

[236] Sloan AW. Thomas Syndenham, 1624-1689. S Afr Med J 1987;72(4):275-8.

[237] Anstey P. The creation of the English Hippocrates. Med Hist 2011;55(4):457-78.

[238] Stochik AM, Zatravkin SN. The contribution of T. Syndenham (16224-1689) to the formation of modern Western medicine (on the occasion of the 390th anniversary of his birth). Ter Arkh 2014;86(8):138-42. [Russian]

[239] Podolsky E. Raymond Vieussens and the affairs of the heart. Med Womans J 1950;57(9):32-5.

[240] Kellett CE. Raymond Vieussens on mitral stenosis. Br Heart J 1959;21:440-4.

[241] No authors listed. Raymond De Vieussens (1641-1715) French neuroanatomist and physician. JAMA 1968;206(8):1785-6.

[242] Loukas M, Clarke P, Tubbs RS, Kapos T. Raymond de Vieussens. Anat Sci Int 2007;82(4):233-6.

[243] Kaiser H, Keitel W. Jean-Baptiste Bouillaud (1796-1881)—rheumatologist, cardiologist and more. Z Rheumatol 2007;66(1):65-8. [German]

[244] Silverman BD. Jean Baptiste Bouillaud. Clin Cardiol 1996;19(10):836-7.

[245] Cheadle WB. Scarlatiniform rashes and scarlatina. Br Med J 1879;1(942):75.

[246] Cheadle WB. Harvarian lectues on the various manifestations of the rheumatic state as exemplified in childhood and early life. Lancet 1889;1:821-827.

[247] Caulfield E. Cheadle on rheumatic fever. Pediatrics 1955;15(5):601-2.

[248] Trimble HG. Award of the 1953 College Medal to Dr Helen Taussig. Dis Chest 1953;24(3):343-7.

[249] Harvey AM. Helen Brooke Taussig. Johns Hopkins Med J 1977;140(4):137-41.

[250] Engle MA. Biographies of great American pediatricians— Helen Brooke Taussig: The mother of pediatric cardiology. Pediatric Ann 1982;11(7):629-31.

[251] Neill CA. Helen Brooke Taussig. J Pediatr 1994;125(3):499-502.

[252] Neubauer K, Murphy AM. Helen Brooke Taussig: Pediatric cardiology leader and innovator. Adv Pediatr 2013;60(1):1-9.

[253] Ferencz C. Maude E Abbott—Physician and scientist of international fame. Can J Cardiol 2000;16(7):889-92.

[254] Cabello CF. Diego Rivera: A great master and a didactic and discerning medical historian. Rev Med Chil 2014;142(11):1458-66. [Spanish]

[255] Wooley CF, Miller PJ. William Osler, Maude Abbott, Paul Dudley White, and Helen Taussig: the origins of congenital disease in North America. Am Heart Hosp J 2008;6(1):5106.

[256] Beattie JM. A contribution to the bacteriology of rheumatic fever. J Exp Med 1907;9(2):186-206.

[257] Branch A. The streptococcus and acute rheumatic fever. Can Med Assoc J 1929;20(1):49-50.

[258] Coburn AF, Pauli RH. Studies on the relationship of streptococcus hemolyticus to the rheumatic process: 1. Observations on the ecology of hemolytic streptococcus in relation to the epidemiology of rheumatic fever. J Exp Med 1932;56(5):609-32.

[259] Fleming A. Penicillin: The Robert Campbell Oration. Ulster Med J 1944;13(2):95-122.

[260] Tan SY, Tatsumura Y. Alexander Fleming (1881-1955): Discover of penicillin. Singapore Med J 2015;56(7):366-7.

[261] Otten H. Domagk and the development of sulphonamides. J Antimicrob Chemother 1986;17(6):689-96.

[262] Oehme J. Gerhard Domagk (1895-1964). Kinderkrankenschwester 1993;12(11):392-3. [German]
[263] Gross RE, Hubbard JP. Surgical ligation of a patent ductus arteriosus: report of first successful case. JAMA 1939;112:729-731.
[264] Castañeda AR. Classics in thoracic surgery. Patent ductus arteriosus: A commentary (Robert E. Gross). Ann Thorac Surg 1981;31(1):92-6.
[265] Chalphin AV, Yeo CJ, Cowan SW, Milan S. Robert Edward Gross (1905-1988): Ligation of a patent ductus arteriosus and the birth of a specialty. Am Surg 2014;80(11);1087-8.
[266] Blalock A, Taussig HB. Surgical treatment of malformations of the heart; in which there is pulmonary stenosis or pulmonary atresia. JAMA 1945;128:189-202.
[267] Toledo-Pereyra LH. Alfred Blalock. Surgeon, educator, and pioneer in shock and cardiac research. J Invest Surg 2005;18(4):161-5.
[268] Hansson N, Schlich T. Why did Alfred Blalock and Helen Taussig not receive the nobel prize? J Card Surg 2015;30(6):506-9.
[269] Moller JH. Alexander S. Nadas Lecture. Fifty years of pediatric cardiology and challenges for the future. Circulation 1994;89(5):2479-83.
[270] Attie F, Buendía Hernández A. Pediatric cardiology from its beginnings to the century that approaches. Arch Inst Cardiol Mex 1998;68(2):101-5. [Spanish]
[271] Freedom RM, Lock J, Bricker JT. Pediatric cardiology and cardiovascular surgery: 1950-2000. Circulation 2000;102(20 Suppl 4):IV58-68.
[272] Castañeda A. Congenital heart disease: a surgical-historical perspective. Ann Thorac Surg 2005;79(6):S2217-20.
[273] Gott VL. Lillehei, Lewis, and Wangensteen: the right mix for giant achievements in cardiac surgery. Ann Thorac Surg 2005;79(6):S2210-3.
[274] Mormile R, Quadrini I, Squarcia U. Milestones in pediatric cardiology: making possible the impossible. Clin Cardiol 2013;36(2):74-6.
[275] Ohye RG, Bove EL. Advances in congenital heart surgery. Curr Opin Pediatr 2001;13(5):473-81.
[276] DeBakey ME. John Gibbon and the heart-lung machine: a personal encounter and his import for cardiovascular surgery. Ann Thorac Surg 2003;76(6):S2188-94.
[277] Paul MH. Alexander Sandor Nadas, M.D. (1913-2000). Pediatric Cardiol 2001;22(3):179-182.
[278] Newburger JW, Fyler DC. Alexander Sandor Nadas: November 12, 1913-May 15, 2000. Cardiol Young 2004;14(1):75-82.
[279] Shumway NE. F. John Lewis, MD: 1916-1993. Ann Thorac Surg 1996;61(1):250-1.
[280] Weisse AB. John W. Kirklin (1917-2004). Clin Cardiol 2005;28(12):585-6.
[281] Shumway N. Clarence Walton Lillehei. BMJ 1999;319(7213):856.
[282] Toledo-Pereyra LH. Innovation according to C. Walton Lillehei. J Invest Surg 2007;20(4):205-9.
[283] Rashkind WH, Miller WW. Creation of an atrial septal defect without thoracotomy: A palliative approach to complete transposition of the great arteries. JAMA 1966;196:991-992.
[284] Squarcia U, Squarcia A. Gianocarlo Rastelli: the scientist, the man. Clin Cardiol 2007;30(9):485-7.
[285] Kulkarni A, Hsu HH, Ou P, Kutty S. Computed tomography in congenital heart disease: Clinical applications and technical considerations. Echocardiography 2015 Dec 16. doi: 10.1111/echo.13147.
[286] Schicchi N, Secinaro A, Muscogiuri G, Ciliberti P, Leonardi B, Santangelo T, et al. Multicenter review: Role of cardiovascular magnetic resonance in diagnostic evaluation, pre-procedural planning and follow-up for patients with congenital heart disease. Radiol Med 2016;121(5):342-51.
[287] Hammerman C. Patent ductus arteriosus. Clinical relevance of prostaglandins and prostaglandin inhibitors in PDA pathophysiology and treatment. Clin Perinatol 1995;22(2):457-79.
[288] Obladen M. History of the ductus arteriosus: 1. Anatomy and spontaneous closure. Neonatology 2011;99(20:83-9.
[289] Benitz WE. Committee on Fetus and Newborn. Patent ductus arteriosus in preterm infants. Pediatrics 2016;137(1):e20153730.
[290] Deen JF, Jones TK. Shunt lesions. Cardiol Clin 2015;33(4):513-20.
[291] Montero JV, Nieto EM, Vallejo IR, Montero SV. Intranasal midazolam for the emergency management of hypercyanotic spells in tetralogy of Fallot. Pediatric Emerg Care 2015;31(4):269-71.

[292] Tsze DS, Vitberg YM, Berezow J, Starc TJ, Dayan PS. Treatment of tetralogy of Fallot hypoxic spell with intranasal fentanyl. Pediatrics 2014;134(1):e266-9.
[293] Bronzetti G, Patrizi A, Giacomini F, Savoia F, Raone B, Brighenti M, et al. A PHACES syndrome unmasked by propranolol interruption in a tetralogy of Fallot patient: case report and extensive review on new indications for beta blockers. Curr Med Chem 2014;21(27):3153-64.
[294] Jamerson KA. Rationale for angiogensin II receptor blockers in patients with low-renin hypertension. Am J Kidney Dis 2000;36(3 Suppl 1):S24-30.
[295] Brady TM. Hypertension. Pediatr Rev 2012; 33(12):541-52.
[296] Banker A, Gupta-Malhotra M, Syamasundar Rao P. Childhood hypertension: A review. J Hypertens 2013;2:128-35.
[297] Mitsnefes MM. Hypertension in children and adolescents. Pediatr Clin North Am 2006; 53(3): 493-512.
[298] Mills KI, Costello JM, Almodovar MC. A review of systemic vasodilators in low cardiac output syndrome following pediatric cardiac surgery. Curr Vasc Pharmacol 2016;14(1):29-36.
[299] Spicer DE, Henderson DJ, Chaudhry B, Mohun TJ, Anderson RH. The anatomy and development of normal and abnormal coronary arteries. Cardiol Young 2015;25(8):1493-503.
[300] Sonesson SE, Acharya G. Hemodynamics in fetal arrhythmia. Acta Obstet Gynecol Scand 2015 Dec 10. doi: 10.1111/aogs.12837.
[301] Behere SP, Weindling SN. Inherited arrhythmias: The cardiac channelopathies. Ann Pediatric Cardiol 2015;8(3):210-20.
[302] Abman SH, Hansmann G, Archer SL, Ivy DD, Adatia I, Chung WK, et al. Pediatric pulmonary hypertension: guidelines from the American Heart Association and American Thoracic Society. Circulation 2015;132(21):2037-99.
[303] Elder RW, Baltimore RS. The changing epidemiology of pediatric endocarditis. Infect Dis Clin North Am 2015;29(3):513-24.
[304] Kawasaki T. Acute febrile mucocutaneous syndrome with lymphoid involvement with specific desquamation of the fingers and toes in children. Arerugi 1967;16(3):178-222. [Japanese]
[305] Rowley AH, Wylie KM, Kim KY, Pink AJ, Yang A, Reindel R. The transcriptional profile of coronary arteritis in Kawasaki disease. BMC Genomics 2015;16(1):1076.
[306] Zhao JY, Chiu PP, Dasgupta R, Jen HC, Rothstein DH. Defining the need for transitional care from pediatric to adult surgery for young adult patients with surgically corrected congenital anomalies. JAMA Surg 2015 Dec 16:1-2. doi: 10.1001/jamasurg.2015.4417.
[307] Wilson B, Jones KB, Weedon D, Bilder D. Care of adults with intellectual and developmental disabilities: Down syndrome. FP Essent 2015;439:20-25.
[308] Gerardin JF, Menk JS, Pyles LA, Martin CM, Lohr JL. Compliance with adult congenital heart disease guidelines: are we following the recommendations? Congenit Heart Dis 2015 Nov 11. doi: 10.1111/chd.12309.
[309] Niwa K. Adults with congenital heart disease transition. Curr Opin Pediatr 2015;27(5):576-80.
[310] Petropoulos A, Ehringer-Schetitska D, Fritsch P, Jokinen E, Dalla Pozza R, Oberhoffer R. Preventing cardiac diseases in childhood. Hell J Nucl Med 2015;18(Suppl 1):148.
[311] Zhu H. Forkhead box transcription factors in embryonic heart development and congenital heart disease. Life Sci 2015 Dec 2. pii: S0024-3205(15)30094-1.
[312] Navar PG, Murugesan R, Mary B, Ahmed SS. CardioGenBase: A literature based multi-omics database for major cardiovascular diseases. PLoS One 2015;10(12):e0143188.
[313] Davies AK, McGale N, Humphries SE, Hirani SP, Beaney KE, Bappa DA, et al. Effectiveness of a self-management intervention with personalized genetic and lifestyle-related risk information on coronary heart disease and diabetes-related risk in type 2 diabetes (CoRDia): study protocol for a randomized controlled trial. Trials 2015;16(1):547.
[314] Spoonamore KG, Ware SM. Genetic testing and genetic counseling in patients with sudden death risk due to heritable arrhythmias. Heart Rhythm 2015 Nov 12. pii:S1547-5271(15)01420-4.
[315] Ingles J, Burns C, Barratt A, Semsarian C. Application of genetic testing in hypertrophic cardiomyopathy for preclinical disease detection. Circ Cardiovasc Genet 2015;8(6):852-9.

[316] Butler MR, Carvan MJ 3rd, Johnson TS. Understanding genetics and pediatric cardiac health. J Pediatr Nurs 2015 Dec 1. pii: S0882-5963(15)00358-9.

[317] Loerakker S, Ristori T, Baaijens FP. A computational analysis of cell-mediated compaction and collagen remodeling in tissue-engineered heart valves. J Mech Behav Biomed Mater 2015 Oct 19. pii: S1751-6161(15)00373-2.

[318] Oomen PJ, Loerakker S, van Geemen D, Neggers J, Goumans MJ, van den Bogaerdt AJ et al. Age-dependent changes of stress and strain in the human heart valve and their relation with collagen remodeling. Acta Biomater 2016;29:161-9.

[319] Moser PT, Ott HC. Recellularization of the organs: what is the future for solid organ transplantation? Curr Opin Organ Transplant 2014;19(6):603-9.

[320] Guyette JP, Charest J, Mills RW, Jank B, Moser PT, Gilpin SE. Bioengineering human myocardium on native extracellular matrix. Circ Res 2015 Oct 25 pii: CIRCRESAHA.115.306874.

[321] Cohen S, Houvel L, Guillemain R, Varnous S, Jannot AS, Ladouceur M. Temporal trends and changing profile of adults with congenital heart disease undergoing heart transplantation. Eur Heart J 2015 Dec 8. pii: ehv628.

[322] Law YM. More lessons learned from the Pediatric Heart Transplant Study. Cardiol Young 2015;25(Suppl 2):131-9.

[323] Colan SD. Review of International Society for Heart and Lung Transplantation Practice guidelines for management of heart failure in children. Cardiol Young 2015;25(Suppl 2):154-9.

[324] Cohen MI, Jacobs JP, Cicek S. The 2017 Seventh World Congress on Paediatric Cardiology and Cardiac Surgery: "The Olympics of our profession." Cardiol Young 2017;27(10):1865-1969.

[325] Karl TR, Martin GR, Jacobs JP, Wernovsky G. Key events in the history of cardiac surgery and paediatric cardiology. Cardiol Young 2017;27(10):2029-2062.

[326] Karl TR. The 2017 Seventh World Congress of Pediatric Cardiology & Cardiac Surgery: week in review--cardiac surgery. Cardiol Young 2017;27(10):2023-2024.

[327] Gursu HA, Cetin II. The history of paediatric cardiology on stamps. Cardiol Young 2018;28(1):1-8.

[328] Jacobs JP, Tchervenkov CI, Stellin G, Kurosawa H, Mavroudis C, Jatene MB, et al. History of the World Society for Pediatric and Congenital Heart Surgery: The first decade. World J Pediatr Congenit Heart Surg 2018;9(4):392-406.

[329] Bovard JM, De Souza AM, Harris KC, Human DG, Hosking MCK, Potts JE, et al. Physiologic responses to exercise in pediatric heart transplant recipients. Med Sci Sports Exerc 2019 Jan 8. doi: 10.1249/MSS.0000000000001889.

[330] Kirk R, Butts RJ, Dipchand AI. The first successful pediatric heart transplant and results from the earliest era. Pediatr Transplant 2019 Jan 1:e13349. doi: 10.1111/petr.13349.

[331] Glotzbach KL, Ward JJ, Marietta J, Eckhauser AW, Winter S, Puchalski MD, et al. The benefits and bias in neurodevelopmental evaluation for children with congenital heart disease. Pediatrc Cardiol 2019 Dec 21. doi: 10.1007/s00246-019-02260-7.

[332] Huang J, Gou B, Rong F, Wang W. Dexmedetomidine improves neurodevelopment and cognitive impairment in infants with congenital heart disease. Per Med 2020;17(1:33-41.

[333] Sarno LA, Misra A, Siddeek H, Kheiwa A, Kobayashi D. Cardiac rehabilitation for adults and adolescents with congenital heart disease: Extending beyond the typical patient population. J Cardiopulm Rehabil Prev 2020;40(1):E1-E4.

[334] Alsoufi B, McCracken C, Kanter K, Shashidharan S, Border W, Kogon B. Outcomes of multistage palliation of infants with single ventricle and atrioventricular septal defect. World J Pediatr Congenit Heart Surg 2020;11(1):39-48.

[335] Law S, Chai P, Ündar A. Outcomes of the Fifteenth International Conference on Pediatric Mechanical Circulatory Support Systems and Pediatric Cardiopulmonary Perfusion. Artif Organs 2020;44(1):5-11.

In: Chronic Disease and Disability
Editors: DE Greydanus, P Anne, JD Rowlett et al.
ISBN: 978-1-53617-656-8

Chapter 2

NEWBORN CARDIOLOGY

Monica Martin Goble[1], MD, Jay Yeh[2], MD, Johannes von Alvensleben[1], MD, Chaitanya Panchangam[3], MBBS and Premchand Anne[4,*], MD, MPH, MBA, FAAP, FACP, FACC

[1]Division of Pediatric Cardiology, Department of Pediatrics, University of Michigan, Ann Arbor, Michigan, United States of America
[2]Department of Pediatrics, University of California, Davis Medical Center, Sacramento, California, United States of America
[3]Department of Pediatrics and Human Development, Sparrow Hospital/Michigan State University, Lansing, Michigan, United States of America
[4]Division of Pediatric Cardiology, Department of Pediatrics, Ascension St John Children's Hospital, Detroit, Michigan, United States of America

ABSTRACT

Approximately eight of every 1,000 newborns have a congenital heart abnormality, ranging from mild to severe. This chapter provides a review of these conditions, beginning with an overview of cardiac embryology, fetal and transitional circulation, newborn cardiac evaluation and principles of newborn cardiac testing. Disorders covered include cyanotic heart defects, persistent pulmonary hypertension of the newborn, acyanotic defects, congestive heart failure and cardiogenic shock, associated congenital heart defects of the dysmorphic newborn, and neonatal arrhythmias. Understanding and appreciation of newborn cardiac physiology is vital for the clinician that is caring for the newborn.

The workings of the human heart are the profoundest mystery of the universe
Charles W. Chesnutt (1858-1932)

---

* Correspondence: Premchand Anne, MD, Pediatric Cardiology, Ascension St John Children's Hospital, 22201 Moross, Suite 275, PB II, Detroit, MI 48236, United States. Email: Premchand.anne@ascension.org.

INTRODUCTION

Approximately eight of every 1,000 newborns have a mild to severe congenital heart abnormality. Congenital cardiac defects can be divided into two major groups based on the presence or absence of cyanosis, which can be determined by physical examination and aided by pulse oximetry. Congenital heart disease (CHD) generally occurs because of incomplete or abnormal development of the fetal heart during the first seven weeks of pregnancy. Some defects are associated with genetic disorders, but the etiology of most congenital heart defects is unknown.

An estimated 90% of children diagnosed with CHD will survive into adulthood (1). Survival rates vary by disease complexity: Long-term (survival over 20 years) rates are estimated to be 95% for *simple CHD* (e.g., isolated semilunar valve disease, atrial and ventricular septal defects), 90% for *moderate-severity CHD* (e.g., coarctation of the aorta, atrioventricular septal defect, ventricular septal defect with comorbidities, tetralogy of Fallot), and 80% for *CHD of great complexity* (e.g., single ventricle, truncus arteriosus, complex transposition of the great arteries. Although specific types of complex CHD (e.g., hypoplastic left heart syndrome) may have lower survival rates, overall rates have increased for even the most complex defects (2).

Since the first open-heart surgery for congenital heart defects over 60 years ago, there have been exciting improvements in outcomes from both surgical and catheter-based interventions. The first successful intracardiac correction of a congenital heart defect using hypothermia was in 1952 by Drs C Walton Lillehei and F John Lewis at the University of Minnesota. In 1954, Dr Lillehei performed a series of open-heart operations using cross-circulation with the patient's parent. Laying the groundwork for this was the 1945 JAMA paper by Alfred Blalock and Helen Taussig reporting the anastomosis of a systemic artery to the pulmonary artery to improve oxygen saturation in 3 cyanotic children (3).

In the US about 40,000 babies are born each year with a heart defect including about 4,800 with a critical heart defect (4). Despite improved detection by fetal ultrasound and surgical advances, CHD remains one of the most important causes of death in infancy. The detection rate by fetal ultrasound is between 15 and 50%. Critical CHD is a potentially life-threatening cardiac abnormality; this term implies that either the systemic or pulmonary circulation is dependent on a patent ductus arteriosus and/or that an invasive procedure is necessary within the first month of life. Stated another way, critical CHD includes heart defects that would result in demise unless neonatal intervention to palliate or correct the defect is undertaken.

CHD can be associated with an underlying chromosomal disorder, and many syndromes are associated with cardiac lesions. Approximately 25% of all infants with CHD have at least one associated extracardiac malformation. Conversely, extracardiac malformations can be associated with cardiac defects. For example, a newborn with a cleft palate has a 20% chance of having a heart defect. For the infant with Down syndrome the risk of CHD is 50%. It is often up to the pediatric provider to connect the dots.

Fetal echocardiography has become a vital tool in the diagnosis of CHD. Prenatal diagnosis of critical CHD avoids the hemodynamic compromise often accompanying postnatal diagnosis. The recommended timing for a fetal echocardiogram is 16-20 weeks gestation. Indications include cardiac or other significant abnormalities noted on prenatal ultrasounds, along with a host of fetal, maternal and familial risk factors. Some cardiac anomalies, such as coarctation of the aorta, small ventricular septal defects, atrial septal defects and anomalous pulmonary venous return may be difficult to detect prenatally.

Advances over the past 20 years have resulted in a dramatic decline in mortality and morbidity for infants requiring early open-heart surgery. The developmental progress of these new survivors remains a concern. Causes contributing to brain injury may include prenatal, preoperative, intraoperative, and postoperative events. Long-term studies suggest that subtle neurological deficits and developmental delay are not uncommon. Exciting areas of focus are early detection, surgical advances, advanced imaging techniques and optimization of developmental outcomes. The implementation of a universal newborn critical congenital heart disease (CCHD) screen using pulse oximetry has contributed to a 33 percent decline in deaths from CCHD and 21 percent decrease in other cardiac deaths; the CCHD screen is expected to save 120 babies nationwide yearly (5).

EMBRYOLOGY OVERVIEW

The cardiovascular system is the first major organ system to develop. It is fully formed and functioning by the eighth week of gestation. Similarities of aspects of heart development across phylogeny have helped elucidate principles underlying cardiac development and cardiac anomalies. Figure 1 below depicts cardiac development.

During the first 20 days post-conception the embryo is without a cardiovascular system. Over the next month, the heart and great vessels develop. Angiogenic cells are transformed into a four-chambered structure. The heart is a mesodermal structure, with precursor cells originating in the lateral plate mesoderm. These precursor cells migrate towards the midline to form a single heart tube. The heart tube differentiates into several fusiform structures. From cranial to caudal, these dilatations include the truncus arteriosus, the bulbus cordis, the primitive ventricles, the primitive atria and the sinus venosus. The tubular heart undergoes rightward looping and grows into a complex, three-dimensional structure with asymmetry along its axes resulting in an asymmetric multi-chambered heart. Rightward looping is essential for proper orientation of the developing cardiac chambers, chamber septation and the development of inflow and outflow tracts. Figure 2 demonstrates cardiac looping.

The heart tube starts beating at 23 days. The primitive heart tube, containing both myocardial and endocardial layers, starts pumping blood through a primitive circulatory system at about four weeks. Blood leaving the lower ventricles enters the truncus arteriosus. Rightward- or d-looping aligns cardiac chambers for morphogenesis into a four-chambered structure. By 30 days, blood circulates throughout the embryo. As the embryo grows and folds on itself, the heart tube undergoes a series of foldings. As a result, the atria align posterior and superior to the ventricles. Septation of atria and the ventricles begins at 27 days. The atrioventricular canal leads to cardiac septation. A spiral septum grows within the truncus arteriosus, dividing it into the pulmonary artery and aorta.

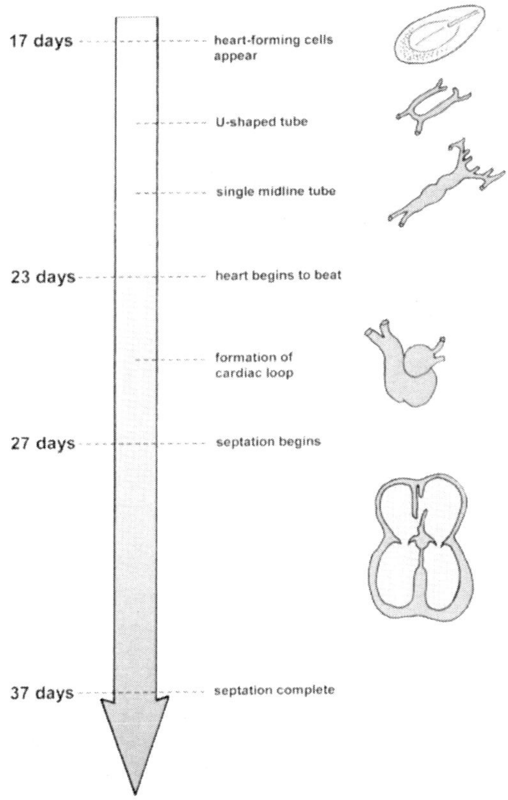

Figure 1. Cardiac development.

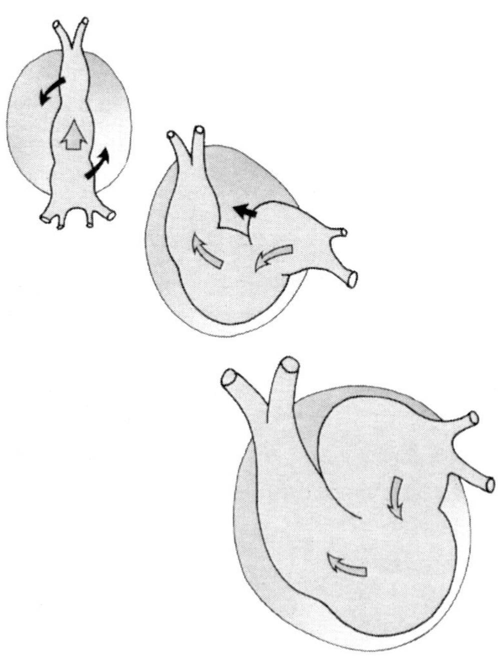

Figure 2. Cardiac looping.

Disruptions of cardiac development are well-recognized. Failure of migration of precursor cells can lead to dextrocardia or situs inversus. Abnormal septation can lead to atrial and ventricular septal defects. Atrioventricular septal defects or tricuspid atresia can result if the endocardial cushion fails to provide normal septation. Failure of the spiral septum to divide the truncus arteriosus into the pulmonary artery and aorta can result in conotruncal defects such as truncus arteriosus, tetralogy of Fallot or transposition of the great arteries (6).

Fetal and Transitional Circulation

After birth, the pulmonary and systemic vascular systems are in series and the systemic vascular resistance is higher than the pulmonary vascular resistance. In utero, the low vascular resistance of the placenta and the high vascular resistance of the fluid-filled fetal lungs result in right-to-left shunting characteristic of the fetal circulation. Figure 3 depicts fetal circulation.

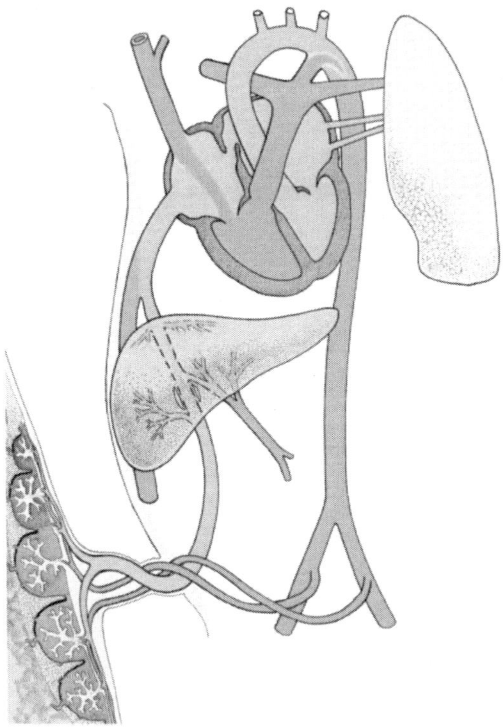

Figure 3. Fetal circulation.

Fetal circulation

A single umbilical vein transports oxygenated blood from the placenta towards the heart via the ductus venosus (bypassing the liver). To bypass the collapsed lungs, the foramen ovale allows for shunting of oxygenated blood from the ductus venosus into the left atrium, left ventricle and to the ascending aorta. The deoxygenated blood from the superior vena cava is directed into the right atrium and ventricle, which then enters the ductus arteriosus which allows shunting into the descending aorta. Two umbilical arteries transport deoxygenated blood back to the placenta.

Some of this oxygen-rich blood, however, travels from the right atrium into the right ventricle and enters the main pulmonary artery, mixing with venous return from the head. The lungs are collapsed, and the pulmonary vascular resistance is therefore high. Because of this high pulmonary vascular resistance most of the blood in the main pulmonary artery crosses the ductus arteriosus and mixes with blood in the aorta supplying the body. In this manner, the right ventricle provides approximately 60% of the total cardiac output. With most of the blood pumped by the right ventricle bypassing the lungs into the descending aorta, the two ventricles are operating in-parallel in utero, rather than in-series as occurs after delivery. The right ventricle is dominant, pumping about twice the output of the left ventricle.

The fetal circulation results in 1) oxygenated blood from the placenta preferentially flowing through the foramen ovale to allow the left heart to pump oxygenated blood into the ascending aorta, aortic arch and, therefore, the brain, and 2) oxygen-poor blood returning from the superior vena cava preferentially flowing into the right ventricle, pulmonary artery, and ductus arteriosus pathway to enter the descending aorta. From the descending aorta blood can flow back to the placenta, via the umbilical arteries, where carbon dioxide and waste products are released in exchange for oxygen and nutrients.

The ascending aorta provides relatively oxygenated blood to the head, myocardium, and upper body, via the carotid, coronary and subclavian arteries; a small portion travels across the aorta to the descending aorta. Intrauterine oxygen tension is low, mostly between 20 and 30 mmHg. The highest oxygen tension is found in the umbilical vein with a PO_2 of only about 55 mmHg. Blood returning to the placenta has a PO_2 between 15 and 25 mmHg.

Transitional circulation

Changes in the fetal circulation occur immediately after birth, beginning with the first breath and the clamping of the umbilical cord. With the clamping of the umbilical cord, there is loss of the low resistance placental circulation, leading to a sudden increase in the systemic vascular resistance. The left ventricular systolic pressure rises in response. Umbilical cord clamping also leads to a sudden loss of flow through the ductus venosus, which then closes. This results in decreased venous return to the right atrium and a drop in the right atrial pressure while the left-sided pressures are rising. An approximation of the septum primum with the septum secundum and functional foramen ovale closure follows. Anatomic closure of the foramen ovale occurs over a period of months to years. In about a third of adults, the foramen ovale remains persistent (7).

When the newborn takes the first few breaths, there is a sudden expansion of the lungs with a fall in pulmonary vascular resistance and increased blood flow through the pulmonary vessels. By then the pressure in the aorta exceeds the pulmonary artery pressure, leading to a reversal in the blood flow across the ductus arteriosus. The musculature of the ductus arteriosus is sensitive to oxygen. As the oxygen tension of the blood increases, the ductus arteriosus constricts and functionally closes during the first few days of life; ductal arteriosus persistency times were 27.4 and 45.1 hours in boys and girls, respectively (8). The pulmonary vascular resistance continues to drop, with the maximal drop occurring within the first few weeks of life.

Newborn Cardiac Evaluation

Symptoms

In newborn and young infants, metabolic demands are highest during feedings. The infant with low cardiac output, most commonly from excessive pulmonary blood flow, will tire easily during feeding, as an older child would with exercise. With congestive heart failure, caloric intake is decreased due to the difficulty of coordinating the suck-swallow mechanism in the presence of tachypnea and general fatigue. Increased sympathetic discharge leads to tachycardia and diaphoresis, especially during feeds. Suboptimal weight gain in infants with congestive heart failure results from both decreased intake and increased caloric demands.

Vital signs

Heart rate

When assessing heart rate, it is important to consider the newborn's activity level, which can result in elevations of heart rate. Resting rates outside the normal range for age should be assessed for normal or abnormal variability or fixed rate, suggesting an underlying dysrhythmia. The newborn heart rate averages about 100 beats per minute, ranging between about 70 and 180 beats per minute. Term newborns may have a resting heart rate towards the lower end especially when sleeping.

More important than the actual heart rate is whether it varies appropriately with activity or stimulation. For newborns with abnormally low heart rates and whose heart rate variability seems blunted, an electrocardiogram may help to exclude complete heart block, as can occur with maternal lupus (diagnosed or undiagnosed). Because neonates have smaller stroke volumes, cardiac output is maintained by higher heart rates. Over time, stroke volume increases and contributes more to the overall cardiac output. Compared with the adult heart, neonatal myocardium has fewer contractile myofibrils and is relatively stiff. Newborns therefore rely primarily on increases in heart rate to increase cardiac output.

Respiratory rate

Tachypnea above 60 breaths per minute with or without retractions suggests a cardiac abnormality. Tachypnea is also evident in pulmonary or metabolic abnormalities. Respiratory distress in the newborn, from cardiac or other causes, may be accompanied by apnea, cyanosis, grunting, stridor, nasal flaring and poor feeding.

Blood pressure

Documentation of blood pressure is essential when assessing the cardiovascular system. Before considering if values are abnormal, record the blood pressures several times when the baby is quiet. For noninvasive measurement, automated Doppler or oscillometric equipment is preferred, along with using the appropriate size cuff (bladder length covering 80 to100% of the arm circumference and inflatable bladder width covering at least 40% of the arm circumference) (9, 10). In newborns, conventional sphygmomanometry is not recommended because the Korotkoff sounds cannot be heard reliably. The same BP cuff selection method as is used in older children applies. An Australian study of 400 term infants showed median systolic, diastolic and mean blood pressures on day 1 of 65 mmHg, 45 mmHg, and 48 mmHg, respectively (11). (The ranges were 46-94, 24-57, and 31-63, respectively.) By day 4, these values had increased slightly to 70 mmHg, 46 mmHg and 54 mmHg.

In the newborn, the systolic arm and leg pressures are expected to be the same (12). In older children systolic amplification in the legs, due to reflected waves, is felt to account for higher pressure in the legs than arms. This absence of a higher systolic pressure in the leg in the newborn may be related to the presence of a normally narrow aortic isthmus. An arm systolic blood pressure more than 10 mmHg above the leg blood pressure suggests an aortic coarctation, aortic arch hypoplasia, or an interrupted aortic arch. If the ductus arteriosus is widely patent, however, a blood pressure difference between upper and lower extremities may not be present with these defects. It is best practice to check the blood pressure "in the right arm for consistency, for comparison with standard tables, and to avoid a falsely low reading from the left arm in the case of coarctation of the aorta (9, 10).

Physical examination

Inspection

The newborn cardiac exam does not start with a stethoscope. It begins with a careful inspection of the infant with these questions in mind: What is the heart rate, respiratory rate, blood pressure? Is the baby unusually small, e.g., from intrauterine growth retardation, or unusually large, e.g., from maternal diabetes? Is the baby dysmorphic? Is the infant comfortable or with increased work of breathing/accessory muscle use? An infant with comfortable tachypnea may have an underlying heart defect, most often a cyanotic defect. If the infant is dysmorphic or syndromic an underlying heart defect is more likely.

Palpation

The cardiac exam begins with palpation to assess precordial activity and pulses. Increased precordial activity may be from an increased right or left ventricular stroke volume, as can be seen with anemia or sepsis. As the weeks pass postnatally, the pulmonary vascular resistance progressively drops. By one to two months of age, increased precordial activity from a left-to-right shunt may be noted. At this age, heart failure symptoms may develop, from a hemodynamically significant ventricular septal defect or a patent ductus arteriosus.

If the murmur is prominent and/or there is marked turbulence, a thrill may be appreciated. If a thrill is not felt on initial palpation, it is advisable in the presence of a loud murmur to go back and palpate the area where the murmur is loudest. The ball of the hand (at the base of the fingers) is most sensitive for detecting thrills. If a thrill is detected, the murmur is at least a Grade IV/VI; if there is no thrill, the murmur is, by definition, a Grade III/VI or less.

Pulses

Palpation of the brachial and femoral pulses in infants should be performed simultaneously. If the timing and intensity of are similar, the diagnosis of coarctation of the aorta is unlikely. Diminished pulses indicate poor cardiac output, peripheral vasoconstriction, or left-sided obstructive heart defects. These include hypoplastic left heart syndrome, severe coarctation of aorta, critical aortic stenosis and an interrupted aortic arch.

Femoral pulses may be difficult to palpate; patience and gentleness are important. If an infant is crying, it's best to try again after the infant relaxes. Absent or diminished femoral pulses suggest coarctation of the aorta. Sometimes in the presence of a coarctation the left radial pulse will be difficult to palpate, along with the femoral pulses, depending on the location of the aortic narrowing.

Auscultation

When listening to the heart sounds, one should be aware of where they are best heard. With dextrocardia, the heart sounds are louder over the right chest, even if audible over the left chest. The precordium should be addressed methodically, encompassing: (1) upper right sternal border, (2) upper left sternal border, (3) mid-left sternal border, (4) lower left sternal border, and (5) the apex (13). The diaphragm of the stethoscope is best for mid and high-pitched sounds and the bell is best for low-pitched sounds. S_1 (first heart sound) is due to closure of the mitral and tricuspid valves and is normally single. It is best heard at the lower left sternal border. S_2 (second heart sound) comes from closure of the aortic and pulmonic valves and is best heard at the upper left sternal border.

The splitting of S_2 should increase with respiration although this is often difficult to appreciate in newborns with their relatively fast heart rates. This splitting occurs because inspiration pulls more blood into the right heart and right ventricular ejection is thereby prolonged, leading to delayed closure of the pulmonary valve. A single S2 may be heard with transposition of the great arteries as the aorta is directly anterior and obscures pulmonary valve closure or with pulmonary atresia when the pulmonary valve is missing.

Systolic ejection clicks are high-pitched sounds that occur with maximal opening of the aortic or pulmonary valves (14). They are heard best with the diaphragm, just after S_1 along the mid-left sternal border. These can occur with a bicuspid or stenotic aortic or pulmonary valve. Aortic valve ejection clicks are constant, i.e., they do not vary with respiration. Pulmonary valve clicks are heard best during expiration.

A murmur does not always signify a heart defect, nor is the absence of a murmur reassuring. Sixty percent of normal newborns can have a murmur. Small ventricular septal defects are common and are not clinically important. Soft systolic flow murmurs (Grade I-III/VI) may occur during the transition from fetal to neonatal circulation, as with transient tricuspid regurgitation.

The most common newborn murmur is a peripheral pulmonic stenosis murmur. The murmur is a soft mid-systolic long ejection murmur heard over the pulmonary area radiating across both sides of the chest and to the axilla and back. This murmur reflects the relative hypoplasia of the branch pulmonary arteries compared to the well-developed main pulmonary artery, and to the branches' sharp angle of origin. There is little flow of blood through the branch pulmonary arteries in utero; as they stretch to accommodate the normal pulmonary blood flow over the first few months of life, this murmur will gradually become softer.

Still's murmur, more common in school-age children, can be heard in infancy. These systolic murmurs have a vibratory or musical quality (like a rubber-band twang) and thought to perhaps be from vibrations of the papillary muscle apparatus of the mitral valve. Pathologic murmurs associated with specific cardiac lesions are discussed separately.

Systolic murmurs are graded on a 6-point scale and diastolic murmurs on a 4-point scale. Systolic murmurs can be characterized as *harsh*, as from high-velocity gradients, *ejection (diamond-shaped)*, best heard at the upper sternal border overlying stenotic pulmonary or aortic valves, or *blowing* or *regurgitant (plateau-shaped),* from a ventricular septal defect or mitral or tricuspid regurgitation, each of which is best heard at the mid- or lower- left sternal border. Diastolic murmurs in the newborn are rare in isolation. Continuous murmurs, most commonly occurring in association with a patent ductus arteriosus, are long systolic murmurs that continue into diastole. Three generalizations concerning auscultatory findings in newborns are:

- Innocent murmurs are heard less frequently in neonates than in older children; if a murmur is heard, take it seriously.
- If a harsh systolic murmur is heard in the first three days, the baby may have an obstructive lesion.
- The murmur of a ventricular septal defect may not be present until a few days of age, appearing only after the pulmonary vascular resistance falls. Parents may wonder why the murmur wasn't detected in the nursery (5).

Liver size

Use the fingertips to work up from right lower quadrant of the abdomen, pressing gently upward. The liver edge is normally 1–2 cm below the right costal margin. If it is enlarged, in the absence of hyperinflated lungs displacing the liver into the abdomen, this suggests heart failure, which may be either right or left sided. Unlike in older children, this is a relatively easy marker to measure. Peripheral edema and rales are rare in infants with heart failure; sacral edema and puffiness of the eyes are more common. Although respiratory distress and tachypnea may be present, subtler signs such as poor feeding and hepatomegaly may be the only manifestations of heart failure. Assessment of the liver edge is thus a critical portion of the physical examination in infants.

NEWBORN CARDIAC TESTING

Hyperoxia test

The hyperoxia test is one way to distinguish cyanotic congenital heart defects from pulmonary disease. Newborns with cyanotic CHD are usually not able to raise their arterial PaO_2 significantly during administration of 100% oxygen. If the PaO_2 rises above 150 mmHg, an intracardiac right-to-left shunt can usually be excluded (although some patients may be able to increase their PaO_2 to >150 mm Hg due to intracardiac streaming patterns). In patients with pulmonary disease on the other hand, PaO_2 generally increases significantly in 100% oxygen, as abnormalities in ventilation-perfusion equilibrate (15). Further, hypoxia with many of the cyanotic heart lesions is consistent, whereas for respiratory disorders and persistent pulmonary hypertension of the newborn (PPHN), arterial oxygen tension varies with time or changes in ventilator settings.

Pulse oximetry screening

In 2011, screening for critical congenital heart disease (CCHD) was added to the Recommended Uniform Screening Panel for newborns in the US and endorsed by the AAP (16, 17). CCHD includes coarctation of the aorta, double outlet right ventricle (DORV), D-transposition of the great arteries (d-TGA), Ebstein's anomaly, hypoplastic left heart syndrome (HLHS), interrupted aortic arch, pulmonary atresia with intact septum, single ventricle, total anomalous pulmonary venous connection (TAPVR), tetralogy of Fallot (TOF), tricuspid atresia, and truncus arteriosus (18). CCHD is often patent ductus arteriosus (PDA)-dependent but is also defined more generally as requiring heart surgery within the first month. Many newborns with CCHD, especially left-sided CCHD, will appear entirely well at the time of routine hospital discharge only to become critically ill within the next few days due to ductal closure. Studies have shown that compared to the physical examination alone, universal neonatal screening with pulse oximetry improves identification of patients with CCHD.

A large Swedish study showed that universal pulse oximetry screening was better than the physical exam at detecting both infants with mild oxygen desaturation and those with CCHD. Six of 16 infants with pulse oximetry saturation between 90 and 94% were not detected by physical examination but were by pulse oximetry. Also noted was a lower rate of missed diagnoses of CCHD in places with universal pulse oximetry screening compared to places without routine oximetry (8 vs 28%). In addition, no newborn died from a ductal-dependent lesion in places utilizing routine pulse oximetry versus five deaths in places without routine oximetry. The investigators concluded that screening seems cost-neutral in the short-term, but it will likely prove cost-effective in the long term, through the prevention of neurological morbidity and a reduced need for pre-operative neonatal intensive care (19).

In a 2012 meta-analysis of 13 studies with data for almost 230,000 newborn infants, the overall sensitivity of pulse oximetry for detection of CCHD was 76% and the specificity was 99.9%, with a false-positive rate of 0.14%. The false-positive rate was particularly low when newborn pulse oximetry was done after 24 hours of age compared to before 24 hours. In contrast, sensitivity is not affected by the timing of the pulse oximetry test. A cutoff SaO_2 <95% is generally used (20).

A number of practical points to consider include:

- Pulse oximetry fails to identify all patients with left-sided obstructive lesions dependent on a PDA and will not detect acyanotic heart defects, such as ventricular septal defects.
- Other conditions, such as transient tachypnea of the newborn, can result in low oxygen saturation readings.
- If the infant is crying or moving, the accuracy of the test will be reduced.
- Training of health care personnel improves reliability and accuracy.
- Post-ductal probe placement is optimal because defects with right-to-left shunting of desaturated blood through the PDA are less likely to be detected with pre-ductal placement only.

Newborn screening is directed towards identifying seven specific lesions. Of note, the undiagnosed conditions most likely to lead to death soon after discharge from hospital are hypoplastic left heart, interruption of the aortic arch and coarctation of the aorta. The seven lesions that are statistically most likely to be detected, however, include only hypoplastic left heart syndrome. The other six are cyanotic lesions. The seven lesions most likely to be detected are:

1) Hypoplastic left heart syndrome
2) Pulmonary atresia
3) Tetralogy of Fallot
4) Total anomalous pulmonary venous return
5) Transposition of the great arteries
6) Tricuspid atresia
7) Truncus arteriosus

The following newborn pulse oximetry screening strategy has been endorsed by the American Academy of Pediatrics (AAP) and the American Heart Association (AHA) (21).

- Screening should be performed at about 24 hours of age, or as late as possible if early discharge is planned.
- A motion-tolerant pulse oximeter should be used, in the right hand and either foot, simultaneously or in direct sequence.
- Screening should be performed by qualified and trained personnel.
- A positive screening test fulfills one of the following three criteria:
    - SaO_2 measurement <90%
    - SaO_2 measurement <95% in both upper and lower extremities on three measurements, each separated by one hour
    - SaO_2 difference >3% between the upper and lower extremities
- Each birthing institution should establish a protocol to ensure a timely evaluation for newborns with a positive screening test. After a careful review of the newborn's condition, medical history and physical exam, assessment of a positive screen most often includes the performance of high-quality echocardiography and interpretation by a clinician with expertise in the diagnosis of CHD. Access to these diagnostic services either at the center, via telemedicine, or via transport is essential.

Electrocardiogram

Note right axis deviation and right ventricular hypertrophy, both of which are normal for age. The negative QRS voltage in lead I, with an overall positive voltage in aVF places the QRS axis in the southwest corner, at about 150 degrees. Across the precordial leads V1and V6, in particular, show right ventricular dominance.

The right ventricle is thicker than the left ventricle in the fetus and newborn as a result of their higher pulmonary pressures. Therefore, the electrocardiogram (ECG) will show right ventricular dominance and right axis deviation. Across the precordium, the R wave amplitude is increased in leads V_1 and V_2 and decreased in leads V_5 and V_6. This is due to stronger right ventricular forces (anterior) compared to left ventricular forces (posterior).

In children, the QRS axis is normally between about 0 and 90 degrees, with the QRS positive in leads I and aVF. Although the PR and QRS intervals tend to be shorter in infants, the corrected QT interval (QTc) is longer than in older children. It is important to note that newborn prolongation of QT interval maybe transient or could indicate a form of long QT syndrome; furthermore, QTc less than 500 milliseconds usually return to normal whereas a QTc greater than 600 milliseconds may remain prolonged and is often associated with severe arrhythmias (22). When there is a question about a long QT interval in newborns, the ECG can be repeated days or weeks later to see if it normalizes. Finally, T wave morphology can be difficult to interpret in neonates and children. At birth, the T wave may be upright, flat, or inverted in V_1. Within a few days after birth, the T wave normally becomes inverted. Upright T waves after a few days of age may indicate right ventricular hypertrophy. Figure 4 demonstrates a normal newborn electrocardiogram.

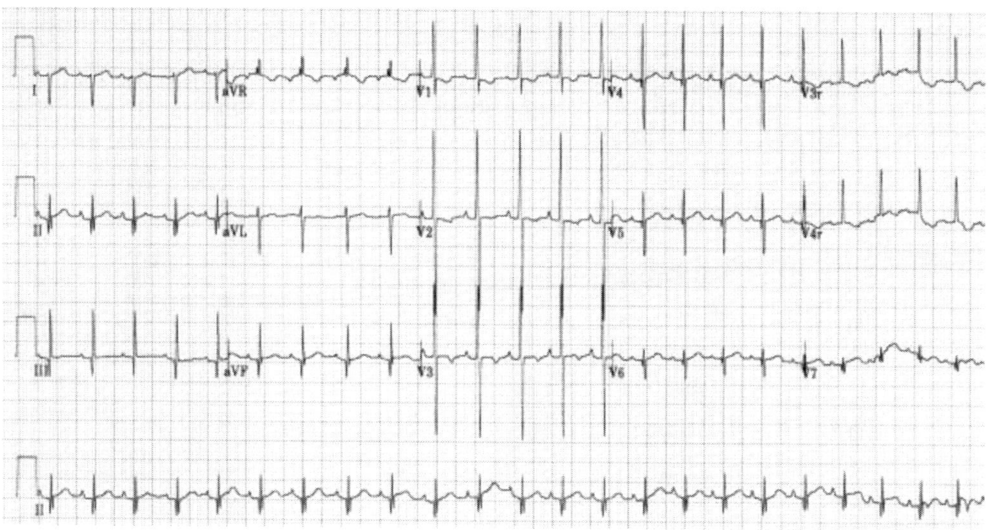

Figure 4. Newborn ECC.

Chest Radiography

A chest X-ray (CXR) in newborns with desaturation or respiratory distress can be helpful in differentiating between pulmonary and cardiac disease. CXR interpretation focuses on heart size, arch sidedness and abdominal situs, pulmonary vascularity and checking for bony abnormalities (e.g., abnormal vertebrae or ribs). In the case of suspected heart disease, it shows whether pulmonary blood flow is increased, normal, or decreased, which can help narrow the cardiac differential diagnosis. The mediastinum and cardiac shadow are relatively large in the newborn. Newborns may therefore appear to have cardiomegaly when in fact the thymus is contributing to the generous "cardio-thymic shadow." The diameter of a normal heart may approach 60% of the thoracic transverse diameter.

A screening CXR for CHD in neonates has a low sensitivity (26–59%) and an even lower specificity for detecting heart defects among neonates under two kilograms (23). Cardiomegaly can be from a congenital heart defect, cardiomyopathy or a pericardial effusion. The atrial and visceral situs can be assessed based on the position of the stomach bubble. If possible, both the side of the aortic arch and the bronchial anatomy can be noted. Vascular rings, although rare, usually occur in association with a right-sided aortic arch; index of suspicion should be high for a vascular ring in infants with a right aortic arch and feeding and/or breathing difficulties.

Regarding pulmonary vascularity, oligemia (dark lung fields) suggests decreased blood flow through the pulmonary circulation. This may result from a right-to-left shunt, as with right ventricular outflow obstruction. Congested pulmonary vasculature, conversely, can represent either increased pulmonary blood flow or increased pulmonary venous pressure from abnormal pulmonary venous return.

Echocardiography

Echocardiography has revolutionized the diagnosis and management of CHD, most notably in the neonatal period. It confirms anatomy and provides information regarding physiology and myocardial function. High-resolution transducers, portability, good neonatal acoustic windows and its safety profile have meant that echocardiography is often the only modality needed to diagnose most neonates with CHD. Strides in fetal ultrasound technology have facilitated prenatal diagnosis of CHD and has improved neonatal management and outcomes, with planned procurement of resources and subspecialists. Specifically, echocardiography is useful to elucidate the following:

- Cardiac anatomy, including venous and arterial connections
- Presence and degree of shunting, for example through a patent ductus arteriosus or ventricular septal defect
- Presence and degree of valvar stenosis and regurgitation
- Atrial and ventricular sizes
- Systolic and diastolic function
- Estimation of right ventricular and pulmonary artery pressures

Echocardiography is the gold standard for diagnosing CHD, but it requires skilled personnel and is not readily available in all hospitals. It is operator-dependent. A sonographer with knowledge of CHD, if available, should obtain the images, ideally with a pediatric cardiologist at the bedside in cases of suspected congenital heart disease. With advances in echocardiography technology and the addition of color Doppler in the late 1980s, most anatomic and hemodynamic information can be obtained from a thorough echocardiogram. This means that cardiac catheterization is reserved for conditions when 1) anatomic detail could not be fully delineated by echocardiography (e.g., distal pulmonary arteries, aortopulmonary collaterals, and aberrant coronary arteries) or 2) transcatheter therapeutic intervention is being considered.

Magnetic resonance imaging

When the information from echocardiography and invasive angiography is insufficient, cardiac magnetic resonance imaging (MRI) can provide detailed information regarding cardiac anatomy, ventricular function and characteristics of the myocardium. MRI studies are typically directed to clarify specific questions about the morphology of known anatomy. MRI offers advantages over other imaging modalities including lack of ionizing radiation, excellent soft tissue contrast and true three-dimensional imaging of anatomy.

Imaging of infants is more demanding than imaging of older children and adults. Sedation is usually needed. Also required are increased spatial resolution because of the subject's smaller size and inability to breath-hold, and increased temporal resolution because of their higher heart rates (24).Neonatal cardiac MRI has a number of advantages over echocardiography:

- Less operator-dependent, enhancing reproducibility
- Provides direct visualization of all areas of the heart.
- More reliable flow measurements and markers of contractility.

Principles of Congenital Heart Disease

Two principles (theories/hypotheses) that determine congenital heart disease are the following:

1) "No flow, no grow" hypothesis (25)
2) Blood follows the path of least resistance.

Understanding these two principles and application of the principles can elucidate/clarify the pathophysiology of congenital heart disease.

Cyanotic Heart Defects and Persistent Pulmonary Hypertension of the Newborn

Cyanosis is a physical finding that is commonly seen in newborns. It is the appearance of a bluish color to the skin and mucous membranes. Newborn cyanosis has become easier to confirm or discount than in the past, as pulse oximeters have become ubiquitous. True cyanosis, or central cyanosis, is best appreciated at the mucous membranes of the eyes and lips, and in the nail beds. Cyanosis represents an increased concentration of reduced hemoglobin, that which is within the red blood cells after the oxygen of oxyhemoglobin has been released to the tissues.

Cyanosis is generally perceptible when 5 grams/100mL of reduced hemoglobin is present in the capillaries (26). The normal amount of reduced hemoglobin is about 2 grams/100mL, although this varies based on the underlying total hemoglobin levels. A polycythemic newborn will have recognizable cyanosis at higher oxygen saturations, while an anemic newborn will not have cyanosis until there is lower oxygen saturation. With a normal hemoglobin level, the degree of reduced hemoglobin (5 g/100mL) necessary to perceive cyanosis in a newborn corresponds to an oxygen saturation of 75-80%. Milder degrees of hypoxemia are not often apparent. Hypoxemia is a biochemical phenomenon in which the systemic arterial partial pressure of oxygen is abnormally low; it is not synonymous with cyanosis for the reasons noted above. *Acrocyanosis* (from the Greek akros meaning extreme or at the end) of the hands and feet is common in the days following delivery, while the circulation to the extremities transitions. It is considered benign. Pulse oximetry readings are reassuringly normal. Similarly, isolated circumoral cyanosis, i.e., around the mouth, is occasionally encountered in children with fair skin and is thought to represent vasoconstriction with resultant sluggish blood flow.

Approach to true cyanosis

When a newborn presents with true cyanosis and hypoxemia, confirmed by pulse oximetry, identifying the cause is paramount to initiate appropriate treatment. The first question to consider is whether the cyanosis is cardiac or non-cardiac (e.g., pulmonary, neurologic or hematologic, such as methemoglobinemia). A cardiac cause of cyanosis can be confirmed with an oxygen challenge or hyperoxia test (see Newborn Cardiac Testing section above). Because the fetus has low oxygen tension by virtue of placental exchange neonatal cyanosis is better tolerated than it would be without this adaptation. Nonetheless, in addition to tracking oxygen levels in infants with cyanotic heart defects it is important to monitor for developing acidosis.

Cyanotic heart defects

These can be divided according to whether pulmonary blood flow is decreased (tetralogy of Fallot, pulmonary atresia with an intact septum, tricuspid atresia and total anomalous pulmonary venous return with obstruction) or increased (transposition of the great vessels, some types of single ventricles, truncus arteriosus and total anomalous pulmonary venous return without obstruction). The chest radiograph is a valuable tool for initial differentiation between these two categories. Many of these defects start with the letter T, to which they may be referred as the "Terrible Ts" or five Ts of CHD.

D-transposition of the great arteries (d-TGA)

The most common cardiovascular cause for cyanosis in the immediate newborn period is d-transposition of the great arteries (d-TGA). There is usually an accompanying patent foramen ovale or atrial septal defect and in one-third of cases there is a ventricular septal defect (as shown in the figure). D-TGA results from abnormal rotation and development of the truncus arteriosus with resulting atrio-ventricular concordance and ventriculo-arterial discordance. This means that the aorta arises from the right-sided morphologic right ventricle and the pulmonary artery arises from the left-sided left ventricle. This alignment results in a circulatory system with two parallel circuits, the systemic circuit being oxygen-poor and the pulmonary circuit being oxygen-rich, rather than in the normal "in-series" arrangement.

The four-chamber views are usually normal in d-TGA; this defect can be difficult to identify prenatally. Along with significant central cyanosis, comfortable tachypnea is a common physical finding. Usually no murmur is present. The second heart sound (S_2) is likely to be single, from the anterior aortic valve. A chest x-ray may show narrowing of the superior mediastinum, related to the orientation of the great vessels, the" egg-on-a-string" shadow; more often the thymus overlies the mediastinum in the newborn, masking this finding that would be more common in older children. A chest x-ray would typically show either normal or increased pulmonary vascularity. The combination of the lack of a murmur and a relatively normal appearing chest x-ray in a significantly cyanotic newborn makes the odds of d-TGA high. Confirmatory diagnosis is made by echocardiogram with attention given to the atrial and ventricular septae, outflow tracts, coronary artery anatomy and size of the PDA.

Delivery of oxygen to the tissues in a newborn with d-TGA depends on communication between the two parallel circuits that allows oxygenated blood to mix with deoxygenated blood; this is the role of the atrial septal defect or patent foramen ovale. If the atrial septum is inadequately small, an emergent atrial septostomy (Rashkind procedure) can be performed at the bedside with echo guidance or as part of a cardiac catheterization - to establish a more reliable communication between the two parallel circuits.

The PDA helps by shunting systemic blood into the lower resistance pulmonary circuit. The PDA is usually kept patent using prostaglandin E_1 (PGE_1) to augment atrial mixing. This is followed by definitive repair with an arterial switch operation, usually done within the first week of life. Figure 5 depicts transposition of the great arteries.

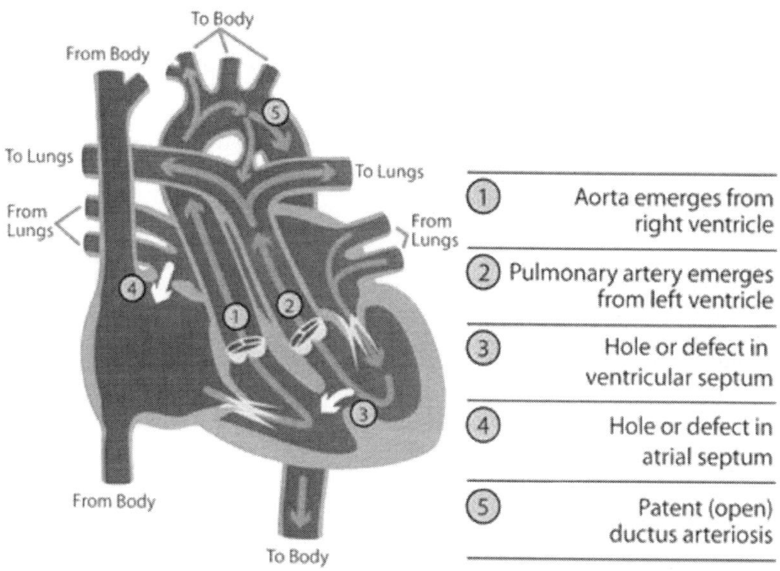

Figure 5. D-transposition of the great arteries with a ventriculoseptal defect (VSD). VSDs are present at birth in half of those with d-transposition, but significant VSDs are present in only a third.

Tetralogy of Fallot

Tetralogy of Fallot (TOF) has a slightly higher prevalence throughout the lifespan than d-TGA, making it the most common cyanotic congenital defect. TOF is a constellation of 4 cardiac abnormalities: large malaligned ventricular septal defect (VSD), aorta overriding the VSD, right ventricular outflow tract (RVOT) obstruction with pulmonary stenosis or infundibular obstruction, and RV hypertrophy. Tetralogy of Fallot ranges from the "pink Tet" with minimal pulmonary stenosis to the most severe form of RVOT obstruction, which is pulmonary atresia. The degree of cyanosis in TOF is roughly related to the degree of antegrade flow across the native pulmonary valve. When the RVOT is more obstructed, less blood passes from RV to pulmonary artery and more "blue" blood is shunted across the VSD and out the overriding aorta.

Most forms of TOF do not require immediate intervention and can be monitored on an outpatient basis prior to surgical intervention at a few months of age. The physical exam may show some cyanosis with a harsh systolic ejection murmur produced by turbulent flow across a narrowed RVOT. A chest x-ray may show a "boot-shaped" heart due to uplifting of the cardiac apex by RV hypertrophy and an absent shadow of the main pulmonary artery. In newborns this may be masked by the overlying thymic shadow. The pulmonary vascularity on chest x-ray is usually reduced. Diagnosis is made by echocardiography that includes detailing the malaligned VSD, RVOT, pulmonary valve leaflets and annulus size (11). A PDA may or may not be present but PGE_1 is generally not needed in management of a "straight-forward" TOF newborn.

Parental education is important for recognizing hypercyanotic ("Tet) spells in the infant, which are more commonly seen after a few weeks of age. These spells can become refractory and life-threatening. They are characterized by paroxysms of hyperpnea (rapid and deep respirations), irritability and prolonged crying with increased cyanosis and decreased intensity of the heart murmur on exam. The medical management of hypercyanotic spells aims to increase systemic vascular resistance, decrease impedance to pulmonary blood flow, and improve the relative balance between the systemic and pulmonary circulations.The knee-to-chest position increases the systemic vascular resistance. Administration of oxygen, intravascular volume expansion, and sedation are used to improve pulmonary blood flow acutely. Similarly, vasopressor agents such as epinephrine, phenylephrine, or norepinephrine can be given acutely to increase systemic vascular resistance and blood pressure. Beta-blocking agents such as propranolol may be used to relax the RVOT obstruction acutely or over the longer term to decrease the occurrence of spells in infants awaiting surgery. The occurrence of hypercyanotic spells is considered an indication for planning surgical intervention, especially given the trend towards earlier surgery. Figure 6 below depicts Tetralogy of Fallot.

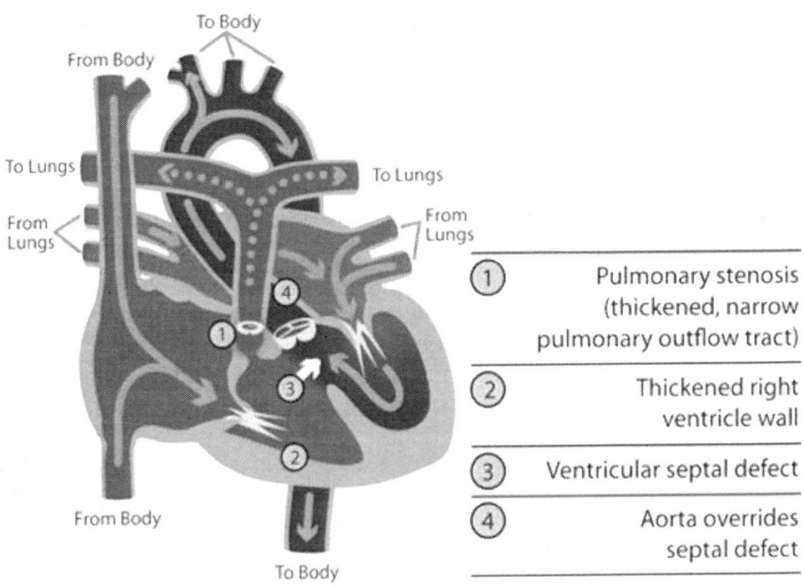

Figure 6. Tetralogy of Fallot.

Tricuspid atresia

Tricuspid atresia is characterized by absence of the tricuspid valve with resultant RV hypoplasia. The diagram resembles that of pulmonary atresia (below) except there are varying degrees of RV outflow tract obstruction and right ventricular hypoplasia. There is an obligatory atrial communication allowing egress of blood from the right atrium. A VSD, if present, may mean that the infant is born with a normal-size right ventricle. That is, the RV is hypoplastic unless there is an associated large VSD.

Cyanosis is common, from decreased pulmonary blood flow. A murmur may or may not be heard depending on the presence of outflow tract obstruction. An ECG typically shows a superior QRS axis and a lack of right-sided forces. (This is a defect for which a newborn ECG may be helpful, as the typical newborn right axis deviation and right ventricular hypertrophy will not be present). Pulmonary vascularity on the chest x-ray is usually reduced.

Initial management for these infants, including the need for PGE_1, depends on the amount of pulmonary blood flow. Surgical treatment aims to establish and control the amount of pulmonary blood flow. These patients will require surgical single-ventricle staged palliation with a Fontan procedure when they are older. The Fontan procedure directs blood flow from both vena cavae to the pulmonary arteries, thus separating the pulmonary and systemic circulations.

Pulmonary atresia with an intact ventricular septum

Pulmonary atresia (PA) with an intact ventricular septum is characterized by complete RVOT obstruction, absence of a VSD (distinguishing it from TOF with pulmonary atresia), and varying degrees of RV and tricuspid valve hypoplasia. The cardiac exam may not be remarkable, other than the single S_2, or there may be a systolic regurgitant murmur if there is tricuspid regurgitation. A chest x-ray typically shows a paucity of pulmonary vascular markings. A PGE_1 infusion is necessary until a reliable source of pulmonary blood flow is surgically provided.

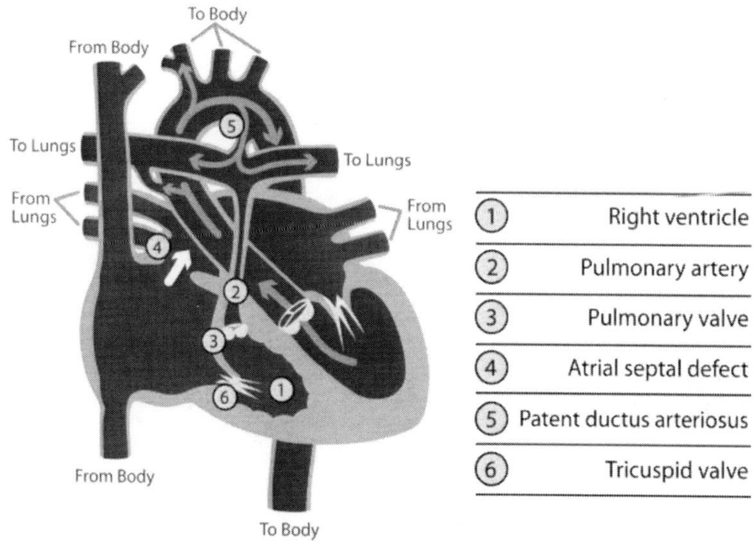

Figure 7. Pulmonary atresia with an intact ventricular septum – the lack of antegrade pulmonary blood flow in utero leads to underdevelopment of other right-sided structures.

Depending on the adequacy of the tricuspid valve, size of the RV, and presence of RV-to-coronary-artery sinusoids, patients may undergo either a 2-ventricle repair or a staged Fontan procedure for single-ventricle type palliation (directing blood flow from both vena cavae to the pulmonary arteries). The Fontan procedure is generally completed by the time the child is 2-4 years of age. Figure 7 depicts pulmonary atresia with intact ventricular septum.

Total anomalous pulmonary venous return

Total anomalous pulmonary venous return (TAPVR) occurs when all four pulmonary veins drain into systemic veins or more directly into the right atrium, with or without pulmonary venous obstruction. Systemic and pulmonary venous blood mixes in the right atrium. Oxygenated blood reaches the systemic circulation only via an ASD or patent foramen ovale, which is essential for survival.

Embryologically, failure of the common pulmonary vein to connect with the pulmonary venous plexus leads to persistence of one or more earlier venous connections to either the superior vena cava, the left vertical vein (innominate vein), or the umbilico-vitelline vein/portal vein (supracardiac, cardiac, infradiaphragmatic or mixed drainage patterns). TAPVR is isolated in two-thirds of patients and is associated with other heart defects (e.g., heterotaxy syndromes) in the remaining one-third of patients. All pulmonary veins frequently converge to a confluence that may sit behind the left atrium but does not communicate with the left atrium. Whether or not there is a "vertical vein" to drain the confluence differentiates the forms of TAPVR. If the vertical vein is unobstructed, patients may have very mild or no cyanosis. Obstructed TAPVR occurs when the vertical vein flow is restricted, leading to pulmonary edema and pulmonary arterial hypertension. Although there is often not a murmur, the physical exam may show, along with cyanosis and tachypnea, a continuous murmur at the location of the obstructed vertical vein. If the pulmonary venous return is obstructed, the chest x-ray will usually show small cardiac silhouette and marked pulmonary edema.

Diagnosis of TAPVR is made by echocardiogram detailing all pulmonary veins and their courses. While PGE_1 is generally helpful for defects with severe cyanosis, it should not be given to patients with TAPVR because it can increase flow into the pulmonary arteries and worsen pulmonary congestion. Obstructed TAPVR is now the only cyanotic congenital heart defect that cannot be aided by medical treatment and is a surgical emergency. Unfortunately, this defect is difficult to diagnose prenatally. Figure 8 depicts totally anomalous pulmonary venous return.

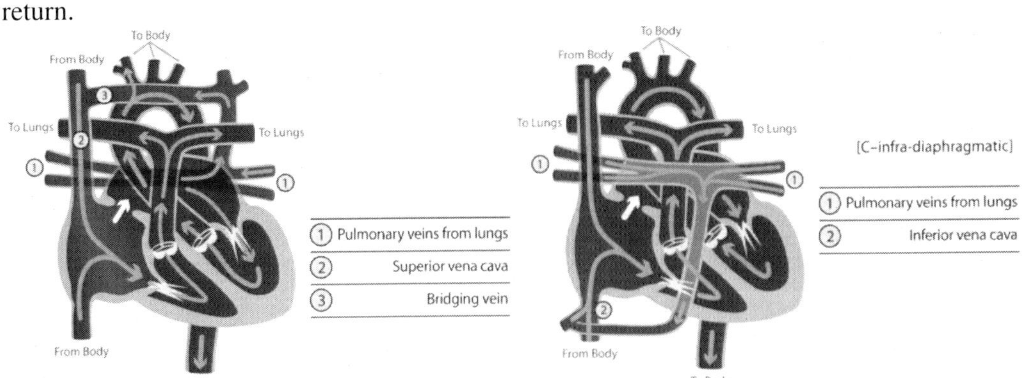

Figure 8. Total anomalous pulmonary venous return (the supracardiac type is shown on the left and infradiaphragmatic on the right).

Truncus arteriosus

Truncus arteriosus comprises only 0.7% of all CHD and 4% of all CCHD cases. One in four cases is associated with a 22q11.2 deletion, suggesting DiGeorge syndrome. In truncus arteriosus there is a common arterial trunk overriding a ventricular septal defect. The truncus arteriosus provides blood for the systemic, pulmonary circulation and coronary arteries. Aortic arch abnormalities are common, including a right aortic arch and an interrupted aortic arch. Cyanosis is relatively mild and is dependent on the size of pulmonary arteries.

Physical exam findings may include a single and loud second heart sound. A systolic ejection click from the large truncal valve may be heard along the left sternal border. There is usually a systolic ejection murmur along the left sternal border. Peripheral pulses may be prominent and may become bounding because of runoff into the pulmonary vascular bed in diastole.

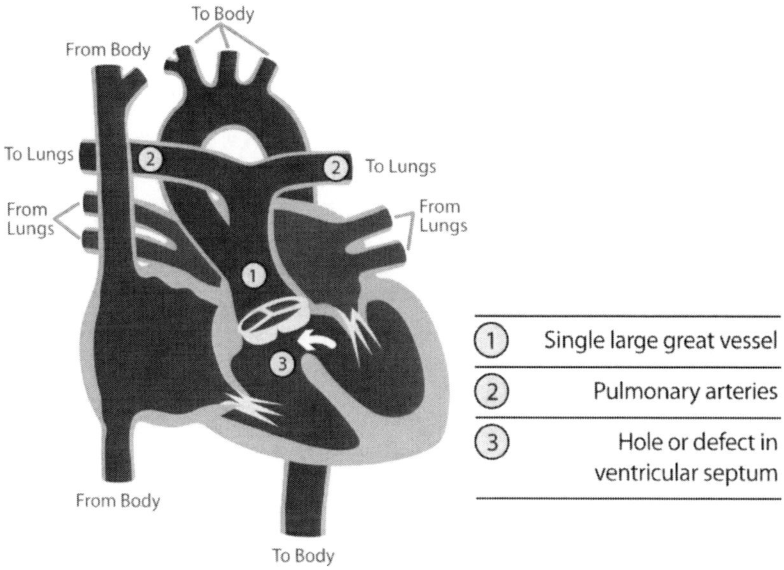

Figure 9. Truncus arteriosus – shown here is type I, wherein the MPA arises from the truncus and then divides into the right and left pulmonary arteries.

There is relatively little left-to-right shunting at birth. Over the first weeks of life, however, the pulmonary vascular resistance drops; left-to-right shunting increases and heart failure symptoms develop. Although the pathophysiology is similar to that of isolated ventricular septal defects, heart failure usually occurs earlier. This is because the systemic and pulmonary circulations are essentially in parallel; with pulmonary blood flow often at least 3-fold higher than systemic blood flow.

The need for surgical repair is dependent on the presence and severity of heart failure symptoms and typically occurs within the first six months of life. Survival rates are 80% or higher. During childhood re-intervention is often necessary, including replacement of the right ventricle to pulmonary artery conduit and/or truncal valve repair or replacement. See Figure 9 for Truncus arteriosus.

Ebstein's anomaly

Ebstein's anomaly is characterized by abnormalities of the tricuspid valve and right ventricle. The tricuspid valve leaflets are malformed and are displaced downwards (atrialization) into the right ventricle, partly attached to the fibrous tricuspid valve annulus and partly to the right ventricular endocardium. The morphology of the tricuspid valve and the clinical presentation are highly variable. Newborns with marked tricuspid leaflet displacement or abnormal leaflet attachment may have severe regurgitation, right-sided heart failure and significant right-to-left inter-atrial shunting resulting in marked cyanosis. Other physical findings may include a prominent "a" wave in the distended jugular veins and hepatomegaly. There may be a palpable prominent parasternal impulse. On auscultation, there may be a widely-split second heart sound from right bundle branch block. A prominent S3 and/or a loud S4 may give the impression of multiple heart sounds. A systolic murmur from tricuspid regurgitation is common. The chest x-ray in severe cases reveals massive cardiomegaly with diminished pulmonary vascularity (27).

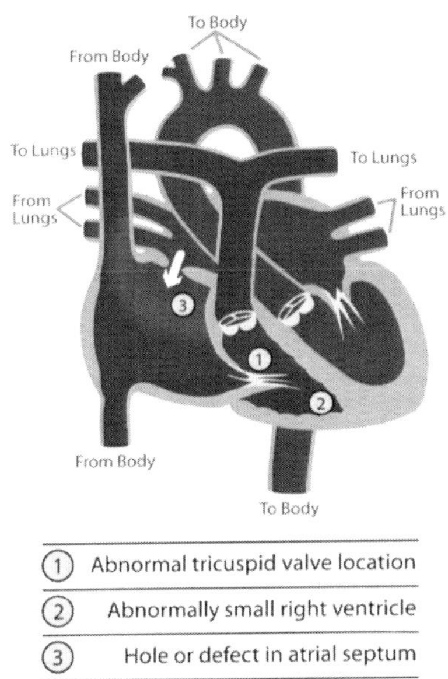

Figure 10. Ebstein's anomaly – note "atrialization" of the right ventricle but the downwardly-displaced tricuspid valve.

In general, surgical therapy is avoided in the newborn period. Neonatal medical management is limited to supportive therapy until the pulmonary vascular resistance drops over time. In case of extreme cyanosis, a PGE_1 infusion may be helpful to keep the ductus arteriosus open for pulmonary blood flow until the pulmonary vascular resistance drops. Inhaled nitric oxide may also help by reducing pulmonary vascular resistance and improving antegrade pulmonary blood flow. Ebstein's anomaly is shown in Figure 10.

Persistent pulmonary hypertension of the newborn

Persistent pulmonary hypertension of the newborn (PPHN), as the name suggests, occurs when the pulmonary vascular resistance (normally high in the fetus and decreasing after birth), remains abnormally elevated after birth. This results in right-to-left shunting through fetal circulatory pathways. The incidence is higher in term and near-term infants and may be as high as 1 in 500. Normally, the decrease in PVR after the first breath results in a 50% decrease in pulmonary artery pressure and in a 10-fold increase in pulmonary blood flow during the first few minutes of life (28). The term originally used to describe this syndrome was persistent fetal circulation. This was changed to PPHN to describe the pathophysiology more accurately. The delayed neonatal transition can lead to severe hypoxemia presenting at or shortly after birth, more often in neonates born at 34 weeks or more of gestation. Severity ranges from mild and transient respiratory distress to severe hypoxemia and cardiopulmonary instability requiring maximal support. Many cases are associated with lung parenchymal disease, such as meconium aspiration syndrome and respiratory distress syndrome, but some have idiopathic PPHN. There is an association with maternal non-steroidal anti-inflammatory agents during the third trimester causing constriction of the PDA.

On cardiac examination, a prominent right ventricular impulse and a loud second heart sound are sometimes apparent. Occasionally, a systolic regurgitant murmur of tricuspid regurgitation may be heard at the lower left sternal border. Hypoxemia is universal and is typically unresponsive to 100% oxygen given by oxygen hood but may respond to hyperoxic ventilation. A PaO_2 gradient between a pre-ductal (right arm) and a post-ductal (umbilical artery or leg) site of blood sampling greater than 20 mm Hg suggests right-to-left shunting through the PDA, as does an oxygenation saturation gradient more than 5% between pre- and post-ductal sites using pulse oximetry. This pre- and post-ductal difference does not reflect shunting at the atrial level, but only across the PDA.

Echocardiography is the most reliable, convenient and noninvasive way to establish the diagnosis, to assess cardiac function, and to exclude an associated structural heart defect. Right-to-left shunting across a patent foramen ovale and/or a PDA may be noted. The right ventricle is usually enlarged, with a flattened ventricular septum that may be displaced into the left ventricle by the elevated right ventricular pressures. It is important to establish that the aortic arch and pulmonary veins are normal, as structural anomalies can masquerade as PPHN. Specifically, a coarctation of the aorta can be associated with right-to-left PDA shunting and anomalous pulmonary venous return with right-to-left foramen ovale shunting. Tricuspid regurgitation may be noted with PPHN and pulsed Doppler interrogation of the tricuspid regurgitation jet velocity can be used to estimate the pulmonary pressure relative to the patient's blood pressure.

Following the discovery of nitric oxide (NO) as the endogenous vasodilator released by blood vessels, it was shown to cause selective pulmonary vasodilation in a sheep model of pulmonary hypertension in 1991 (29). The introduction of inhaled NO therapy has been the most significant milestone in the era of vasodilator therapy for PPHN and is a remarkable example of bench-to-bedside translational advances. With the advent of nitric oxide, the need for extracorporeal membrane oxygenation (a procedure that uses a machine to bypass the lungs and sometimes the heart) in these infants has declined by about 40%. NO is scavenged by hemoglobin (Hb) after diffusing into the blood and is rapidly inactivated. The vasodilatory effect of inhaled NO is therefore limited mostly to the lung. This is in contrast to formerly used intravenous vasodilators that caused systemic vasodilation and hypotension.

Survival of patients with PPHN varies by severity and underlying diagnoses. Newborns with mild PPHN who respond quickly to therapy have a good long-term outlook. Survival rates for PPHN in general exceed 90%. Infants with severe PPHN requiring extracorporeal membrane oxygenation have a 70-80% survival rate. These survivors are at risk for developmental delay, cerebral palsy and sensorineural hearing loss (30).

ACYANOTIC DEFECTS

Non-obstructive lesions

Atrial septal defect

After ventricular septal defects, an atrial septal defect (ASD) is the second most common congenital heart defect, accounting for 10-15% of all CHD. ASDs occur almost twice as frequently in girls. There are three types of atrial septal defects: ostium primum (10-15%) in the lower portion of the atrial septum near the mitral and tricuspid valves, ostium secundum (70-80%), central and in the region of the fossa ovalis, and sinus venosus (10-15%), posterior, near the orifice of the superior vena cava and frequently associated with partial anomalous pulmonary venous return. Right-sided chamber enlargement can develop after the newborn period.

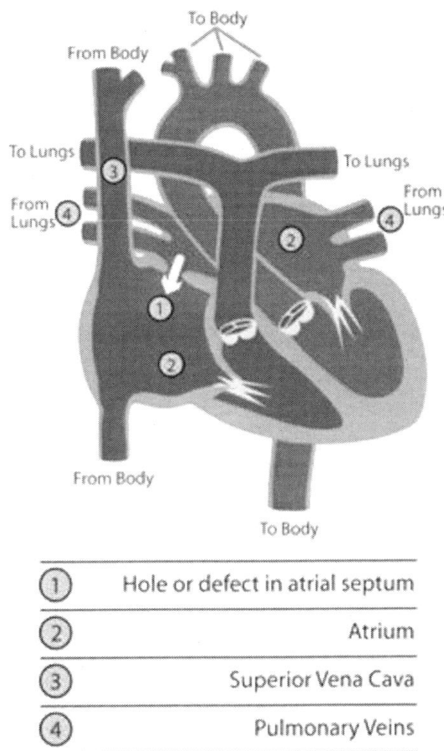

Figure 11. Atrial septal defect – secundum-type.

The exam is characterized by wide and fixed splitting of the second heart sound and a soft pulmonary flow murmur. Even if the ASD is large, there are usually no symptoms during infancy and childhood. Symptoms resulting from increased pulmonary blood flow generally do not develop until the second or third decade.

Elective repair for ASDs with significant shunting is recommended at about 3-4 years of age. This can be done surgically. For many secundum ASDs device closure at that age or older is also an option. Figure 11 illustrates an atrial septal defect.

Ventricular septal defect

A ventricular septal defect (VSD) is the most common congenital heart defect and accounts for 20-30% of CHD. Small VSDs often close spontaneously. Moderate and large defects are less likely to close and may result in congestive heart failure at about a month of age. The terms restrictive and non-restrictive describe whether or not the right ventricular pressure is the same as the systemic blood pressure, i.e., a significant left ventricle to right ventricle gradient among restrictive VSDs and an absence of a gradient among, non-restrictive (predominantly large) VSDs.

VSDs may be muscular (trabecular), perimembranous, inlet or outlet. Sometimes, a ventricular septal aneurysm is seen on the echocardiogram. This thin flap of tissue may increase the chances that the defect will close spontaneously.

Symptoms from a large VSD are not seen before a few weeks of age, at which time diuretics may be used to control them and optimize weight gain. Surgery may follow weeks or months later for larger defects especially if weight gain is compromised. Figure 12 demonstrates ventricular septal defect.

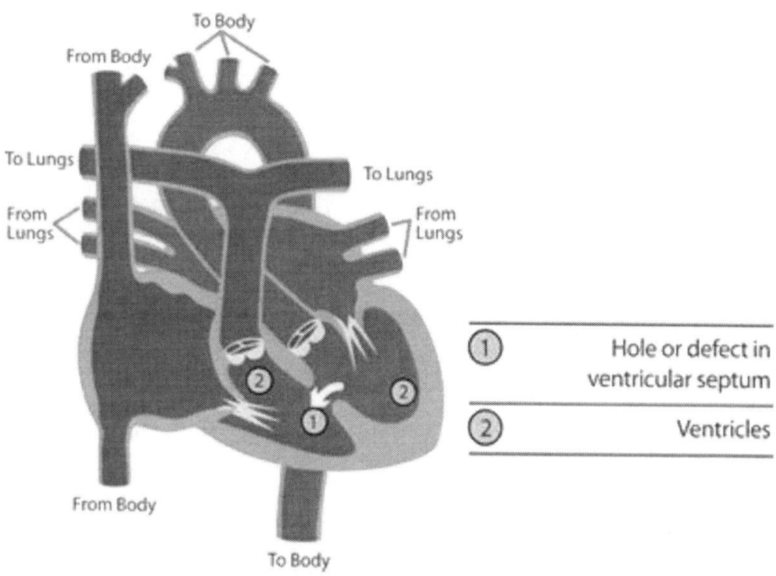

Figure 12. Ventricular septal defect - muscular type.

Atrioventricular canal defects

The term atrioventricular canal defect (AVCD), also called endocardial cushion or atrioventricular septal defects, refers to a spectrum of lesions that have improper development of the atrioventricular junction as the underlying abnormality. An ACVD can be considered a failure of chamber septation. In these cases, the atrioventricular junction fails to undergo normal septation and formation of separate atrioventricular valves, leaving a common atrioventricular valve providing inflow to both ventricles. The atrioventricular cushion contributions to atrial and ventricular septation are abnormal, resulting in an ASD of the ostium primum type, and/or a VSD of the inlet type.

Although ACVDs comprise only 7% of congenital malformations, they occur in about 40% of patients with Down syndrome. To date, no single gene on chromosome 21 has been implicated in causing ACVDs.

Surgical repair is necessary unless the defect is very small or is mostly occluded by aneurysmal valve tissue. Defects with significant ventricular shunting are typically closed at a few months of age. Those with only atrial shunting (so-called partial ACVDs) may be closed, in the absence of symptoms, at the recommended time for ASD closures, that is, at 3-4 years of age. See Figure 13 for a depiction of atrial septal defect.

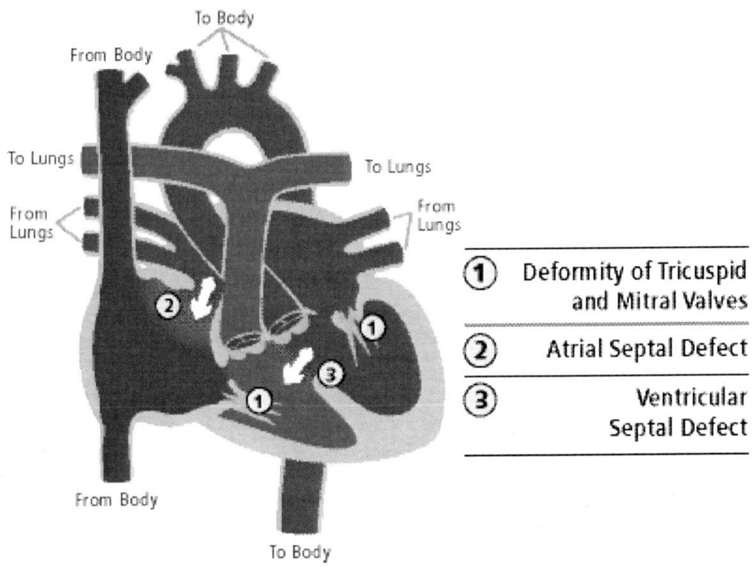

Figure 13. Atrioventricular septal defect – complete and balanced.

Patent ductus arteriosus (PDA)

In infancy, a PDA is most often seen in the setting of preterm delivery. The ductus arteriosus (DA) is thought to derive from the embryonic left sixth aortic arch. The aortic end of the DA arises distal to the left subclavian artery and the pulmonary end inserts at the junction of the main and left pulmonary arteries. The clinical manifestations of a PDA are determined by the degree of left-to-right shunting, which is dependent upon the size and length of the PDA, and the difference between pulmonary and systemic vascular resistances. Physical-exam findings include a continuous murmur and bounding pulses, including the presence of palmar pulses in the newborn. Precordial palpation may reveal a dynamic left ventricular impulse; an apical mid-diastolic rumble induced by increased flow across the mitral valve may also be present.

Non-steroidal agents (ibuprofen, indomethacin) are effective in closing the PDA in premature infants. Traditionally, surgical PDA ligation may be necessary when pharmacotherapy is either contraindicated or fails. In early January 2019, the Food and Drug Administration (FDA) approved a duct occluder device for premature babies weighing more than 700 grams (31). In older children, coil embolization is the method of choice. Figure 14 below demonstrates a PDA.

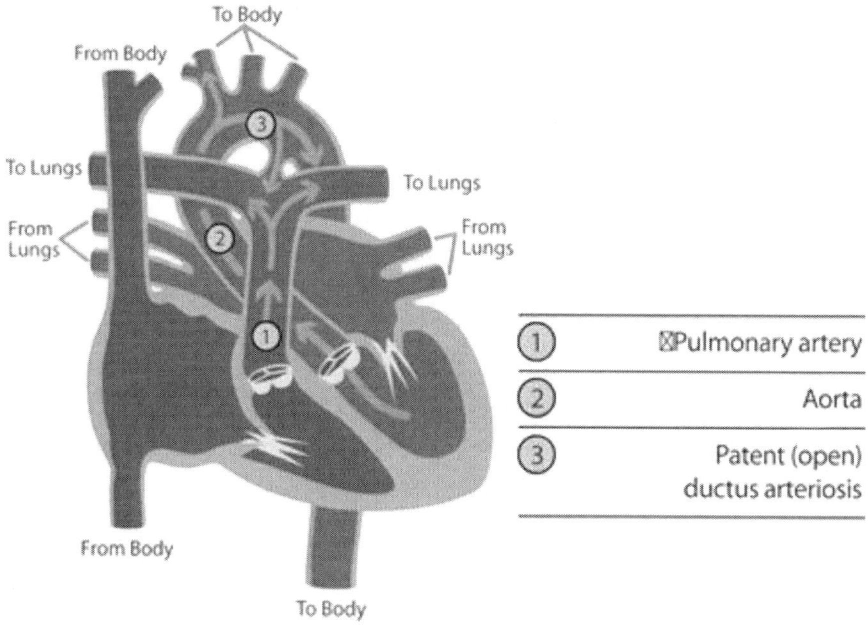

Figure 14. Patent ductus arteriosus. A patent ductus arteriosus allows blood to flow from the aorta back into the pulmonary artery, to recirculate to the lungs. Left-sided dilatation may develop.

Left-sided obstructive lesions

Coarctation of the aorta and interrupted aortic arch

Coarctation of the aorta is a discrete narrowing of the aorta. It accounts for 4 to 6% of all CHD. On physical examination, a clinical diagnosis is made if the femoral pulses are absent or delayed (especially when compared with the right brachial pulse). Four-limb blood pressure measurements may show a higher systolic pressure in the right arm compared to the legs. The cardiac exam is usually otherwise unremarkable. A murmur/bruit may be auscultated in the mid-scapular region of the back. Prenatal diagnosis is challenging as the ductus arteriosus may overlie the narrowing and it provides much of the descending aortic flow. Because patients with Turner syndrome have about a 10% risk of coarctation, female patients with a coarctation should be examined for features of Turner syndrome. Once coarctation of aorta is diagnosed, the mode of repair can be surgical, balloon arterioplasty, or stent placement. The mode of repair of the native coarctation is determined by age at diagnosis and the complexity of the defect, with the newborns and young children requiring surgical repair and the older children, adolescents and adults being amenable to stenting of the lesion (32). See Figure 15 below that demonstrates coarctation of the aorta.

The most extreme form of coarctation is an interrupted aortic arch. Complete interruption usually occurs between the left carotid and left subclavian arteries (as shown in Figure 16); it can also occur either distal to the left subclavian artery or between the innominate and left carotid artery. It is usually associated with a large ventricular septal defect. Surgical correction is required for both the arch obstruction and the ventricular septal defect. Figure 16 below depicts interrupted aortic arch.

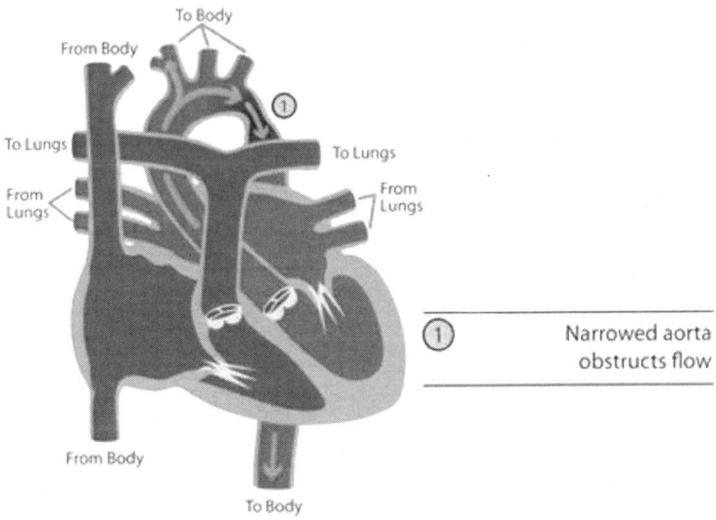

Figure 15. Coarctation of the aorta.

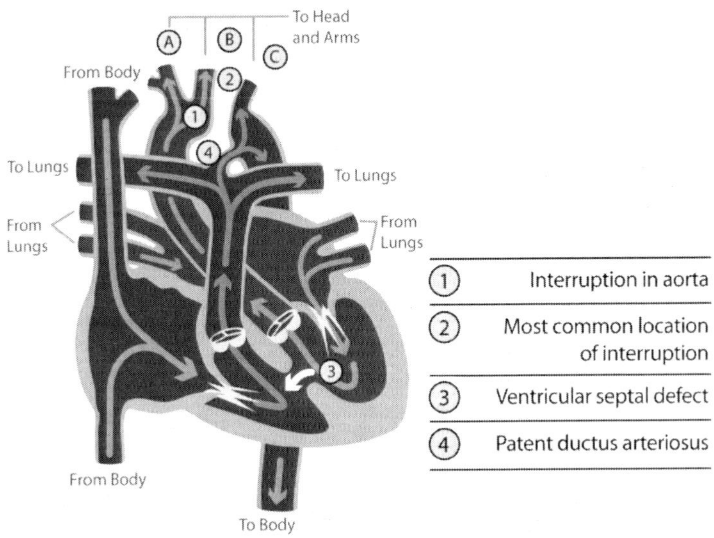

Figure 16. Interrupted aortic arch – the most common site of interruption is between the left carotid and left subclavian arteries, as shown here.

Hypoplastic left heart syndrome

Hypoplastic left heart syndrome (HLHS) and related functional single right-ventricle conditions remain the highest risk and costliest group of lesions among commonly-occurring CHD. Hypoplastic left heart syndrome accounts for 2 to 3% of all CHD. HLHS is characterized by hypoplasia of the left heart and the aorta, with compromised cardiac output. Untreated, 95% will die within the first few weeks of life. Syndromes occurring with HLHS include Turner syndrome, trisomy 13, trisomy 18, Holt-Oram, Smith-Lemli-Opitz and Jacobsen syndrome. HLHS patients with a genetic disorder and/or extracardiac abnormality have a worse prognosis (33).

As the PDA begins to close and pulmonary vascular resistance decreases, infants become symptomatic from a decrease in systemic perfusion with diminished peripheral pulses and increasing pulmonary blood flow. They may appear tachypneic and poorly perfused. Usually, there is no murmur, but the second heart sound may be noted to be single. Untreated, infants soon develop hypotension, acidosis, and respiratory distress and finally cardiogenic shock. Hepatomegaly helps distinguish infants with this type of shock from infants in shock from sepsis or dehydration. Establishing a PDA with PGE1 can reverse this process. The PDA provides vital flow from the right ventricle to the systemic circulation. While this is not considered a cyanotic defect, the degree of cyanosis is determined by the relative amount of pulmonary versus systemic blood flow. Infants with high pulmonary blood flow may have only minimal cyanosis.

Infants generally undergo a three-stage reconstruction culminating in the Fontan procedure. The first operation (stage I) is the Norwood procedure, in which the right ventricle is connected to a reconstructed aorta with the use of the proximal main pulmonary artery for systemic outflow. Pulmonary blood flow is reestablished using a shunt from the aorta or a conduit from the right ventricle, to the pulmonary arteries. In the second operation (stage II), generally performed by six months, the shunt is removed, and pulmonary blood flow is supplied by an anastomosis between the superior vena cava and the pulmonary artery. The Fontan procedure (stage III) generally occurs when the child is age 2 to 4 years. In this operation, blood flow through the inferior vena cava is directed to the pulmonary artery, thus separating the pulmonary and systemic circulations. After Fontan palliation, only coronary sinus blood mixes with the pulmonary venous blood.

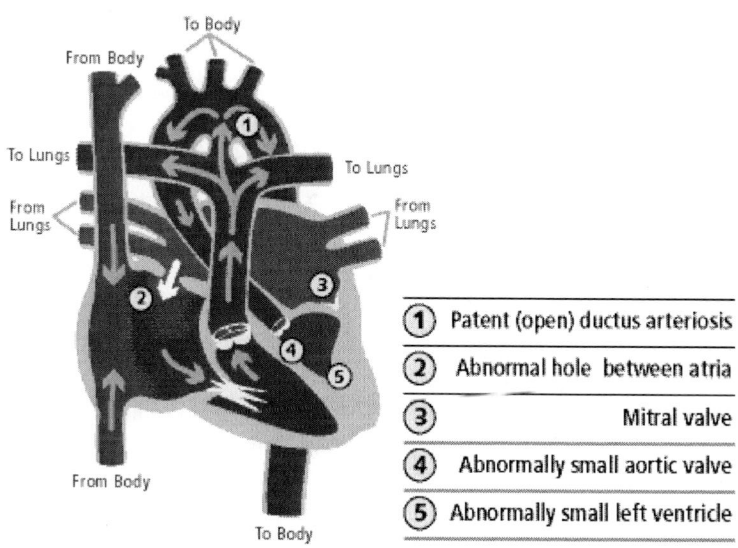

Figure 17. Hypoplastic left heart syndrome - note underdevelopment of the left heart with hypoplasia of the left ventricle including atresia, stenosis or hypoplasia of the aortic or mitral valve (or both valves), hypoplasia of the ascending aorta and aortic arch and PDA-dependent systemic blood flow.

Mortality associated with the Norwood procedure remains the highest among common congenital heart procedures, ranging from 7 to 19% and is associated with the highest cost and the third longest length of stay. Between the Norwood procedure and the stage II procedure, 4 to 15% of infants die; this mortality rate is expected to improve with recent quality-improvement initiatives directed at outpatient interstage monitoring. A newer option, called the hybrid approach, uses a combination of surgical and transcatheter techniques to accomplish the goals of the Norwood repair but without cardiopulmonary bypass and circulatory arrest (34). This approach also culminates in the Fontan procedure. See Figure 17 for hypoplastic left heart features. A good review of acyanotic heart lesions is found in Marino et al. (35).

CONGESTIVE HEART FAILURE AND CARDIOGENIC SHOCK

Congestive heart failure (CHF) is a clinical syndrome that manifests as tachypnea, tachycardia, hepatosplenomegaly, and cardiomegaly. It represents a physiologic state where the heart is unable to adequately meet the metabolic demands of the body. The newborn with CHF frequently presents with tachypnea or diaphoresis during feeding leading to failure to thrive.

A chest x-ray may reveal pulmonary edema and cardiomegaly. Although generally less useful, an ECG may demonstrate an arrhythmia (if this is the cause) or chamber enlargement due to excessive volume load. An echocardiogram is helpful in confirming impaired ventricular function or structural heart defects that may cause of CHF. If CHF goes unrecognized and untreated, inadequate tissue perfusion may lead to hypoxemia and acidosis, with progression to cardiogenic shock. In most cases, repair or palliation of the underlying cardiac defect provides the most effect treatment for CHF.

Hydrops fetalis is the presentation of CHF in the fetus. It is characterized by abnormal amounts of fluid in two or more body spaces. Fluid accumulation can lead to skin edema, pericardial or pleural effusions, and ascites. Hydrops fetalis is classified as immune versus non-immune. Cardiovascular disorders represent about 20% of non-immune cases. In the fetus or immediate newborn period, the most likely structural problems are severe atrioventricular valve regurgitation, Ebstein's anomaly of the tricuspid valve, any type of severe atrioventricular valve regurgitation, and a large arteriovenous malformation.

CHF in the newborn period may be caused by non-structural heart disease. Non-structural causes include birth asphyxia with myocardial ischemia, hypoglycemia, hypocalcemia, hypothyroidism, severe anemia, sepsis, and arrhythmias. Myocarditis and different types of cardiomyopathy should also be considered in the differential of CHF in the newborn period.

An approach to evaluating CHF in the newborn is assessment of the age at presentation. While functional closure of the ductus arteriosus may happen by several hours, ductal-dependent lesions predominate within the first postnatal week. The most likely structural problems at this time are HLHS, interrupted aortic arch and a severe coarctation of the aorta. Patients with these defects may present with cardiogenic shock. Another cause of CHF that is more common in preterm infants is a PDA. Arrhythmias such as complete heart block, supraventricular tachycardia, or much less often, ventricular tachycardia can cause hydrops fetalis or newborn CHF. Other causes include severe anemia and myocardial dysfunction such as from a cardiomyopathy or myocarditis.

By a month of age, the pulmonary vascular resistance of a newborn reaches its nadir. This leads to a predominance of left-to-right shunt lesions causing CHF around that time, with the most likely lesions being VSDs and AVCDs.

The Dysmorphic Newborn and Associated Congenital Heart Defects

The percentage of heart defects related to an abnormal chromosome is estimated to be 5%, single gene defects about 4%, and environmental factors about 2%. In 85 to 90% of cases, however, there is no identifiable cause. Some genetic conditions, such as Down syndrome, Turner syndrome, and 22q11.2 deletion syndrome, result from changes in the number or structure of particular chromosomes. Other conditions, including Noonan syndrome and Alagille syndrome, result from mutations in single genes. Potential environmental risk factors include exposures to maternal viral infections (e.g., rubella), medications, diabetes and phenylketonuria.

Dysmorphic features in a newborn can lead to the diagnosis of CHD and additional congenital malformations. Nearly 25% of those with CHD have one or more extracardiac malformations. It is not uncommon for a cardiac defect to raise suspicion of an associated syndrome, such as pulmonary stenosis leading to a diagnosis of Noonan syndrome or fetal heart block revealing maternal lupus. It is important to be familiar with frequently-encountered syndromes or teratogenic exposures and their associated cardiac defects. Patients often require a comprehensive and coordinated approach among various subspecialty areas. The following is a brief summary of major syndromes and exposures commonly associated with CHD.

Down syndrome (Trisomy 21)

Down syndrome is commonly associated with advanced maternal age and is the most frequently encountered chromosomal abnormality affecting live births. The estimated incidence is 1 in 1,000 live births. This syndrome is characterized by cognitive, motor, and growth delays. Patients have a recognizable and abnormal flat facial appearance with slanted palpebral fissures, small eyes, small ears and macroglossia. They also may have other findings such as hypotonia, short and broad necks, shortened limbs, single transverse palmar crease, Brushfield spots of the iris, and clinodactyly (a bend or curvature of the fifth finger). A karyotype analysis identifies cases due to translocation or mosaicism. Down syndrome is considered non-hereditary, except for rare cases of translocation. The majority of cases (95%), are caused by non-disjunction.

About 50% will have CHD, most often an atrioventricular septal defect (formerly called an endocardial cushion defect), ventricular septal defect, atrial septal defect and/or a patent ductus arteriosus. Due to the high incidence of CHD in this population, an echocardiogram is recommended at the time of suspected diagnosis (either in utero and/or in the newborn period).

An echocardiogram in an asymptomatic newborn with suspected Down syndrome is ideally done after 24-hours of age but before hospital discharge, to allow time for spontaneous patent ductus arteriosus and patent foramen ovale closure. Not all newborns will have undergone this transition by hospital discharge; however, waiting to do the echocardiogram allows a day for this to occur. Similarly, a normal fetal echocardiogram does not rule out a patent ductus arteriosus or secundum atrial septal defect, both common in Down syndrome patients.

22q11.2 deletion syndrome (DiGeorge Syndrome)

This syndrome is associated with microdeletions of chromosome 22 and has an estimated incidence of 1 in 4,000. It is the most common microdeletion syndrome and the inheritance pattern is autosomal dominant. The deletion occurs near the middle of the chromosome at a location designated q11.2. Over 70% have congenital heart defects with the most common defects being truncus arteriosus, interrupted aortic arch, and tetralogy of Fallot. The presentation can be variable, even among members of the same family, and it can be subtle. Because the phenotype is so varied, different combinations of features were once identified by different names, including DiGeorge syndrome, velocardiofacial syndrome and CATCH 22 (Cardiac defects, Abnormal facial features, Thymic hypoplasia, Cleft palate, and Hypocalcemia).

DiGeorge syndrome was described in 1968 by a pediatric endocrinologist from Philadelphia, Angelo DiGeorge. The pattern of malformations was recognized as early as 1671, when Nicolai Stensen described a patient with cleft palate and truncus arteriosus. Others had reported the association of the various findings with hypoplasia of the thymus and parathyroid glands. DiGeorge syndrome has been used for patients with a cardiac anomaly, hypocalcemia and poor T-cell production. Confusion exists because there are those who have the deletion but not the clinical syndrome and there are those considered to have DiGeorge syndrome who do not carry the deletion. The preferred term is 22q11.2 deletion syndrome.

Diagnosis can be confirmed with targeted FISH (fluorescent in-situ hybridization) testing or chromosomal microarray analysis. Unique facial characteristics include a prominent nose, hypertelorism, short philtrum, down-slanting eyes and auricular abnormalities. Infants may have palatal abnormalities, conductive hearing loss, feeding problems, developmental and growth delay, learning disabilities, hypoplasia or absent thymus and parathyroid, hypocalcemia and T-cell dysfunction. Later in life, they are at an increased risk for schizophrenia, depression, anxiety and bipolar disorder.

Associated cardiac defects are ventricular septal defects and conotruncal malformations. Conotruncal malformations include truncus arteriosus, interrupted aortic arch and other aortic arch anomalies, tetralogy of Fallot, double outlet right ventricle, and d-transposition of the great arteries. Of truncus arteriosus patients, 34.5-35.5% will have the 22q11.2 microdeletion, as will 50-56% of interrupted aortic arch (type B) patients, and 13-16% of tetralogy of Fallot patients (36, 37). In these studies, 0-0.4% of the d-TGA patients had the 22q11.2 deletion.

Turner syndrome

Turner syndrome is a chromosomal syndrome with features of short stature, primary amenorrhea, webbed neck, barrel-shaped chest, congenital lymphedema, and cubitus valgus (the elbow deviates away from the body when extended). The chromosomal aberration is the presence of a single X sex chromosome leading to the 45, XO karyotype. Turner syndrome affects approximately 1 in 2,500 newborn girls worldwide and is more common among pregnancies that lead to miscarriages and stillbirths.

Diagnosis is confirmed by a karyotype. The cardiac defects associated with Turner syndrome are coarctation of the aorta, aortic stenosis, bicuspid aortic valve (BAV), hypoplastic left heart syndrome, aortic dilation and hypertension. Approximately 11% have coarctation and

16% have BAV. Aortic coarctation and BAV are more frequent in patients with webbed necks (38).

Noonan syndrome

Noonan syndrome is single gene disorder affecting multiple organ systems. The estimated prevalence is 1 in 1,000-2,500. The major features are short stature, developmental delay, a characteristic facial appearance (hypertelorism, epicanthal folds, ptosis, and low-set ears), short webbed neck, chest deformity, cubitus valgus, peripheral lymphedema and cryptorchidism. Multiple gene mutations (all involving proteins in the RAS-MAPK pathway) have been identified as causing Noonan syndrome, with about half due to mutations of the *PTPN11* gene.

Diagnosis is confirmed with widely available genetic testing. Several congenital heart defects are associated with Noonan syndrome, including pulmonary stenosis (dysplastic pulmonary valve), hypertrophic cardiomyopathy and secundum ASDs. The inheritance pattern is autosomal dominant.

Williams syndrome

Williams syndrome is another single gene disorder affecting multiple organ systems. Williams syndrome results from a defect in the *ELN* gene on chromosome 7 that codes for the protein elastin and can be confirmed with genetic testing. Although it is considered autosomal dominant, most cases are not inherited.

Cognitive delay, distinctive facial features, unique personality traits, hypercalcemia, and CHD characterize the condition. Early case reports gave it the nickname "elfin facies syndrome" due to the distinctive facial features of broad forehead, periorbital fullness, rounded cheeks, flattened nasal bridge, upturned nose, long philtrum, wide mouth, full lips, and a pointed chin. Affected children have outgoing and engaging "cocktail" personalities. They have difficulty with visual-spatial tasks but perform well in tasks that involve spoken language and music. Some may have hyperacusis (acuteness of hearing with intolerance for normal sound levels).

Supravalvar aortic stenosis is commonly associated with Williams syndrome. Due to the ubiquitous nature of elastin, other forms of arterial stenosis (pulmonary, coronary and systemic) can also be seen.

Marfan syndrome

Marfan syndrome is caused by a defect in the fibrillin-1 gene (*FBN1*) on chromosome 15 that codes for the extracellular matrix protein fibrillin-1. It has autosomal dominant inheritance. The incidence is approximately 1 in 5,000 (39). Marfan syndrome is a connective-tissue disorder with a wide variability of phenotypic expression involving the musculoskeletal, ocular, dura, pulmonary and cardiovascular systems. Neonatal Marfan syndrome is the severest phenotype of this disease and has a poor prognosis. The main reason for death in the neonatal type is congestive heart failure from mitral regurgitation. This is, in contrast, to classic Marfan syndrome, in which death is more often from aortic root disease and dissection. Individuals with Marfan syndrome are usually tall and slender, have arachnodactyly, and increased arm-span to height ratio. Other common features include scoliosis or kyphosis, pectus deformities, dural ectasia, spontaneous pneumothorax, myopia, ocular lens dislocation (ectopia lentis) and early cataracts or glaucoma. Nearly all patients have some cardiovascular involvement, most commonly mitral valve prolapse and aortic root dilation. As the aortic root enlarges, these patients are at risk for aortic regurgitation, dissection, and rupture. Diagnosis is based on a set of established criteria focused on family history and physical findings involving more than one organ system (40).

Ehlers-Danlos syndrome

Ehlers-Danlos syndrome (EDS) is a group of connective-tissue disorders with variable presentation from mildly loose joints to life-threatening aneurysms. Multiple mutations in genes coding for collagen have been discovered to cause EDS. The incidence is similar to Marfan syndrome, i.e., approximately 1 in 5,000. The pathogenetic etiology of EDS depends on the type of EDS. There are 13 types of EDS and the inheritance pattern varies by type (classical, classical-like, cardiac-vascular, vascular, brittle cornea, spondylodysplastic, musculocontractural, myopathic, arthrochalasia, dermatosparaxis, hypermobility, kyphoscoliosis, and periodontal types). Most EDS patients have hypermobile joints. Infants have joint laxity that can delay the development of gross motor skills such as sitting, standing, and walking. The skin is often soft, highly elastic, with easy bruising, poor wound healing. EDS can be associated with mitral valve prolapse, aortic aneurysm and rupture. Diagnosis is confirmed via molecular testing of skin biopsy or genetic testing for EDS-associated pathogenic variants (41).

CHARGE Association

CHARGE association is an acronym for a group of congenital anomalies including **C**oloboma, **H**eart defects, choanal **A**tresia, **R**etardation of **g**rowth and development, **G**enitourinary anomalies, and **E**ar anomalies. Of those with CHD, conotruncal anomalies (tetralogy of Fallot, double-outlet right ventricle, truncus arteriosus) and aortic arch anomalies (vascular ring, interrupted aortic arch) are common. Other associated defects include PDAs, VSDs, and ASDs. Mutations in the *CHD7* gene have been found in cases of CHARGE syndrome; mode of transmission in some cases is noted to be autosomal dominant, although majority of the cases are due to *de novo* mutations (42).

VACTERL Association

VACTERL is an acronym for **V**ertebral defects, **A**nal **a**tresia, **C**ardiac defects, **T**racheo-**E**sophageal fistula, **R**enal anomalies, and **L**imb abnormalities. In this syndrome, VSDs, ASDs and tetralogy of Fallot are the most common heart defects. The etiology is unknown and there is no clear pattern of inheritance. Although diagnostic criteria vary, the incidence is estimated to be about 1 in 10,000 to 1 in 40,000 live-born infants (43).

Trisomy 13 (Patau's) syndrome

Trisomy 13 occurs in 1 in 5000 to 1 in 20,000 births (44). The syndrome's major features are cleft lip and palate, holoprosencephaly, polydactyly, and cutis aplasia congenita (a localized scalp skin defect). CHD occurs in approximately 80% of cases, including PDAs, VSDs, ASDs, polyvalvular disease, coarctation of the aorta, conotruncal defects, and dextrocardia. The overall prognosis is poor, and rare long-term survivors are profoundly impaired.

Trisomy 18 (Edward's) syndrome

Trisomy 18 occurs in 1 in 8,000 births (44). The syndrome is characterized by microcephaly, micrognathia, rocker-bottom feet and closed fists with overlapping fingers. Nearly all patients with Trisomy 18 syndrome have some form of CHD. The most common defect is a VSD. Other common defects are PDAs, polyvalvular disease, TOF, and DORV. As with Trisomy 13, the prognosis is poor, with high infant mortality within the first week. Survival into teen and adult ages has been reported but long-term survivors are profoundly impaired.

Alagille syndrome

These infants frequently present with acholic stools with jaundice due to a paucity of intrahepatic bile ducts. The prevalence of Alagille syndrome is approximately 1 in 70,000 newborns, which is underestimated due to absence of symptoms in some newborns. Mutations in the *JAG1* gene on chromosome 20 (89 percent) and/or *NOTCH2* gene on chromosome 1 (seven percent) lead to Alagille syndrome and inheritance is autosomal dominant (45). Affected infants have a broad forehead, long straight nose, prominent chin, and small malformed ears. The associated heart defect is branch pulmonary artery stenosis.

Tuberous sclerosis complex (TSC)

TSC is characterized by benign tumors affecting the brain, skin, kidneys, lungs and heart. The cardiac finding frequently encountered in infants and children with TSC is rhabdomyoma (50-70 percent). These are often multiple, variable in size and involve the ventricles. Large rhabdomyomas may obstruct the intracavitary space or cardiac valves, but more often they are small and not hemodynamically significant.

In the fetus, TSC may be suspected if cardiac rhabdomyomas are seen. Infants may present with seizures (infantile spasms). With a careful examination of the skin and brain, it is possible to diagnose TSC in a very young infant. Facial angiofibromas, appear later. Mutations in the *TSC1* on chromosome 9 or *TSC2* gene on chromosome 16 can cause TSC and inheritance is autosomal dominant (46). The incidence is estimated to be 1 in 6,000.

Maternal systemic lupus erythematosus (SLE) and Sjögren's syndrome

SLE and Sjögren's syndrome are autoimmune diseases associated with anti-SSA/Ro and anti-SSB/La anti-nuclear autoantibodies. The congenital heart block associated with neonatal lupus is considered a form of passively acquired autoimmune disease in which maternal autoantibodies to these intracellular ribonucleoproteins cross the placenta and injure the previously normal fetal heart.

Complete heart block occurs in about 1-2% of babies born to these mothers and 10% have an associated cardiomyopathy at the initial diagnosis or develop it later. Cases may occur in infants of mothers who have these autoantibodies; typically, these mothers are not aware and are asymptomatic. About half of these mothers proceed to develop SLE or Sjögren's.

Fetal alcohol syndrome

Fetal alcohol syndrome develops in a fetus exposed to high levels of maternal alcohol consumption during pregnancy. Affected children have variable cognitive delays and abnormal facies (small eyes, smooth philtrum, thin upper lip and microcephaly. CHD occurs in 30-50%. The most common defects are VSDs, PDAs, ASDs, and d-transposition of the great arteries. In a recent meta-analysis investigating association between prenatal exposure to alcohol and congenital heart defects, there was marginal association between prenatal alcohol exposure and conotruncal defects but significant association with d-TGAs (47). However, there is significant association between heavy prenatal drinking and binge drinking and overall CHD (OR: 3.76 and 2.49, respectively). Prenatal moderate drinking was associated with conotruncal defects (OR: 1.35) and d-TGA (OR: 1.86) (47).

Maternal diabetes mellitus

Maternal diabetes is a recognized teratogen affecting numerous organ systems including the fetal heart. Studies estimate a relative risk of approximately 4 to 5 for fetal CHD in mothers having diabetes. Cardiac anomalies are the most common malformations with IDM, with VSDs and complex lesions such as double outlet right ventricle, truncus arteriosus, and transposition of the great vessels predominating. Woman most at risk for fetal CHD are those with poor periconceptional control, long-standing diabetes, insulin-dependence, and vascular disease. Ventricular hypertrophy (predominantly asymmetric septal hypertrophy) is the most common cardiac abnormality (38%) with left ventricular outflow tract obstruction can also be seen (48). Although most infants with this are asymptomatic, respiratory distress or signs of cardiac failure can occur. This cardiac hypertrophy likely results from fetal exposure to maternal hyperinsulinemia, leading to fat and glycogen deposition in the myocardium. Thus, it generally occurs in poorly-controlled pregnancies with resultant macrosomia. Symptoms improve over several weeks with supportive care, and echocardiographic changes are transient and resolve typically over the first six months (49).

ARRHYTHMIAS

Rhythm disturbances are important causes of pediatric cardiac disease and can occur in children with either heart disease or an otherwise normal heart. Recognition of arrhythmias has increased because of the routine use of obstetrical ultrasonography and perinatal heart rate monitoring, thereby improving the prenatal diagnosis of congenital cardiac disease. Neonatal arrhythmias may be either benign or malignant, depending on their potential to cause death or morbidity. Some helpful general references are cited in the reference section (50-52). Common pediatric arrhythmias will be discussed in Chapters 4A and 4B.

Ectopy

Premature atrial beats

Premature atrial beats (APBs) are common atrial ectopies that occur when atrial tissue other than the sinoatrial node depolarizes prematurely. In the otherwise healthy infant, they rarely suggest an underlying abnormality and are unlikely to be symptomatic. They are frequently an incidental finding on cardiac monitoring, ECGs or Holter monitors. APBs may trigger arrhythmias in patients predisposed to atrial tachyarrhythmias such as atrioventricular reentrant tachycardia and atrial flutter.

On the ECG, associated p-wave morphology may appear different from normal sinus. The APB may be conducted normally, conducted with aberrancy, or blocked, depending on the refractory period of the AV node. They are common in premature infants whose respiration is compromised by respiratory distress syndrome and on a ventilator support. Blocked APBs are often confused for a primary bradycardia and can be recognized by discovering a blocked p-wave buried within the preceding T-wave (usually able to note a change in T-wave morphology).

Premature ventricular beats

Premature ventricular beats (VPBs) are less common in neonates than APBs but are also infrequently associated with serious heart disease. They are usually seen in an otherwise healthy infant. An echocardiogram may be helpful in infants with greater than 25-30% ectopy to rule out cardiomyopathy or structural heart disease.

Bradyarrhythmias

Bradycardia in the term newborn is defined as a heart rate <90 bpm; it increases to <110 bpm by the first month of age. The etiology of infant bradycardia ranges from suppression of the sinus node to complete atrioventricular (AV) block, with various clinical presentations. Each component of the formation and propagation of the electrical impulse from atria to ventricles (sino-atrial node, atrial tissue, AV node, and His-Purkinje system) may be implicated in bradyarrhythmias.

While the cardiac conduction system is strongly influenced by the autonomic nervous system throughout life, sympathetic innervation dominates in infancy and bradycardia is frequently due to sympathetic withdrawal and increased parasympathetic tone. It is very common to note sinus bradycardia in sleeping infants with the heart rate dropping into mid to high 70s to low 80s; the heart rate recovers with minimal activity or upon awaking.

Atrioventricular block

Careful study of the atrioventricular (AV) node has revealed that this structure is much more complex than previously thought with multiple conduction fibers. First degree AV block is characterized by a PR interval above the normal range for age. In neonates, this ranges from 0.14-0.16 ms, although it is strongly influenced by the underlying heart rate.

PR prolongation in association with normal heart rates is likely secondary to AV-nodal dysfunction whereas prolongation with bradycardia is more suggestive of increased parasympathetic tone. First degree AV block is rarely symptomatic; it usually only progresses to higher grade block in the presence of heart disease. Treatment is not necessary; when it is present, the use of known AV blocking agents should be avoided.

Second degree AV block is divided into Mobitz I (Wenckebach) and Mobitz II. With typical Wenckebach, there is gradual prolongation of the PR interval until non-conduction of a p-wave. Conversely in Mobitz II, there is no prolongation of the PR interval prior to the non-conducted p-wave. The greatest increment of PR prolongation in Wenckebach occurs during the first several beats, after which the change is minimal. This can lead to the incorrect diagnosis of Mobitz II because the non-conducted beat appears to come suddenly. Careful examination of the first conducted beat, however, will reveal shortening of the PR interval in Wenckebach and no change in Mobitz II and can be confirmed in classic cases to a shortening of the corresponding R-R interval prior to the dropped beat.

Complete heart block, or third degree, reflects complete interruption of electrical activity between the atria and ventricles. The most common etiology is neonatal lupus, accounting for 60-90% of congenital complete heart block; its presence is frequently the first indication of maternal disease. Among women with anti-Ro/SSA or anti La/SSB, roughly 1-2% of pregnancies will develop heart block, crossing the placenta to the fetus in the first trimester. Antibodies (Anti-Ro and anti-La) were present in 95% of those with in-utero diagnosis, 90% in neonatal diagnosis and 5% in those with childhood diagnosis (53). That risk increases to 16-18% in subsequent pregnancies once a child is born with heart block (54). The pathophysiology is likely immune mediated injury of the AV node, release of tumor necrosis factor causing fibrosis, and targeted inhibition of the cardiac calcium channels. Other causes of congenital complete heart block include tumors, myocarditis, and long QT Syndrome (LQTS). Complex congenital heart disease, specifically L-looped ventricles, heterotaxy, and single ventricle physiology, account for 25-33% of cases.

The clinical presentation depends on the underlying ventricular heart rate, which is typically a narrow complex escape rhythm arising from the AV junction; ventricular rates less than 50 beats per minute are more likely to cause symptoms. Treatment is dictated by whether a pacemaker is necessary or not. For congenital complete heart block in a structurally normal heart, a pacemaker is indicated in the presence of failure to thrive, marked bradycardia, decreased ventricular function, long pauses, widened QRS or associated ventricular arrhythmias. Remarkably, infants can do quite well with heart rates even in the 40s and careful observation may be the best initial course of action. Infants with structural heart disease or post-surgical block, on the other hand, should receive a pacemaker. Steroids have been used for complete heart block secondary to maternal autoantibodies including prenatally in-utero. The prognosis is poor in neonates with a fetal diagnosis of complete heart block, fetal hydrops, endocardial fibroelastosis and prematurity less than 32 weeks (53).

Tachyarrhythmias

Supraventricular tachycardia

Supraventricular tachycardia (SVT) is the most common tachyarrhythmia in children, occurring in as many as 1:1,000, with most presenting within the first year of life. While this category encompasses a number of tachycardia mechanisms, the vast majority (90%) involve a reentrant circuit between the atria and ventricles (AV). These include AV reentrant tachycardia (AVRT), AV node reentrant tachycardia (AVNRT), and persistent junctional reciprocating tachycardia (PJRT). Children less than a year old are most likely to have SVT secondary to AVRT (85%) while the other mechanisms are more common later in childhood.

Atrioventricular reentrant tachycardia may be facilitated by a concealed or manifest accessory pathway. These strands of myocardium (accessory pathway) bridge the electrically insulated AV valve annuli and allow for anterograde or retrograde conduction independent of the AV node-His-Purkinje system. In young children, ventricular rates during tachycardia are typically 240-300 bpm and characterized by absent or retrograde p-waves. Anterograde conduction through the accessory pathway results in ventricular preexcitation and the characteristic delta wave seen on a surface ECG (manifest conduction). Manifest pathways are able to conduct in antegrade and retrograde directions. Ventricular preexcitation in the presence of palpitations or documented SVT describes the Wolff-Parkinson-White (WPW) syndrome which occurs with an incidence of 1.6:1000. A small subset of these accessory pathways have the ability to rapidly conduct atrial depolarizations to the ventricles during atrial fibrillation, making WPW a rare, and even rarer in newborn (but known), cause of sudden death in the young.

Atrioventricular nodal reentrant tachycardia is supported by a circuit that revolves around AV nodal tissue. While its clinical presentation is similar to that of AVRT, it is uncommon in the newborn.

PJRT is a rare reentrant tachycardia that is supported by retrograde conduction through a concealed accessory pathway with decremental conduction properties. It is implicated in less than 1% of SVT in children but usually presents during the first year of life. Criteria for diagnosis of PJRT are a narrow complex tachycardia, a long R-P interval, and inverted p-waves in leads II, III, and aVF.

Typical atrial flutter is a common arrhythmia in adults but comprises less than 1% of SVT in children with a structurally normal heart, which is the majority in infancy. Although a fetus may be symptomatic in-utero, the infant (if not diagnosed in-utero) will have a benign course; the flutter may spontaneously terminate, or it can be converted with either DC cardioversion (0.5 j/kg) or by transesophageal overdrive pacing. Recurrence is rare. Anti-arrhythmic medications are of little value.

Atrial fibrillation is exceptionally rare in children; the small atrial chamber size cannot adequately support the multiple reentrant waves that continuously circulate through the atrium causing disorganized activation and contraction. Two rare chromosomal abnormalities have been linked to fetal atrial fibrillation.

Multifocal atrial tachycardia (MAT), ectopic atrial tachycardia (EAT), and junctional ectopic tachycardia (JET) are arrhythmias characterized by disorders of impulse formation, i.e., abnormal automaticity in the newborn and infant. MAT, also known as chaotic atrial tachycardia, is by far the most common in neonates. It is usually detected in an otherwise healthy newborn or infant who presents with a fast and irregular heart rate. MAT is characterized by p-waves of at least three morphologies, irregular p-p intervals with an isoelectric period between them, and a ventricular rate greater than 100 bpm. Unlike its presentation in adults, MAT can be seen in otherwise asymptomatic children. Treatment is frequently not required as the arrhythmia is typically self-limited unless there is underlying congenital heart disease.

JET occurring in the neonatal period presents as either a congenital form (rare) or in the post-operative period (most common). It originates from the AV node or His bundle and the heart rate may be extremely rapid, ranging from 150-240 bpm. In the post-operative period, therapy is geared toward lowering the ventricular rate such that atrial pacing can be performed to reestablish AV synchrony. It is typically transient and long-term therapy is rarely required.

Ventricular tachycardia

The diagnosis of VT implies an arrhythmia that arises distal to the upper part of the His bundle, typically within the ventricular myocardium. The differential diagnosis of wide QRS complex tachycardia in the young child includes several other forms of tachyarrhythmias other than ventricular tachycardia (VT) and is beyond the scope of this chapter as they rarely pertain to a wide QRS tachycardia in a newborn. However, certain ECG findings should be used to distinguish it from other tachycardias. First, the QRS duration must be longer than the normal duration for age. Thus, it is important to recognize that QRS duration is an age-related finding and > 80 ms is considered prolonged in infants. Secondly, dissociation between atrial and ventricular beats may be observed but can be difficult to distinguish at the high rates typically seen in infants. P-waves can be seen buried in the QRS or the abnormal ST-T wave complex and may present as polymorphic QRS and/or ST-T wave complexes. A transesophageal electrogram recording can often helpful in differentiating the atrial from the ventricular electrogram.

Various descriptive terms are often used incorrectly to classify VT. Non-sustained VT describes VT greater than three consecutive ventricular beats that self-terminates before 30 seconds and does not cause hemodynamic compromise. Sustained VT refers to an episode lasting longer than 30 seconds. In repetitive or recurrent VT, multiple episodes of non-sustained VT are separated by periods of sinus rhythm. Finally, incessant VT describes long periods of sustained VT typically requiring intervention to terminate.

A patient with repetitive/recurrent or incessant VT is not necessarily symptomatic; thus, these terms only describe time course and onset pattern. Additionally, the morphology of VT is divided into monomorphic and polymorphic types. In polymorphic VT, there is beat to beat variability in the QRS axis and shape. This has clinical implications as polymorphic VT is more likely to degenerate into ventricular fibrillation. An important and most common form of VT in the newborn is accelerated idioventricular rhythm; in this arrhythmia, the wide QRS rhythm is approximately 125% of the sinus rate. As is seen with SVT, infants may manifest symptoms as irritability, decreased feeding, or pallor. Infants who present in congestive heart failure or complete cardiovascular collapse and shock are more likely to have had surgery for congenital heart disease or myocarditis after an infectious or inflammatory insult.

The clinical presentation of VT varies and is dependent on the ventricular rate, and presence of concomitant heart disease. Infants can frequently tolerate higher heart rates although significant atrio-ventricular dissociation may compromise overall cardiac output. Asymptomatic patients are more likely to have non-sustained VT and/or slower ventricular rates (< 150 bpm).

Genetic disorders

Advances in our understanding of molecular genetics have led to developments in the diagnosis and characterization of heritable cardiac arrhythmias. These disorders include channelopathies such as the long QT syndrome (LQTS). In LQTS, multiple genes (with seven being primary) have been identified that can produce distinct manifestations of the disease. The majority of genes encode potassium channel subunits although sodium channels may also be affected. Inheritance patterns may be autosomal dominant or recessive and recent studies have suggested an incidence of 1:2,000 live births. These newborns can rarely present with life threatening ventricular arrhythmias (torsade de points) and even degrees of heart block. Diagnosis is based on measurements of the QT interval on a 12-lead ECG and corrected for the heart rate using Bazett's formula. It is clear that LQTS mutations are incompletely penetrant and genetic testing is now recommended for first-degree relatives of genotype-positive individuals.

Another channelopathy, the Brugada syndrome, is characterized by specific ST-segment elevations in the right precordial leads in the absence of cardiac ischemia or other structural heart disease. It is an autosomal dominant disorder with an incidence of up to 66 per 10,000 individuals. The risk is highest in males (8:1) and in areas of Southeast Asia. Especially important for the infant, the ECG findings of Brugada syndrome, including life threatening ventricular arrhythmias, can be enhanced by fever. Thus, the concomitant findings of fever (even induced by a vaccination) and VT should prompt the consideration of this genetic disorder.

Conclusion

Approximately eight in 1,000 newborns have a congenital heart defect that can range from mild to severe and from asymptomatic to life-threatening phenotypes. Identification of congenital heart disease is a vital component of the pediatric clinician's responsibility in caring for the newborn in collaboration with experts in pediatric cardiology. This discussion considers various aspects in this potentially complex task and provides a practical review of cyanotic heart defects, persistent pulmonary hypertension of the newborn, acyanotic defects, congestive heart failure as well as cardiogenic shock, associated congenital heart defects of the dysmorphic newborn, and cardiac arrhythmias. The newborn is a marvelous human being fueled by a remarkable organ—the newborn heart.

REFERENCES

[1] Moons P, Bovijn L, Budts W, Belmans A, Gewillig M. Temporal trends in survival to adulthood among patients born with congenital heart disease from 1970 to 1992 in Belgium. Circulation 2010;122:2264-72.

[2] Marino BS, Lipkin PH, Newburger JW, Peacock G, Gerdes M, J Gaynor, JW, et al. Neurodevelopmental outcomes in children with congenital heart disease: Evaluation and management. A scientific statement from the American Heart Association. Circulation 2012; 126(9):1143-72.

[3] Blalock A, Taussig HB. The surgical treatment of malformations of the heart: In which there is pulmonary stenosis or pulmonary atresia. JAMA 1945;128:189-202.

[4] Hoffman JL, Kaplan S. The incidence of congenital heart disease. *J Am Coll Cardiol* 2002; 39(12):1890-1900.

[5] Rahi A, Grosse SD, Ailes EC, Oster ME. Association of US State Implementation of Newborn Screening Policies for Critical Congenital Heart Disease with Early Infant Cardiac Deaths. *JAMA* 2017;318(21):1-8.

[6] Fetal circulation and embryology diagrams used with permission from Richard Dryden PhD. URL: www.bionalogy.com.

[7] Purvis JA, Morgan DR, Hughes SM. Prevalence of patent foramen ovale in a consecutive cohort of 261 patients undergoing routine "coronary" 64-multi-detector cardiac computer tomography. Ulster Med J 2011;80(2):72-5.

[8] Nagasawa H, Hamada C, Wakabayashi M, Nakagawa Y, Nomura S, Kohno Y. Time to spontaneous ductus arteriosus closure in full-term neonates. Open Heart, 2016;3:e000413. doi: 10.1136/openhrt-2016-000413.

[9] Flynn JT, Kaelber DC, Baker-Smith CM, Blowey D, Carroll AE, Daniels SR, et al. Clinical practice guideline for screening and management of high blood pressure in children and adolescents. Pediatrics 2017;140(3):e20171904.

[10] Pickering TG, Hall JE, Appel LJ, Falkner BE, Graves J, Hill MN, et al. Recommendations for blood pressure measurement in humans and experimental animal: part 1: Blood pressure measurement in humans: A statement for professionals from the Subcommittee of Professional and Public Education of the American Heart Association Council on High Blood Pressure Research. Circulation 2005;111(5):697-716.

[11] Kent AL, Kecskes Z, Shadbolt B, Falk MC: Normative blood pressure data in the early neonatal period. Pediatr Nephrol 2007;22(9):1335-41.

[12] Park MK, Lee DH. Normative arm and calf blood pressure values in the newborn. Pediat, 1989; 83(2): 240-3.

[13] Goldbloom R, ed. Pediatric clinical skills, 4th edition. Philadelphia, PA: Saunders Elsevier, 2010:137-47.

[14] Jacobs WR. Ejection clicks. In: Walker HK, Hall WD, Hurst JW, eds. Clinical methods: The history, physical, and laboratory examinations, 3rd ed. Boston, MA: Butterworths, 1990.

[15] Bernstein D. Cyanotic congenital heart disease: Evaluation of the critically ill neonate with cyanosis and respiratory distress. In: Kleigman RM, Stanton BM, St Geme J, Schor NF, eds. Nelson textbook of pediatrics, 20th ed. Philadelphia, PA: Elsevier Health Sciences, 2015.

[16] Secretary of Health and Human Services letter to the Secretary's Advisory Committee on Heritable Disorders in Newborns and Children (SACHDNC). URL: https://www.hrsa.gov/sites/default/files/hrsa/advisory-committees/heritable-disorders/reports-recommendations/response-congenital-cyanotic.pdf.

[17] Mahle WT, Martin GR, Beekman III RH, Morrow R, Rosenthal GL, Snyder C, et al.. Endorsement of Health and Human Services recommendation for pulse oximetry screening for critical congenital heart disease. Pediatrics 2012;129:190-2.

[18] Centers for Disease Control and Prevention. Critical congenital heart defects, 2018. URL: https://www.cdc.gov/ncbddd/heartdefects/cchd-facts.html.

[19] De-Wahl Granelli A, Wennergren M, Sandberg K, Mellander M, Bejlum C, Inganäs L, et al. Impact of pulse oximetry screening on the detection of duct dependent congenital heart disease: a Swedish prospective screening study in 39,821 newborns. BMJ 2009;338:a3037.
[20] Thangaratinam S, Brown K, Zamora J, Khan KS, Ewer AK. Pulse oximetry screening for critical congenital heart defects in asymptomatic newborn babies: A systematic review and meta-analysis. Lancet 2012;379:2459-64.
[21] Mahle WT, Newburger JW, Matherne GP, Smith FC, Hoke TR, Koppel R, et al. Role of pulse oximetry in examining newborns for congenital heart disease: A scientific statement from the AHA and AAP. Pediatrics 2009;124(2):823-36.
[22] Villain E, Levy M, Kachaner J, Garson A Jr. Prolonged QT interval in neonates: benign, transient, or prolonged risk of sudden death. Am Heart J 1992;124(1):194-7.
[23] Fonseca B, Chang RK, Senac M, Knight G, Sklansky MS. Chest radiography and the evaluation of the neonate for congenital heart disease. Pediatr Cardiol 2005;26:367–72.
[24] Manning, WJ, Pennell DJ. Cardiovascular magnetic resonance, Second edition. Philadelphia, PA: SB Saunders, 2010:111-28.
[25] Andelfinger G. Genetic factors in congenital heart malformation. Clin Genet 2008;73(6): 516-27.
[26] Martin L, Khalil H. How much reduced hemoglobin is necessary to generate central cyanosis? Chest 1990;97(1):182-5.
[27] Ramaciotti C, Chin AJ. Non-invasive evaluation of newborns with congenital heart disease. J Intensive Care Med 1993;8(3):130-43.
[28] Cassin S, Dawes GS, Mott JC, Ross BB, Strang LB. The vascular resistance of the foetal and newly ventilated lung of the lamb. J Physiol 1964;171:61-79.
[29] Ichinose F, Roberts Jr JD, Zapol W. Inhaled nitric oxide A selective pulmonary vasodilator: current uses and therapeutic potential. Circulation 2004;109:3106-11.
[30] Konduri GG, Kim UO. Advances in neonatology: advances in the diagnosis and management of persistent pulmonary hypertension of the newborn. Pediatr Clin North Am 2009;56:579-600.
[31] The Food and Drug Administration. URL: https://www.accessdata.fda.gov/scripts/cdrh/cfdocs/cfpma/pma.cfm? id=P020024S052.
[32] Torok RD, Campbell MJ, Fleming GA, Hill KD. Coarctation of the aorta: Management from infancy to adulthood. World J Cardiology 2015;7(11):765-75.
[33] Feinstein JA, Benson DW, Dubin AM, Cohen MS, Maxey DM, Mahle WT, et al. Hypoplastic left heart syndrome: Current considerations and expectations. J Am Coll Cardiol 2012;59(1):S1-S42.
[34] Baba K Kotani Y, Chetan D, Chaturvedi RR, Lee KJ, Benson LN, Grosse-Wortmann L, et al. Hybrid versus Norwood strategies for single ventricle palliation. Circulation 2012;126(11) Suppl 1: S123.
[35] Marino BS, Bird GL, Wernovsky G. Diagnosis and management of the newborn with suspected congenital heart disease. Clin Perinatol 2001;28(1):91-136.
[36] Goldmuntz E, Clark BJ, Mitchell LE, Jawad AF, Cuneo BF, Reed L, et al. Frequency of 22q11 deletions in patients with conotruncal defects. J Am Coll Cardiol 1998;32(2):492-8.
[37] Peyvandi S, Lupo PJ, Garbarini J, Woyciechowski S, Edman S, Emanuel BS, et. al. 22q11.2 deletions in patients with conotruncal defects: Data from 1610 consecutive cases. Pediatr Cardiol 2013;34(7):1687-94.
[38] Loscalzo ML, Van PL, Ho VB, Bakalov VK, Rosing DR, Malone CA, et al. Association between fetal lymphedema and congenital cardiovascular defects in Turner syndrome. Pediatrics 2005;115:732–5.
[39] Marian AJ, Brugada R, Roberts R. Cardiovascular diseases caused by genetic abnormalities. In: Fuster V, Walsh RA, Harrington RA, eds. Hurst's the heart, Vol 1, 13th ed. New York: McGraw-Hill, 2011:1783-1826.
[40] Loeys BL, Dietz HC, Braverman AC, Callewaert BL, De Backer J, Devereux RB, et al. The revised Ghent nosology for the Marfan syndrome. J Med Genet 2010;4 (7):476-85.
[41] Shalhub S, Byers PH, Hicks KL, Coleman DM, Davis FM, De Cardi G, et al. A multi-institutional experience in vascular Ehlers-Danlos syndrome diagnosis. J Vasc Surg 2019; doi: 10.1016/j.jvs.2019.04.487.

[42] Bergman JE, Janssen N, Hoefsloot LH, Jongmans MC, Hofstra RM, van Ravenswaaij CM. CHD7 mutations and CHARGE syndrome: The clinical implications of an expanding phenotype. J Med Genet 2011;48(5):334-42.

[43] Khoury MJ, Cordero JF, Greenberg F, James LM, Erickson JD. A population study of the VACTERL association: evidence for its etiologic heterogeneity. Pediatrics 1983;71:815–20.

[44] Brown DW, Fulton DR. Congenital heart disease in children and adolescents. In: Fuster V, Walsh RA, Harrington RA, eds. Hurst's the heart, Vol 1, 13th ed. New York: McGraw-Hill, 2011:1827-83.

[45] Spinner NB, Leonard LD, Krantz ID. Alagille syndrome. In: Adam MP, Ardinger HH, Pagon RA, eds. GeneReviews®. Seattle, WA: University of Washington, 1993-2019. URL: https://www.ncbi.nlm.nih.gov/books/NBK1273/.

[46] Crino PB, Nathanson KL, Henske EP. The tuberous sclerosis complex. New Eng J Med 2006;355:1345-56.

[47] Yang J, Qiu H, Qu P, Zhang R, Zeng L, Yan H. Prenatal alcohol exposure and congenital heart defects: A meta-Analysis. PLoS One 2015;10(6):e0130681. doi:10.1371/journal.pone.0130681.

[48] Abu-Sulaiman RM, Subaih B. Congenital heart disease in infants of diabetic mothers: echocardiographic study. Pediatr Cardiol 2004;25(2):137-40.

[49] Gutgesell HP, Speer ME, Rosenberg HS. Characterization of the cardiomyopathy in infants of diabetic mothers. Circulation 1980;61:441-50.

[50] Dick M 2nd. Clinical cardiac electrophysiology in the young. New York: Springer, 2006.

[51] Deal BJ, Wolff GS, Gelband H. Current concepts in diagnosis and management of arrhythmias in infants and children. Armonk, NY: Futura, 1998.

[52] Dumaine R, Antzelevitch C. Molecular mechanisms underlying the long QT syndrome. Curr Opin Cardiol 2002;17(1):36-42.

[53] Jaeggi ET, Hamilton RM, Silverman ED, Zamora SA, Hornberger LK. Outcome of children with fetal, neonatal or childhood diagnosis of isolated congenital atrioventricular block. J Am Coll Cardiol 2002;39:130–7.

[54] Buyon JP, Heibert R, Copel J. Autoimmune-associated congenital heart block: Mortality, morbidity, and recurrence rates obtained from a national neonatal lupus registry. J Am Coll Cardiol 1998; 31:1658–66.

In: Chronic Disease and Disability
Editors: DE Greydanus, P Anne, JD Rowlett et al.
ISBN: 978-1-53617-656-8

Chapter 3

CARDIOLOGY: AN OVERVIEW

Thomas Austin Melgar*, MD and Elizabeth Doherty, MD
Department of Pediatrics, Adolescent and Internal Medicine, Western Michigan University School of Medicine, Kalamazoo, Michigan, United States of America

ABSTRACT

Problems of cardiology are important concerns for pediatric patients throughout the world including those in tropical climates. This discussion reviews physical skills needed to differentiate cardiac problems that require expertise beyond the primary care clinician. It also reviews common cardiac conditions including issues that are unique to children in developing areas. Early recognition of cardiac problems can lead to improved outcomes in these children and adolescents.

INTRODUCTION

The intent of this chapter is to help the primary care physician working in the tropics or resource poor areas to assess and manage common issues in infants, children and adolescents with known or suspected cardiology problems. It is not the intent of this chapter to be a comprehensive resource on pediatric cardiology. We will cover three main areas:

- Physical exam skills to help the reader distinguish those murmurs that require further investigation from the vast majority of murmurs in children that should not require any additional attention.
- Cardiac problems that are common to children in both the developed and developing world

* Correspondence: Professor Thomas A Melgar, MD, Department of Pediatrics and Adolescent Medicine and Internal Medicine, Western Michigan University Homer Stryker MD School of Medicine, Oakland Drive Campus, 1000 Oakland Drive, Kalamazoo, Michigan 49008-1284, United States. Email: Thomas.melgar@med.wmich.edu.

- Problems that are unique to children in developing areas or are very uncommon in developed areas.

This chapter will not cover hypertension, obesity, diabetes, and ischemic heart diseases although these are important and growing problems in tropical regions in children. There is insufficient space and these topics are covered in great detail in other sources.

The practice of pediatrics in the tropics will vary widely depending on local disease patterns and resources available. In some cases the same resources of developed countries are available to care for patients and in others few if any resources are available. This chapter will assume that all resources of best practice are available. The practitioner without those resources will need to adjust their practice based on those resources available.

Some of these problems may ultimately require the help of a pediatric cardiologist or a pediatric cardiovascular surgeon, although many problems discussed in this chapter should not. The threshold for making a referral to a pediatric cardiologist or cardiovascular surgeon will vary depending the skill and confidence of the primary care physician and on the access for each patient and each location. Those practicing in locations with no access to specialists will need to read a more in depth text on pediatric cardiology. We recommend that the reader have a good understanding of pediatric cardiology including and especially excellent physical exam skills.

Ultrasonography if available can be an enormously useful tool in resource poor environments but is also too great a topic to be covered in this chapter. Physicians practicing in a setting where the technology is available may find it beneficial to develop basic echocardiography skills.

HEART SOUNDS AND MURMURS

Murmurs occur in up to 77% of neonates and up to 72% of older children and as high as 87% with exercise. Congenital heart disease occurs in only 0.4-1.2% of children. In developing countries in the tropics acquired heart disease from rheumatic fever increases the incidence of significant murmurs but anemia from hookworm, nutritional deficiencies and malaria will increase the incidence of innocent murmurs as well. This disparity between the incidence of murmurs and the prevalence of real heart disease reflects the benign nature of heart murmurs in the vast majority of pediatric patients. It is impractical and not cost effective for primary care physicians to order testing such as echocardiography for all children with murmurs or to refer all of them to pediatric cardiologists.

It is imperative that physicians caring for children become highly skilled at confidently distinguishing innocent murmurs from pathologic murmurs. Studies have shown that primary care physicians historically have not been very proficient at identifying pathologic murmurs in children but knowledge, practice and interest can improve these skills (1).

A great variety of different pathologic cardiac conditions exist and some of these are exceedingly rare. The pediatrician is unlikely to be familiar with the specific physical findings for each of these relatively uncommon entities. It is impractical to approach the patient with a murmur by attempting to rule in or rule out each of these specific pathologic conditions and then referring those with suspected pathology to a pediatric cardiologist.

It is more practical for the primary care physician practicing in a tropical location to begin by becoming an expert in diagnosing innocent murmurs that do not need further evaluation and then investigate all others that do not fit the usual innocent patterns. In this section we focus on how to identify the five innocent or functional murmurs in childhood as well as some basic pathologic murmurs such as those of ventricular and atrial septal defects, aortic, mitral and tricuspid regurgitation, and mitral, pulmonic and aortic stenosis.

Common symptoms which suggest the presence of cardiac disease include unexplained tachypnea, cyanosis, squatting, syncope, chest pain, palpitations and excessive sweating and difficulty feeding in the newborn. When auscultating murmurs the child should be examined in a quiet room with the stethoscope in direct contact with the skin since many murmurs are softer than the ambient noise of many if not most tropical clinic settings. Innocent murmurs may be present, but unrelated, in symptomatic children and pathologic murmurs may be present in the absence of symptoms. The age of the patient at murmur presentation, the tonal quality and loudness may all be helpful in determining the significance of the murmur.

Age may be the most important discriminator for the majority of murmurs. Most pathologic congenital heart disease will be discovered early in life and many forms present with a murmur. Therefore, the earlier in childhood a murmur is heard, the more likely it is to have pathological implications. The pitch of the murmur may also be a reflection of pathology with low pitched murmurs more likely to be benign in nature. Determination of pitch does require some instruction and practice over time, as does the interpretation of the relative loudness. Louder, easily heard murmurs are more likely to represent pathology.

Innocent murmurs

We summarize innocent murmurs in Table 1.

- Stills murmur – This murmur is most common in toddlers and young children although it may still be present in some young adults. The sound is produced by blood flow across the chordae tendinae in the left ventricle as it enters the aortic outflow tract. It is estimated that as many as 60% of children have this murmur at some point in their childhood. It is located midway between the left lower sternal boarder and the apex. It is systolic and typically, a crescendo-decrescendo murmur or ejection type murmur. Since it occurs during aortic outflow, it must not begin before the closure of the mitral valve and completion of isovolumetric contraction and therefore S1 should be separate from the murmur and easily heard.
- The quality is very low-pitched and vibratory as would be expected from a vibrating tendon. It is this low-pitched, vibratory tonal quality which truly distinguishes this common murmur. Recognizing this as a unique sound should be the key to the clinical recognition. There is little radiation of the murmur although it can occasionally extend to the carotid arteries. The murmur will typically become louder in the supine position but may simply change with position changes.
- Venous hum – This murmur is also common in pre-school and school aged children. The murmur often disappears during or before early school age (3-6 years). It is common to detect a Still's murmur and a venous hum in the same healthy patient. The

sound is produced by venous turbulence of blood returning from the jugular and subclavian veins and mixing in the innominate vein and superior vena cava. Consistent with continuous venous blood flow, the murmur is higher pitched, heard continuously although varying in intensity throughout the cycle. It is best heard over the medial aspect of the clavicles, usually on the right, but can occur on the left.

It is loudest in the sitting position with the patient looking forward. Turning the head to the left usually extinguishes the murmur as does lying down or occluding the jugular flow with the examiners thumb. The murmur may mimic a patent ductus arteriosus. If the murmur does not diminish with these maneuvers, the patients require further evaluation.

Table 1. Innocent murmurs

Type of innocent murmur	Timing, location	Character, Pitch	Helpful maneuvers	Common Clinical Setting	Cause
Still's	Systolic ejection. Heard midway between left lower sternal boarder and apex	Low-pitched, Vibratory Crescendo-Decrescendo	Changes in intensity with position and breathing	Common in pre-school - school age children.	Vibration of the cordae tendonae as blood flows across on the way out the aorta
Venous Hum	Continuous. Heard on or below the medial third of the clavicle usually on the right	High pitched, very "musical" in intensity varying during the cardiac cycle	Disappears with supine positioning, turning the head away from the side of the murmur and gentle pressure on the jugular vein	Pre-school age children	Turbulence of venous return at the junction of the jugular and subclavian veins.
Peripheral Pulmonary Branch Stenosis	Systolic ejection. Heard at right and left upper sternal boarder with radiation to one or both axillae	Intermediate pitch, soft, may be loudest in the axilla	None	Infants up to six months of age.	Turbulence at branch points of the pulmonary arteries due to differences in cross sectional area.
Pulmonary Flow Murmur	Systolic ejection. Heard at the left upper sternal boarder	Intermediate pitch, soft	Diminished with decreased pulmonary blood flow (sitting or standing)	All age groups. Louder with high cardiac output (fever, hyperthyroidism, anemia)	Turbulence in the normal pulmonary outflow tract and valve
Mammary Souffle	Continuous or systolic. Heard at the left and/or right sternal boarder at 2nd -4th intercostal spaces		Elimination of the murmur with compression by the stethoscope of the area of maximal intensity	Pregnant and lactating teens	Caused by increased blood flow the the mammary arteries

- Peripheral pulmonary branch stenosis – This is the most common murmur in the neonate and young infant. It most often present in the first 3 months of life. It is due to turbulence at the branch points of the pulmonary arteries. As a result, a systolic crescendo-decrescendo murmur is audible over the left second intercostal space and radiates to one or both lungs depending on which branch points are involved. Distinguishing this murmur from the murmur of pulmonary valvular stenosis can be difficult.

One important clinical clue may be that the murmur of peripheral pulmonary branch stenosis is louder in one or both axilla when compared to the sound over the precordium. An opening snap heard immediately after S1 in the second intercostal space can be a clue to pulmonary valvular stenosis, but an opening snap like splitting of the first heart sound is a difficult distinction given the typical heart rates in this age group. Growth of the pulmonary arteries in the first year causes the angle of the branches of the pulmonary arteries to change and the murmur of pulmonary branch stenosis lessens and then usually resolves by six months of age.

Additionally, this murmur may become more prominent at 2-3 months due to the development of normal physiologic anemia in some infants. A reasonable approach to this murmur in the absence of symptoms or an opening snap is to observe the infant until six months of age and evaluate further if the murmur persists beyond this age. In situations where referral for further evaluation is difficult and the patient is asymptomatic it is reasonable to wait until 12 months of age since some PPBS murmurs may persist up to a year.

- Pulmonary flow murmur - This murmur occurs at any age but typically occurs in adolescents and adults. It is due to flow over a normal pulmonary valve. The murmur is heard best over the pulmonary outflow tract at the left second intercostal space. It typically does not radiate to the lungs and is rarely greater than a 2/6 in intensity. Non-cardiac causes for increased blood flow such as anemia and hyperthyroidism should be considered. Another very important cause for a very similar murmur in this location is an atrial septal defect (ASD). Whenever a pulmonary flow murmur is diagnosed the examiner should listen carefully over the pulmonic area for a wide and fixed (not varying with respiration) split S2, as these may be the only clues to an ASD.
- Mammary souffle – This murmur only appears in pregnant teens and women in the second and third trimester and the post-partum periods. It is caused by increased blood flow to the mammary arteries and is located on the left and/or right sternal boarders between the 2nd, 3rd and/or 4th intercostal spaces. The murmur is easily extinguished when pressure is applied with the stethoscope over the area of maximal intensity (2).

Pathologic findings

There are some general characteristics of murmurs, as well as other clinical findings which should prompt further evaluation: Purely diastolic murmurs other than those that are part of continuous murmurs or a venous hum, are always indicative of pathology and should be referred. However, the pathology which produces diastolic murmurs is relatively rare in pediatrics and, when present, are frequently accompanied by a more obvious systolic murmur.

Holosystolic murmurs occur in three situations

Mitral and tricuspid regurgitation and ventricular septal defects. In children almost all of these require further evaluation. Mitral and tricuspid regurgitation which produces an audible murmur in children is virtually always significant. In children, these murmurs require further evaluation for severity and associated anomalies. The most common holosystolic murmur in children will be from a ventricular septal defect. These murmurs are usually loud and obvious and require some type of advanced testing or referral to determine the clinical significance.

Many small muscular VSDs do not require any intervention

These murmurs usually have harsh high pitched crescendo-decrescendo murmurs and are asymptomatic. However, it can be difficult for the primary care physician to determine the size and significance of the VSD on physical examination alone.

Second heart sound

It is worthwhile to perform a focused examination of this sound over the 2nd left intercostal space during the physical exam. The normal S2 should vary with respiration. In children, splitting of S2 is audible with practice and careful examination at heart rates less than 120 bpm. The splitting should be more easily detectable during inspiration and more narrowly split or single on expiration. In a child who is old enough to cooperate, asking the child to inspire slowly and deeply may make it easier to detect. A loud, fixed, widely or paradoxically split S2 (Split on expiration rather than inspiration) may be the only finding in some congenital heart disease.

A loud P2 suggests pulmonary hypertension

P2 is loud when splitting of the S2 can be heard as far from the pulmonary valve as the apex. Normally pulmonary pressures are not high enough to generate a sound that is audible at that distance. Fixed splitting of S2 suggests an atrial septal defect and wide and paradoxically split S2 may be a result of conduction abnormalities, outflow obstruction, or poor contractility. The physician should develop competence and confidence in listening to S2 since patients may need to go to great lengths for further evaluation based on this finding alone and anomalies may progress to life-threatening and irreversible disease if not recognized and treated.

Pathologic murmurs

- *Ventriculoseptal defects* – This murmur can vary in presentation depending on the size of the defect and the age of the patient. Large VSD's may not have a murmur during the first month of life when elevated pulmonary pressures prevent significant shunting and low resistance from a wide VSD result in little if any turbulence. As the pulmonary pressures drop more shunting occurs and symptoms and a blowing holosystolic murmur at the left lower sternal boarder become apparent. Small muscular VSD's are often heard earlier in life because the pulmonary pressures can drop earlier and there is more resistance. The murmur may be holosystolic or shorter crescendo-decrescendo in nature.

- *Atrial septal defects* – Flow across the defect may not be heard directly. Increased pulmonary blood flow typically creates a pulmonary flow murmur in the right upper sternal boarder exactly like the innocent murmur with the same name. The distinguishing feature is the fixed split S2 caused by the compensatory left to right shunting during expiration keeping the right ventricular output constant during the respiratory cycle. Prevention of Eisenmenger's syndrome depends on early recognition of the fixed split S2 and correction of the defect.
- *Mitral regurgitation* – The murmur of mitral regurgitation is systolic. Although classically holosystolic at the apex with radiation to the left axilla, there is considerable variation in the characteristics of the murmur of mitral regurgitation depending on the cause and severity of the murmur and may be decrescendo, crescendo or crescendo-decrescendo. The intensity does not correlate well with severity unless a thrill is felt. S1 is often diminished due to ineffective closing of the valve or absent or obliterated by the murmur which may begin before the valve is approximated and the onset of isovolumetric contraction. S2 may be widely split because of shortened left ventricular ejection time.
- *Tricuspid regurgitation* – Like mitral regurgitation the murmur of tricuspid regurgitation is usually holosystolic. It is heard closer to the left lower sternal boarder and occasionally the right lower sternal boarder. It may vary with respiration and may be accompanied by very right ventricular heave, pulsatile neck veins, edema and hepatomegaly. Since pulmonary pressures tend to be lower tricuspid regurgitation murmurs may be softer. With increased venous return during inspiration the listener may appreciate variation in the intensity of the murmur with respiration.
- *Aortic stenosis* – The murmur of aortic stenosis is high pitched crescendo-decrescendo and radiates to the carotids. It can never interfere with S1 since it cannot begin before the end of isovolumetric contraction. In critical aortic stenosis the sound may radiate down to the apex and may be inaudible between the aortic region and the apex mimicking a second murmur of mitral regurgitation also known as the Gallavardin phenomenon. The lower pitched apical murmur does not radiate to the axilla in the Gallavardin phenomenon whereas in mitral regurgitation it does. Other supporting findings may include diminished carotid upstroke, thrill over the aortic region, increased left ventricular impulse and an ejection systolic click heard immediately after S1.
- *Pulmonary stenosis* – The murmur of pulmonary stenosis is systolic ejection murmur in at the right base and may be mistaken for a pulmonary flow murmur and pulmonary branch stenosis. Distinguishing features include and opening snap after S1 and a widely split S2.
- *Aortic regurgitation* – Aortic regurgitation along with mitral stenosis are diastolic murmurs and much harder to hear. In many settings such as crowded clinics or large hospital wards in developing countries it may not be possible to reduce the ambient noise level to be able to detect diastolic murmurs. To increase the chances of detecting it the patient should be upright and leaning forward and holding his breath in expiration. The classic finding in aortic regurgitation of a wide pulse pressure or water hammer pulse is due to the rapid rise in systolic pressure from increased stroke volume

and rapid drop off in diastolic pressure due to regurgitation. This finding is uncommon in young children because aortic regurgitation is usually not severe in children.

- *Mitral stenosis* – The murmur of mitral regurgitation may be the most difficult of all murmurs to hear yet it is very important. Mitral stenosis is a major cause of morbidity due to rheumatic heart disease. Because of the low pressure gradient across the mitral valve during diastole the intensity and pitch of the murmur is very low. Under ideal circumstances a 1-2/6 diastolic rumble can be heard in a quiet room using the bell of the stethoscope resting lightly on the chest overlying the apex with the patient in the left lateral decubitus position. Even in a quiet setting with the stethoscope in the ears the background noise of a fairly quiet air vent in the exam room is usually louder than the diastolic rumble. S1 should be louder than normal because the mitral valve leaflets are still widely separated at the onset of systole.
  An mitral opening snap immediately after S2 may be heard at the apex and can be confused with a split S2 with a loud P2 component which may also be present in mitral stenosis because of pulmonary hypertension but the opening snap can be distinguished by the absence of the sound at the base. Mitral stenosis tends to progress more rapidly in developing countries and late supporting findings of MS may be present in young children. These include: atrial fibrillation and pulmonary hypertension with a loud P2 and narrowly split S2.

Cardiology testing in heart murmur evaluation

Chest x-ray and EKG

Studies have shown that chest x-rays are neither sensitive nor specific enough to be helpful to the clinician trying to distinguish innocent murmurs from the most common congenital cardiac diseases. It is not advisable to obtain a chest x-ray in the evaluation of murmurs and its use has been largely abandoned as routine by cardiologists. A chest x-ray has its greatest utility in cardiology in evaluating overall heart size and pulmonary vascularity and should be used when those clinical questions are important. The EKG has limited sensitivity and specificity for the diagnosis of structural congenital heart disease. It would be hazardous to conclude from either a normal chest x-ray or normal EKG or both that a murmur is innocent.

Echocardiography

In the hands of technicians and physicians experienced in pediatric examinations, echocardiography is exquisitely sensitive in detecting congenital heart disease. The yield of echocardiography for the detection of structural heart disease is inversely related to the age of the patient. In almost every case, it is more cost effective to refer patients with suspicious murmurs to an experienced pediatric cardiologist. Pediatric cardiologists have approximately 95% sensitivity and specificity for discriminating heart disease from innocent murmurs on clinical grounds with missed disease being only trivial or minor lesions.

This approach must be tailored to the physician's practice environment including the availability of a pediatric cardiologist, ability of the cardiologist, the cardiologist's selectiveness for echocardiography and the ability of the patient, particularly neonates, to be transported if necessary. Although not optimal, in areas where pediatric cardiologists and echo technicians are not available the primary care physician may want to develop skills in echocardiography.

CONGENITAL HEART DISEASE IN DEVELOPING COUNTRIES

Prevalence data from developing countries is lacking, but congenital heart disease (CHD) is thought to affect approximately 0.4-1% of live births worldwide (3-6). Management through advanced cardiothoracic surgery has saved lives and greatly limited morbidity for patients with CHD in developed nations. In developing countries, however, CHD often goes undetected or is detected too late to avoid complications such as growth failure, heart failure, irreversible pulmonary hypertension, and early death (7-9).

Barriers to better pediatric cardiac care in developing countries include lack of education on signs and symptoms for families and primary health care workers, home deliveries far from health care facilities, and severe deficits of specialists and specialty centers to diagnose and manage both congenital and acquired cardiac disease (5, 6). In 2003, it was reported that Children's Hospital of Boston alone employed more than twice the number of pediatric cardiologists in all of India (10). In Ethiopia, 1600 doctors serve 83 million people (11). And in sub-Saharan Africa, 3% of the global health workforce attempts to treat 24% of the global disease burden (5).

One report out of a referral center in Guatemala illustrates the issues above (6). CHD detection rates were estimated based upon the center's number of new referrals in 2006 and Guatemala's calculated country-wide CHD incidence (using the approximation of 1% live births affected and birth rates from the National Ministry of Health). In addition to overall low detection rates (14% of calculated incidence), only 11.5% of CHD cases detected were in neonates. This is in contrast to 33-60% of CHD patients detected in the neonatal period in developed countries.

This illustrates the predictable conclusion that more severe congenital lesions cause a far greater number of deaths in developing versus developed countries based on ability to detect and treat. One statistic cited was 95% mortality by age one year for untreated children with transposition of the great arteries versus 95% long-term survival rate for those patients with TGA who have the arterial switch procedure (6).

Within Guatemala, regions with lower human development indices – a composite measure of life expectancy, literacy, education, and standard of living developed by the United Nations to study the underserved – had lower CHD detection rates (6). Guatemala is of particular interest to study since there exists within the country an affordable (and relatively accessible) comprehensive pediatric cardiac center, the only one in Central America. Despite this local expertise, only 14% of predicted cardiac defects reached this referral center, and older children with simple lesions were "over-represented" (6).

In recent years, pediatric cardiologists and cardiothoracic surgeons have written a great deal on the need to address huge disparities in the identification and care of children with cardiac disease throughout the world. For many poor countries, governments do not invest enough in health care or assure health care access for the population. Most efforts addressing illness focus on communicable disease (5, 12). Some argue that surgery needs to be recognized as a component of public health when it comes to congenital lesions that - left uncorrected -

leave children vulnerable to infectious endocarditis, stroke, pulmonary hypertension, and heart failure among other sequelae (8, 13, 14).

Three strategies to address the need for CHD repair in developing nations are widely recognized (15, 16): 1) Transport affected children to countries with specialty facilities, 2) Transport specialists and technology from ther countries to sites of need periodically and 3) Create more sustainable pediatric cardiac care facilities in developing nations. The third has been accomplished in multiple countries through collaborative efforts between well-established programs from Western nations and programs within a host country.

Some examples are Boston, MA and Cochin, India (10); Belgium and Kigali, Rwanda (12); and Shanghai and Project HOPE (5, 9). Often these collaborations occur outside of government involvement/support, with the onus on the "medical fraternity" to develop and sustain them. Millions of children with correctable CHD – many of whom in developing countries will die from complications by age 20 (8, 9) - provide motivation for international efforts.

With regards to "choosing whom to fix," some of the surgical contraindications cited by a center in Mozambique, one that uses the second strategy, were fixed pulmonary hypertension, neurological impairment, severe malnutrition, and HIV infection (14). Selection criteria included potential for complete repair and ability to avoid use of prosthetic material (14). Long term anticoagulation is often seen as impractical in resource-poor settings (15).

Authors of the Mozambique center study reported that almost 7% of patients presenting to the center had Eisenmenger syndrome (14), the practically inoperable consequence of uncorrected intracardiac shunt in which pulmonary hypertension from strain of left to right shunting ultimately reverses the shunt and causes cyanosis. Culprit lesions are simple lesions (typically ventricular septal defects or persistent ductus arteriosus) that can wreak havoc when uncorrected.

The goal of the center is to address simple lesions early (ASD, VSD, persistent ductus) as well as to fix some lesions of moderate complexity such as Tetralogy of Fallot, aortic stenosis, pulmonary stenosis, and ostium primum ASD. For reasons of efficient resource allocation, cases of complex (double outlet RV, tricuspid or pulmonary atresia, TGA, complete AV septal defect, TA, and other single ventricle or cyanotic CHD) and complicated CHD were less likely to be selected for surgical intervention (14).

In addition to the obvious need for increased neonatal and pediatric CHD screening and management, other interventions in developing countries bear mention as well. These include the need for counseling of adolescent girls and women with CHD who are planning pregnancies (14, 17) as well as specialist services for post-operative patients (14). Much effort now, however, remains focused on improving morbidity and mortality in the very young by increasing CHD detection rates and accessible management options.

CONGESTIVE HEART FAILURE

Pediatric patients differ significantly from adult patients in the usual etiology of congestive heart failure. The majority of pediatric patients with symptoms of congestive heart failure (HF) have excessive pulmonary blood flow from structural lesions resulting in left to right shunting as opposed to primary pump failure. These patients have normal ventricular contractile function. A smaller subset of pediatric patients in the tropics have impaired ventricular function from congenital or acquired cardiomyopathies, rheumatic heart disease, endomycardial fibrosis or previously palliated or repaired congenital heart disease. The distinction between these groups is important when considering the symptoms, physical exam findings, and management.

Table 2. Ross classification of pediatric heart failure

Class	Symptoms and Signs
I	None
II	Mild tachypnea/diaphoresis with feedings in infants. Exertional dyspnea in children
III	Marked tachypnea/diaphoresis with feedings in infants. Marked exertional dyspnea in children
IV	Symptoms at rest (diaphoresis, tachypnea, tachycardia, retractions)

Also see: Modified Ross Criteria: Ross RD. The Ross classification for heart failure in children after 25 years: A review and an age-stratified revision. Pediatr Cardiol 2012;33(8):1295-300. doi: 10.1007/s00246-012-0306-8.

Table 3. Causes of congestive heart failure in pediatrics

	Fetus	Neonate/Infant	Childhood/Adolescent
Normal Cardiac Structure	Anemia Arrhythmia Cardiomyopathies Extracardiac shunts Hyperthyroidsism	Anemia Arrhythmia Cardiomyopathies Endocrinopathies Extracardiac shunts Hypertension Hypoxic ischemic events Kawasaki Disease Metabolic (Hypoglycemia) Sepsis	Anemia Arrhythmia Cardiomyopathy HIV Kawasaki disease Myocarditis Hypertension Renal failure Cardiotoxin exposure Inherited diseases Muscular dystrophies Mitochondial diseases
Congenital Heart Disease	AV valve regurgitation Inflow/Outflow Obstruction Premature PDA closure Premature closure of foramen ovale	Systemic outflow obstruction Valvular aortic stenosis Subvalvular aortic stenosis Coarctation of aorta Systemic inflow obstruction Mitral stenosis Cor triatriatum Pulmonary vein stenosis Anomalous left coronary TAPVR Systemic volume overload Aortic/mitral regurgitation Patent ductus arteriosus Ventricular septal defect Aortopulmonary window Single ventricle Truncus arteriosus	Aortic regurgitation Mitral regurgitation Mitral stenosis Pulmonary vein stenosis Failed palliation procedures

Symptoms and physical findings in children are dependent on both the age of the patient and the etiology of the HF. Infants present with prolonged feeding time associated with diaphoresis and tachypnea or dyspnea due to increased metabolic demand from sucking effort, respiratory effort and sustaining adequate blood flow to the digestive tract. Pallor and tachycardia are present. Feeding intolerance and vomiting may be present due to hepatic and intestinal congestion. Growth failure, especially poor weight gain, may be present from the combination of decreased intake and increase energy requirements. Physical exam almost universally shows tachypnea and tachycardia and often reveals irritability, pallor, cachexia, diaphoresis, retractions, nasal flaring, prominent cardiac impulse and hepatomegaly.

Older children and adolescents will more often present with history and physical findings similar to adults. Symptoms of HF in this age group includes decreased exercise tolerance, dyspnea on exertion, weight gain from fluid retention or weight loss from nausea and edema of the digestive tract, peripheral edema and orthopnea. Physical findings include jugular venous distention, tachycardia, rales, hepatomegaly edema and ascites. See the Ross criteria in Table 2 for classification of HF in children as well as Table 3 for etiologies of HF in children.

TREATMENT OF CONGESTIVE HEART FAILURE

Since much of heart failure in pediatrics is due to underlying conditions such as systemic illness or structural heart disease identifying the cause is essential. Treatment of the underlying cause by cardiac catheterization, surgical correction or palliation or by medical therapy may result in resolution of congestive heart failure. Often the medical treatment directed at congestive heart failure will control symptoms until there is definitive care of the underlying condition.

The October 2007 cardiovascular medicines section of the WHO Essential Medicines List for Children (EMLc) contains digoxin, furosemide, spironolactone and dopamine (18). In practice many drugs not on the list are used including ACE inhibitors and beta blockers and many of these both on the list and not on the list are not licensed for use in the management of children with congestive heart failure. Support of a pediatric cardiologist is beneficial.

Salt and fluid restriction in older children with congestive heart failure is generally reserved for patient with pump failure. Since the majority of pediatric patients with heart failure have high output failure it is usually inadvisable to restrict fluids in infants because of the competing demands for calories which are increased 20% or more over baseline requirements. Sodium is potentially harmful in heart failure as it may cause fluid overload and lead to acute decompensation. Restriction of sodium reduces exacerbations and allows the reduction of diuretic dose. In advanced stages of heart failure water restriction may be useful in older patients.

Diuretics

Loop diuretics such as Furosemide are preferred to reduce venous congestion, hepatomegaly and respiratory distress from fluid overload. Aldosterone blocking potassium sparing diuretics such as spironolactone are useful in augmenting diuretic therapy while reducing or eliminating the need for potassium supplementation. Use caution with patients who are also on ACE inhibitors since life-threatening hyperkalemia may occur.

ACE inhibitors (ACEi)

ACEi have been associated with reduction of symptoms, reduced progression and improved survival in adults. Pediatric data is more limited but there are some findings, which are unique to infants and children, including reduction of left to right shunts and reduction of pulmonary artery pressures (19). Another large study did not show any improvement in survival, transplant, growth or episodes of CHF (20). None-the less the use of these medications in pediatric heart failure is now common. It is important to monitor renal function and potassium in children treated with an ACEi. Chronic cough is a common side effect, which may be intolerable. Adult patients who develop ACEi associated cough can be treated with angiotensin receptor blockers (ARBs) however there is no evidence to support its use in children with CHF.

Digitalis glycosides (digoxin)

Digoxin is used less frequently in children relative to adults. Little data exists to support its use in children. Use of digoxin for children with poor cardiac contractility may be justified. Patients with volume overload lesions and shunts have normal contractility and are not likely to benefit from digoxin.

Beta blockers

Data in adults shows clear evidence of benefit from beta-blockers in heart failure but in pediatrics, the data is very limited. Small studies suggest improved cardiac function, exercise tolerance, symptoms and reduction of neurohormonal activation in children with cardiomyopathies. However, the only large multicenter study in children to date did not show any clinical benefit (21). Among the beta blockers there is more data supporting the use of Carvedilol but direct comparison to other commonly used beta blockers in children has not been done.

Refractory heart failure

Potentially beneficial non-pharmacologic treatments include resynchronization therapy using biventricular pacing, implantable cardioverter-defibrillator and ventricular assist devices. Heart transplantation provides good outcomes with 90% and 80% one and five-year survival rates with good quality of life for children with end-stage HF or inoperable congenital defects. Transplantation may be an option for patients who in spite of optimal medical therapy have heart failure that is progressive, continued growth failure, life-threatening arrhythmias, or require intravenous inotropic support and have an unacceptable poor quality of life.

Endomyocardial fibrosis

Endomyocardial fibrosis (EMF) is also known by several other names including: Davies' disease. idiopathic mural endocarditis, obliterative cardiomyopathy, eosinophilic carditis, tropical endomyocardial fibrotic restrictive cardiomyopathy. It was first described by in 1938 on pathologic specimens and identified in Nigerian soldiers during WWII by Davies (22). It affects an estimated 10-12 million people and has a high morbidity and mortality. It is usually seen in children and adolescents but may also be seen in infants and adults (23-25).

EMF is a progressive cardiac disease which is most common in children and young adults beginning as early at two years of age. It is characterized by swelling and thickening of the ventricular endocardial connective tissue with mucopolysaccharides resulting in dense and white fibrous tissue that extends as deep as the inner third of the myocardium, causing cavity obliteration and restriction of ventricular filling (22). It may affect one (right 45%, left 10%) primarily or both (45%) ventricles. It is not accompanied by lesions in any other part of the body and the etiology is not known. It is endemic in most of Africa while rare in other parts of Africa.

It is present in South America and Asia and short term visitors to endemic areas may acquire it suggesting an infectious etiology. The incidence has been stable in some areas. It has dropped 500 fold in some areas of Nigeria over the last 30-40 years in along with the improvements in hygiene and health care in those areas (26). Hypereosinophilia is present in up to 30% of cases suggesting a parasitic or allergic etiology however this is an inconsistent finding in blood or tissues (27).

Fibrosis begins at the apex and may involve papillary muscles and the posterior wall near the tricuspid and mitral valves. The fibrosis decreases compliance leading to restrictive cardiomyopathy. Mitral and/or tricuspid valve regurgitation ultimately develops. Unlike rheumatic heart disease the valves leaflets in endomyocardial fibrosis are normal. Atrial enlargement is common leading to atrial arrhythmias. Fibrosis of the ventricles also leads to impaired conduction and activation of contractions as well as ventricular arrhythmias.

Clinical manifestations depend on whether it is an acute presentation or a more advanced chronic presentation as well as the side of the heart that is predominantly involved.

Acute endomyocardial fibrosis may present with fever, itching, rash, eosinophilia and signs of myopericarditis. Up to 40% present with pericardial effusions further complicating poor cardiac function. Most patients are likely asymptomatic during the acute phase and not diagnosed until they have signs of chronic disease. Chronic features include signs of heart failure and of chronic disease such as, clubbing, growth failure and failure of development of secondary sex characteristics.

Right sided involvement results in the development of increased systemic venous pressure with distended neck veins, hepatic congestion, pleural effusions, ascites but pedal edema is not common. Left sided involvement results in dyspnea and pulmonary congestion. Atrial fibrillation is common and atrial and ventricular thrombi on either side may develop, embolize and result in stroke or death.

EKG findings vary depending on the chronicity, location and extent of the endomyocardial fibrosis. Those with pericarditis and or pericardial effusions will show low voltage or electrical alternans. Right sided EMF will manifest as right atrial anomaly. Left sided EMF may show left atrial anomaly, T wave inversions, and ST segment depressions in the lateral leads. Chest x-rays usually show cardiomegaly in a pattern consistent with the predominant side involved and maybe massive.

Echocardiogram may be necessary to rule out pericardial effusion. Echo typically shows significant chamber enlargement and shows hyperdynamic outflow tracks and dilated pulmonary arteries. MRI is the gold standard for diagnosing EMF however it is not available to the vast majority of the population where EMF is endemic (28, 29). Echo is an accurate non-invasive investigation. It has an 82.8% agreement with intraoperative findings (27). In endemic areas clinical history and physical exam along with a chest x-ray are usually sufficient to make the diagnosis and echocardiogram may be used for confirmation when readily available or in non-endemic areas when the EMF is suspected.

The differential diagnosis includes those disorders with valvular and restrictive heart diseases including rheumatic heart disease, endocardial fibroelastosis, infiltrative diseases such as sarcoidosis, amyloidosis, hemochromatosis, Loeffler's endocarditis, hypertrophic and dilated cardiomyopathies, and malignancies. Pericardial disease such as constrictive pericarditis and tuberculosis should be considered but should be distinguishable on careful echocardiogram evaluation of the pericardium and endocardium.

Management of chronic EMF is that of congestive heart failure due to pump failure including diuretics, beta blockers and ACE inhibitors. Anticoagulation may be considered but must be weighed against the risks. Rate control for atrial fibrillation can be achieved with beta blockers, calcium channel blockers or digitalis. For acute EMF a short course of corticosteroids has been recommended but should be weighed in light of the potential for reactivation of TB and other infections endemic to the tropics as well as exacerbation heart failure (30).

RHEUMATIC FEVER AND RHEUMATIC HEART DISEASE

Rheumatic heart disease incidence has fallen dramatically in developed countries thanks to improved living conditions and aggressive treatment of group A beta-hemolytic streptococcal (GABHS) pharyngitis (31, 32). If acute rheumatic fever (ARF) is diagnosed, prompt echocardiogram, treatment with anti-inflammatory and antibiotics, and relative accessibility of cardiology follow-up care is to be expected. This is in stark contrast to the natural history of non-suppurative sequelae of GABHS pharyngeal infection in developing countries.

There are 15-20 million people with rheumatic heart disease (RHD) globally (33, 34) with 2.4 million children affected (34); 42% of the latter live in sub-Saharan Africa (34). The annual death toll of RHD is about 230,000-295,000 with burden of disease falling on developing nations (34, 35). RHD is the main cause of cardiac morbidity and mortality in children and young adults in Africa, and it is the leading cause of acquired heart disease in young people worldwide (33, 36).

Though prevalence data obtained through clinical screening in primary and secondary schools already shows a greater rheumatic heart disease burden in developing versus developed countries, a 2007 Lancet report (37) illustrates that inclusion of subclinical disease (detected by echocardiography) may increase prevalence rates by a factor of ten (37). The study was conducted in Mozambique and Cambodia. It is not clear whether subclinical disease is also more widespread in places like the US, but presumably it is not, and the disease-burden divide widens. Of note, RHD screening by murmur detection, even when the primary physician auscultates a pathologic murmur, is not sensitive.

One study found sensitivity of auscultation to detect a pathologic murmur to be just 46% (38). This deficiency in detection means that RHD is often first diagnosed when a child, adolescent, or young adult presents with heart failure. Using clinical assessment, prevalence rates in developing countries range from about 1-5 per 1000, with sub-Saharan Africa reporting among the highest (34, 37). With echocardiography, disease rates reach 30-50 per 1,000 (37).

Pathophysiology

Clinical descriptions of ARF date back to the 1500's, but only in the 19th century was it definitively linked to carditis (31). Today the etiology of acute rheumatic fever and subsequent rheumatic heart disease remain active areas of research. Currently, the diseases are understood as delayed autoimmune responses to GABHS pharyngitis, with latency of 1-5 weeks to development of multi-organ symptoms (34).

In particular, carditis is attributed to molecular mimicry whereby cardiac myosin is attacked for its resemblance to the M-protein on GABHS cell membranes (31). The risk of development of ARF is about 3% in untreated GABHS pharyngitis, with much higher risk in subsequent infections (up to 75%) (34). That said, there are still genetic and other host factors affecting susceptibility that are yet to be fully understood.

Table 4. Jones Criteria for rheumatic fever

Two Major OR One Major and Two Minor Criteria AND Evidence of a Recent Strep Infection	
Major	**Minor**
Migratory Polyarthritis Erythema Marginatum Subcutanous Nodules Carditis Sydenham's Chorea	Arthralgias Fever First Degree Heart Block Elevated Inflammatory Markers

Diagnosis

The Jones (Thomas Duckett Jones, MD, 1899-1954) criteria were first put forth in 1944 and have since undergone modifications (31, 34). The major criteria, Table 4, are migratory polyarthritis, rash (erythema marginatum), subcutaneous nodules, carditis and Sydenham chorea. Minor criteria are arthralgia, fever, first degree heart block, and elevated inflammatory markers (31). Diagnosis of ARF is made if two major criteria or one major and two minor criteria are present along with evidence of recent strep infection. Of note, these criteria are not sensitive enough in developing nations to address the public health burden of acute rheumatic fever (34).

In addition, the requisite GABHS infection preceding symptoms is difficult to prove in developing countries where rapid strep assays, throat cultures, and anti-streptolysin-O titers are not always readily obtained. Some researchers propose primary prevention of rheumatic heart disease through empiric treatment of febrile pharyngitis, approximately 20% of which may be the result of GABHS infection (34, 39).

Treatment

Primary prevention of ARF entails treating GABHS pharyngitis with antibiotics – starting within nine days of symptoms onset (31). Antibiotic options for GABHS pharyngitis include oral penicillin V (first line), benzathine penicillin G IM, amoxicillin, first generation cephalosporins, clindamycin, clarithromycin, and azithromycin (31). Some physicians in areas where RHD is endemic opt to treat empirically those children 5-15 years of age with fever and pharyngitis (31).

This may be an important means of eradicating ARF globally. Of note, "primordial" prevention – improving socioeconomic conditions, hygiene, and housing – would ideally emerge and obviate the need for primary and secondary prophylaxis (40), but as social change is slow and dependent on so many factors, the focus remains on relatively more feasible intervention strategies.

If ARF is diagnosed, therapy with high-dose salicylates is also given until evidence of inflammation resolves (4-6 weeks typically). The significant and rapid (24-48 hours) improvement in joint symptoms with salicylate therapy supports a diagnosis of ARF over other forms of arthritis (31).

Approximately 60% of people with ARF will go on to develop RHD (31, 35). In secondary prevention (i.e., treatment after an episode of carditis), IM benzathine penicillin G is given every 3-4 weeks. Alternatively, penicillin V is taken orally twice daily. Sulfadiazide or macrolides are alternatives (31). Per American Heart Association guidelines, those who have had ARF without carditis should receive antibiotic therapy through age 21 or 5 years after the last ARF episode, whichever period is longer.

If diagnosed with RHD, a patient should be treated until age 40 or 10 years after the last ARF episode (again, whichever period is longer) (31, 41). Those who have continued high-risk exposure may need lifelong prophylaxis. Without secondary prophylaxis, annual mortality in RHD is about 1.5% (35). In addition, 3-7.5% of strokes in less developed countries are attributed directly to RHD (35).

Since the mitral valve is most often involved in RHD, the mainstay of treatment once heart failure occurs is valve repair or replacement. Mitral valve stenosis may be treated percutaneously via commisurotomy or balloon valvuloplasty. Concurrent medical management of heart failure is generally indicated. Surgical intervention costs around $25,000, so one can imagine that funding of ARF and RHD screening programs would be more cost-effective than managing failing rheumatic valves (31, 42). Since at least the early 1970's, the World Health Organization has attempted to facilitate surveillance of GAS related disease via registries in developing nations, but general consensus is that under-reporting is the norm (34, 43-45).

Regarding valve replacement, as RHD is largely seen in the young in developing nations, bioprostheses are likely to deteriorate or simply be outgrown. Mechanical prostheses carry the risk of thromboembolic events, and adherence to anticoagulation can be low and erratic (31). In addition, with RHD in adolescents and women of child-bearing age, the goal is to avoid a need for anticoagulation, therefore valvuloplasty is preferred (33).

No vaccine yet exists for GABHS, though there are candidates in development. None of the four vaccines that target the M-protein are yet in phase II trials (33), and one major concern is that the vaccine itself could prompt immune-mediated destruction of heart valves (considering myosin's resemblance to the targeted antigen) (31). That said, vaccine development remains an important element in addressing the burden of GAS related morbidity and mortality. Combining the suppurative and non-suppurative sequelae of GAS infection (both pharyngeal and skin), this pathogen is responsible for at least half a million deaths per year around the world (35). As individual pathogens, only HIV, Mycobacterium tuberculosis, Plasmodium falciparum, and Streptococcus pneumoniae take more lives (35).

Complications

Complications of RHD include heart failure, infective endocarditis (IE), and stroke. Of note, rheumatic disease accounts for nearly 90% of cardiac disorders in women of child-bearing age in developing countries (46).

Regarding IE, the American Heart Association put forward revised recommendations in 2007 addressing "cardiac conditions associated with the highest risk of adverse outcome from endocarditis for which prophylaxis is recommended." These consist of prosthetic cardiac valve, previous IE, congenital heart disease (unrepaired cyanotic CHD including palliative shunts and conduits, completely repaired CHD with prostheses during the first 6 post-procedure months, and repaired CHD with residual defects), and cardiac transplant recipients who develop cardiac valvulopathy. Further studies on IE in RHD are warranted as unrepaired RHD itself may well qualify as a condition of "highest risk" especially in resource-poor settings like sub-Saharan Africa.

KAWASAKI DISEASE

Kawasaki disease is the leading cause of acquired pediatric heart disease in North America and in Japan. Cardiac complications including coronary aneurysms and coronary artery stenosis with subsequent myocardial infarction, myocarditis, pericarditis and valvular heart disease occur in roughly 20-25% of untreated children (47, 48). There is significant reduction (to about 5%) of the frequency of these complications when treated early in the course (within 10 days of onset of the fever). Prompt recognition and diagnosis is essential in early initiation of treatment. Table 5 illustrates the criteria for diagnosis of Kawasaki disease. Table 6 reviews risks for cardiac sequelae. Kawasaki disease recurs in about 3% of patients (49).

Table 5. Diagnostic criteria for Kawasaki syndrome

Complete Kawasaki Syndrome – Must meet each of the following criteria:		
a.	Fever of at least 5 days duration	
b.	4 of the 5 following criteria	
	i.	Bilateral conjunctival injection without exudate
	ii.	Mucous membrane changes: strawberry tongue, injected fissured lips
	iii.	Polymorphous rash
	iv.	Changes of the extremities: peripheral edema, peripheral erythema and periungal desquamation.
	v.	Cervical lymphadenopathy (>1.5 cm diameter)
c.	Lack of another known disease process to explain the illness	
Incomplete (atypical) Kawasaki Syndrome: Must meet each of the following criteria:		
a.	Fever of at least 5 days duration	
b.	At least two of the clinical criteria for Kawasaki syndrome (or evidence of coronary artery abnormalities on 2D echo if <4 criteria met)	
c.	Lack of another known disease process to explain the illness	
d.	Laboratory findings consistent with severe systemic inflammation*	

*ESR, CRP, Neutrophil leukocytosis, Pyuria, Elevated platelet count.

Table 6. Risk factors for cardiac sequelae in Kawasaki disease

Male sex
Age < 1 year or > 5 years
Longer duration of fever prior to treatment
IVIG resistance
Incomplete KD
CRP > 10.0 mg/dl
WBC count > 30,000/mm^3
Low serum albumen (<3g/L)

The majority of cases of Kawasaki disease (~75%) present in children between one and five years old (49). Those younger than one and older than five tend to have incomplete presentations and thus delayed diagnosis with subsequent increased risk for coronary complications (47, 49). Up to a third of patients with Kawasaki disease (KD) have concurrent infections whose symptoms can confound and delay diagnosis (49). The differential for KD includes viral and bacterial infections as well as rheumatologic conditions. The list includes adenovirus, measles, toxic shock syndrome, scarlet fever, idiopathic juvenile arthritis, Rocky Mountain spotted fever, and Stevens-Johnson syndrome.

The etiology of KD is not known, but is thought to encompass an exaggerated immune response to some infectious trigger in a genetically susceptible host (48, 49). One identified susceptibility gene is ITPKC, a T-cell activity modulator (48). No one infection is the definitive culprit to trigger abnormal T cell activity and subsequent KD. With respect to genetic influence, sibling risk of an affected child is ten times greater than the general population (48). That said, there are numerous genes and environmental interactions under study and no defined way to counsel families on individuals' risk.

First described in 1967 by Dr. Tomisaku Kawasaki (1925-) in Tokyo, KD has since been reported world-wide – in at least 60 countries in Asia, the Middle East, the Americas, Africa, and Europe – though with higher prevalence in people of Asian descent. (47, 50, 51) Global incidence varies from 1 to >200 cases per 100,000 children annually, with Japan reporting the highest numbers and India on the lower end, though that reflects in part a younger surveillance system in India. In the US, the incidence is around 20:100,000. KD and Henoch-Schonlein purpura are the most common multi-system vasculitides of infancy and childhood.

MANAGEMENT

IVIG

Treatment with IVIG and aspirin shortens the duration of clinical symptoms and decreases the frequency of coronary artery abnormalities. Treatment with IVIG (2 gm/kg given IV infused over 10-12 hours) should be given within the 10 days after the onset of fever and if possible within the first 7 days. Patients treated prior to five days are more likely to require retreatment with IVIG. There is some evidence that treatment after 10 days may still be beneficial if there is evidence of ongoing inflammation.

Aspirin

Currently the American Heart Association and the American Academy of Pediatrics guidelines recommends high dose aspirin (80 -100 mg/kg/d divided in four doses) during the acute phase (52). It is not clear that high dose aspirin is better than medium dose (30-50 mg/kg/d in four divided doses). It is also not clear whether it is more effective in combination with IVIG as compared to IVIG alone for the acute inflammatory symptoms or the prevention of coronary artery disease. Once the patient is afebrile for 48 hours the aspirin dose can be changed to low dose therapy at 3-5 mg/kg/d. Use low dose for 8 weeks if no coronary artery disease is present.

Continue low dose aspirin until laboratory evidence of inflammation (ESR and platelet count) has returned to normal unless aneurysms are present. If large aneurysms (>8mm diameter) are still present three months after the acute illness treatment with antiplatelet therapy with aspirin or dipyramadole AND anticoagulation with low molecular weight heparin or warfarin may be needed to prevent thrombosis within the aneurysm.

Refractory cases

A refractory case is failure to become afebrile within 24 hours. 13% of cases fail to respond to initial IVIG and aspirin. It is important to wait at least 36 hours after the initial IVIG dose before retreating since fever prior to that time may be related to the IVIG. Half of refractory cases respond to a second dose of IVIG. Corticosteroids do not add benefit when added to conventional first line treatment. Advanced therapies beyond IVIG and aspirin should be referred to specialists familiar with their delivery.

Echocardiograms

An echocardiogram is required the time of diagnosis, at two weeks and at six to eight weeks following the acute illness. Repeat echocardiography in patients without coronary involvement after this time is considered to be optional. Patients who have demonstrated coronary involvement with dilation or aneurysm are classified by the degree of involvement. Follow-up and prescribed treatment occurs with greater frequency and intensity based upon the degree of involvement. All of these patients need to be seen and followed by a pediatric cardiologist. Patients should not receive live immunizations for at least 11 months after treatment for Kawasaki disease because IVIG may interfere with the effectiveness of the vaccines. Patients receiving long-term aspirin should receive flu vaccine and varicella vaccine because of the risk of Reye syndrome.

Chagas' disease

Chagas' disease represents an important cause of cardiac morbidity and mortality in the tropics. The protozoa trypanasoma cruzi causes gastrointestinal and cardiac disease including acute myocarditis, arrhythmias and conduction abnormalities, thromboembolism and stroke and chronic myocardial fibrosis with congestive heart failure. Acquired in South America, Chagas' disease is seen worldwide because of its' chronic nature and increasing global migration. Because of the low parasitic load children typically are asymptomatic during the acute phase of the disease or present with a nonspecific febrile illness with malaise. Hepatosplenomegaly, morbilliform rash, lymphadenopathy and unilateral lid edema (Romaña's sign) may be present. When they do have cardiac symptoms they are those of myocarditis and pericarditis.

Chronic Chagas cardiomyopathy can occur as early as 5 years after infection but typically occurs decades later and rarely occurs in children. Chronic cardiovascular manifestations includes heart failure, arrhythmias, thromboembolism, stroke and chest pain. Findings of chronic Chagas' cardiomyopathy may include those of congestive heart failure, wide splitting of S2 due to right bundle branch block disease presents. Because treatment of chronic disease is of modest benefit it is important to recognize that this it is a pediatric disease and prevention of chronic Chagas' cardiomyopathy should begin in childhood.

Schistosomiasis

Schistosomiasis induced pulmonary artery hypertension is a progressive and fatal complication of schistosoma mansoni infections affects only 1% of those infected with schistosoma mansoni yet is the most common cause of pulmonary hypertension world-wide affecting 2-5 million people (53). The pathophysiology is not known but is likely multifactorial from egg embolization and the resultant local and systemic host immune response and increased portocaval shunting from portal hypertension. Infections acquired in childhood may take decades to develop. With the exception of a single case report antiparasitic treatment including successful elimination of parasites in childhood has not been shown to improve or prevent the development of schistosomiasis induced pulmonary hypertension later in adulthood (53, 54). Therefore it is imperative that education about the disease include children living or traveling to areas where schistosomiasis is endemic.

Filariasis

Filariasis affects more than 120 million people world wide along equitorial regions of Africa, Turkey, India, the East Indies, Southeast Asia, Philippines, Oceanic Islands, Haiti and parts of South America. It is caused predominantly by Wuchereria bancrofti and Brugia malayi. In addition to the well-known symptoms of elephantiasis filariasis may cause tropical pulmonary eosinophilia (TPE) and severe pulmonary hypertension in teenagers, particularly in girls. In persons susceptible to the development of TPE, the microfilariae released into the circulation from adult worms in the lymphatics are rapidly opsonized with antifilarial antibodies and these are then cleared in the pulmonary vasculature (55-57).

Symptoms of cough, wheezing and eosinophil counts in excess of 3,000 in a patient from an area where filariasis is endemic. Embolization by circulating microfilaria or the antigenic response this elicits or both are thought to be the cause. Decades later fibrosis occurs. The right sided pressures rise as the right atrial and pulmonary arterial pressures rise, the foramen ovale opens, leading to right to left shunting and central cyanosis. If this release mechanism does not operate, fatal right-sided cardiac failure develops. The radiological features are those expected of any form of pulmonary hypertension. Most filarial infections do not cause pulmonary hypertension at this young age.

Nutritional issues

Endemic cardiomyopathy (Keshan's disease)

In 1935, an outbreak of rapidly progressive and fatal cardiomyopathy was reported in Keshan and surrounding areas in the Heilongjiang province of China (58). Autopsy specimens from patients with Kashan's disease were found to be similar to white muscle disorder in seen sheep which was related to selenium deficiency (58, 59). Blood levels and diets low in selenium was correlated with low local selenium levels in the soil. Supplementation of diets with selenium in these regions virtually eliminated the disease from those areas. The mechanism of action of selenium is thought to be due to decreased production of glutathione peroxidases resulting in increased oxidative stress and damage to the heart leading to cardiomyopathy (60, 61).

Beriberi

Thiamine is present in many food sources including cereals, legumes, rice, yeast and meat, especially pork. It is absent in milk, fruits, white rice, and most vegetables. Processing foods rich in thiamine by cooking, baking or canning may destroy thiamine. Tannins in coffee and tea can react with thiamine, converting it to a form that is difficult for the body to take in. In some areas where thiamine deficiency is already prevalent consumption of large quantities of tea or coffee may precipitate symptoms of beriberi. Chronic furosemide therapy for congestive failure promotes renal wasting of thiamine and may further exacerbate the congestive heart failure due to any cause (62).

High-output, hyperkinetic heart failure with plethoric pulmonary vasculature from thiamine deficiency is no longer frequent in the majority of tropical areas although it is still prevalent in some regions in Africa. When it does occur it is usually associated with alcoholic malnutrition. Beriberi occurs in infants between one and four months of age who have protein-energy malnutrition, are receiving unsupplemented hyperalimentation fluid or boiled milk, or are breastfed by mothers who are themselves deficient in thiamine (63).

Most patients are symptomatic and the clinical features for the majority of patients deficient in thiamine who have symptoms may be subtle. More severe symptoms may include a fulminant high output cardiac failure with cardiomegaly, tachycardia, a loud piercing, aphonic or hoarse cry due to vocal cord paralysis, cyanosis, dyspnea, and vomiting (64, 65). A form of aseptic meningitis has also been described in which the affected infants exhibit vomiting, nystagmus, purposeless movements, and seizure, despite a "normal" cerebrospinal fluid. The cardiac symptoms and cardiomegally typically improve or resolve completely within hours of thiamine administration although neurologic symptoms ranging from moderate to severe intellectual disability, delays in language and motor development and chronic epilepsy may be permanent (60, 64).

Recommened replacement doses of thiamine for children are not clear. 10 to 25 mg IM or IV daily (if critically ill), or 10 to 50 mg orally every day for 2 weeks, then 5 to 10 mg orally daily for 1 month. If collapse occurs: 25 mg IV. Administer with caution.

Daily dietary suppliments for prevention of thiamine deficiency are as follows: infants 0-6 months, 0.2 mg; infants 7-12 months, 0.3 mg; children 1-3 years, 0.5 mg; children 4-8 years, 0.6 mg; children 9-13 years, 0.9 mg; men 14 years and older, 1.2 mg; women 14-18 years, 1 mg; women over 18 years, 1.1 mg; pregnant women, 1.4 mg; and breast-feeding women, 1.5 mg (66).

SYNCOPE

Syncope is a common event in childhood in the tropics and nontropical areas alike, particularly in teens and pre-teens. Fortunately, the vast majority of these episodes have benign causes. Up to 75% are neurocardiogenic syncope mediated by hypotension or bradycardia, which are triggered by a variety of stimuli such as pain, emotion, surprise, cough, urination or defecation. Another 11% are orthostatic syncope from volume depletion, autonomic insufficiency or medications and drugs. The distinction between neurocardiogenic and orthostatic related syncope is not always clear. Regardless of the trigger or etiology, the patient is most frequently in an upright position when the event occurs and may have a variable period of prodrome.

In rare cases, syncope may be the presenting symptom of seizure or cardiac arrhythmias. These episodes raise concerns that they are predecessors to future sudden cardiac death. In children, cardiac causes are rare but important because of the potential for future morbidity or mortality. The physician's task is to differentiate the benign forms of syncope from those that are associated with an increased risk of sudden cardiac death.

The history and physical examination are sufficient to define the cause of syncope in up to 77% of pediatric cases. A complete description of the events before, during and after the event is essential in making the diagnosis. This should include a detailed timing of the event including any prodromal sensations such as dizziness. A dietary history including what was consumed the day of the event (particularly fluids) as well as gastrointestinal and urinary losses and excessive sweating may be revealing for a relatively hypovolemic state.

The history should include evidence of infections including those contributing to anemia such as hook worm and malaria, cardiac, neurologic, endocrine and psychiatric diseases, eating disorders, drug and alcohol abuse. Interview witnesses if they are available. Exercise related syncope should be considered to be distinctly abnormal, although syncope occurring after the cessation of exercise can be common.

The physical exam is often normal, but should include a search for findings suggestive of Marfan syndrome, orthostatic blood pressure changes and an abnormal neurological exam. A careful dynamic cardiovascular examination with the patient in different positions will help identify abnormalities including murmurs, which may not be present in one position. A systolic ejection murmur that increases when rising from supine or squatting position suggests hypertrophic cardiomyopathy.

The harsh high-pitched systolic murmur radiating to the carotids with a diminished carotid upstroke suggests aortic stenosis. Evaluate the rhythm carefully. A right ventricular heave, loud P2 or narrowly or paradoxically split S2 indicates pulmonary hypertension. A mid-systolic click with or without a systolic murmur suggests mitral valve prolapse, although its relationship to syncope is questionable.

An EKG is useful in identifying several conditions including Wolff-Parkinson-White syndrome, long QT syndrome, Brugada syndrome, arrhythmogenic right ventricular dysplasia, ischemia, myocarditis, heart block and ectopy but is not sufficiently sensitive to rule these conditions out completely.

A normal diagnostic screen (reassuring history, benign physical examination and normal EKG) is generally sufficient to exclude the possibility of cardiac disease without further workup. Tables 7-10 below outline salient history and physical examination points regarding syncope.

Echocardiography is not recommended in the routine evaluation of syncope unless the history is atypical or physical exam suggests a structural lesion. In a study of 322 children and adolescents who underwent screening echocardiography for syncope, only two had findings that were related to the syncope. Both had cardiomyopathies and both had markedly abnormal ECGs.

If the history is suggestive of an arrhythmia as in the case of perceived palpitations or exercise related syncope, a monitor if available such as a Holter monitor or event monitor may help identify the etiology. Because the Holter monitor records continuously for a few days, symptoms which occur less frequently than several times a day may be missed on the recording. Event monitors may be necessary for a longer period and are more practical for infrequent symptoms. However, event monitors are useful only when the patient is having perceptible symptoms.

Table 7. Causes of syncope

Noncardiac	Cardiac - Structural	Cardiac - Arrhythmia
Vasodepressor – simple faint	Obstruction	Long QT syndrome
Excess vagal tone	Hypertropic obstructive cardiomyopathy	SVT
Reflex-	Aortic stenosis	Wolff-Parkinson-White Syndrome
Breath holding	Atrial myxoma	Brugada syndrome
Cough	Pulmonary Hypertension	Ventricular tachycardia
Swallow	Cyanotic heart disease	Third degree heart block
Carotid sinus stimulation	Tamponade	Arrhythmogenic right ventricular dysplasia
Orthostatic hypotension	Myocardial dysfunction	Ebstein's anomaly
Hypovolemia	Myocarditis	Atrial tachycardia
Drugs	Cardiomyopathy	Drug induced
Autonomic insufficiency	Anomalous origin of the coronary arteries	
Seizure		
Hyperventilation		
Migraine		
Metabolic		
Hysterical		

Table 8. Syncope history

- Triggering factors - pain, fear, surprise, anger, loud noise, cough, urinating, hyperventilating, exercise, hypodermic needles
- Atmosphere - hot, crowded
- Position - stable, changing, lying, standing sitting
- Activity – crying, urinating, defecating, tantrum, breath holding,
- Set up - hungry, ill, hot, dehydrated, exercise or exertion, prolonged standing, anxiety
- Warning symptoms – nausea, vomiting, diarrhea, fever, lightheadedness, diaphoresis, visual changes, warmth, aura, headaches, palpitations, dizziness, perioral paresthesias or no warning at all
- Event – duration, motor activity, eye deviation, color changes, incontinence, tongue biting,
- Recovery - confusion, headache, fatigue, weakness, nausea, diaphoresis, neurologic signs
- Medical history – syncope, headache, seizures, trauma, diabetes, heart disease
- Drugs and toxins – prescription, nonprescription, illicit drugs, alcohol, carbon monoxide
- Family History – sudden death, heart disease, dyslipidemia, diabetes, seizures, syncope

Table 9. Syncope warning symptoms, refer for further work-up

• Recurrent syncope
• Seizure activity
• Syncope during exercise
• Syncope while in supine position
• Syncope in sitting position
• Family history of sudden death in person younger than 30
• Family history of conditions associated with sudden death
• Personal history of cardiac disease
• Precipitated by loud noise or fright

*Nonsustained palpitations are frequent with neurocardiogenic syncope.

Table 10. Evaluation of syncope

Initial Evaluation	Secondary Studies
• History	• U/A
• Physical examination	• Electrolytes
• Blood glucose	• Mg, Ca, Phos
• Pulse oxymetry	• Drug tox screen
• Orthostatic vital signs	• Carboxyhemoglobin
• 12 lead EKG	• ABG
• Rhythm monitor	• EEG
• Hemoglobin	• Chest Cray
• Pregnancy tests	• BUN, Creat
	• Echocardiogram
	• Tilt table
	• Stress test
	• Coronary angiography

History should dictate laboratory testing which may include electrolytes, magnesium, calcium, phosphate, CBC, glucose, pregnancy test. However, the real need for laboratory tests is low, as is the yield.

Treatment of syncope depends upon the etiology. Since the vast majority of childhood syncope is either neurocardiogenic or orthostatic, there are several underlying treatment principles which should be helpful in relieving symptoms in the vast majority of patients. The patient must understand that most syncopal episodes occur because of diminished cerebral perfusion.

Therefore, sitting and assuming a head down position quickly is the first suggestion. Regardless of the cause, syncopal patients are usually very sensitive to fluid balance and vigorous fluid intake, particularly in the morning, should be advised. Increased sodium intake with sport drinks may also be helpful. If these simple steps fail to alleviate the problem, then referral to a cardiologist may be helpful for further testing or therapy. In children with typical childhood syncope in an upright position, referral to neurology is unnecessary.

CHEST PAIN

Chest pain is a common pediatric symptom, particularly in the adolescent age group. It can also occur in younger school-aged children. Chest pain in children is very rarely due to cardiac causes. Typical childhood chest pain is brief, sharp, mid-sternal and primarily non-exertional. Most childhood chest pain is due to a benign muscular or skeletal cause. It may not be entirely correct to label it as "costochondritis," since much of the pain does not produce reproducible tenderness at the time of physical exam. However, the majority of the pain may be exacerbated by movement, breathing or pressure, when the pain is occurring, leading to the conclusion of a chest wall pain, unrelated to cardiac issues although not necessarily benign.

Pain which is typical for chest wall origin as outlined above does not require advanced testing or cardiology referral. Exertional pain, unrelenting pain or unusual radiation may be an indication for further evaluation. Chest pain is very unusual as a presenting symptom for structural heart disease or cardiomyopathy. Chest pain due to pericarditis is typically worse in a supine position and relieved with sitting forward. A friction rub may be heard. Large effusions from TB pericarditis may be painless since there is little contact between the heart and the pericardium.

SBE PROPHYLAXIS

The guidelines regarding antibiotic prophylaxis were updated in 2007. This updated guideline removed the recommendation for routine endocarditis prophylaxis for a wide variety of relatively simple and common heart defects including simple shunts and simple valvular obstructions (69). High Risk patients who should receive prophylaxis (see Table 11 for medication schedules):

- Prosthetic heart valves including bioprosthetic and homograft valves
- A prior history of infective endocarditis
- Unrepaired cyanotic congenital heart disease including palliative shunts and conduits
- Completely repaired congenital heart disease with prosthetic material or device, whether placed by surgery or catheter intervention during the first six months after the procedure
- Repaired congenital heart disease with residual defects at the site or adjacent to the site of the prosthetic device.
- Cardiac valvulopathy in a transplanted heart

High-risk procedures for which high-risk patients should receive prophylaxis

- Dental procedures that involve manipulation of either gingival tissue or the periapical region of teeth or perforation of the oral mucosa
- Procedures of the respiratory tract which involve incision or biopsy of the respiratory mucosa
- Procedures in patients with ongoing GI or GU tract infections
- Procedures on infected skin, skin structures or musculoskeletal tissue
- Surgery to place prosthetic heart valves or prosthetic intravascular or intracardiac materials

Table 11. Endocarditis antibiotic choice

Procedure	Antibiotic prophylaxis given 30-60 minutes prior to the procedure.
Dental	Amoxicillin 50 mg/kg (Max 2 gm) Ampicillin 2 gm IM or IV Altenatives: Azithromycin or Clarithromycin 15 mg/kg (Max 500mg) Clindemycin 20mg/kg (Max 600mg) PO or 600mg IV Cephalexin 50mg/kg (Max 2gm) Cefazolin or Ceftriaxone 1 gm IV or 600mg IV
Genitourinary or Gastrointestinal	Amoxicillin 50 mg/kg (Max 2 gm) Ampicillin 2 gm IM or IV Vancomycin IV
Skin Or Musculoskeletal	Amoxicillin 50 mg/kg (Max 2 gm) Ampicillin 2 gm IM or IV Clindemycin 20 mg/kg PO or IV (Max 600mg) Vancomycin – 15 mg/kg IV (Max 1 g)

GENERAL PEDIATRIC CARE OF CHILDREN WITH COMPLEX HEART DISEASE

In children who have undergone surgical correction of cardiac disease, the general pediatric care does not differ significantly from normal children. The majority of pediatric cardiac operations will restore normal four-chamber cardiac anatomy and relieve symptoms. Most corrective operations are performed in the first few months of life. Children with very complex single ventricle physiology will undergo a series of operations in the first two years of life and will be at increased risk for morbidity and mortality from growth and nutritional issues, infection risk and sudden death.

NUTRITIONAL ISSUES

In children with congenital heart diseases, nutritional support in all age groups is of great importance. This is especially true in all stages of HF, which increase metabolic demand. Symptoms of HF include anorexia, nausea and vomiting resulting in growth failure. Metabolic demand increases from increased cardiac work to meet volume and pressure demands and respiratory work from tachypnea and dyspnea. Gastrointestinal symptoms are a result of bowel wall edema, decreased absorption, altered motility, reduced gastric capacity from hepatomegaly and anorexia from proinflamatory cytokines.

As a result, malnutrition is common among young children with congenital heart disease and most of the malnutrition can be accounted for by decreased calorie intake. Proper nutrition is critical in order for other surgical and medical therapies for cardiac diseases to be successful. Nutritional causes of anemia such as iron deficiency should be avoided to reduce unnecessary work on the heart. The optimal caloric intake is approximately 110-125% of the estimated energy requirement (EER) for their age, height and weight.

For infants this amounts to 140-150 kcal/kg/d. This is achievable in infants using high-density formulas or adding polycose or rice cereal to the formula. If adequate calories cannot be ingested orally and severe growth failure (BMI< 5% or weight/height < 5%) has occurred, then the nutritional support plan should include consideration of nasogastric feedings as a temporary enhancement until surgical correction can take place (70). Rarely, prolonged nutritional support is required which may make a semi-permanent gastrostomy tube a preferred option.

Physical activity in congenital heart disease: In general, aerobic exercise is beneficial for all but a small minority of patients with congenital heart diseases. Most patients with repaired congenital heart disease without significant anatomic or functional abnormalities can participate in unrestricted physical activity.

INFECTIOUS DISEASES IN PATIENTS WITH COMPLEX CARDIAC DISORDERS

Primary basic precautions such as prevention from smoke exposure and exposure to infection such as respiratory syncitial virus (RSV) during the winter season are most important.

Palivizumab (murine monoclonal RSV antibody) is indicated for children less than two years of age at the start of the RSV season with hemodynamically significant congenital heart disease (CHD) including those receiving medication for congestive heart failure, those with moderate to severe pulmonary artery hypertension, and those with unrepaired cyanotic heart disease. It is very expensive and may not be available for the majority of children with congenital heart diseases in tropical countries.

Patients with hemodynamically insignificant heart disease (secundum ASD, small VSD, pulmonary stenosis, uncomplicated aortic stenosis, mild coarctation of the aorta and PDA) should not receive prophylaxis. Treatment with Palivizumab is given IM once monthly during RSV season. RSV-IGIV (human polyclonal RSV antibody) is beneficial in premature infants and children with chronic lung disease but is not indicated in children with congenital heart disease.

Immunizations

Children with congenital heart disease should receive all routine vaccinations. Patients who have undergone heart transplantation cannot receive live virus vaccines such as MMR and Varicella but should receive all other routine childhood vaccines. In addition to the patient, family members should have full immunization. The immunization schedule may need to be temporarily altered to accommodate surgical repair. It is not advisable for practical purposes (development of low grade fever) to administer routine immunizations within two weeks of a scheduled cardiac operation.

Influenza

Patients with unrepaired congenital heart disease should have annual influenza immunization as generally recommended. After repair, the risk should be no different than the general population assuming normal cardiac function and four chamber anatomy. Single ventricle physiology or persistent heart failure may warrant regular influenza vaccination.

CONCLUSION

Cardiac problems are common in children of all lands including those in tropical areas. A careful evaluation is necessary to make the proper diagnosis and management should be according to accepted guidelines. Attention to nutrition and immunizations are important. The primary care clinicians can be of significant help to pediatric patients with cardiac conditions.

REFERENCES

[1] Pelech AN. The cardiac murmur – when to refer? Pediatric Clin North Am 1998;45:107-22.
[2] Tabatznik B, Randall TW, Hersch C. The mammary souffl? of pregnancy and lactation. Circulation 1960;22:1069-73.
[3] van der Linde D, Konings EE, Slager MA, Witsenburg M, Helbing WA. Birth prevalence of congenital heart disease worldwide: a systematic review and meta-analysis. J Am Coll Cardiol 2011;58:2241-7.
[4] Jonas RA. Congenital heart surgery in developing countries. Semin Thorac Cardiovasc Surg Pediatr Card Surg Annu 2008:3-6. doi: 10.1053/j.pcsu.2007.12.001.
[5] Saxena A. Congenital cardiac surgery in the less privileged regions of the world. Expert Rev Cardiovasc Ther 2009;7:1621-9.
[6] Trucco SM, Barnova J, Larraabal LA, Cantaneda A, Teitel DF. Detection rates of congenital heart disease in Guatemala. Cardiol Young 2011;21(2):153-60.
[7] Palacios-Macedo A. Birth of a new program in Mexico City: The Kardias experience. Semin Thorac Cardioavasc Surg Pediatr Card Surg Ann 2008;11:7-10.
[8] Cohen AJ, Tamir A, Houri S, Abegaz B, Gilad E, Omohkdion S, et al. Save a child's heart: we can and we should." Ann Thorac Surg 2001;71(2):462-468.
[9] Liu J. Challenges and progress of the pediatric cardiac surgery in Shanghai children's medical center. Semin Thorac Cardioavasc Surg Pediatr Card Surg Ann 2009;12:12-18.
[10] Kumar R. Letter to editor: "Congenital heart disease management in developing countries. Pediatr Cardiol 2003;24:311.
[11] Zühlke L, Mirabel M, Marjon E. Congenital heart disease and rheumatic heart disease in Africa: recent advances and current priorities. Heart 2013;99 (21):1554-61.
[12] Senga J, Rusingiza E, Mucumbitsi J, Binaqwaho A, Suys B, Lys C, et al. Catheter interventions in congenital heart disease without regular catheterization laboratory equipment: the chain of hope experience in Rwanda Pediatr Cardiol 2013;34(1):39-45.
[13] Pezzella, AT. Global Aspects of Cardiothoracic Surgery with Focus on Developing Countries. Asian CardiovascThor Ann 2010;18:299-310.
[14] Mocumbi AO, Lameira E, Yaksh A, Paul L, Ferreira MB, Sidi D. Challenges on the management of congenital heart disease in developing countries. Int J Cardiol 2011;148 (3):285-8.
[15] Saxena A. Strategies for the improvement of cardiac care services in developing countries: what does the future hold? Future Cardiol 2012;8(1):29-38.
[16] Giamberti A, Mele M, Di Terlizzzi M, Abella R, Carminata M, Cirri S, et al. Association of children with heart disease in the world: 10-Year experience. Pediatr Cardiol 2004;25(5):492-4.
[17] Madazli R, Sal V, Cift T, Guralp O, Goymen A. Pregnancy outcomes in women with heart disease. Arch Gynecol Obstet 2010;281(1):29-34.
[18] Beggs S, Thompson A, Nash R, Tompson A, Peterson G, 17th expert committee on the selection and use of essential medicines: cardiac failure in children. Geneva, March 2009.

[19] Margossian R. Contemporary management of pediatric heart failure. Expert Rev Cardiovasc Ther 2008;6:187-96.
[20] Hsu DT, Zak L, Mahony L, Sleeper LA, Atz AM, Levine JC, et al. Enalapril in infants with single ventricle: results of a multicenter randomized trial. Circulation 2010;122(4):333-40.
[21] Shaddy RE, Boucek MM, Hsu DT, Boucek RJ, Canter CE, Mahony L, et al. Carvedilol for children and adolescents with heart failure: a randomized controlled trial. JAMA 2007;298(10):1171-9.
[22] Mocumbi AO, Falase AO. Recent advances in the epidemiology, diagnosis and treatment of endomyocardial fibrosis in Africa. Heart 2013;99(20):1481-7.
[23] Cilliers AM, Adams PE, Mocumbi AO. Early presentation of endomyocardial fibrosis in a 22-month-old child: a case report Cardiol Young 2011;21:101–3.
[24] Jatene MB, Contreras IS, Lameda L. Endomyocardial fibrosis in Infancy. Arq Bras Cardiol 2003;80:442–5.
[25] Mocumbi AO, Ferreira MB, Sidi D. A population study of endomyocardial fibrosis in a rural area of Mozambique. N Engl J Med 2008;359:43.
[26] Akinwusi PO, Odeyemi AO. The changing pattern of endomyocardial fibrosis in South-West Nigeria. Clin Med Insights Cardiol 2012;6:163– 8.
[27] Mocumbi AO, Carrilho C, Sarathchandra P, Ferreira MB, Yacoub M, Burke M. Echocardiography accurately assesses the pathological abnormalities of chronic endomyocardial fibrosis. Int J Cardiovasc Imaging 2011;27(7):955–64.
[28] Leon D, Martin M, Corros C, Santamarta E, Costilla S, Lambert JL. Usefulness of cardiac MRI in early diagnosis of endomyocardial fibrosis. Rev Port Cardiol 2012;31(5):401–2.
[29] Estornell J, Lopez MP, Dicenta F, Iqual B, Martonez V, Sonileva A. Usefulness of magnetic resonance imaging in the assessment of endomyocardial disease. Rev Esp Cardiol 2003;56(3):321–4.
[30] Mocumbi AO, Falase AO. Recent advances in the epidemiology, diagnosis and treatment of endomyocardial fibrosis in Africa. Heart 2013;99(20):1481-7.
[31] Seckeler MD, Hoke TR. The worldwide epidemiology of acute rheumatic fever and rheumatic heart disease Clin Epidemiol 2011;3:67– 84.
[32] Bryant PA, Robins-Browne R, Carpetis JR, Curtis N. Some of the people, some of the time: susceptibility to acute rheumatic fever. Circulation 2009;119(5):742-53.
[33] Zuhlke L, Mirabel M, Jarijon E. Congenital heart disease and rheumatic heart disease in Africa: recent advances and current priorities. Heart 2013;99(21):1554-61.
[34] Nkomo VT. Epidemiology and prevention of valvular heart diseases and infective endocarditis in Africa. Heart 2007;93:1510-9.
[35] Carapetis JR, Steer AC, Mulholland EK, Weber M. The global burden of group A streptococcal disease. Lancet Infect Dis 2005;5(11):685-94.
[36] Diller GP, Uebing A. Predicting the risks of pregnancy in congenital heart disease: the importance of external validation. Heart 2014;100(17):1311-2.
[37] Marijon E, Ou P, Celermajer DS, Ferreira B, Mocumbi AO, Jani D, et al. Prevalence of rheumatic heart disease detected by echocardiographic screening. N Engl J Med 2007;357(5):470-6.
[38] Carapetis JR, Hardy M, Fakakovikaetau t, Taib R, Wilkinson L, Penny DJ, et al. Evaluation of a screening protocol using auscultation and portable echocardiography to detect asymptomatic rheumatic heart disease in Tongan schoolchildren Nat Clin Pract Cardiol Med 2008;5(7):411-7.
[39] Irlam J, Mayosi BM, Engel M Gaziano TA. Primary prevention of acute rheumatic fever and rheumatic heart disease with penicillin in South African children with pharyngitis: a cost-effectiveness analysis. Circ Cardiovasc Qual Outcomes 2013;6(3):343-51.
[40] Marijon E, Mirabel M, Celermajer DS, Jouven X. Rheumatic heart disease. Lancet 2012;379(9819):953-64.
[41] Gerber MA, Baltimore RS, Eaton CB, Gewitz M, Rowley AH, Shulman ST, et al. Prevention of rheumatic fever and diagnosis and treatment of acute Streptococcal pharyngitis: a scientific statement from the American Heart Association Rheumatic Fever, Endocarditis, and Kawasaki Disease Committee of the Council on Cardiovascular Disease in the Young, the Interdisciplinary Council on Functional Genomics and Translational Biology, and the Interdisciplinary Council on Quality of Care

and Outcomes Research: endorsed by the American Academy of Pediatrics. Circulation 2009;119(11):1541-51.
[42] Karthikeyan G, Mayosi BM. Is primary prevention of rheumatic fever the missing link in the control of rheumatic heart disease in Africa? Circulation 2009;120:709-13.
[43] Thakur JS. Integrated community-based screening for cardiovascular diseases of childhood. World Health Forum 1997;18:24-27.
[44] Saxena A. Strategies for the improvement of cardiac care services in developing countries: what does the future hold? Future Cardiology 2012;8:29-38.
[45] McDonald M, Brown A, Noonan S, Carpetis JR. Preventing recurrent rheumatic fever: the role of register based programmes Heart 2005;91(9):1131-3.
[46] Nanna M, Stergiopoulos K. Pregnancy complicated by valvular heart disease: an update. J Am Heart Assoc 2014;3(3):e000712.
[47] Uehara R, Belay ED. Epidemiology of Kawasaki disease in Asia, Europe, and the United States. J Epidemiol 2012;222:79-85.
[48] Rowley AH. Kawasaki disease: novel insights into etiology and genetic susceptibility. Annu Rev Med 2011;62:69-77.
[49] Jamieson N, Singh-Grewal D. Kawasaki disease: a clinician's update. Int J Pediatr 2013;2013:645391.
[50] Kawasaki T, Naoe S. History of Kawasaki disease. Clin Exp Nephrol 2014;18:301-4.
[51] Signh S, Kawasaki T. Kawasaki disease. An Indian perspective. Indian Pediatrics 2009;46:563-571.
[52] Newberger JW, Takahashi M, Gerber MA, Gewitz MH, Tani LY, Burns JC, et al. American Academy of Pediatrics. Diagnosis, treatment and long-term management of Kawasaki disease: A statement for health professionals from the committee on rheumatic fever, endocarditis, and Kawasaki disease, Council on Cardiovascular Disease in the Young, American Heart Association. Circulation 2004;110(17):2747-71.
[53] Fernandes CJ, Jardim CV, Hovnanian A, Hoette S, Morinaga LK, Souza R. Schistosomiasis and pulmonary hypertension. Expert Rev Respir Medicine 2011;5(5):675-81.
[54] Bouree P, Piveteau J, Gerbal, JL, Halpen G. Pulmonary arterial hypertension due to bilharziasis. apropos of a case due to schistosoma haematobium having been cured by praziquantel. Bull Soc Pathol Exot 1990;83(1):66-71.
[55] Ong RKC, Doyle RL. Tropical pulmonary eosinophilia. Chest 1998;113(6):1673-9.
[56] Teo SK. Tropical pulmonary eosinophilia. Singapore Med J 1991; 32:118-9.
[57] Mullerpattan JB, Udwadia ZF, Udwadia FE. Tropical pulmonary eosinophilia: A review. Indian J Med Res 2013;138(3):295-302.
[58] Yang GQ, Ge KY, Chen JS, Chen XS. Selenium-related endemic diseases and the daily selenium requirement of humans. World Rev Nutr Diet 1988;55:98-152.
[59] Yang GQ, Chen JS, Wen ZM, Ge KY, Zhu LZ, Chen XC et al. The role of selenium in Keshan disease. Adv Nutr Res 1984;6:203-31.
[60] Loscalzo J. Keshan disease, selenium deficiency, and the selenoproteome. N Engl J Med 2014;370;18:1756-60.
[61] Marinescu V, McCullough PA. Nutritional and micronutrient determinants of idiopathic dilated cardiomyopathy: diagnostic and therapeutic implications. Expert Rev Cardiovasc Ther 2011;9(9):1161-70.
[62] Seligmann H, Halkin H, Rauchfleisch S, Kaufmann N, Motro M, Vered Z, et al. Thiamine deficiency in patients with congestive heart failure receiving long-term furosemide therapy: a pilot study. Am J Med 1991;91(2):151-5.
[63] Seear M, Lockitch G, Jacobson B, Quigley G, MacNab A. Thiamine, riboflavin, and pyridoxine deficiencies in a population of critically ill children. J Pediatr 1992;121(4):533.
[64] Porter SG, Coats D, Fischer PR, Ou K, Frank EL, Sreang P, et al. Thiamine deficiency and cardiac dysfunction in Cambodian infants J Pediatr 2014;164(6):1456-61.
[65] Chaitiraphan S, Tanphaichitr V, Cheng TO. Nutritional heart disease. In: Cheng TO, ed. The international textbook of cardiology. New York: Pergamon Press, 1986:864.
[66] Fattal-Valevski A, Bloch-Mimouni A, Kivity S, Heyman E, Brezner A, Strausberg R, et al. Epilepsy in children with infantile thiamine deficiency. Neurology 2009;73(11):828.

[67] Yates AA, Schlicker SA, Suitor CW. Dietary reference intakes: The new basis for recommendations for calcium and related nutrients, B vitamins, and choline. J Am Diet Assoc 1998;98:699-706.

[68] Feinberg AN, Lane-Davies A. Syncope in the adolescent. State Art Rev Adolesc Med 2002;13(3):553-67.

[69] Wilson LL, Taubert KA, Gewitz M, Lockhart PB, Baddour LM, Levison M, et al. Prevention of infective endocarditis: guidelines from the American Heart Association, Rheumatic Fever, Endocarditis and Kawasaki Disease Committee, Council on Cardiovascular Disease in the Young, Council on Clinical Cardiology, Council on Cardiovascular Surgery and Anesthesia and the Quality of Care and Outcomes Research Interdisciplinary Working Group. Circulation 2007;116:1736-54.

[70] Miller TL, Neri D, Extein J, Somarriba G, Stickman-Stein N. Nutrition in pediatric cardiomyopathy. Prog Pediatr Cardiol 2007;24:59-71.

In: Chronic Disease and Disability
Editors: DE Greydanus, P Anne, JD Rowlett et al.

ISBN: 978-1-53617-656-8

Chapter 4

HYPERTENSION IN CHILDREN: CURRENT CONCEPTS

Vimal Master Sankar Raj*[1,*]*, MD
and Donald E Greydanus*[2]*, MD, DrHC(Athens)
[1]Department of Pediatric Nephrology, University of Illinois College of Medicine at Peoria, Peoria, Illinois, United States of America
[2]Department of Pediatric and Adolescent Medicine, Western Michigan University Homer Stryker M.D. School of Medicine,Kalamazoo, Michigan, United States of America

ABSTRACT

Hypertension in children and adolescents has significant short-term and long-term adverse effects leading to complications in adulthood. After confirming elevated blood pressure in children, a through work up is needed to rule out secondary causes of hypertension. The younger the child, the more likely is the probability of finding an etiology for the hypertension. Management should include lifestyle modifications that involves dealing with obesity if present. If these measures are unsuccessful, pharmacologic intervention is needed. Continued monitoring in the outpatient setting is essential to ensure adequate control of blood pressure in the pediatric patient. Monitoring (i.e., ABPM) and controlling elevated blood pressure are important roles of primary care clinicians caring for children, adolescents, and young adults.

INTRODUCTION

Pediatric hypertension is on the rise and constitutes a major health burden with morbidity and mortality extending into adulthood. It has been shown that hypertension in children predicts cardiovascular risk factors in adults such as atherosclerosis and metabolic syndrome (1-3). The National Health and Nutrition Examination Survey (NHANES) data revealed an increase in both systolic and diastolic blood pressure in United States (US) children over the past decades (4). This increase in blood pressure (BP) is more prevalent among non-Hispanic blacks and

[*] Corresponding Author's Email: vraj@uic.edu.

Mexican American children than white children (5). The estimated prevalence of pediatric hypertension is estimated at 2% to 5% from screening studies in children and adolescents (6).

Notably the increase in prevalence of pediatric hypertension has paralleled the increase in childhood obesity (7, 8). The prevalence of childhood obesity and overweight has almost increased three-fold in American children over the past 30 years. Current obesity estimates are at 20% in children aged 6 to 11 years of age (9). Obese adolescents were also found to have a three-fold greater chance of being hypertensive when compared to their non- obese peers (10). With its increasing prevalence and associated healthcare burden, it becomes of paramount importance for the clinician to properly recognize, evaluate, and treat pediatric hypertension (11, 12).

DEFINITION

Pediatric hypertension is defined as sustained elevation of BP either systolic or diastolic at or above the 95 percentile specific for the patient's age, sex, and height. The current normative data on BP in children and adolescents is based on "The fourth report on the diagnosis, evaluation and treatment of high blood pressure in children and adolescents" by the US National Heart, Lung and Blood Institute (13). In September of 2017, the American Academy of Pediatrics (AAP) published updated screening guidelines with new normative BP tables based on normal weight children from the Fourth Report excluding patients with overweight and obesity (14-18).

Table 1. Updated BP definition and stages in Pediatric population

	Age (1 to 13 years)	**≥ 13 years**
Normal BP	< 90th percentile	< 120/<80 mm Hg
Elevated BP	≥ 90th percentile to < 95th percentile or 120/80 to < 95th percentile (whichever is lower)	120 -129/< 80 mm Hg
Stage 1 Hypertension	≥ 95th percentile to < 95th percentile+ 12 mm Hg or 130/80 to 139/89 mm Hg (whichever is lower)	130 -139/80 -89 mm Hg
Stage 2 Hypertension	≥ 95th percentile + 12 mm Hg or ≥ 140/90 mm Hg (whichever is lower)	> 140/90 mm Hg

Table 2. Simplified BP screening parameters

Age in years	**Boys**		**Girls**	
	Systolic	**Diastolic**	**Systolic**	**Diastolic**
1	98	52	98	54
2	100	55	101	58
3	101	58	102	60
4	102	62	103	62
5	103	63	104	64
6	105	66	105	67
7	106	68	106	68
8	107	69	107	69
9	107	70	108	71
10	108	72	109	72
11	110	74	111	74
12	113	75	114	75
≥13	120	80	120	80

The decision to create a new screening table is to exclude bias as both overweight and obesity have shown strong association with elevated BP and hypertension. Excluding overweight patients has caused the normal BP values to be several millimeters lower than similar tables in the Fourth Report. Simplified tables are available that provides the new data to give screening BP parameters requiring further evaluation (see Tables 1 and 2). A height-specific table for blood pressure has also been developed internationally as well (19).

SCREENING FOR HYPERTENSION

The importance of accurate screening for hypertension in pediatric patients becomes if growing importance as one views current data on their health, such as end-organ damage with the development of increased stiffness of arteries, left ventricular hypertrophy, cognitive dysfunction and others (14, 20-22). All children older than 3 years of age and all adolescents should have their BP checked during each physician visit with minimum one measurement every year.

In addition, children with other comorbid conditions should have their BP measured even if they are younger than 3 years of age; these conditions include prematurity, low birth weight, prolonged neonatal intensive care stay, recurrent urinary tract infections, protein or blood in urine, family history of congenital kidney problems and those with any organ transplant (23, 24).

It is essential to use proper technique to identify and diagnose hypertension in children. The first step is to choose the correct cuff size for a specific child's bare arm. The inflatable bladder width on the BP cuff should cover at the least 40% of the child's mid-arm circumference and the bladder length should encircle 80% to 100% of the same (25). When in doubt a larger cuff should be used. The child should be sitting quietly for 5 minutes before BP measurement with his back as well as right arm supported and feet touching the floor. In infants and small children, a supine position can be used for BP measurement. BP should then be recorded in the right arm with the cubital fossa positioned at heart level using the appropriate-sized cuff.

Automated or oscillometric devices are preferable as screening tools especially in neonates and infants; also, in those with BP greater than the 90th percentile, the recordings must be rechecked using manual auscultatory methods using a clinical sphygmomanometer. Automated devices do not measure systolic and diastolic BP directly but rather estimate them on the point of maximal oscillation (mean intra-arterial pressure) as the cuff gets deflated. The algorithms for BP measurement in these automated devices vary with different manufacturers and hence are not uniform across devices.

Also, the normative data on the Fourth Report reference table were obtained by auscultation and hence, every BP elevation picked up by automated devices should be confirmed by manual auscultatory technique. Once BP is found to be elevated (greater than the 90th percentile or $\geq$120/80 mm Hg), an average of three measurements are need to be obtained and hypertension staged as per guidelines. Research continues on 21st century technology to collect and assess blood pressure data (26-28).

Ambulatory Blood Pressure Monitoring (ABPM) can be a very useful tool to monitor BP changes at home environment especially if there are concerns that BP elevation is related to the stress of clinic visits (i.e., white coat hypertension). For ABPM, patients are asked to wear a portable monitor that records blood pressure every 20 minutes over a 24-hour period. The recorded BP readings are downloaded using custom software; then, the mean day and night systolic BP (SBP) as well as diastolic BP (DBP) values are compared against gender and height specific normative ambulatory BP data.

Systolic BP load, defined as percentage of SBP readings exceeding the 95th percentile during the whole 24-hour period, is also calculated. Mean ambulatory SBP or DBP > 95th percentile with SBP load >25% will constitute ambulatory hypertension. The various definitions and stages of ambulatory BP levels in children are shown in Table 3 (29). ABPM is helpful not only for initial evaluation but could also be used to assess responsiveness to treatment.

Etiology

Hypertension can be classified into primary or essential hypertension with an unknown underlying cause or secondary hypertension. Although primary hypertension has been on the rise especially in adolescents, it is very important to investigate and rule out secondary causes of hypertension in children of all age groups. The likelihood of finding a secondary cause for hypertension is much higher in children less than 12 years of age with a reported incidence of 70% to 85% when compared to children 12 years and above where primary hypertension contributes to the majority of presentation (30).

The role of the intestinal microbiome in the development and/or maintenance of hypertension and many other disorders remains under active research in this part of the 21st century (31, 32). The increased risk of hypertension in those with a history of imbalanced maternal nutrition, intrauterine growth retardation (IUGR) and prematurity, consistent with the Barker hypothesis, remains under study (33, 34). The links between sedentary lifestyles and hypertension phenotypes remain under active study (35). Clinicians should be valiant regarding so-called *white-coat* hypertension and underlying causes of *masked* hypertension (36, 37). Links with dyslipidemia for screening and management must also be considered (38).

Primary hypertension

The true cause for primary hypertension is unknown but considered multifactorial. A family history of hypertension or obesity is often seen in children with essential hypertension indicating the interplay of multiple genetic and environmental factors (39, 40). A positive family history for first degree relatives with hypertension is almost present in 80% of all children with essential hypertension (41). The prevalence of primary hypertension is higher in children of Native American, Hispanic and African American race in contrast to Caucasian children (42-44)

Obesity is present in 35% to 50% of hypertensive adolescents and involves factors such as insulin resistance, hyperuricemia and increased sympathetic activity as the possible triggering mechanisms. Obesity is an independent risk factor for metabolic syndrome and strong predictor for cardiovascular events in adults with essential hypertension (45). Obstructive sleep apnea is associated with primary hypertension in obese children and should be evaluated as well as treated.

Secondary hypertension

The etiology for secondary hypertension varies with the age of the child and renal vascular or parenchymal causes account for almost 70% to 90% of all cases. In the neonatal intensive care unit (NICU), the most common cause is renal vascular related to umbilical artery catheterization (46, 47). From age 1 to 6 years renal parenchymal, renal vascular causes and coarctation of the aorta predominates. Between 6 and 10 years of age renal parenchymal disorders predominates; these include glomerulonephritis, obstructive uropathy and renal scarring (48, 49).

Other etiologies for secondary hypertension should be evaluated based on clues obtained from the history and physical examination; these include endocrine causes, iatrogenic-related causes, neurologically-induced causes or rarer forms of monogenic hypertension (see Table 4). Premature cardiovascular disease, including hypertension, is found in pediatric persons surviving chemotherapy and radiation treatment for cancer in childhood and adolescence (50).

A brief discussion is discussed below regarding some of the secondary etiologies for hypertension and their clinical features.

Table 4. Etiology for secondary hypertension based on organ systems

Kidney Parenchymal abnormalities – Dysplasia, Hypoplasia, Glomerulonephritis, Cystic kidney disease, renal scarring with pyelonephritis, solitary kidney, oligonephropathy Obstructive uropathy Reflux nephropathy Mutations affecting solute reabsorption in tubules – Liddle syndrome, Gordon Syndrome
Vascular Renovascular – Renal artery stenosis (main or branched artery) Coarctation of aorta Mid aortic syndrome Vasculitis
Central Increased intracranial pressure Seizures Dysautonomia Gullian barre syndrome Vasomotor abnormalities
Endocrine Hyper or hypothyroidism Congenital adrenal hyperplasia Cushing syndrome, pituitary tumors Pheochromocytoma Adrenal adenoma or carcinoma causing excess mineralocorticoid production Glucocorticoid remediable aldosteronism Syndrome of apparent mineralocorticoid excess
Miscellaneous Medications – NSAIDS, Erythropoietin, Oral contraceptives, Sympathomimetic drugs Cocaine, Amphetamines Food – caffeine, tyramine and licorice

Several medications used therapeutically can have an adverse effect of increasing blood pressure. Some of the most commonly used medications, such as non-steroidal anti-inflammatory drugs (NSAIDs), can inhibit prostaglandin production and cause adverse renal effects. NSAIDs can also increase systemic vascular resistance by altering arachidonic metabolism affecting blood pressure (51).

Medications used to treat attention-deficit/hyperactivity disorder (ADHD) have been shown to cause elevated BP; these include methylphenidate, amphetamine, and dextroamphetamine (52, 53). Increased blood pressure may be seen from taking sympathomimetics routinely used in over-the- counter decongestants containing phenylephrine and pseudoephedrine (54). Medications such as systemic steroids and oral contraceptives can also elevate BP. Illicit medications, such as cocaine, can cause severe acute increase in blood pressure leading to hypertensive emergencies (55).

Hypertension with Renal Parenchymal Abnormalities

Children with renal parenchymal disorders have concomitant features of renal involvement in addition to hypertension; these include blood or protein in urine, anemia secondary to erythropoietin deficiency, disorders of bone and mineral metabolism due to secondary hyperparathyroidism and easy fatigability. Rarely, hypertension could be the only first indication of an occult renal disease. (56). Renal scarring secondary to chronic pyelonephritis and reflux nephropathy is a major cause for elevated blood pressure in children. This is especially true if there is an underlying renal abnormality (such as dysplasia or hyperplasia) or if the renal insult occurred at a very young age in life (57).

Both acute and chronic glomerulonephritis can present with hypertension. Hypertension is a key component of nephritic syndrome including acute post streptococcal glomerulonephritis (APSGN), crescentic glomerulonephritis of any cause and focal segmental glomerulosclerosis (FSGS). Polycystic kidney disease, both recessive and dominant (ARPKD and ADPKD), can present with resistant hypertension (58, 59).

Chronic kidney disease of any etiology will usually have hypertension with declining glomerular filtration rate (stage 3 and above) secondary to impaired sodium excretion and volume overload (60). Proposed additional factors contributing to high blood pressure in chronic kidney disease (CDK) include an increase in renal sympathetic activity along with vasoconstrictors such as endothelin, thromboxane, angiotensin II and a decrease in vasodilators (such as nitric oxide and prostacyclin) (61).

Renal tumors, such as Wilms tumor, are associated with hypertension either due to mass effect of impinging on the renal blood flow or secondary to increased renin production (62, 63). Small tumors, such as reninomas, can result in resistant hypertension due to increased renin production (64, 65).

Renovascular Hypertension

Renovascular hypertension is one of the important etiologies in childhood hypertension and should be considered in the evaluation of all childhood hypertension (66-68). Decreased blood flow to one or both kidneys or even portion of a single kidney results in renovascular hypertension secondary to elevated renin production (69, 70).

Certain risk factors should increase the suspicion for hypertension secondary to renovascular etiology; these include prolonged neonatal stay with history of umbilical artery catheterization, predisposing factors such as neurofibromatosis type 1 (NF1), and history of systemic vasculitis (such as Kawasaki disease (71-73), Takayasu disease and Moyamoya syndrome) (74-78). Fibromuscular dysplasia is the most common form of renovascular disease in the pediatric age group (79-82). Also, NF1 has a propensity for intimal hyperplasia and is usually progressive.

The clinical presentation can vary from asymptomatic hypertension picked up on routine clinic visit to a life-threatening hypertensive crisis with end organ involvement. Flank or abdominal bruits may be heard on physical examination but these are not always present. Evaluation for renal artery stenosis (RAS), if suspected, can start with a duplex renal ultrasound; however, this is neither sensitive nor specific for detection of RAS. Intra-arterial angiography still remains the gold standard though less invasive technologies also becoming more available across various centers; these include magnetic resonance angiography and 3-dimensional computerized tomography (3D-CT) (83). Renal vein renin determination could also provide useful clues to the diagnosis based on available expertise to perform this procedure.

COARCTATION OF AORTA (COA)

CoA involves narrowing of a segment of aorta most commonly just distal to the origin of the left subclavian artery (84-88). Depending on the severity of narrowing, the presentation can be detected in the neonatal period or can remain asymptomatic for many years. In the less severe forms, patients might present with exercise intolerance, headaches, and shortness of breath, cold feet or leg pain after exercise.

Depending on the site of obstruction, BP gradient between upper extremities and/or between upper and lower extremities should increase the suspicion for CoA. Brachio-femoral pulse delay in infants and radio-femoral pulse delay in children will also be a good clinical sign to elicit, again depending on the site of narrowing. Certain syndromes have an increased association with CoA; these include Turner syndrome and Shone's Complex or Syndrome (series of left-sided obstructions/hypoplasia), William Beuren syndrome, and extremely rare in Williams syndrome (89-98).

Mid-aortic syndrome can be seen with extensive narrowing of the abdominal aorta often with narrowing of renal arteries, as well as celiac, superior and inferior mesenteric arteries; it is a rare but resistant hypertension condition that requires extensive surgical repair (99-101). Presentation can be asymptomatic with high blood pressures picked up on routine examination to severe abdominal pain, leg claudication, and other evidence of end organ damage. CT angiogram or MR angiogram are typically used to establish the diagnosis.

MONOGENIC HYPERTENSION

Measuring serum renin levels or plasma renin activity (PRA) could be a useful tool in identifying the rarer but well established etiology of monogenic hypertension. Renin levels are usually elevated in renovascular causes of hypertension but also in essential hypertension limiting its usefulness as a screening tool. Many children with renovascular hypertension can have totally normal renin levels as well. However, in children with monogenic hypertension, a condition which usually involves the adrenal gland or its response to an aberrant gene, low PRA or renin levels are usually seen. Monogenic hypertension should be considered in any young children especially if there is a strong family history of resistant and early onset hypertension coupled with urinary finding of sodium retention (102).

In monogenic forms of hypertension, the final pathway is that of increased sodium reabsorption leading to volume expansion and subsequent low renin activity. Three distinct mechanisms can all lead to this final common pathway:

1. Excessive aldosterone activity secondary to escape from normal regulatory mechanism (glucocorticoid remediable aldosteronism (GRA);
2. Abnormalities in enzymes that regulate adrenal steroid metabolism and
3. activity (congenital adrenal hyperplasia (CAH) and apparent mineralocorticoid excess (AME);
4. Mutations leading to hyperactivity of sodium and chloride transporters in the distal tubules (Liddle and Gordon syndrome)

GLUCOCORTICOID REMEDIABLE ALDOSTERONISM (GRA)

GRA, also known as familial hyperaldosteronism type 1, occurs secondary to unequal crossing between the gene for aldosterone synthase (CYP11B2) and the gene for corticosterone synthesis (CYP11B1) with both the genes closely neighbored on chromosome 8 (103-106). The hybrid gene ends up carrying the promoter part under control of adrenocorticotrophic hormone (ACTH) resulting in ACTH stimulated aldosterone production. This has an autosomal dominant pattern of inheritance and can present with severe infantile hypertension. Milder phenotypes exist as well where hypertension can be the presenting feature alone later in life. Use of glucocorticosteroids is used to normalize the blood pressure (104).

Children with GRA usually have hypokalemia as well as metabolic alkalosis and can present with muscle weakness. Plasma renin activity is suppressed and elevated aldosterone to renin ratio is an important clue to trigger suspicion of primary aldosteronism. GRA patients are at increased risk for cerebral aneurysm as well as intracranial bleeding and a screening MR is recommended at the beginning of puberty (107). Testing for chimeric gene is available and can help identify GRA (108).

CONGENITAL ADRENAL HYPERPLASIA (CAH)

Congenital adrenal hyperplasia (CAH) is a variety of conditions with disordered cortisol production due to different enzyme deficiencies that are part of the mechanism for adrenal steroid development (steroidogenesis) (109-111).

The most common variety of CAH with 21-hydroxylase deficiency results in hypotension due to its salt-losing state (112). However, in two other CAH subtypes – namely 11 β-hydroxylase deficiency (CAH type IV) and 17 α-hydroxylase deficiency (CAH type V) – there is overproduction of precursors with potent mineralocorticoid activity.

Typically, renin and aldosterone levels are both low in these patients and depending on the site of blockage, type IV has increased sex hormone with androgenic action while the reverse is true for type V. In type IV, virilization occurs in girls and precocious puberty occurs in boys; however, in type V, girls have delayed sexual development while boys have ambiguous genitalia (113).

SYNDROME OF APPARENT MINERALOCORTICOID EXCESS (AME)

This is an autosomal recessive disease resulting in inactivating mutation of 11 β-hydroxysteroid dehydrogenase (HSD) type 2 enzyme (114-117). 11 β-HSD type 2 plays an important role in inactivating cortisol and hence, it's binding to the mineralocorticoid receptor (MR). In the absence of inhibitory action, cortisol binds to MR receptor leading to severe arterial hypertension. Depending on the amount of enzyme defect, presentation can be in infancy with end organ damage or in later adulthood with a milder phenotype (118). Urinary steroid profiling shows an increased ratio of tetrahydrocortisol to tetrahydrocortisone while free cortisol/free cortisone is elevated in a 24-hour urine sample.

LIDDLE SYNDROME

Liddle syndrome is probably the most common type of monogenic hypertension. It is an autosomal dominant disorder that is characterized by an increased activity of epithelial sodium channels (ENaC) leading to sodium retention secondary to a gain of function mutation (119-123). The usual presentation is an early-onset hypertension with hypokalemia and metabolic alkalosis; plasma renin and aldosterone levels are markedly depressed.

GORDON SYNDROME

Though the genetic background of Gordon syndrome remains unclear, mutations in kinases WNK1 and WNK4 have been found in some cases (124). The mode of inheritance is autosomal dominant causing abnormal function of the thiazide-sensitive distal convoluted tubule. In contrast to other forms of monogenic hypertension, hyperkalemia, hyperchloremic metabolic acidosis and hypertension are the presenting feature (125-127). Plasma renin activity is suppressed but aldosterone levels may remain elevated as hyperkalemia can stimulate its secretion.

PHEOCHROMOCYTOMA

Pheochromocytomas are rare neuroendocrine tumors that secrete catecholamine arising from adrenal medullary chromaffin cells. Eighty to 85% of pheochromcytomas are adrenal in origin while the rest being extra-adrenal paraganglioma (128, 129). They are rare but potentially lethal cause for secondary hypertension with a prevalence between 0.1 to 0.5% (130). Pheochromocytoma can occur as part of hereditary genetic syndromes (such as neurofibromatosis, multiple endocrine neoplasia Type 2, von Hippel-Lindau) or can be sporadic spontaneous mutations. With up to a quarter of sporadic cases having known genetic mutations, it is recommended to do genetic screening especially if the incidence is at a younger age (131).

The classic presentation is that of paroxysmal episodes of palpitations, anxiety, diaphoresis, headaches with elevated blood pressure as the catecholamine secretion is episodic; episodes appear very much similar to a panic attack. Those with a hereditary mutation tend to present at younger age. In patients with predominant epinephrine or dopamine secretion, symptoms of orthostatic hypotension, such as presyncope, predominate.

Rare presentations can present that include epigastric pain mimicking acute abdomen, urological symptoms with episodic hematuria, syncope or blurred vision after voiding with urinary bladder paraganglioma (132). In addition to catecholamine secretion, atypical presentations include increased production of hormones such as ACTH causing Cushing's syndrome, vasoactive intestinal polypeptide (VIP) causing diarrhea, and parathyroid hormone-related peptide (PTHrP) causing hypercalcemia (133-135).

GENETIC SYNDROMES ASSOCIATED WITH PHEOCHROMOCYTOMA

Both types of multiple endocrine neoplasia (MEN type 1 and type 2) have an autosomal dominant pattern of inheritance with variable penetration (136). MEN type 1 is caused by a mutation in the tumor suppressor gene MEN1; it is characterized by pituitary tumors, pancreatic islet tumor, and primary hyperparathyroidism. MEN type 2 occurs secondary to mutation in the RET protooncogene with a very high incidence of medullary thyroid carcinoma. Pheochromocytoma occurs much more predominantly in MEN type 2 over type 1 with incidence as high as 50% (137-139).

Neurofibromatosis type 1 (NF1)

NF1 is caused by inactivating mutation of the NF1 tumor suppressor gene which encodes for neurofibromin. NF1 is characterized by multiple neurofibromas, café-au-lait spots, Lisch nodules in the iris, and axillary as well as inguinal freckling (140-143). Two percent of patients with NF1 develop pheochromocytoma (144). Hypertension is common in patients with NF1 (145).

von Hippel –Lindau disease (VHL)

VHL occurs secondary to mutation in the VHL tumor suppressor genes and presents with a variety of benign and malignant neoplasms; these include retinal angiomas, pancreatic neuroendocrine tumors, endolymphatic sac tumors of middle ear and clear cell renal carcinoma (146-152).

Succinate dehydrogenase (SDH) mutations

SDH are a group of enzymes involved in oxidative phosphorylation and electron transport chain. Mutations in SDH and its subunit genes (SDHA, SDHB, SDHC, SDHD and SDHAF2) can result in various familial paraganglioma syndromes (153-159). The inheritance is autosomal dominant with worse penetrance if the mutation is of maternal origin (maternal imprinting). Plasma fractionated metanephrine has a better sensitivity and comparable specificity to urine metanephrine but levels can be affected by medication (i.e., β blockers, levodopa, sympathomimetic, tricyclic antidepressants) and physical as well as emotional stress of the patient.

Due to the high sensitivity of this test, a normal metanephrine level can make the diagnosis of pheochromocytoma very unlikely. Twenty-four hour urinary measurements can also be done for metabolites of catecholamine and catecholamine itself. Once a biochemical diagnosis is established, imaging studies may be used to identify the exact anatomic location of the tumor; these studies include computerized tomography (CT), magnetic resonance imaging (MRI) or radiolabeled studies such as metaiodobenzylguanidine (MIBG scan).

Laboratory and Imaging Evaluation

Evaluation of hypertension should include a thorough history and physical examination looking for secondary causes of hypertension and conditions associated with hypertension (160). Initial evaluation in all children with hypertension must include a urinalysis (looking for proteinuria, hematuria), serum electrolytes, complete blood count, renal function studies and a renal as well as bladder ultrasound (161).

A duplex renal ultrasound, though not sensitive or specific, is a noninvasive testing modality for renal arterial stenosis. Echocardiography is a useful screening tool to detect congenital anomalies of the heart such as coarctation of aorta that can present with elevated blood pressure. In addition, it can also assess end organ damage such as left ventricular hypertrophy that can give clues on the chronicity of hypertension.

Serum renin and aldosterone levels can give important clues to genetic forms of hypertension (161). Fasting lipid profile and glucose levels are indicated especially in obese children to assess for metabolic syndrome and other comorbidities, including nephrotic syndrome (162). Specific testing for secondary forms of hypertension are based on the index of clinical suspicion.

TREATMENT

Initial approach for children and adolescents with mild hypertension who are asymptomatic (prehypertension or stage 1) would be to incorporate therapeutic lifestyle changes that include focus on dietary modifications, physical activity, reduction in screen time, and emphasis on weight loss if needed. DASH (Dietary Approach to Stop Hypertension) emphasizes the importance of a low fat diet with increased intake of vegetables and fruits in addition to reduced intake of sodium (1 to 1.5 g/day for children), high saturated fat and refined sugars (163).

Table 5. Preferred antihypertensive agents based on specific medical condition

Medical condition	Preferred	Avoid
Kidney disease/proteinuria	ACE inhibitors, Angiotensin receptor blockers (can reduce proteinuria and offer renoprotection)	
Bilateral renal artery stenosis		ACE inhibitors, ARB can precipitously drop glomerular filtration rate (GFR)
Asthma/chronic lung disease		β blockers (causes bronchospasm)
Coarctation of aorta	B blockers preferred	
Migraine	β blockers and calcium channel blockers (might provide symptomatic relief for migraines)	
Diabetes	ACE inhibitors, Angiotensin receptor blockers (can reduce proteinuria and offer renoprotection)	B blockers (can mask hypoglycemia, abnormal lipid profile) Diuretics (can worsen insulin resistance and dyslipidemia)
Sexually active females		ACE inhibitors (teratogenic, recommend birth control if need to be used)
Hypercalciuria, kidney stones	Use thiazide diuretic which can also lower calcium excretion in urine	Avoid furosemide which can worsen hypercalciuria
GRA	Glucocorticoids to suppress ACTH production	
AME	Mineralocorticoid antagonist such as spironolactone or eplerenone. Epithelial sodium channel (ENaC) blockers such as amiloride or triamtrene	
Liddle syndrome	Epithelial sodium channel (ENaC) blockers such as amiloride or triamtrene	
Gordon's syndrome	Low dose Thiazide diuretic	
Pheochromocytoma	Irreversible nonspecific α- blocker such as phenoxybenzamine first. Once adequate α blocking is established a β blocker such as propronalol	Do not start β blockers first due to uncontrolled α adrenergic activation. Avoid αβ blockers such as labetalol for preferentially more action on the β blockers

Increased physical activity (minimum 30 to 60 minutes per day) and other behavioral measures are recommended, especially in children who are overweight or obese with or without hypertension (14, 164-167). Sedentary screen time should be limited to less than 2 hours a day (this varies by age). Continued research on obesity genetics and the interplay of cardiovascular health will allow improved management and prognosis in both areas (168). Community-wide quality improvement (QI) efforts can also improve hypertension in pediatric patients as well (169).

Pharmacologic intervention is indicated in patients in whom conservative management is not successful as well as those with stage 2 hypertension, symptomatic hypertension, diabetes, target organ damage, and secondary forms of hypertension (170-173). The choice of initial medication is largely based on physician preference though certain medical conditions warrant a specific antihypertensive class.

For instance, it would be wise to avoid β blockers in asthmatics since they can cause bronchospasm. In athletes, β blockers and diuretics can negatively impact their athletic performance. ACE inhibitors are a preferred medication in children with diabetes, and those with kidney disease as well as proteinuria for its renal protective effect. For patients with secondary hypertension, a specific medication class can be more effective than others depending on the underlying mechanism of hypertension (see Table 5).

The initial approach is based on the Fourth Report in children and adolescents with uncomplicated hypertension and includes starting low dose of a single medication (monotherapy) along with continued lifestyle modifications (13, 14). The medication dose should be gradually increased to maximal dosage until target blood pressures (less than 95th percentile for height, age and gender) are achieved, while closely monitoring for possible side effects. If the target BP is not achieved, a second drug from a different class should be started at a low dose and titrated up (174).

If blood pressure control requires more than two medications, a referral should be made to an expert on hypertension. In patients with underlying chronic kidney disease, a much tighter control of BP is recommended–under the 50th percentile for height, age, and gender (175, 176). The different classes of antihypertensive medications, dose recommendations, and possible adverse effects are presented in Table 6.

Patients with symptomatic hypertension or those in hypertensive urgency/emergency need inpatient hospital admission to lower their blood pressure in a controlled setting, usually utilizing intravenous infusions. Some of the commonly used anti-hypertensive medications in continuous infusion form include sodium nitroprusside, labetalol, esmolol, and nicardipine (177-179).

Current recommendations advise no more than a 25% reduction in systolic BP over the first 8 hours followed by a gradual reduction to normal blood pressures over a period of 24 to 48 hours (180). Acute drop in blood pressure, especially in patients with underlying chronic hypertension, can dramatically decrease blood flow to the brain and cause irreversible neurological damage (181). Once blood pressures are adequately controlled, patients should be monitored closely in the outpatient setting. Potential problems that need to be monitored include noncompliance to medication and tolerance to a particular anti-hypertensive class.

Table 6. Different classes of anti-hypertensive medications, dosage and commonly encountered adverse effects*

Class	Drug	Starting dose	Maximal dose	Adverse effects
ACE inhibitor	Captopril	0.3 to 0.5 mg/kg/day	6 mg/kg/day	Hyperkalemia, renal impairment, cough, angioedema, hypotension, teratogenicity and congenital malformation in utero exposure
	Lisinopril	0.07 mg/kg/day	5 mg/day	
	Enalapril	0.08 mg/kg/day	5 mg/day	
	Fosinopril	5 to 10 mg oral daily	40 mg/day	
ARB	Candesartan	4 to 8 mg (6-17 years)	16 mg (6-17 years)	Hypotension, hyperkalemia, renal impairment, angioedema, rhabdomyolysis, fetal/neonatal harm in utero exposure
	Losartan	0.75 mg/kg/day	1.4 mg/kg/day	
	Valsartan	1.3 mg/kg/day (6-17 years)	2.7 mg/kg/day (6-17 years)	
Calcium channel blocker	Amlodipine	0.05 to 0.1 mg/kg/day	0.3 mg/kg/day (max 10 mg)	Peripheral edema, palpitations, fatigue, dizziness, nausea, flushing, hypersensitivity reaction
	Isradipine	0.1 to 0.2 mg/kg/day	0.8 mg/kg/day	
	Nifedipine ER	0.5 mg/kg/day	3 mg/kg/day	
	Nicardipine	IV dose 1-4 mcg/kg/min		
Diuretics	Furosemide	0.5 to 2 mg/kg/dose	6 mg/kg/day	Electrolyte imbalance, ototoxicity, interstitial nephritis, hypovolemia, hypercalciuria, metabolic alkalosis
	Hydrochlorothi azide	0.5 to 1 mg/kg/day	3 mg/kg/day	Electrolyte imbalance, hypercalcemia, hyperuricemia, hyperlipidemia, hypotension, SLE exacerbation
α blocker	Phenoxyben-zamine	0.2 mg/kg/day	1 mg/kg/day	Orthostatic hypotension, reflex tachycardia, nasal congestion, ejaculatory dysfunction
	Prazosin	0.5 to 1 mg three times a day	7 mg/day	
β blocker	Propronalol	1 mg/kg/day	8 mg/kg/day	Bradycardia, heart block Raynaud phenomenon, bronchospasm, weakness
	Metaprolol	1-2 mg/kg/day	6 mg/kg/day	
	Atenolol	0.5 -1 mg/kg/day	2 mg/kg/day	
α and β blocker	Labetalol	IV dose 0.4 to 1 mg/kg/hr		Bradycardia, syncope, heart block, bronchospasm
		2 to 3 mg/kg/day (oral dose)	10 to 12 mg/kg/day	
Central α agonist	Clonidine	5 to 20 mcg/kg/day	25 mcg/kg/day	Hypotension, somnolence, headache, depression, rebound hypertension on abrupt discontinuation
Vasodilators	Hydralazine	1 mg/kg/day	7.5 mg/kg/day	Blood dyscrasias, neutropenia, lupus erythematosus, reflex tachycardia
	Minoxidil	0.1 to 0.2 mg/kg/day	1 mg/kg/day	Hypertrichosis, edema, tachycardia, breast tenderness, pericardial effusion
	Sodium nitroprusside	IV dose 3 to 5 mcg/kg/min		Cyanide toxicity, methhemoglobinemia, thiocyanate toxicity
Mineralocor-ticoid receptor blockers/antago nists	Spironolactone	1 mg/kg/day	3 mg/kg/day	Electrolyte imbalance, renal failure, metabolic acidosis, muscle cramps, arrhythmias, hepatotoxicity, vasculitis
	Amiloride	0.4 to 0.6 mg/kg/day	20 mg daily	

* All indicated doses for oral administration unless indicated as IV.
IV – intravenous.

Conclusion

Hypertension in children and adolescents is on the rise, often under-diagnosed, and has significant short term as well as long term adverse effects leading into adulthood (3, 182-186). The American Academy of Pediatrics provided new guidelines for pediatric blood pressure in 2017 (183, 184, 187). After confirming elevated blood pressure in children, a through work up must be done to rule out secondary causes of hypertension. The younger the children, the more likely is the probability of finding a secondary etiology for hypertension. Treatment should include lifestyle modifications including exercise and if unsuccessful, must proceed with pharmacologic intervention (187-189).

Continued monitoring in the outpatient setting is essential to ensure adequate control of blood pressures. Twenty four-hour ambulatory blood pressure monitoring (ABPM) is increasingly used in young adults/adolescents to establish diagnosis and can also be used to assess the efficacy of therapy. Though the difficulty for some patients to utilize ABPM, must be considered by clinicians as well, the importance of home blood pressure monitoring must also be remembered by patients and clinicians alike along with guidance of the pediatric patient's health care professional (190-192).

In addition, the reality of pediatric and adult hypertension reminds all to understand the key role of nutrition in human health as well as disease prevention with regard to obesity, obesity complications, and associated conditions (193-201). Research continues to explore various factors in hypertensive status including pulse wave velocity, drug use (i.e., binge drinking), fetotoxic effects of gestational use of angiotensin-converting enzyme inhibitors (as well as other chemicals), factors of pregnancy, the mysteries of sleep effects and many others (202-208).

As the 21st century continues, researchers and clinicians will compare, contrast, and correlated hypertension guidelines for all age groups with the need for ensuring accuracy of blood pressure measurements in various settings (i.e., home, office, other) (209-211). The complexities of hypertension management continue to unraveled that include crisis treatment, dealing with cardiopulmonary crises, understanding why treatment non-compliance remains a serious issue, and unraveling the relationships between diabetes mellitus and hypertension (212-215).

References

[1] Sun SS, Grave GD, Siervogel RM, Pickoff AA, Arslanian SS, Daniels SR. Systolic blood pressure in childhood predicts hypertension and metabolic syndrome later in life. Pediatrics 2007;119(2):237-46.

[2] Berenson GS, Srinivasan SR, Bao W, Newman WP 3rd, Tracy RE, Wattigney WA. Association between multiple cardiovascular risk factors and atherosclerosis in children and young adults. The Bogalusa Heart Study. N Engl J Med 1998;338(23):1650-6.

[3] Kaelber DC, Liu W, Ross M, Localio AR, Leon JB, Pace WD, et al. Diagnosis and medication treatment of pediatric hypertension: A retrospective cohort study. Peditrics 2016;138(6). pii: e20162195.

[4] Muntner P, He J, Cutler JA, Wildman RP, Whelton PK. Trends in blood pressure among children and adolescents. JAMA 2004;291(5):2107-13.

[5] Din-Dzietham R, Liu Y, Bielo MV, Shamsa F. High blood pressure trends in children and adolescents in national surveys, 1963 to 2002. Circulation 2007;116:1488-96.

[6] Lande MB, Kupferman JC. Pediatric hypertension: the year in review. Clin Pediatr (Phila) 2014;53(4):315-9.
[7] Greydanus DE, Agana M, Kamboj MK, Shebrain S, Soares N, Eke R, et al. Pediatric obesity: Current concepts. Dis Mon 2018;64(4):98-156.
[8] Larkins NG, Teixeira-Pinto A, Kim S, Burgner DP, Craig JC. The population-based prevalence of hypertension and correlates of blood pressure among Australian children. Pediatr Nephrol 2019 Feb 18. doi: 10.1007/s00467-019-04206-w.
[9] Ogden CL, Carroll MD, Curtin LR, McDowell MA, Tabak CJ, Flegal KM. Prevalence of overweight and obesity in the United States, 1999-2004. JAMA 2006;295(13):1549-55.
[10] Sorof JM, Poffenbarger T, Franco K, Bernard L, Portman RJ. Isolated systolic hypertension, obesity, and hyperkinetic hemodynamic states in children. J Pediatr 2002;140(6):660-6.
[11] Lalji R, Tullus K. What's new in paediatric hypertension? Arch Dis Child 2018;103(1):96-100.
[12] Tiu AC, Bishop MD, Asico LD, Jose PA, Villar VAM. Primary pediatric hypertension: Current understanding and emerging concepts. Curr Hypertens Rep 2017;19(9):70. doi: 10.1007/s11906-017-0768-4.
[13] National High Blood Pressure Education Program Working Group on High Blood Pressure in Children and Adolescents. The fourth report on the diagnosis, evaluation, and treatment of high blood pressure in children and adolescents. Pediatrics 2004;114(2 Suppl 4th Report):555-76.
[14] Flynn JT, Kaelber DC, Baker-Smith CM, Blowey D, Carroll AE, Daniels SR, et al. Clinical practice guideline for screening and management of high blood pressure in children and adolescents. Pediatrics 2017;140(3). pii: e20171904. doi: 10.1542/peds.2017-1904.
[15] Sharma AK, Metzger DL, Rodd CJ. Prevalence and severity of high blood pressure among children based on the 2017 American Academy of Pediatrics guidelines. JAMA Pediatr 2018;172(6):557-65.
[16] Baker-Smith CM, Flynn JT, Kaelber DC. Systematic reviews: a small fraction of the evidence used to generate the 2017 clinical pediatric hypertension clinical practice guideline. J Hypertens 2019;37(2):451-2.
[17] Bell CS, Samuel JP, Samuels JA. Prevalence of hypertension in children. Hypertension 2019;73(1):148-52.
[18] Liu Q, Hou Y, Yang L, Zhao M, Li S, Xi B. Diagnostic effect of the single BP cut-offs for identifying elevated BP and hypertension in adolescents aged 13-17 years. Pediatr Cardiol 2019 Feb 1. doi: 10.1007/s00246-019-02058-7.
[19] Hou Y, Bovet P, Kelishadi R, Litwin M, Khadilkar A, Hong YM, et al. Height-specific blood pressure cutoffs for screening elevated and high blood pressure in children and adolescents: An international study. Hypertens Res 2018 Dec 26. doi: 10.1038/s41440-018-0178-2.
[20] Lande MB, Kupferman JC. Blood pressure and cognitive function in children and adolescents. Hypertension 2019;73(3):532-40.
[21] Urbina EM, Lande MB, Hooper SR, Daniels SR. Target organ abnormalities in pediatric hypertension. J Pediatr 2018;202:14-22.
[22] Khoury M, Urbina EM. Cardiac and vascular target organ damage in pediatric hypertension. Front Pediatr 2018;6:148. doi: 10.3389/fped.2018.00148.
[23] Frankfurt JA, Duncan AF, Heyne RJ, Rosenfeld CR. Renal function and systolic blood pressure in very-low-birth-weight infants 1–3 years of age. Pediatr Nephrol 2012;27(12):2285–91.
[24] Hsu CW, Yamamoto KT, Henry RK, De Roos AJ, Flynn JT. Prenatal risk factors for childhood CKD. J Am Soc Nephrol 2014;25(9):2105–11.
[25] Falkner B, Daniels SR. Summary of the Fourth Report on the Diagnosis, Evaluation, and Treatment of High Blood Pressure in Children and Adolescents. Hypertension 2004;44(4):387-8.
[26] O'Brien E, Alpert BS, Stergiou GS. Assessing blood pressure measuring devices: Influencing users in the 21st century. J Clin Hypertens (Greenwich) 2018;20(7):1138-41.
[27] Bussenius H, Zeck AM, Williams B, Haynes-Ferere A. Surveillance of pediatric hypertension using smartphone technology. J Pediatr Health Care 2018;32(5):e98-e104.
[28] Stergiou GS, Alpert BS, Mieke S, Wang J, O'Brien E. Validation protocols for blood pressure measuring devices in the 21st century. J Clin Hypertens (Greenwich) 2018;20(7):1096-9.

[29] Urbina E, Alpert B, Flynn J, Hayman L, Harshfield GA, Jacobson M, et al. Ambulatory blood pressure monitoring in children and adolescents: recommendations for standard assessment: a scientific statement from the American Heart Association Atherosclerosis, Hypertension, and Obesity in Youth Committee of the council on cardiovascular disease in the young and the council for high blood pressure research. Hypertension 2008;52(3):433-51.

[30] Brady TM. Hypertension. Pediatr Rev 2012;33(12):541-52.

[31] Morris DJ, Brem AS. The role of gut metabolism of adrenal corticosteroids and hypertension– clues gut cleansing antibiotics give us. Physiol Genomics 2019 Jan 25. doi: 10.1152/physiolgenomics.00115.2018.

[32] Knauf F, Brewer JR, Flavell RA. Immunity, microbiota and kidney disease. Nat Rev Nephrol 2019 Feb 22. doi: 10.1038/s41581-019-0118-7.

[33] Chatmethakul T, Roghair RD. Risk of hypertension following perinatal adversity: IUGR and prematurity. J Endocrinol 2019 Jan 1. pii: JOE-18-0687.R1. doi: 10.1530/JOE-18-0687.

[34] Hsu CN, Tain YL. The double-edged sword effects of maternal nutrition in the developmental programming of hypertension. Nutrients 2018 Dec 4;10(12). pii: E1917. doi: 10.3390/nu10121917.

[35] Karatzi K, Moschonis G, Botelli S, Androutsos O, Chrousos GP, Lionis C, et al. Physical activity and sedentary behavior thresholds for identifying childhood hypertension and its phenotypes: The Healthy Growth Study. J Am Soc Hypertens 2018;12(10):714-22.

[36] Martin CA, McGrath BP. White-coat hypertension. Clin Exp Pharmacol Physiol 2014;41(1):22-9.

[37] Tang H, Gong WY, Zhang QZ, Zhang J, Ye ZC, Peng H, et al. Prevalence, determinants, and clinical significance of masked hypertension and white-coat hypertension in patients with chronic kidney disease. Nephrology (Carlton) 2016;21(10):841-50.

[38] Herrington L, Susi A, Gorman G, Nylund CM, Hisle-Gorman E. Factors affecting pediatric dyslipidemia screening and treatment. Clin Pediatr (Phila) 2019 Feb 22:9922819832068. doi: 10.1177/0009922819832068.

[39] Manios Y, Karatzi K, Moschonis G, Ioannou G, Androutsos O, Lionis C, et al. Lifestyle, anthropometric, socio-demographic and perinatal correlates of early adolescence hypertension: The Healthy Growth Study. Nutr Metab Cardiovasc Dis 2019;29(2):159-69.

[40] Kuciene R, Dulskiene V, Medzioniene J. Associations between high birth weight, being large for gestational age, and high blood pressure among adolescents: a cross-sectional study. Eur J Nutr 2018;57(1):373-81.

[41] Banker A, Gupta-Malhotra M, Syamasundar Rao P. Childhood hypertension: A review. J Hypertens 2013;2:128. doi: 10.4172/2167-1095.1000128.

[42] Harshfield GA, Wilson ME. Ethnic differences in childhood blood pressure. In: Portman RJ, Sorof JM, Ingelfinger JR, eds. Pediatric hypertension. Clinical hypertension and vascular diseases. Totowa, NJ: Humana Press, 2004:293-305.

[43] Cornoni-Huntley J, LaCroix AZ, Havlik RJ. Race and sex differentials in the impact of hypertension in the United States. The National Health and Nutrition Examination Survey I Epidemiologic Follow-up Study. Arch Intern Med 1989;149(4):780-8.

[44] Kit BK, Kuklina E, Carroll MD, Ostchega Y, Freedman DS, Ogden CL. Prevalence of and trends in dyslipidemia and blood pressure among US children and adolescents, 1999-2012. JAMA Pediatr 2015;169(3):272-9.

[45] Schillaci G, Pirro M, Vaudo G, Gemelli F, Marchesi S, Porcellati C, et al. Prognostic value of the metabolic syndrome in essential hypertension. J Am Coll Cardiol 2004;43(10):1817-22.

[46] Flynn JT. Neonatal hypertension: diagnosis and management. Pediatr Nephrol 2000;14(4):332-41.

[47] Harer MW, Kent AL. Neonatal hypertension: an education review. Pediatr Nephrol 2018 Jul 5. doi: 10.1007/s00467-018-3996-1.

[48] Mitsnefes MM. Hypertension in children and adolescents. Pediatr Clin North Am 2006;53(3):493-512,viii.

[49] Sethna CB, Merchant K, Reyes A. Cardiovascular disease risk in children with kidney disease. Semin Nephrol 2018;38(3):298-313.

[50] Chow EJ, Leger KJ, Bhatt NS, Mulrooney DA, Ross CJ, Aggarwal S, et al. Pediatric cardio-oncology: Epidemiology, screening, prevention, and treatment. Cardiovasc Res 2019 Feb 15. pii: cvz031. doi: 10.1093/cvr/cvz031.
[51] Aronow WS, Fleg JL, Pepine CJ, Artinian NT, Bakris G, Brown AS, et al. ACCF/AHA 2011 expert consensus document on hypertension in the elderly: a report of the American College of Cardiology Foundation Task Force on Clinical Expert Consensus documents developed in collaboration with the American Academy of Neurology, American Geriatrics Society, American Society for Preventive Cardiology, American Society of Hypertension, American Society of Nephrology, Association of Black Cardiologists, and European Society of Hypertension. J Am Coll Cardiol 2011;57(20):2037-114.
[52] Cortese S, Holtmann M, Banaschewski T, Buitelaar J, Coghill D, Danckaerts M, et al. Practitioner review: current best practice in the management of adverse events during treatment with ADHD medications in children and adolescents. J Child Psychol Psychiatry 2013;54(3):227-46.
[53] Grisaru S, Yue M, Samuel SM, Chaput KH, Hamiwka LA. Blood pressure in children with attention deficit/hyperactivity disorder. Paediatr Child Health 2018;23(6):e102-8.
[54] Chiong JR, Aronow WS, Khan IA, Nair CK, Vijayaraghavan K, Dart RA, et al. Secondary hypertension: current diagnosis and treatment. Int J Cardiol 2008;124(1):6-21.
[55] Grossman E, Messerli FH. Drug-induced hypertension: an unappreciated cause of secondary hypertension. Am J Med 2012;125(1):14-22.
[56] Adelman RD, Coppo R, Dillon MJ. The emergency management of severe hypertension. Pediatr Nephrol 2000;14(5):422-7.
[57] Zhang Y, Bailey RR. A long term follow up of adults with reflux nephropathy. NZ Med J 1995;108(998):142-4.
[58] Sweeney WE, Avner ED. Polycystic kidney disease, autosomal recessive. In: GeneReviews. Seattle, WA: University of Washington, 1993-2019. 2001 Jul 19.
[59] Harris PC, Torres VE. Polycystic kidney disease, autosomal dominant. In: GeneReviews. Seattle, WA: University of Washington, 1993-2019. 2002 Jan 10.
[60] Pugh D, Gallacher PJ, Dhaun N. Management of hypertension in chronic kidney disease. Drugs 2019 Feb 13. doi: 10.1007/s40265-019-1064-1.
[61] D'Amico M, Locatelli F. Hypertension in dialysis: pathophysiology and treatment. J Nephrol 2002;15(4):438-45.
[62] Anderson TE, Conran RM. Educational case: Wilms tumor (nephroblastoma). Acad Pathol 2019 Jan 15;6:2374289518821381. doi: 10.1177/2374289518821381.
[63] Charlton J, Irtan S, Bergeron C, Pritchard-Jones K. Bilateral Wilms tumour: a review of clinical and molecular features. Expert Rev Mol Med 2017;19:e8. doi: 10.1017/erm.2017.8.
[64] Maas MH, Cransberg K, van Grotel M, Pieters R, van den Heuvel-Eibrink MM. Renin-induced hypertension in Wilms tumor patients. Pediatr Blood Cancer 2007;48(5):500-3.
[65] Shao L, Manalang M,Cooley L. Juxtaglomerular cell tumor in an 8-year-old girl. Pediatr Blood Cancer 2008;50(2):406-9.
[66] Humbert J, Roussey-Kesler G, Guerin P, LeFrançois T, Connault J, Chenouard A, et al. Diagnostic and medical strategy for renovascular hypertension: report from a monocentric pediatric cohort. Eur J Pediatr 2015;174(1):23-32.
[67] Samadian F, Dalili N, Jamalian A. New insights into pathophysiology, diagnosis, and treatment of renovascular hypertension. Iran J Kidney Dis 2017;11(2):79-89.
[68] Ilivitzki A, Glozman L, Lopez Alfonso R, Ofer A, Beck Razi N, Rotman Shapira M. Sonographic evaluation of renovascular hypertension in the pediatric population: State-of-the-art. J Clin Ultrasound 2017;45(5):282-292.
[69] Deal JE, Snell MF, Barratt TM, Dillon MJ. Renovascular disease in childhood. J Pediatr 1992;121(3):378-84.
[70] Dillon MJ. The diagnosis of renovascular disease. Pediatr Nephrol 1997;11(3):366-72.
[71] Singh S, Jindal AK, Pilania RK. Diagnosis of Kawasaki disease. Int J Rehum Dis 2018;21(1):36-44.
[72] Saguil A, Fargo M, Grogan S. Diagnosis and management of Kawasaki disease. Am Fam Physician 2015;91(6):365-71.

[73] Williams K. Preventing long-term cardiac damage in pediatric patients with Kawasaki disease. J Pediatr Health Care 2017;31(2):196-202.
[74] Hiner LB, Falkner B. Renovascular hypertension in children. Pediatr Clin North Am 1993;40(1):123-40.
[75] Fan L, Zhang H, Cai J, Yang L, Liu B, Wei D, et al. Clinical course and prognostic factors of childhood Takayasu's arteritis: over 15-year comprehensive analysis of 101 patients. Arthritis Res Ther 2019;21(1):31. doi: 10.1186/s13075-018-1790-x.
[76] Horino T, Ichii O, Matsumoto T, Terada Y. Takayasu arteritis presenting as renovascular hypertension. J Clin Rheumatol 2018 Dec 18. doi: 10.1097/RHU.0000000000000936.
[77] Choi Y, Kang BC, Kim KJ, Cheong HI, Hwang YS, Wang KC, et al. Renovascular hypertension in children with moyamoya disease. J Pediatr 1997;131(2):258-63.
[78] Guo J, Guo L, Zeng G, Tong Z, Gao X, Gu Y. An infant case of renovascular hypertension in moyamoya disease treated by angioplasty. Turk J Pediatr 2018;60(3): 331-4.
[79] Khoury MH, Gornik HL. Fibromuscular dysplasia (FMD). Vasc Med 2017;22(3):248-52.
[80] Green R, Gu X, Kline-Rogers E, Froehlich J, Mace P, Gray B. Differences between the pediatric and adult presentation of fibromuscular dysphasia: results from the US Registry. Pediatr Nephrol 2016;31(4):641-50.
[81] Narula N, Kadian-Dodov D, Olin JW. Fibromuscular dysplasia: Contemporary concepts and future directions. Prog Cardiovasc Dis 2018;60(6):580-5.
[82] Kadian-Dodov D. Fibromuscular dysplasia: Beginning to see the forest through the trees. Vasc Med 2019 Feb 10:1358863X19826346. doi: 10.1177/1358863X19826346.
[83] Vo NJ, Hammelman BD, Racadio JM, Strife CF, Johnson ND, Racadio JM. Anatomic distribution of renal artery stenosis in children: implications for imaging. Pediatr Radiol 2006;36(10):1032-6.
[84] Boris JR. Primary-care management of patients with coarctation of the aorta. Cardiol Young 2016;26(8):1537-42.
[85] Nguyen L, Cook SC. Coarctation of the aorta: Strategies for improving outcomes. Cardiol Clin 2015;33(4):521-30.
[86] Doshi AR, Chikkabyrappa S. Coarctation of aorta in children. Cureus 2018 Dec 5;10(12):e3690. doi: 10.7759/cureus.3690.
[87] Francis CM. Coarctation of the aorta: are genes relevant? J Cardiovasc Surg (Torino) 2016;57(4):545-56.
[88] Ing FF, Starc TJ, Griffiths SP, Gersony WM. Early diagnosis of coarctation of the aorta in children: a continuing dilemma. Pediatrics 1996;98(3 Pt 1):378-82.
[89] Davis SM, Geffner ME. Cardiometabolic health in Turner syndrome. Am J Med Genet C Semin Med Genet 2019 Feb 18. doi: 10.1002/ajmg.c.31678.
[90] Freel EM, Mason A. Turner syndrome. Hypertension 2019;73(1):42-44.
[91] Allybocus ZA, Wang C, Shi H, Wu Q. Endocrinopathies and cardiopathies in patients with Turner syndrome. Climacteric 2018;21(6):536-41.
[92] Ganju NK, Kandoria A, Thakur S, Ganju SA. A constellation of cardiac anomalies: Beyond Shone's complex. Heart Views 2016;17(1):23-6.
[93] Nicholson GT, Kelleman MS, De la Uz CM, Pignatelli RH, Ayres NA, Petit CJ. Late outcomes in children with Shone's complex: a single-centre, 20-year experience. Cardiol Young 2017;27(4):697-705.
[94] True A, Baidya M, Lui C, Kilimnik G, Sadler M. Computed tomography imaging characteristics of shone syndrome. Radiol Case Rep 2018;14(2):164-7.
[95] Furusawa EA, Esposito CSL, Honjo RS, Suzuki L, Leal GN, Kim CA, et al. Diagnosis and management of systemic hypertension due to renovascular and aortic stenosis in patients with Williams-Beuren syndrome. Rev Assoc Med Bras (1992) 2018;64(8):723-8.
[96] Pober BR. Williams-Beuren syndrome. N Engl J Med 2010;362(3):239-52.
[97] Das KM, Momenah TS, Larsson SG, Jadoon S, Aldosary AS. Lee EY. Williams-Beuren syndrome: computed tomography imaging review. Pediatr Cardiol 2014;35(8):1309-20.
[98] Royston R, Waite J, Howlin P. Williams syndrome: recent advances in our understanding of cognitive, social and psychological functioning. Curr Opin Psychiatry 2019;32(2):60-6.

[99] Kadoya Y, Zen K, Saburi M, Matoba S. Mid-aortic syndrome: A rare cause of juvenile hypertension. Intern Med 2018;57(3):447. doi: 10.2169/internalmedicine.9337-17.

[100] Harmon CM, Azzuga AA, Ranganathan S, Mahmood B, Good M. Mid-aortic syndrome in a premature infant: A rare cause of hypertension. J Pediatr 2015;167(2):492-e1. doi: 10.1016/j.jpeds.2015.05.007.

[101] Lin YJ, Hwang B, Lee PC, Yang LY, Meng CC. Mid-aortic syndrome: A case report and review of the literature. Int J Cardiol 2008;123(3):348-52.

[102] Yiu VW, Dluhy RP, Lifton RP, Guay-Woodford LM. Low peripheral plasma renin activity as a critical marker in pediatric hypertension. Pediatr Nephrology 1997;11(3):343-6.

[103] Lifton RP, Dluhy RG, Powers M, Rich GM, Cook S, Ulick S, et al. A chimaeric 11 beta-hydroxylase/aldosterone synthase gene causes glucocorticoid-remediable aldosteronism and human hypertension. Nature 1992;355(6357):262-5.

[104] Shahrrava A, Moinuddin S, Boddu P, Shah R. A case of glucocorticoid remediable aldosteronism and thoracoabdominal aneurysms. Case Rep Endocrinol 2016;2016:2017571. doi: 10.1155/2016/2017571.

[105] Methe H, Pehlivanli S. Glucocorticoid-remediable aldosteronism in a young adult with a family history of Conn's syndrome. Clin Case Rep 2018;6(2):416-9.

[106] Kamrath C, Maser-Gluth C, Haag C, Schulze E. Diagnosis of glucocorticoid-remediable aldosteronism in hypertensive children. Horm Res Paediatr 2011;76(2):93-8.

[107] Litchfield WR, Anderson BF, Weiss RJ, Lifton RP, Dluhy RG. Intracranial aneurysm and hemorrhagic stroke in glucocorticoid-remediable aldosteronism. Hypertension 1998;31(1 Pt 2):445-50.

[108] Zennaro MC, Jeunemaitre X. SFE/SFHTA/AFCE consensus on primary aldosteronism, part 5: Genetic diagnosis of primary aldosteronism. Ann Endocrinol (Paris) 2016;77(3):214-9.

[109] El-Maouche D, Arlt W, Merke DP. Congenital adrenal hyperplasia. Lancet 2017;390(10108):2194-2210.

[110] Witchel SF. Congenital adrenal hyperplasia. J Pediatr Adolesc Gynecol 2017;30(5):520-34.

[111] Nermoen I, Husebye ES, Myhre AG, Løvås K. Classic congenital adrenal hyperplasia. Tidsskr Nor Laegeforen 2017;137(7):540-543. [English, Norwegian]

[112] Tajima T. Health problems of adolescent and adult patients with 21-hydroxylase deficiency. Clin Pediatr Endocrinol 2018;27(4):203-13.

[113] Milford DV. Investigation of hypertension and the recognition of monogenic hypertension. Arch Dis Child 1999;81(5):452-5.

[114] Wilson RC, Krozowski ZS, Li K, Obeyesekere VR, Razzaghy-Azar M, Harbison MD. A mutation in the HSD11B2 gene in a family with apparent mineralocorticoid excess. J Clin Endocrinol Metab 1995;80(7):2263-6.

[115] Tapia-Castillo A, Baudrand R, Vaidya A, Campino C, Allende F, Valdivia C, Vecchiola A. Clinical, biochemical, and genetic characteristics of "nonclassic" apparent mineralocorticoid excess syndrome. J Clin Endocrinol Metab 2019;104(2):595-603.

[116] Yau M, Haider S, Khattab A, Ling C, Mathew M, Zaidi S, et al. Clinical, genetic, and structural basis of apparent mineralocorticoid excess due to11β-hydroxysteroid dehydrogenase type 2 deficiency. Proc Natl Acad Sci USA 2017;114(52):E11248-56.

[117] Carvajal CA, Tapia-Castillo A, Valdivia CP, Allende F, Solari S, Lagos CF, et al. Serum cortisol and cortisone as potential biomarkers of partial 11β-hydroxysteroid dehydrogenase type 2 deficiency. Am J Hypertens 2018;31(8):910-8.

[118] Morineau G, Sulmont V, Salomon R, Fiquet-Kempf B, Jeunemaître X, Nicod J, et al. Apparent mineralocorticoid excess: report of six new cases and extensive personal experience. J Am Soc Nephrol 2006;17(11):3176-84.

[119] Shimkets RA, Warnock DG, Bositis CM, Nelson-Williams C, Hansson JH, Schambelan M, et al. Liddle's syndrome: heritable human hypertension caused by mutations in the beta subunit of the epithelial sodium channel. Cell 1994;79(3):407-14.

[120] Mubarik A, Aeddula NR. Liddle syndrome. StatPearls. Treasure Island, FL: StatPearls Publishing, 2018.

[121] Tetti M, Monticone S, Burrello J, Matarazzo P, Veglio F, Pasini B, et al. Liddle syndrome: Review of the literature and description of a new case. Int J Mol Sci 2018;19(3). pii: E812. doi: 10.3390/ijms19030812.

[122] Cui Y, Tong A, Jiang J, Wang F, Li C. Little syndrome: Clinical and genetic profiles. J Clin Hypertens (Greenwich) 2017;19(5):524-9.

[123] Mumford E, Unwin RJ, Walsh SB. LIquorice, Liddle, Bartter or Gitelman-how to differentiate? Nephrol Dial Transplant 2019;34(1):38-9.

[124] Yang CL, Angell J, Mitchell R, Ellison DH. WNK kinases regulate thiazide-sensitive Na-Cl cotransport. J Clin Invest 2003;111(7):1039-45.

[125] O'Shaughnessy KM. Gordon syndrome: a continuing story. Pediatric Nephrol 2015;30(11):1903-8.

[126] Alisch F, Weichert A, Kalache K, Paradiso V, Longardt AC, Dame C, et al. Familial Gordon syndrome associated with a PIEZO2 mutation. Am J Med Genet A 2017;173(1):254-9.

[127] McMillin MJ, Beck AE, Chong JX, Shively KM, Buckingham KJ, Gildersleeve HI, et al. Mutations in PIEZO2 cause Gordon syndrome, Marden-Walker syndrome, and distal arthrogryposis type 5. Am J Hum Genet 2014;94(5):734-44.

[128] Lenders JW, Eisenhofer G, Mannelli M, Pacak K. Phaeochromocytoma. Lancet 2005;366(9486):665-75.

[129] Jain A, Baracco R, Kapur G. Pheochromocytoma and paraganglioma-an update on diagnosis, evaluation, and management. Pediatr Nephrol 2019 Jan 2. doi: 10.1007/s00467-018-4181-2.

[130] Omura M, Saito J, Yamaguchi K, Kakuta Y, Nishikawa T. Prospective study on the prevalence of secondary hypertension among hypertensive patients visiting a general outpatient clinic in Japan. Hypertens Res 2004;27(3):193-202.

[131] Neumann HP Bausch B, McWhinney SR, Bender BU, Gimm O, Franke G, et al. Germ-line mutations in nonsyndromic pheochromocytoma. N Engl J Med 2002;346(19):1459-66.

[132] Pahwa HS, Kumar A, Srivastava R, Rai A. Unsuspected pheochromocytoma of the urinary bladder: reminder of an important clinical lesson. BMJ Case Rep 2012:Aug 8;2012. doi. 10.1136/bcr-2012-006377.

[133] O'Brien T, Young WF Jr, Davila DG, Scheithauer BW, Kovacs K, Horvath E, et al. Cushing's syndrome associated with ectopic production of corticotrophin-releasing hormone, corticotrophin and vasopressin by a phaeochromocytoma. Clin Endocrinol (Oxf) 1992;37(5):460-7.

[134] Onozawa M, Fukuhara T, Minoguchi M, Takahata M, Yamamoto Y, Miyake T, et al. Hypokalemic rhabdomyolysis due to WDHA syndrome caused by VIP-producing composite pheochromocytoma: a case in neurofibromatosis type 1. Jpn J Clin Oncol 2005;35(9):559-63.

[135] Mune T, Katakami H, Kato Y, Yasuda K, Matsukura S, Miura K. Production and secretion of parathyroid hormone-related protein in pheochromocytoma: participation of an alpha-adrenergic mechanism. J Clin Endocrinol Metab 1993;76(3):757-62.

[136] Castinetti F, Waguespack SG, Machens A, Uchino S, Hasse-Lazar K, Sanso G, et al. Natural history, treatment, and long-term follow up of patients with multiple endocrine neoplasia type 2B: an international, multicentre, respective study. Lancet Diabetes Endocrinol 2019;7(3):213-20.

[137] Peczkowska M, Januszewicz A. Multiple endocrine neoplasia type 2. Fam Cancer 2005;4(1):25-36.

[138] Pomares FJ, Cañas R, Rodriguez JM, Hernandez AM, Parrilla P, Tebar FJ. Differences between sporadic and multiple endocrine neoplasia type 2A phaeochromocytoma. Clin Endocrinol (Oxf) 1998;48(2):195-200.

[139] Makri A, Akshintala S, Derse-Anthony C, Del Rivero J, Widemann B, Stratakis CA, et al. Pheochromocytoma in children and adolescents with multiple endocrine neoplasia type 2B. J Clin Endocrinol Metab 2019;104(1):7-12.

[140] Karaconji T, Whist E, Jamieson RV, Flaherty MP, Grigg JRB. Neurofibromatosis type 1: Review and update on emerging therapies. Asia Pac J Ophthalmol (Phila) 2018 Nov 2. doi: 10.22608/APO.2018182.

[141] Evans DGR, Salvador H, Chang VY, Erez A, Voss SD, Schneider KW, et al. Cancer and central nervous system tumor surveillance in pediatric neurofibromatosis 1. Clin Cancer Res 2017;23(12):e46-e53.

[142] Hirbe AC, Gutmann DH. Neurofibromatosis type 1: a multidisciplinary approach to care. Lancet Neurol 2014;13(8):834-43.

[143] Liu P, Li M, Guan X, Yu A, Xiao Q, Wang C, et al. Clinical syndromes and genetic screening strategies of pheochromocytoma and paraganglioma. J Kidney Cancer VHL 2018;5(4):14-22.

[144] Bausch B, Borozdin W, Mautner VF, Hoffmann MM, Boehm D, Robledo M, et al. Germline NF1 mutational spectra and loss-of-heterozygosity analyses in patients with pheochromocytoma and neurofibromatosis type 1. J Clin Endocrinol Metab 2007;92(7):2784-92.
[145] Stabouli S, Vargiami E, Maliachova O, Printza N, Dotis J, Kyriazi M. Arterial stiffness in a toddler with neurofibromatosis type 1 and refractory hypertension. Case Rep Pediatr 2018 Oct 31;2018:5957987. doi: 10.1155/2018/5957987.
[146] van Leeuwaarde RS, Ahmad S, Links TP, Giles RH. Von Hippel-Lindau syndrome. In: Adams MP, Ardinger HH, Pagon RA, Wallace SE, Bean LJH, Stephens K, et al. (eds). GeneReviews. Seattle, WA: University of Washington, 1993-2019. 2018 Sep 6.
[147] Tsang SH, Sharma T. Von-Hippel-Lindau disease. Adv Exp Med Biol 2018;1085:201-3.
[148] Sivaskandarajah GA, Arnason TG. Unsuspected Von Hippel-Lindau syndrome in acute-onset resistant hypertension. BMJ Case Rep 2018;2018. pii: bcr-2018-225162. doi: 10.1136/bcr-2018-225162.
[149] Igaki J, Nishi A, Sato T, Hasegawa T. A pediatric case of pheochromocytoma without apparent hypertension associated with von Hippel-Lindau disease. Clin Pediatr Endocrinol 2018;27(2):87-93.
[150] Rednam SP, Erez A, Druker H, Janeway KA, Kamihara J, Kohlmann WK, et al. Von Hippel-Lindau and hereditary pheochromocytoma/paraganglioma syndromes: Clinical features, genetics, and surveillance recommendations in childhood. Clin Cancer Res 2017;23(12):e68-e75.
[151] Wang Y, Liang G, Tian J, Wang X, Chen A, Liang T, et al. Pedigree analysis, diagnosis and treatment in Von Hippel-Lindau syndrome: A report of three cases. Oncol Lett 2018;15(4):4882-90.
[152] Varshney N, Kebede AA, Owusu-Dapaah H, Lather J, Kaushik M, Bhullar JS. A review of Von Hippel-Lindau syndrome. J Kidney Cancer VHL 2017;4(3):20-9.
[153] Baysal BE, Ferrell RE, Willett-Brozick JE, Lawrence EC, Myssiorek D, Bosch A, et al. Mutations in SDHD, a mitochondrial complex II gene, in hereditary paraganglioma. Science 2000;287(5454):848-51.
[154] Settas N, Faucz FR, Stratakis CA. Succinate dehydrogenase (SDH) deficiency, Carney triad and the epigenome. Mol Cell Endocrinol 2018;469:107-111.
[155] Gill AJ. Succinate dehydrogenase (SDH)-deficient neoplasia. Histopathology 2018;72(1):106-16.
[156] Wong MY, Andrews KA, Challis BG, Park SM, Acerini CI, Maher ET, et al. Clinical practice guidance: Surveillance for phaeochromocytoma and paraganglioma in paediatric succinate dehydrogenase gene mutation carriers. Clin Endocrinol (Oxf) 2018 Dec 27. doi: 10.1111/cen.13926.
[157] Cavenagh T, Patel J, Nakhla N, Elstob A, Ingram M, Barber B, et al. Succinate dehydrogenase mutations: paraganglioma imaging and at-risk population screening. Clin Radiol 2019;74(3):169-77.
[158] Rasheed MRHA, Tarjan G. Succinate dehydrogenase complex: An updated review. Arch Pathol Lab Med 2018;142(12):1564-70.
[159] Bayley JP, Devilee P, Taschner PE. The SDH mutation database: an online resource for succinate dehydrogenase sequence variants involved in pheochromocytoma, paraganglioma and mitochondrial complex II deficiency. BMC Med Genet 2005;16(6):39.
[160] Riley M, Hernandez AK, Kuznia AL. High blood pressure in children and adolescents. Am Fam Physician 2018;98(8):486-94.
[161] Lee S, Choi YH, Cho YJ, Cheon JE, Park JE, Kim WE, et al. Diagnostic role of renal Doppler ultrasound and plasma renin activity as screening tools for renovascular hypertension in children. J Ultrasound Med 2019 Feb 18. doi: 10.1002/jum.14966.
[162] Franke I, Aydin M, Kurylowicz L, Lopez CEL, Ganshow R, Lentze MJ, et al. Clinical course & management of childhood nephrotic syndrome in Germany: a large epidemiological ESPED study. BMC Nephrol 2019;20(1):45. doi: 10.1186/s12882-019-1233-1.
[163] Chiavaroli L, Viguiliouk E, Nishi SK, Blanco Mejia S, Rahelić D, Kahleová H, et al. DASH dietary pattern and cardiometabolic outcomes: An umbrella review of systematic reviews and meta-analyses. Nutrients 2019;11(2). pii: E338. doi: 10.3390/nu11020338.
[164] Appel LJ, Brands MW, Daniels SR, Karanja N, Elmer PJ, Sacks FM. Dietary approaches to prevent and treat hypertension: a scientific statement from the American Heart Association. Hypertension 2006 47(2):296-308.
[165] Martin A, Booth JN, Laird Y, Sproule J, Reilly JJ, Saunders DH. Physical activity, diet and other behavioural interventions for improving cognition and school achievement in children and adolescents

with obesity or overweight. Cochrane Database Syst Rev 2018;3:CD009728. doi: 10.1002/14651858.CD009728.pub4.

[166] Binka E, Brady TM. Real-world strategies to treatment hypertension associated with pediatric obesity. Curr Hypertens Rep 2019;21(2):18. doi: 10.1007/s11906-019-0922-2.

[167] Köchli S, Endes K, Steiner R, Engler L, Infanger D, Schmidt-Trucksäss A. Obesity, high blood pressure, and physical activity determine vascular phenotype in young children. Hypertension 2019;73(1):153-61.

[168] Sanghera DK, Bejar C, Sharma S, Gupta R, Blackett PR. Obesity genetics and cardiometabolic health: Potential for risk prediction. Diabetes Obes Metab 2019 Jan 22. doi: 10.1111/dom.13641.

[169] Fortuna RJ, Rocco TA, Freeman J, Devine M, Bisognano J, Williams GC. A community-wide quality improvement initiative to improve hypertension control and reduce disparities. J Clin Hypertens (Greenwich) 2019;21(2):196-203.

[170] Wühl E. Hypertension in childhood obesity. Acta Paediatr 2019;108(1):37-43.

[171] Chrysaidou K, Stabouli S. Treatment of hypertension induced target organ damage in children and adolescents. Curr Pharm Des 2018 Nov 26. doi: 10.2174/1381612825666181127095450.

[172] Miyashita Y, Hanevold C. Evaluation and management of Stage 2 hypertension in pediatric patients. Curr Hypertens Rep 2018;20(9):73. doi: 10.1007/s11906-018-0873-z.

[173] Burrello J, Erhardt EM, Saint-Hilary G, Veglio F, Rabbia F, Mulatero P, et al. Pharmacological treatment of arterial hypertension in children and adolescents: A network meta-analysis. Hypertension 2018;72(2):306-313.

[174] Stotter BR, Ferguson MA. Should ACE inhibitors and ARBs be used in combination in children? Pediatr Nephrol 2018 Aug 15. doi: 10.1007/s00467-018-4046-8.

[175] Kidney Disease: Improving Global Outcomes (KDIGO) CKD-MBD Work Group. KDIGO clinical practice guideline for the diagnosis, evaluation, prevention, and treatment of Chronic Kidney Disease-Mineral and Bone Disorder (CKD-MBD). Kidney Int Suppl 2009;113:S1-130. doi: 10.1038/ki.2009.188.

[176] Kidney Disease: Improving Global Outcomes (KDIGO) CKD-MBD Update Work Group. KDIGO 2017 clinical practice guideline update for the diagnosis, evaluation, prevention, and treatment of Chronic Kidney Disease-Mineral and Bone Disorder (CKD-MBD). Kidney Int Suppl 2017;7(1):1-59. doi: 10.1016/j.kisu.2017.04.001.

[177] Patel NH, Romero SK, Kaelber DC. Evaluation and management of pediatric hypertensive crises: hypertensive urgency and hypertensive emergencies. Open Access Emerg Med 2012;4:85-92. doi: 10.2147/OAEM.S32809. eCollection 2012.

[178] Seeman T, Hamdani G, Mitsnefes M. Hypertensive crisis in children and adolescents. 2018 Oct 1. doi: 10.1007/s00467-018-4092-2.

[179] MacNeill E. Pediatric hypertension and hypertensive emergencies recognition and management in the emergency department. Pediatr Emerg Med Pract 2019;16(3):1-16.

[180] Flynn JT, Tullus K. Severe hypertension in children and adolescents: pathophysiology and treatment. Pediatr Nephrol 2009;24(6):1101–12.

[181] Vaughan CJ, Delanty N. Hypertensive Emergencies. Lancet 2000;356(9227):411–7.

[182] Matossian D. Pediatric hypertension. Pediatr Ann 2018;47(12):e499-e503.

[183] Flynn JT. Childhood blood pressure matters. Hypertension 2019;73(2):296-8.

[184] Lande MB, Batisky DL. New American Academy of Pediatrics Hypertension Guideline. Hypertension 2019;73(1):31-32.

[185] Guzman-Limon M, Samuels J. Pediatric hypertension: diagnosis, evaluation and treatment. Pediatr Clin North Am 2019;66(1):45-57.

[186] Jackson SL, Zhang Z, Wiltz JL, Loustalot F, Ritchey MD, Goodman AB, et al. Hypertension among youths—United States, 2001-2016. MMWR 2018;67(27):758-62.

[187] Baker-Smith CM, Flinn SK. Flynn JT, Kaelber DC, Blowey D, Carroll AE, et al. Diagnosis, evaluation, and management of high blood pressure in children and adolescents. Pediatrics 2018;142(3). pii: e20182096. doi: 10.1542/peds.2018-2096.

[188] Connolly SD, Ward KM. The role of exercise prescription in pediatric preventive cardiology programs. Pediatr Ann 2018;47(12):e494-8.

[189] Nerenberg KA, Zarnke KB, Leung AA, Dasgupta K, Butalia S, McBrien K, et al. Hypertension Canada's 2018 guidelines for diagnosis, risk assessment, prevention, and treatment of hypertension in adults and children. Can J Cardiol 2018;34(5):506-25.

[190] Hamdani G, Flynn JT, Daniels S, Falkner B, Hanevold C, Ingelfinger J, et al. Ambulatory blood pressure monitoring tolerability and blood pressure status in adolescents: the SHIP AHOY study. Blood Press Monit 2019;24(1):12-7.

[191] Liyanage-Don N, Fung D, Phillips E, Kronish IM. Implementing home blood pressure monitoring into clinical practice. Curr Hypertens Rep 2019;21(2):14. doi: 10.1007/s11906-019-0916-0.

[192] Bismar N, Barlow SE, Brady TM, Turer CB. Pediatrician communication about high blood pressure in children with overweight/obesity during well-child visits. Acad Pediatr 2019 Nov 26. pii: S1876-2859(19)30467-X. doi: 10.1016/j.acap.2019.11.012.

[193] James WPT, Johnson RJ, Speakman JR, Wallace DC, Frühbeck G, Iverson PL, et al. Nutrition and its role in human evolution. J Intern Med 2019;285(5):533-49.

[194] Zafarmand MH, Spanjer M, Nicolaou M, Wijnhoven HAH, van Schaik BDC, Uitterlinden AG, et al. Influence of dietary approaches to stop hypertension-type diet, known genetic variants and their interplay on blood pressure in early childhood: ABCD Study. Hypertension 2019 Dec 2:hypertensionaha.11812292. doi: 10.1161/hypertensionaha.118.12292.

[195] Keung V, Lo K, Cheung C, Tam W, Lee A. Changes in dietary habits and prevalence of cardiovascular risk factors among school students in Macao, China. Obes Res Clin Pract 2019 Nov 25. pii: S1871-403X(19)30376-X. doi: 10.1016/j.orcp.2019.10.007.

[196] Zhao M, Caserta CA, Medeiros CCM, López-Bermejo A, Kollias A, Zhang Q, et al. Metabolic syndrome, clustering of cardiovascular risk factors and high carotid intima-media thickness in children and adolescents. J Hypertens 2019 Nov 28. doi: 10.1097/HJH.0000000000002318.

[197] Avnieli Velfer Y, Phillip M, Shalitin S. Increased prevalence of severe obesity and related comorbidities among patients referred to a pediatric obesity clinic during the last decade. Horm Res Paediatr 2019 Dec 5:1-10. doi: 10.1159/000504540.

[198] Barrett T, Jalaludin MY, Turan S, Hafez M, Shehadeh N; Novo Nordisk Paediatr Type 2 Diabetes Global Expert Panel. Rapid progression of type 2 diabetes and related complications in children and young people – a literature review. Pediatr Diabetes 2019 Dec 5. doi: 10.1111/pedi.12953.

[199] Hoorn EJ, Gritter M, Cuevas CA, Fenton RA. Regulation of renal NaCl cotransporter and its role in potassium homeostasis. Physiol Rev 2020;100(1):321-356.

[200] Braconnier P, Milani B, Loncle N, Lourenco JM, Brito W, Delacoste J, et al. Short-term changes in dietary sodium intake influence sweat sodium concentration and muscle sodium content in healthy individuals. J Hypertens 2020;38(1):159-66.

[201] Del Pinto R, Wright JT, Monaco A, Pietropaoli D, Ferri C. Vitamin D and blood pressure control among hypertensive adults: results from NHANES 2001-2014. J Hypertens 2020;38(1):150-8.

[202] Safar ME. Current assessment of pulse wave velocity: comprehensive review of validation studies. J Hypertens 2020;38(1):178. doi: 10.1097/HJH.0000000000002261.

[203] Hwang CL, Piano MR, Thur LA, Peters TA, da Silva ALG, Phillips SA. The effects of repeated binge drinking on arterial stiffness and urinary norepinephrine levels in young adults. J Hypertens 2020;38(1):111-17.

[204] Stabouli S. Renin-angiotensin system blockers exposure in utero: a life-long risk for the offspring health. J Hypertens 2020;38(1):35-7.

[205] Weber-Schoendorfer C, Kayser A, Tissen-Diabaté T, Winterfeld U, Eleftheriou G, Te Winkel B, et al. Fetotoxic risk of AT1 blockers exceeds that of angiotensin-converting enzyme inhibitors: an observational study. J Hypertens 2020;38(1):133-41.

[206] Bello NA, Jaeger BC, Booth JN 3rd, Abdalla M, Anstey DE, Pugliese DN, et al. Associations of awake and asleep blood pressure and blood pressure dipping with abnormalities of cardiac structure: the Coronary Artery Risk Development in Young Adults study. J Hypertens 2020;38(1):102-10.

[207] Mo M, Shen Y, Si S, Xin X, Shao B, Wang S, et al. Feature of trajectory of blood pressure among pregnant women with gestational hypertension. J Hypertens 2020;38(1):127-32.

[208] Grau-Perez M, Redon J. Unraveling new factors associated with hypertension: the Mendelian randomization approach. J Hypertens 2020;38(1):30-2.

[209] Jensen GB. Hypertension guidelines in children should be universal. Eur J Prev Cardiol 2019 Nov 21:2047487319887463. doi: 10.1177/2047487319887463.

[210] Feitosa ADM, Mota-Gomes MA, Barroso WS, Miranda RD, Barbosa ECD, Pedrosa RP, et al. Correlation between office and home blood pressure in clinical practice: a comparison with 2017 American College of Cardiology/American Heart Association Hypertension Guidelines recommendations. J Hypertens 2020;38(1):179-81.

[211] Sharman JE, O'Brien E, Alpert B, Schutte AE, Delles C, Hecht Olsen M, et al. Lancet Commission on Hypertension group position statement on the global improvement of accuracy standards for devices that measure blood pressure. J Hypertens 2020;38(1):21-9.

[212] Tocci G, Presta V, Volpe M. Hypertensiv e crisis management in the emergency room: time to change? J Hypertens 2020;38(1):33-4.

[213] Marra AM, Benjamin N, Cittadini A, Bossone E, Grünig E. When pulmonary hypertension complicates heart failure. Heart Fail Clin 2020; 16(1):53-60.

[214] Rea F, Mella M, Monzio Compagnoni M, Cantarutti A, Merlino L, Mancia G, et al. Women discontinue antihypertensive drug therapy more than men. Evidence from an Italian population-based study. J Hyperten 2020;38(1):142-9.

[215] Holtrop J, Spiering W, Nathoe HM, De Borst GJ, Kappelle JL, De Valk HW, et al. Apparent therapy-resistant hypertension as a risk factor for the development of type 2 diabetes mellitus. J Hypertens 2020; 38(1): 45-51.

In: Chronic Disease and Disability
Editors: DE Greydanus, P Anne, JD Rowlett et al.
ISBN: 978-1-53617-656-8

Chapter 5

COMMON PEDIATRIC ARRHYTHMIAS: PART I

Premchand Anne[1], MD, MPH, MBA, FAAP, FACP, FACC and Harinder R Singh[2,*], MD, FHRS, CEPS-P, CCDS

[1]Pediatric Cardiology, Ascension St John Children's Hospital, Detroit, Michigan, United States of America

[2]Associate Professor, Pediatric Electrophysiology, The Children's Hospital of San Antonio, San Antonio, Texas, United States of America

ABSTRACT

Electrocardiogram interpretation in pediatrics is based on the evolutionary changes with maturation, and clinical manifestations. Systematic approach is warranted for precise interpretation during baseline rhythm and in arrhythmia. The knowledge and detection of normal variants and abnormal findings is of utmost importance and can guide pediatric cardiology referrals for consultations. In this chapter on pediatric arrhythmias, the epidemiology, natural history, clinical manifestations, diagnosis and management options of common arrhythmias and ectopies will be discussed.

INTRODUCTION

An electrocardiogram (ECG) is a vital tool in detection and management of electrical disturbances of the heart. These electrical changes can be normal, normal variants or abnormal findings. The interpretation of the pediatric ECG is unique and different than the adult ECG as the findings are related to the maturational and physiological changes from birth to adulthood. Awareness of these transitional ECG changes is important for a pediatric care provider. Correlation of clinical manifestations with the electrical changes on the ECG will provide opportunities for adequate management.

---

* Correspondence: Harinder Singh, MD, Pediatric Electrophysiology, The Children's Hospital of San Antonio, 333 North Santa Rosa Street, San Antonio, Texas, 78207, United States. Email: Harinder.Singh@bcm.edu.

STEPS FOR INTERPRETING A PEDIATRIC ELECTROCARDIOGRAM

Using a systematic approach will help avoid missing important findings as well as aid in interpreting normal variants from abnormal ECGs during interpretation. Below are the steps to guide clinicians in interpreting a pediatric ECG:

a) Determine age of the patient to identify normal values for age.
b) Make sure ECG has normal standardization (10 millimeters/millivolt- mm/mV).
c) Evaluate paper speed (normal is 25 millimeters/second- mm/sec).
d) Calculate heart rate and determine normal values for age.
    a. Divide 300 by number of large boxes between 2 consecutive R-R complexes
    b. Divide 15,000 by number of small boxes between 2 consecutive R-R complexes
    c. If rhythm is irregular, count the number of QRS complexes on a standard ECG sheet (paper speed of 25 mm/sec) and multiply by 6
e) Determine rhythm and variability: Normal sinus rhythm is presumed if
    d. P-wave precedes every QRS complex and
    e. P wave axis is normal
f) Define QRS frontal plane axis
g) Evaluate individual complexes and intervals: P wave, Q wave, QRS complex, T wave, U wave, PR interval, ST segment, and QT/QTc intervals.

COMMON ARRHYTHMIAS

Sinus arrhythmia

Sinus arrhythmia is a normal variation in the sino-atrial (SA) node activity that is associated with the phase of respiration. It is common in children and the incidence decreases with age (1). Inspiration is associated with an increase heart rate due to decreased parasympathetic activity while expiration is associated with decreased heart rate due to increased parasympathetic tone (2). Conditions leading to decreased parasympathetic activity (e.g., heart failure) leads to absence of sinus arrhythmia. Auscultation reveals increased heart rate with inspiration and lower heart rate with expiration.

ECG reveals normal sinus rhythm with variation in the P-P interval preceding the change in R-R intervals (see Figure 1). The prognosis is excellent and does not require any further investigations as it is a normal variant.

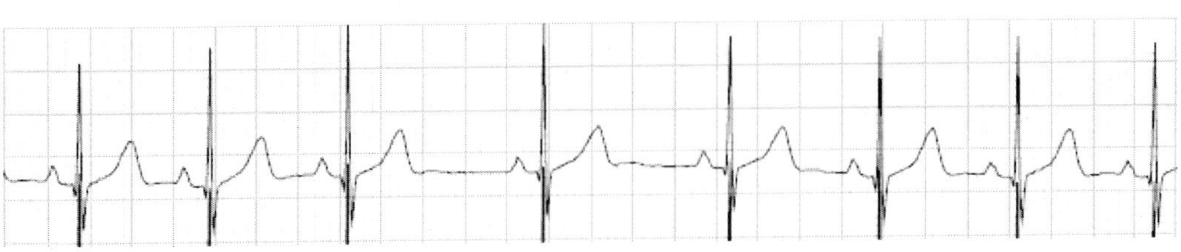

Figure 1. Sinus arrhythmia.

Ectopic Complexes (Premature Beats)

Premature Atrial Contractions

Premature atrial contraction (PAC), is a premature atrial depolarization arising from an atrial focus other than the SA node. Premature atrial contractions are the most common arrhythmia in fetal life and is common in infants and children on 24-hour ECGs (14% and 13%, respectively) (3, 4). Majority of children have at least one PAC over 24-hours, with frequency increasing through teenage years (5). Primary causes of PACs include a reentrant circuit or a focus other than the SA node, atrial dilation (obstructive process, heart failure, volume overload), surgical scarring and trauma (6). Common secondary causes of PACs include electrolyte abnormalities, caffeine intake, stimulant use (including medications used for management of attention deficit and hyperactivity disorder), nicotine use and alcohol use. Typical management of the PACs includes correcting the underlying etiology. Patients with PACs maybe be symptomatic or incidentally detected. Prognosis for PACs is excellent although PACs may be the trigger for supraventricular tachycardia, intra-atrial reentrant tachycardia in post-surgical patients, or atrial fibrillation (7).

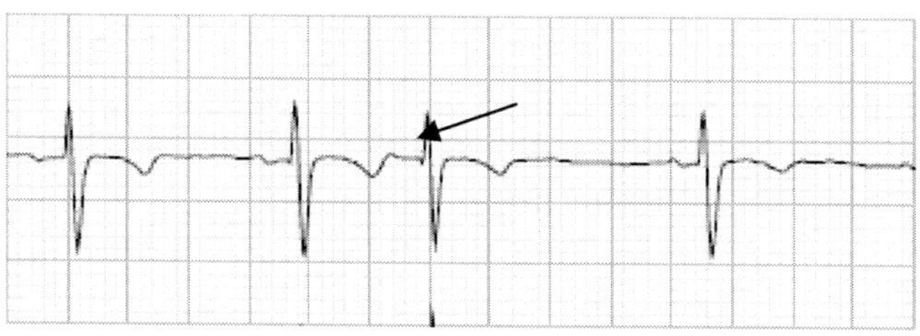

Figure 2A. Premature atrial complex that is normally conducted.

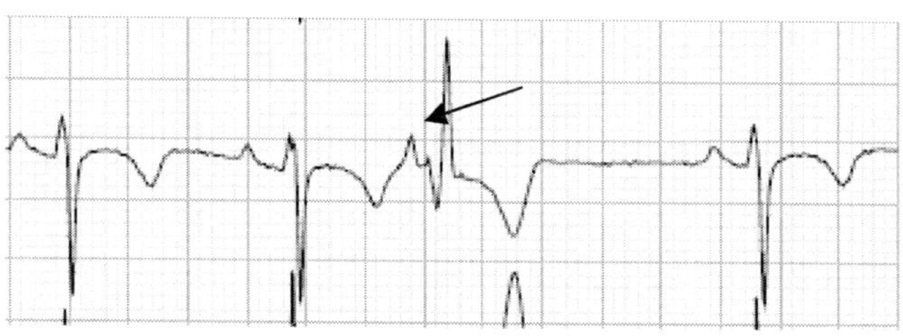

Figure 2B. Premature atrial complex that is conducted with aberrancy.

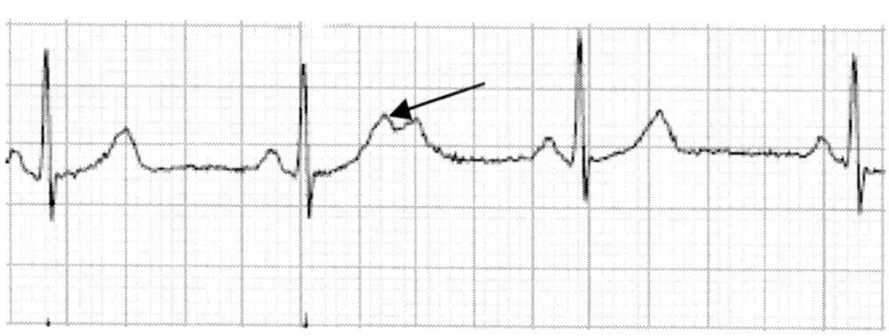

Figure 2C. Premature atrial complex that is blocked.

On ECG, a PAC appears with a markedly shortened P-P interval, typically with a P-wave of different morphology and different P-wave axis. They may be conducted normally if it presents after the AV refractory period (see Figure 2A), conducted with aberrancy if PAC presents during the partial refractory period (see Figure 2B), or blocked if it occurs during the effective refractory period (see Figure 2C). There is an incomplete compensatory pause as the sinus node is reset. Diagnosis of PACs can occur with the aid of a 12-lead ECG if the PACs are frequent; however, a Holter monitor (monitor which tracks every heart beat) or an event monitor (monitors actively when triggered, or unless abnormal rhythm is detected) may be of use when the symptoms are infrequent or unable to be captured on an ECG.

Prognosis for patients with PACs is excellent in those with normal hearts and do not require pharmacotherapy. Very often, lifestyle management, including avoidance of caffeine and stimulants, is more than adequate to control the symptoms. Sugimoto et al. (8) reported a decrease in PACs by 50% with bisoprolol, although 25% of these patients had adverse reactions (8).

Premature ventricular contractions

A premature ventricular contraction (PVC) is a premature ventricular beat that originates from below the His bundle bifurcation, and thereby characterized by a wide-QRS complex without a preceding P-wave. Typically, the QRS morphology during a PVC is wider and different from the baseline complexes. It occurs in all pediatric age groups and may occur without an underlying etiology; most are benign, paroxysmal and resolve without intervention in those with normal cardiac anatomy. He etiologies of PVCs include electrolyte abnormalities, chest trauma, anesthesia, cardiac tumors, myocarditis, hypoxia, caffeine use, and history of congenital cardiac surgery with the surgical scar as the focus (9). The rate of PVCs can vary depending on the etiology and increase in frequency with age and in the male gender (10). A benign etiology of PVCs is associated with increased vagal tone in athletes. Increased sympathetic tone can also cause PVCs (stimulant medications, caffeine, nicotine).

On an ECG, a ventricular complex must meet four criteria to be considered a PVC: 1) an early QRS without a preceding P wave, 2) prolonged QRS duration for age, 3) different QRS morphology compared to baseline QRS complexes and 4) opposite net QRS and T wave deflections. There is a complete "compensatory pause" as the sinus node is not reset after a PVC. (see Figure 3). The sinus node timing is fixed; the normally-timed P-wave following a PVC (during ventricular refractory period) does not conduct; therefore, the P-wave after the non-conducted P-wave should conduct normally. PVC morphology can be monomorphic (unifocal) or polymorphic (multifocal). PVCs can occur as singlets, couplets, short runs, or in bigeminy and trigeminy patterns. A right bundle branch morphology indicates a left ventricular origin and a left bundle branch morphology indicates a right ventricular origin of the PVC.

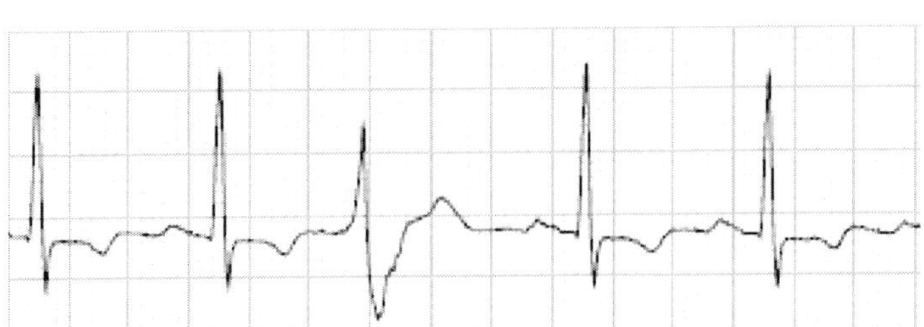

Figure 3. Premature ventricular complex with a compensatory pause.

In establishing a diagnosis, a thorough history and physical are vital. When obtaining the history, typically reported symptoms include palpitations-irregular, "pounding", and/or fast heart rate, lightheadedness, abdominal discomfort, chest pain and shortness of breath. History of congenital heart disease repair is critical; surgical scars may serve as a focus for PVCs. Reports of increased palpitations with activity are concerning and requires further testing, including an echocardiogram, Holter monitor to evaluate PVC burden, and an exercise stress test to assess response to increasing heart rates (11-13). Prognosis of single and infrequent PVCs is generally very good. In structurally normal hearts, uniform PVCs have good prognosis (14). PVCs may present as malignant ventricular tachyarrhythmias; in the context of congenital heart disease, electrophysiologic testing is warranted, with possibility of ablation.

Management of PVCs in pediatric patients with normal cardiac anatomy is dependent on the frequency and morphology of PVCs, symptoms and whether the PVCs decrease or increase with exercise. Children with single uniform PVCs that disappear with exercise are usually not pharmacologically treated. The patients should avoid caffeine, pseudoephedrine and other stimulants. On the other hand, patients with more frequent PVCs, ventricular triplets or non-sustained ventricular tachycardia, multiform PVCs, persistent or worse with exercise and surgically-corrected congenital heart disease are at increased risk for ventricular tachycardia and sudden cardiac death and require pediatric cardiology expertise (9). In these patients, beta-blockers can reduce frequency of PVCs in symptomatic patients; catheter ablation is the invasive option if a need arises (15, 16). Athletes with repaired structural heart disease with PVCs should be restricted to low-intensity sports (17).

Premature junctional complexes

A premature junctional complex (PJC) or beat (PJB), is a premature discharge that originates in the AV junction either at the level of the AV node or the bundle of His, in the absence of a prior atrial discharge. PJCs may occur in structurally normal or abnormal hearts and in all age groups. The incidence and prevalence are not well known. Among 16-19-year-old males, 0.21% had premature junctional complexes on 12-lead ECG and similar in other age groups (18). PJCs arise due to increased automaticity or triggered activity due to after-depolarizations within the AV junction (19, 20). PJCs may predispose the patient to ventricular tachycardia. Potential causes include normal variants, stimulant use, alcohol use, hypokalemia, hypoxemia, ischemia, and digitalis toxicity (21). It may be incidentally detected or may produce symptoms like palpitations, syncope, or dizziness.

ECG shows QRS complex morphology similar to sinus node originated activation, without preceding P-wave. A PJC conducting to the ventricle with aberrancy has a QRS complex comparable to a PVC. A retrograde P-wave may appear before, during, or after the QRS complex (Figure 4) (21). Depending on the frequency of the PJCs, an ECG can identify the premature complexes. If unsuccessful, a 24-hour Holter monitor may be used. An electrophysiology study may be needed to identify the location of the origin of the PJCs; origin distal to the AV node can initiate ventricular tachycardia (21). Patients with PJCs are usually managed conservatively. If symptoms are severe, medical management and pacing may be warranted to increase the heart rate. The management of underlying etiology is essential to decrease symptomatic PJCs.

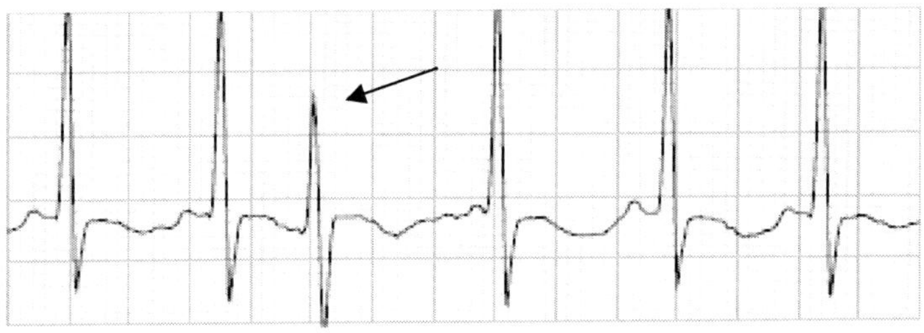

Figure 4. Premature junctional complex.

Bradyarrhythmias

Bradyarrhythmia is a heart rate less than low normal rate for age and physiological state. The etiologies can be of sinus node, atrial, and junction origins or secondary to atrioventricular (AV) blocks. Sinus node etiologies include sinus bradycardia, non-conducted atrial PACs (bigeminy and trigeminy patterns) and sinus node dysfunction. Atrial escape rhythm and junctional escape rhythms are often noted on pediatric ECGs. Finally, first degree, second degree types I and II, and third degree (complete) AV blocks can be consequential.

Bradycardia may be incidentally detected or can present with symptoms of lightheadedness, chest pain, syncope, fatigue and difficulty breathing. The management of symptomatic bradycardia depends on the etiology of the bradycardia, ranging from atropine, temporary pacing to permanent pacemaker implantation.

Sinus bradycardia

Sinus bradycardia is due to slower SA nodal activity. The criteria described above for sinus rhythm must be met. One of the most common presentations of sinus bradycardia is an asymptomatic, well-trained athlete, in whom further workup is not required (22). In the neonatal population, apnea is a major association with sinus bradycardia. In the older children, few conditions associated with sinus bradycardia include increased vagal tone (increased parasympathetic activity), acute infections, hypoxia, hypoglycemia, hyperkalemia, hypothermia, hypothyroidism, anorexia, sleep apnea, increased intracranial pressure, medications or drugs (9, 23); relief and management of these conditions will alleviate the sinus bradycardia. Diagnosis is established with an ECG, Holter monitor, event monitor and an exercise stress test. Symptomatic patients benefit from a pacemaker.

Sinus node dysfunction (SND)

Sinus node dysfunction (SND) is an uncommon rhythm disturbance in pediatric population with normal hearts and is characterized by bradycardia. Inherited forms of SND are associated with mutations in multiple genes, in particular, channelopathies or cardiomyopathies (24). Malignancies, inflammatory conditions and medications are other etiologies. In SND, the sinus node is unable to discharge an impulse or inappropriately discharge, leading to sinus pauses or tachy-brady syndrome, respectively. It is an age-dependent progressive fibrosis of SA nodal tissue and surrounding atrial myocardium (25). SND, when present in infants, can present with decreased feeding and poor weight gain; older children and adolescents (more than 70%) may be asymptomatic due to atrial and junctional escape activity that occurs in the presence of sinus pause or arrest (26, 27). Symptomatic children report inability to keeping up with their peers, fatigue, syncope and shortness of breath. Sudden death maybe the initial presentation if a channelopathy is responsible for SND. Sinus node dysfunction is a common problem in surgically-repaired congenital heart disease (CHD) patients, especially those involving atrial surgery as in Fontan procedure (28). As the time from surgery and the age of the patient increases, the frequency of sinus node dysfunction increases.

A comprehensive history and physical examination should be performed (Class I recommendation) (25). ECG may show severe sinus bradycardia, sinus pause, atrial or junctional escape rhythm, and/or atrial fibrillation/flutter. A 24-hour Holter monitor can document various manifestations of SND and the frequency. Once established, it is important to assess maximal heart rate response with an exercise stress test. Secondary etiologies must be investigated (drug screen, inflammatory markers, thyroid function testing, and metabolic etiologies). Further evaluation, if needed, will be undertaken by a pediatric electrophysiologist, with the possibility of pacemaker implantation based on the severity and history of symptomatic SND. Due to the lack of a minimal heart rate or pause criteria for permanent pacing, correlation between symptoms and bradycardia must determine the necessity of pacemaker implantation (25). Once the pacemaker is implanted, there is resolution of symptoms (29).

Atrio-ventricular heart blocks

First-degree atrio-ventricular heart block

First-degree heart block is defined as 1:1 atrioventricular conduction with a prolonged PR interval for age attributed to conduction delay within the atrium, AV node, and/or the His-Purkinje system. (30). It has been noted in neonates through adolescents (4, 31). Increased vagal tone is the most common mechanism in pediatric patients. Common secondary etiologies of first-degree heart block include intrinsic AV node disease, drugs (digoxin, beta blockers, calcium channel blockers), electrolyte abnormalities (hyper- and hypokalemia, hyper- and hypocalcemia, hypomagnesemia), hypothyroidism, hypothermia, myocarditis, Lyme disease, congenital heart disease (Ebstein's anomaly, atrial septal defect and atrioventricular canal defect), and less frequently, acute rheumatic fever in developed countries (9). Four sites for first degree AV block with a normal QRS include: atrium (3-20%), AV node (35-90%), Bundle of His (15%), and infra-Hisian conduction system (32). When accompanied with a wide QRS complex, conduction in the AV node or the bundle of His is delayed; bilateral bundle branch conduction is slowed in most cases; two levels of conduction delay are also seen (33). Normal P-R interval naturally varies with age in the pediatric population and prolongation of the P-R interval should be viewed in this context (see Figure 5). An ECG can detect first degree block with or without infranodal disease based on QRS pattern.

First-degree AV block does not require further evaluation in children who are otherwise asymptomatic; however, there is increased tendency to progress to higher degree AV block with myocarditis, especially in those with markedly prolonged PR interval (>300 msec) (34). Progression of first degree heart block to higher degree heart block is associated with spinal anesthesia (35). As the heart rate increases, it is expected that the PR interval shortens; in the absence of shortening of markedly prolonged PR intervals with activity and/or if the patient is symptomatic, further workup with an electrophysiologist may be needed (36). Indications for a pacemaker include first degree block with symptoms suggestive of a pacemaker syndrome

(Class IIa), and presence of first degree block in neuromuscular diseases and LV dysfunction (Class IIb) (37).

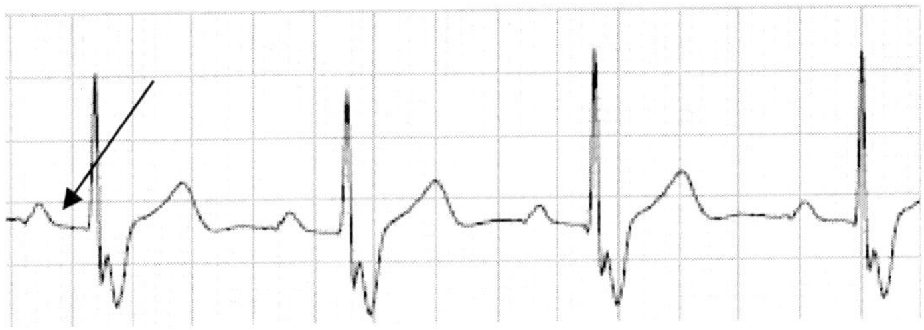

Figure 5. First degree AV block.

Second-degree atrio-ventricular heart block

Second-degree heart block is atrio-ventricular block characterized by intermittent dropped beats due to failure of conduction of atrial impulses. Second-degree AV block is of two types: Mobitz type I (Wenkebach) and Mobitz type II. Of the two types, Wenkebach-type is the most common. The location of the block determines the QRS duration; normal QRS duration implies block at the AV node and prolonged QRS duration indicates block within or below the His bundle (38). Von Burneth et al. detected 2% of infants, 7% of toddlers, and 6% of children to have second degree atrio-ventricular block type I at rest (39). Wenkebach occurs in infants, toddlers, and young children at rest and maybe mediated by increased vagal influence in athletes (39, 40). Wenkebach typically does not occur when awake except in elite athletes at rest. Myocarditis, cardiomyopathies, congenital heart disease, digoxin, beta blockers, and calcium channel blockers can cause Wenckebach phenomenon (9). Surgical repair of congenital heart disease is a risk factor for Wenkebach type and may progress to complete heart block (41). Mobitz type I block is usually benign. However, in pediatric population without heart disease, Mobitz type I block may rarely serve as intermediary prior to development of idiopathic complete heart block (41). In adults, second degree AV-nodal block proximal to the His bundle has a benign course in those without heart disease; but is associated with poor prognosis in those with underlying heart disease (42).

ECG criteria to be met for Mobitz type I include: 1) progressive prolongation of the PR intervals, 2) PR interval prolongation at progressively decreasing increments, 3) progressive shortening of the RR interval, and 4) eventual failure to conduct an atrial beat to the ventricle (43) (see Figure 6a). It is due to increased refractory period at the level of the AV node. In Wenkebach, a routine echocardiogram, therapy, or follow-up is not indicated.

Mobitz type II AV block is characterized by constant P-P interval and PR interval with intermittent non-conducted P-wave, with the ventricular rate being dependent on the conducted atrial beats (see Figure 6b). It is an "all or none" phenomenon. It is characterized by enhanced refractory period in the His-Purkinje system, which leads to conduction failure (9). It is considered a higher-degree block and is not considered normal in the pediatric population. Myocarditis, post-operative complication, and post-transplant coronary artery disease are the most common etiologies of Mobitz type II block in the pediatric population. It can progress to symptomatic complete heart block and is associated with Stokes-Adams attacks and sudden death (44). An electrophysiology study is indicated if there is unexplained syncope, and AV block distal to the AV node to identify the location of the block (45). In complete or high second-degree AV block, an echocardiogram is indicated (46). In patients with Mobitz type II, syncope is a poor prognostic factor (44). Symptomatic chronic bradycardia in Mobitz type I and type II (Class I), Mobitz type II with bifascicular or trifascicular block (Class I), Mobitz type II with wide QRS (Class I), asymptomatic Mobitz type II (Class IIa), and neuromuscular disease with AV block (Class IIb) are all indications for permanent pacemaker implantation (37).

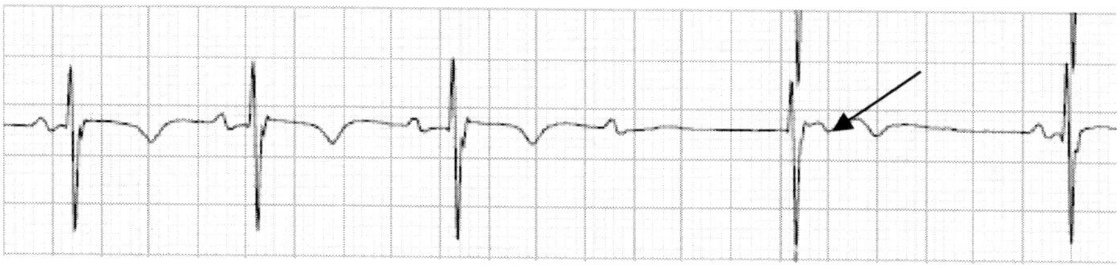

Figure 6A. Second degree Type I AV block (Wenkebach).

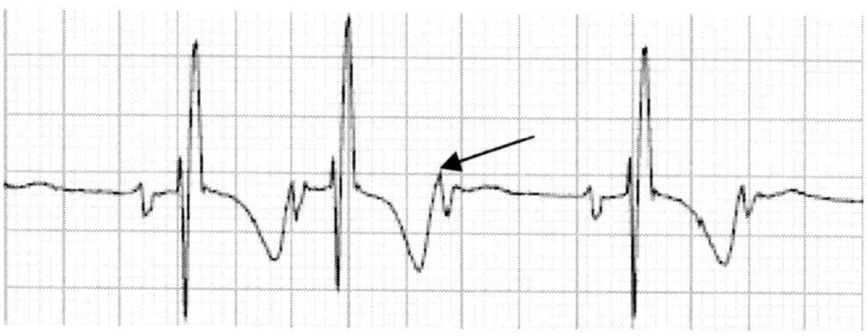

Figure 6B. Second degree Type II (Mobitz) AV block.

Third-degree (complete) atrio-ventricular heart block

Third degree or complete heart block is due to complete atrio-ventricular dissociation (see Figure 7). To establish the diagnosis of complete heart block, there is complete absence of conduction of atrial impulses to the ventricles (23). The ventricular complexes are independent of the atrial complexes, and the atrial rate is faster than the ventricular rate. Third-degree heart block may be acquired or congenital. The most common cause of acquired complete heart block in pediatric patients is surgical repair of congenital heart disease, in particular, left ventricular outflow tract obstruction, corrected transposition of the great arteries, AV canal defect repair, TOF or VSD repair (24). Lyme disease, Kawasaki disease, Chagas disease, diphtheria, rheumatic fever, Rocky Mountain Spotted Fever, myocarditis, cardiomyopathies, hypothyroidism, infiltrative diseases and metabolic diseases are other acquired etiologies (9, 24). Congenital complete heart block can be isolated or is often associated with structural heart disease (e.g., left atrial isomerism and L-transposition of the great arteries (2% per year incidence)), and maternal connective tissue disease (50%) including systemic lupus erythematosus, sarcoidosis, Sjogren syndrome, rheumatoid arthritis, and scleroderma (24, 47-49). Genetic causes have been identified as a cause of complete AV block. Cardiac transcription factor (*NKX2.5*), which leads to familial atrial septal defects, Holt-Oram syndrome (*TBX5*, hand-heart syndrome), and *SCN5A* sodium ion channel responsible for long QT and Brugada syndromes are three examples (24, 50, 51).

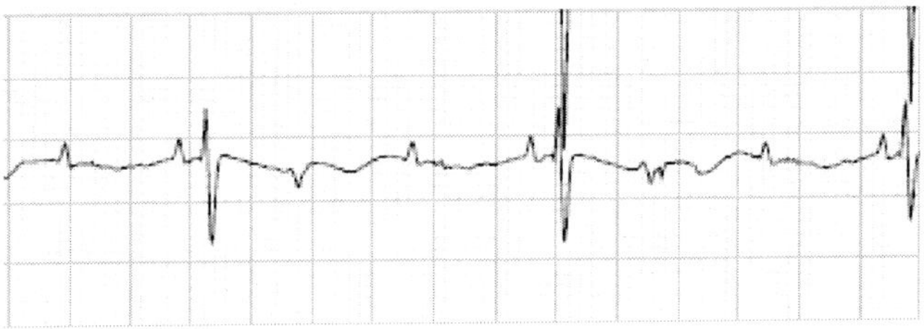

Figure 7. Third degree (complete) AV block.

Symptoms range from none to confusion, fatigue, weakness, syncope, exercise intolerance, lightheadedness, congestive heart failure, and sudden cardiac death in congenital complete heart block (9, 52). Symptoms are usually dependent on ventricular rate, form of escape rhythm, myocardial systolic and diastolic function, QT interval and atrio-ventricular synchrony. Ventricular rate is dependent on the level of origination of the escape rhythm which is at or below the level of the block; the more proximal the block, the higher the ventricular rate. Poor prognosis in the newborn period is associated with structural heart disease, hydrops in the postnatal period, ventricular rate less than 55 beats per minute, dilated ventricles, decreased ventricular function, prematurity and prolonged QT interval. In older children, syncope, presyncope, prolonged corrected QT interval, mitral regurgitation, heart rate less than 50 beats per minute, marked ventricular dilation and impaired systolic dysfunction (compensatory mechanism for slow heart rates), multifocal ventricular ectopy, low-Hisian/ventricular escape rhythm, and ventricular tachycardia are associated with poor prognosis and also indications for pacing (53, 54).

On ECG, there is complete atrioventricular dissociation. The QRS complexes can be narrow to wide depending on the level of the block. It is important to differentiate between complete heart block versus 2:1 AV block. With prognostic factors including ECG and structural criteria, a Holter monitor and an echocardiogram must be part of the evaluation, prior to consideration of a pacemaker; the indications for pacing are stated above. The echocardiogram must evaluate any structural defects, atrioventricular valve regurgitation, ventricular systolic and diastolic function, and ventricular dimensions. If echo is unsatisfactory due to poor imaging windows, a cardiac MRI should be considered. Exercise stress testing is necessary to assess exercise tolerance and potential for arrhythmias when deciding activity restrictions. For postoperative complete heart block, pacing is indicated if there is no return of sinus rhythm for at least 7-10 post-operative days. Management of complete heart block is with implantation of a permanent pacemaker for the indications stated above. Post pacemaker implantation for CAVB, there is a decrease in heart size and normalization of shortening fraction in most patients (55).

Escape rhythms

Escape rhythms can arise at various levels of the conduction based on the level of a conduction block and/or dysfunction of a more proximal pacemaker. Pediatric heart rates for atrial, junctional, and ventricular escape rhythms range from 60-80 beats per minute, 40-60 beats per minute, and 20-40 beats per minutes, respectively (56, 57).

Atrial escape rhythm

Atrial escape rhythm arises from ectopic atrial foci during periods of severe sinus bradycardia or significant sinus node dysfunction. These atrial ectopic foci have slower spontaneous rates and are unstable. The exact incidence of atrial escape rhythm is not known. The automaticity of an ectopic atrial focus generates a faster rate than the dysfunctional sinus node by escaping overdrive suppression of the SA node. Atrial escape rhythm rate is between 60-80 beats per minute (58). The P-wave morphology differs from the sinus P-wave. The P-wave is smaller and shorter in duration with the P-wave axis dependent on the location of the ectopic focus. The PR interval may be shorter than the normal PR interval due to the proximity of the ectopic atrial focus to the AV node. The atrial escape rhythm is slower than the normal sinus rate. Resolution or treatment of a slow underlying sinus rhythm resolves the atrial escape rhythm. Automaticity in ectopic foci is more responsive to autonomic control compared to the SA node (59). Most symptoms are secondary to underlying rhythm abnormalities such as sinus node dysfunction with severe sinus bradycardia, sinus pause and/or sinus arrest. This will manifest as lightheadedness, activity intolerance and syncope. Although stimulants/sympathomimetic agents increase the ventricular rate, symptoms refractory to medical therapy likely require pacemaker implantation. Work-up is focused on identifying the underlying abnormality leading to increased automaticity or suppression of the sinus node.

Atrio-ventricular junctional escape rhythm

AV junctional escape rhythm is defined as an ectopic rhythm originating from the AV node or the proximal His bundle at the junction of the atrium and the ventricle (56, 60). Southall et al. reported 19% of full-term neonates with episodes of junctional escape rhythm (3). Due to the lack of overdrive suppression from the higher pacemakers, the AV junction has its intrinsic automaticity with an escape rate ranging between 40-60 beats per minute (58). Nodal escape rhythm is associated with apnea (61). The rate of AV junctional escape rhythm varies with underlying conditions, such as sick sinus syndrome, complete heart block, ablation of AV node, congenital heart surgery including Fontan palliation, hypertrophic cardiomyopathy, and ischemia (60, 62-67). It is common in athletes with heightened vagal tone, primarily during rest, and equally in both genders. Secondary causes can include anorexia nervosa, congestive heart failure, myocarditis, digoxin toxicity, medications (beta blockers, calcium channel blockers), Lyme disease, muscular dystrophy, ventricular noncompaction, inflammation, hypoxia, metabolic, drugs, electrolyte disturbances and channelopathies (68-70). Junctional escape rhythm can occur intermittently during sinus pauses, atrial "standstill", and intermittent AV block (71). Symptoms pertaining to AV junctional escape rhythm are related to suppression of the sino-atrial tissues and or failure to conduct to the junction. Symptoms include lightheadedness, palpitations, dyspnea, exercise intolerance, or syncope.

In AV junctional escape rhythm, there are no P-waves before the QRS complexes; they may occur simultaneously or follow the QRS complexes. The QRS complex is narrow if the focus is closer to the AV node or wide if proximal to the His bundle bifurcation. In the case of complete AV block, P-waves of sinus origin are dissociated from the QRS complexes. ECG may identify the rhythm; if unsuccessful, a Holter monitor can help identify the rhythm abnormality. Workup should also include identifying the causes listed above. Pacemaker implantation may be needed in symptomatic bradycardia due to junctional escape rhythm.

Idioventricular escape rhythm

Ventricular escape (idioventricular) rhythm arises in the absence/suppression of pacemaker activity or a conduction block at or above the level of the His bundle. The ventricular escape results when the higher pacemaker systems are unable to generate and/or conduct an impulse to the ventricles. It is rare, and incidence is not known. Idioventricular rate ranges from 20-40 beats per minute (58). A diagnosis that should be considered in the differential diagnosis of idioventricular escape rhythm is sinus bradycardia with a complete bundle branch block, although the ventricular rate would differentiate the two rhythms. Multiple etiologies result in idioventricular rhythm, including enhanced parasympathetic stimulation (athletes), complete heart block, myocarditis, hypothermia, drugs (adrenaline, digoxin toxicity, cocaine), and ischemic conditions (72). Stokes-Adams syncopal attacks are more prevalent in ventricular escape rhythm than atrial or junctional escape rhythms. This is also accompanied by hypotension, dizziness, syncope and exercise intolerance.

The ECG shows wide QRS complexes with a rate of 20-40 beats per minute, with atrioventricular dissociation. If P-waves exist, they occur independently and are dissociated from the ventricular beats. ECG is the first step in diagnosing ventricular escape rhythm. Holter and event recorders are alternatives when ECG is not diagnostic. Electrophysiology study is indicated (class IIA) in patients with suspected bradyarrhythmias with syncope (31). An EP study can establish the level of the AV block. Symptomatic relief is important in patients with ventricular escape rhythm. Pacemaker implantation with ventricular pacing is essential to avoid Stokes-Adams attacks (73).

Pacemaker indications

Class 1 indications for permanent pacemaker implantation include: symptomatic high second-degree and third-degree atrioventricular block (level C); symptomatic sinus node dysfunction (level B); postoperative complete or high second-degree AV block that is not expected to resolve or persisting more than 7-10 days (level B); CCHB with wide QRS escape rhythm, complex ventricular ectopy, or ventricular dysfunction (level B); and CCHB in an infant with ventricular rate is less than 55 bpm, or with congenital heart disease with a ventricular rate less than 70 bpm (level C) (74).

Conclusion

An important goal for pediatric care providers is to identify whether a rhythm is normal or abnormal. Interpretation of an ECG appropriately in the context of clinical manifestations is an essential skill. It helps to differentiate arrhythmias that need further evaluation, follow up or management from benign variants. Sinus arrhythmia is a normal variation in the heart rate associated with phasic variation in respiration, which is benign and does not require additional work-up. Hypervagotonia manifesting as sinus bradycardia, first degree AV block or second degree type I AV block and premature complexes in the presence of structurally normal heart are usually benign. Athletes with intense physical conditioning demonstrate lower resting heart rates. Symptomatic sinus node dysfunction manifested as sinus bradycardia, escape rhythms, and atrial fibrillation/flutter warrants evaluation and treatment. Referral to pediatric cardiology should be considered when the arrhythmia is associated with symptoms, is complex, has unclear etiology or requires further evaluation and/or intervention.

Using a systematic approach to ECG interpretation will allow the clinician to reassure the parents and/or guardians or to seek further evaluation and management by the pediatric cardiology service. A number of common normal variants and pathological rhythms were presented in the chapter. There are primary and secondary etiologies for rhythm abnormalities and the ability to recognize the rhythms will insure appropriate patient care. *Scientia est potentia*-knowledge is power!

REFERENCES

[1] Kaushal P, Taylor JA. Inter-relations among declines in arterial distensibility, baroreflex function and respiratory sinus arrhythmia. J Am Coll Cardiol 2002;39:1524-30.

[2] Coker R, Koziell A, Oliver C, Smith SE. Does the sympathetic nervous system influence sinus arrhythmia in man? Evidence from combined autonomic blockade. J Physiol 1984; 356:459-64.

[3] Southall DP, Richards J, Mitchell P, Brown DJ, Johnston PG, Shinebourne EA. Study of cardiac rhythm in healthy newborn infants. Br Heart J 1980;43:14-20.

[4] Scott O, Williams GJ, Fiddler GI. Results of 24-hour ambulatory monitoring of electrocardiogram in 131 healthy boys aged 10 to 13 years. Br Heart J 1980;44:304-8.

[5] Nagashima M, Matsushima M, Ogawa A, Ohsuga A, Kaneko T, Yazaki T, et al. Cardiac arrhythmias in healthy children revealed by 24-hour ambulatory ECG monitoring. Pediatr Cardiol 1987;8(2):103-8.

[6] Wallace AG, Daggett WM. Re-Excitation of the Atrium. "the Echo Phenomenon". Am Heart J 1964; 68:661-6.

[7] Jideus L, Kesek M, Joachimsson PO, Ericson M, Nilsson L, Blomstrom-Lundqvist C. The role of premature atrial contractions as the main triggers of postoperative atrial fibrillation. J Electrocardiol 2006;39:48-54.

[8] Sugimoto T, Hayakawa H, Osada H, Yamazaki N, Mori H, Yasuda H, Sakamoto A. Clinical evaluation of bisoprolol in the treatment of extrasystoles and sinus tachycardia: an interim report. J Cardiovasc Pharmacol 1986;8(Suppl 11):S171-4.

[9] Doniger SJ, Sharieff GQ. Pediatric dysrhythmias. Pediatr Clin North Am 2006;53(1):85-105.

[10] Silka MJ, Garson A, Jr. Ventricular Arrhythmias. In: Gillette PC, Garson A Jr, eds. Clinical pediatric arrhythmias. Philadelphia, PA: WB Saunders, 1999:121-45.

[11] Frolkis JP, Pothier CE, Blackstone EH, Lauer MS. Frequent ventricular ectopy after exercise as a predictor of death. N Engl J Med, 2003;348:781-90.

[12] Paridon S. Clinical stress testing in the pediatric age group. A statement from the American Heart Association Council on Cardiovascular Disease in the Young, Committee on Atherosclerosis, Hypertension, and Obesity in Youth. Circulation 2006;113:1905-20.

[13] Zipes D. ACC/AHA/ESC 2006 Guidelines for management of patients with ventricular arrhythmias and the prevention of sudden cardiac death. J Am Coll Cardiol 2006;48:e247-e346.

[14] Dickinson DF, Scott O. Ambulatory electrocardiographic monitoring in 100 healthy teenage boys. Br Heart J 1984;51(2):179-83.

[15] Alexander M. Ventricular arrhythmias in children and young adults. In: Walsh E, Saul J, Triedman J, eds. Cardiac arrhythmias in children and young adults with congenital heart disease. Philadelphia, PA: Lippincott Williams Wilkins, 2001:219.

[16] Zhu DW, Maloney JD, Simmons TW, Nitta J, Fitzgerald DM, Trohman RG, et al. Radiofrequency catheter ablation for management of symptomatic ventricular ectopic activity. J Am Coll Cardiol 1995;26:843-9.

[17] Zipes DP, Garson A, Jr. 26th Bethesda conference: recommendations for determining eligibility for competition in athletes with cardiovascular abnormalities. Task Force 6: arrhythmias. J Am Coll Cardiol, 1994; 24:892-9.
[18] Hiss RG, Lamb LE. Electrocardiographic findings in 122,043 individuals. Circulation 1962; 25:947-61.
[19] Hoffman BF, Cranefield PF. The physiological basis of cardiac arrhythmias. Am J Med 1964;37:670-84.
[20] Rosen MR, Fisch C, Hoffman BF, Danilo P, Jr., Lovelace DE, Knoebel SB. Can accelerated atrioventricular junctional escape rhythms be explained by delayed afterdepolarizations? Am J Cardiol 1980;45:1272-84.
[21] Olgin J, Zipes D. Specific arrhythmias: Diagnosis and treatment: Premature ventricular complexes. In: Zipes D, Braunwald E, Libby P, Bonow R, eds. Braunwald's heart disease: A textbook of cardiovascular medicine. Philadelphia, PA: Saunders, 2005:838-41.
[22] Sharma S, Whyte G, Elliott P, Padula M, Kaushal R, Mahon N, et al. Electrocardiographic changes in 1000 highly trained junior elite athletes. Br J Sports Med 1999;33(5):319-24.
[23] Jat KR, Lodha R, Kabra SK. Arrhythmias in children. Ind J Ped 2011;78:211-8.
[24] Baruteau AE, Perry JC, Sanatani S, Horie M, Dubin AM. Evaluation and management of bradycardia in neonates and children. Eur J Pediatr 2016;175(2):151-61.
[25] Kusumoto FM, Schoenfeld MH, Barrett C, Edgerton JR, Ellengogen KA, Gold MR, et al. 2018 ACC/AHA/HRS Guideline on the evaluation and management of patients with bradycardia and cardiac conduction delay: Executive summary: A report of the American College of Cardiology/American Heart Association Task Force on Clinical Practice Guidelines, and the Heart Rhythm Society. J Am Coll Cardiol 2018. pii: S0735-1097(18)38984-8.
[26] Yabek SM, Swensson RE, Jarmakani JM. Electrocardiographic recognition of sinus node dysfunction in children and young adults. Circulation 1977;56(2):235-9.
[27] Yabek SM, Jarmakani JM. Sinus node dysfunction in children, adolescents, and young adults. Pediatrics 1978;61(4):593-8.
[28] Fishberger S. Sinus node dysfunction. In: Walsh E, Saul J, Triedman J, eds. Cardiac arrhythmias in children and young adults with congenital heart disease. Philadelphia, PA: Lippincott Williams Wilkins, 2001:271-83.
[29] Kardelen F, Celiker A, Ozer S, Ozme S, Oto A. Sinus node dysfunction in children and adolescents: treatment by implantation of a permanent pacemaker in 26 patients. Turk J Ped 2002;44:312-6.
[30] Alimurung MM, Massell BF. The normal PR interval in infants and children. Circulation 1956;13:257-62.
[31] Ferrer P. Arrhythmias in the neonate, infant, and child. In: Roberts N, Gelband H, eds. Arrhythmias in the neonate. New York: Appleton-Century-Crofts, 1977:265-316.
[32] Sherron P, Torres-Arraut E, Tamer D, Garcia OL, Wolff GS. Site of conduction delay and electrophysiologic significance of first-degree atrioventricular block in children with heart disease. Am J Cardiol 1985;55:1323-7.
[33] Peuch P, Groileau R, Guimond C. Incidence of different types of A-V block and their localization by His bundle recordings. In: Wellens HJ, Lie KI, Janse MJ, eds. The conduction system of the heart. Leiden: Stenfert, 1976:467.
[34] Mymin D, Mathewson FA, Tate RB, Manfreda J. The natural history of primary first-degree atrioventricular heart block. N Engl J Med 1986;315:1183-7.
[35] Bernards CM, Hymas NJ. Progression of first degree heart block to high-grade second degree block during spinal anesthesia. Can J Anaest 1992;39(2):173-5.
[36] Barold SS, Ilercil A, Leonelli F, Herweg B. First-degree atrioventricular block. Clinical manifestations, indications for pacing, pacemaker management and consequences during cardiac resynchronization. J Interv Card Electrophysiol 2006;17(2):139-52.
[37] Gregaratos G, Abrams J, Epstein AE, Freedman RA, Hayes DL, Hlatky MA, et al. ACC/AHA/NASPE 2002 Guideline update for implantation of cardiac pacemakers and antiarrhythmia devices. Circulation 2002;106(16):2145-61.

[38] Gilette P, Reitman M, Gutgesell H, Vargo TA, Mullins CE, McNamara DG, et al. Intracardiac electrophysiology in children and young adults. Am Heart J 1975;89:36-44.

[39] von Bernuth G, Toussaint R, Mund C, Rabe P, Timbul K. [Heart rate and heart rhythm in healthy infants and children]. Klin Pädiatr 1989;201:98-103. [German]

[40] Stein R, Medeiros CM, Rosito GA, Zimerman LI, Ribeiro JP. Intrinsic sinus and atrioventricular node electrophysiologic adaptations in endurance athletes. J Am Coll Cardiol 2002;39:1033-8.

[41] Young D, Eisenberg R, Fish B, Fisher JD. Wenckebach atrioventricular block (Mobitz type I) in children and adolescents. Am J Cardiol 1977;40:393-9.

[42] Strasberg B, Amat YLF, Dhingra RC, Palileo E, Swiryn S, Bauernfeind R, Wyndham C, Rosen KM. Natural history of chronic second-degree atrioventricular nodal block. Circulation 1981;63:1043-9.

[43] Denes P, Levy L, Pick A, Rosen KM. The incidence of typical and atypical A-V Wenkebach periodicity. Am Heart J 1975;89:26-31.

[44] Dhingra RC, Denes P, Wu D, Chuquimia R, Rosen KM. The significance of second degree atrioventricular block and bundle branch block. Observations regarding site and type of block. Circulation 1974;49:638-46.

[45] Zipes DP, DiMarco JP, Gillette PC, Jackman WM, Myerburg RJ, Rahimtoola SH, Ritchie JL, Cheitlin MD, Garson A, Jr., Gibbons RJ, et al. ACC/AHA Guidelines for clinical intracardiac electrophysiological and catheter ablation procedures. A report of the American College of Cardiology/American Heart Association Task Force on Practice Guidelines (Committee on Clinical Intracardiac Electrophysiologic and Catheter Ablation Procedures), developed in collaboration with the North American Society of Pacing and Electrophysiology. J Am Coll Cardiol 1995;26:555-73.

[46] Cheitlin MD, Armstrong WF, Aurigemma GP, Beller GA, Bierman FZ, Davis JL, Douglas PS, Faxon DP, Gillam LD, Kimball TR, Kussmaul WG, Pearlman AS, Philbrick JT, Rakowski H, Thys DM. ACC/AHA/ASE 2003 guideline update for the clinical application of echocardiography–summary article: a report of the American College of Cardiology/American Heart Association Task Force on Practice Guidelines (ACC/AHA/ASE Committee to Update the 1997 Guidelines for the Clinical Application of Echocardiography). J Amer Coll Cardiol 2003;42:954-70.

[47] Tan E. Antinuclear antibodies: diagnostic markers for autoimmune diseases and probes for cell biology. Adv Immunol 1989;44:93-152.

[48] Meilof J, Smeenk R. Autoantibodies and their target antigens in Sjogren's Syndrome. Neth J Med 1992;40(3-4):140-7.

[49] Waltuck J, Buyon J. Autoantibody-associated congenital heart block: outcome in mothers and children. Ann Intern Med 1994;120:144-51.

[50] Elliott DA, Kirk EP, Yeoh T, et al. Cardiac homeobox gene NKX2.5 mutations and congenital heart disease: associations with atrial septal defect and hypoplastic left heart syndrome. J Am Coll Cardiol 2003;41:2072-76.

[51] Probst V, Hoorntje T, Hulsbeck M, et al. Cardiac conduction defect associated with mutation in SCN5A. Nature Genet 1999;23:20-1.

[52] Gomes J, Sherif NE. Atrioventricular block: mechanism, clinical presentation, and therapy. Med Clin North Am 1984;68:955-67.

[53] Kertesz NJ, Fenrich AL, Friedman RA. Congenital complete atrioventricular block. Tex Heart Inst J 1997 24:301-7.

[54] Michaelsson M, Riesenfeld T, Jonzon A. Natural history of congenital complete atrioventricular block. Pacing Clin Electrophysiol 1997;20(8 pt 2):2098-101.

[55] Bruer JM, Udink Ten Cate FE, Kapusta L, Cohen MI, Crosson JE, Boramanand N, et al. Pacemaker therapy in isolated congenital complete atrioventricular block. Pacing Clin Electrophysiol 2002;25(12):1685-91.

[56] Hafeez Y, Grossman SA. Junctional rhythm. StatPearls 2018. URL: https://www.ncbi.nlm.nih.gov/books/NBK507715/.

[57] Grimm W, Hoffmann J, Maisch B. Accelerated idioventricular rhythm. Z Kardiol 1994;83 (12):898-907.

[58] Dubin D. Rapid Interpretation of EKGs. Fort Meyers, FL: COVER, 2000:112-21.

[59] Randall WC, Wehrmacher WH, Jones SB. Hierarchy of supraventricular pacemakers. J Thorac Cardiovasc Surg 1981;82:797-800.

[60] Alison JF, Yeung-Lai-Wah JA, Schulzer M, Kerr CR. Characterization of junctional rhythm after atrioventricular node ablation. Circulation 1995;91:84-90.

[61] Valimaki I, Tarlo PA. Heart rate patterns and apnea in newborn infants. Am J Obstet Gynecol 1971;110:343-9.

[62] Shepard RK, Natale A, Stambler BS, Wood MA, Gilligan DM, Ellenbogen KA. Physiology of the escape rhythm after radiofrequency atrioventricular junctional ablation. Pacing Clin Electrophysiol 1998;21:1085-92.

[63] Pattoneri P, Astorri E. Junctional rhythm in hypertrophic cardiomyopathy: A case report. Int J Cardiol 2006;113:E117-8.

[64] Levy AM, Camm AJ, Keane JF. Multiple arrhythmias detected during nocturnal monitoring in patients with congenital complete heart block. Circulation 1977;55:247-53.

[65] Kleinfeld MJ, Boal BH. Junctional escape rhythm in the sick sinus syndrome. Cardiol 1978; 63:193-8.

[66] Momma K, Takao A, Shibata T. Characteristics and natural history of abnormal atrial rhythms in left isomerism. Am J Cardiol 1990;65(3):231-6.

[67] Aresman FW, Bostock J, Radley-Smith R, Yacoub MH. Cardiac rhythm and conduction before and after anatomic correction of transposition of the great arteries. Am J Cardiol 1983; 52(7):836-9.

[68] Fisch C, Knoebel SB. Junctional rhythms. Prog Cardiovasc Dis 1970;13:141-58.

[69] Kossaify A. management of sinus node dysfunction with junctional escape rhythm in a case of anorexia nervosa. Turk Kardi Dern Ars 2010;38(7):486-8.

[70] Kim D, Shinohara T, Joung B, Maruyama M, Chol EK, On YK, et al. Calcium dynamics and the mechanisms of atrioventricular junctional rhythm. *J Am Coll Cardiol* 2010;56(10):805-12.

[71] Disertori M, Guarnerio M, Vergara G, Del Favero A, Bettini R, Inama G, et al. Familial endemic persistent atrial standstill in a small mountain community: Review of eight cases. Eur Heart J 1983;4(5):354-61.

[72] Talbot S, Greaves M. Association of ventricular extrasystoles and ventricular tachycardia with idioventricular rhythm. Br Heart J 1976;38:457-64.

[73] Sigurd B, Sandoe E. Management of Stokes-Adams syndrome. Cardiology 1990;77(3):195-208.

[74] Epstein AE, DiMarco JP, Ellenbogen KA, Estes NAM III, Freedman RA, Gettes LS, et al. ACC/AHA/HRS 2008 guidelines for device-based therapy of cardiac rhythm abnormalities: executive summary: a report of the American College of Cardiology/American Heart Association Task Force on Practice Guidelines (Writing Committee to Revise the ACC/AHA/NASPE 2002 Guideline Update for Implantation of Cardiac Pacemakers and Antiarrhythmia Devices). J Am Coll Cardiol 2008;51:2085–105.

In: Chronic Disease and Disability
Editors: DE Greydanus, P Anne, JD Rowlett et al.

ISBN: 978-1-53617-656-8

Chapter 6

COMMON PEDIATRIC ARRHYTHMIAS: PART II

Premchand Anne[1,*], MD, MPH, MBA, FAAP, FACP, FACC and Harinder R Singh[2], MD, FHRS, CEPS-P, CCDS

[1]Pediatric Cardiology, Ascension St John Children's Hospital, Detroit, Michigan, United States of America

[2]Associate Professor, Pediatric Electrophysiology, The Children's Hospital of San Antonio, San Antonio, Texas, United States of America

ABSTRACT

In part I of common pediatric arrhythmias, we discussed normal variants and brady-arrhythmias in detail with attention to definition, epidemiology, natural history, mechanism and management. In part II of this evidence-based review article, we will focus our attention on most common pediatric tachy-arrhythmias. The objective is to familiarize pediatricians with electrocardiogram (ECG) interpretation, assist the pediatrician in recognition and management of common pediatric tachy-arrhythmias.

INTRODUCTION

Sinus tachycardia is an automatic rhythm characterized by rapid discharge from the sinus node due to physiologic influences (1, 2). The rate of sinus tachycardia is dependent on age and on the body's increased sympathetic response to physiologic phenomena, such as fever, pain, anxiety, dehydration, medications, anemia, hyperthyroidism and heart failure. It occurs due to increased automaticity with rate variability associated with increased sympathetic response or vagal withdrawal. Decreasing the underlying enhanced sympathetic tone or increasing the vagal tone will decrease the sinus tachycardia. Most of the patients are asymptomatic from the cardiovascular standpoint. However, very high rate of sinus tachycardia can compromise

* Correspondence: Premchand Anne, MD, Pediatric Cardiology, Ascension St John Children's Hospital, 22201 Moross, Suite 275, PB II, Detroit, MI 48236, United States. Email: Premchand.anne@ascension.org.

cardiac output by decreasing the ventricular filling time. The inciting factor for sympathetic response or vagal withdrawal is the usual presenting symptom.

On the ECG, there is a normal P-wave axis and a P-wave precedes each QRS complex (3). P-waves may have larger amplitude and become peaked (2). It is important to identify the extrinsic factors causing the tachycardia and treat them; it is also necessary to rule out inappropriate sinus tachycardia (see below). Prognosis depends on the nature of the underlying cause. No specific treatment is required for physiologic sinus tachycardia except treatment of the underlying cause(s). Beta-adrenergic receptor blockers have occasionally been used for treatment of symptomatic physiologic sinus tachycardia (2).

Inappropriate Sinus Tachycardia (IST)

It is defined by elevated resting heart rate and/or an exaggerated heart rate response to exercise or stress (2, 4). IST often follows a viral illness or physical trauma, usually in women (90%) who are generally healthy physically and emotionally (5). Etiology is not known. The mechanism may involve a primary sino-atrial (SA) node disorder with increased automaticity, a dysautonomia with increased sympathetic tone, decreased parasympathetic tone, increased SA node beta-adrenergic sensitivity, impaired baroreflex control or a combination of the above (4-7). Another mechanism is stimulation of the beta-adrenergic receptors by anti-beta-adrenergic receptor autoantibodies (8). IST is more common in women in the 20s and 30s, who are otherwise healthy. It is likely to improve over time and tends to have a benign course (5, 9). Palpitations, lightheadedness, exercise intolerance, and fatigue are common symptoms. Patients may also have orthostatic intolerance, chest pain, anxiety, depression, headache, myalgia, gastro-intestinal disturbances, and diaphoresis (5, 10). Only consistent finding on physical exam is tachycardia (5, 10).

On ECG, P-wave morphology is similar to that of normal sinus rhythm (10). There is sinus tachycardia at rest on ECG. Criteria for diagnosis include: 1) persistent sinus tachycardia during the day with increased rate in response to activity and normalization during sleep per 24-hour Holter recording, 2) non-paroxysmal tachycardia and symptoms, 3) P-wave morphology and activation similar to sinus rhythm, and 4) exclusion of secondary causes of sinus tachycardia (2). Secondary causes of sinus tachycardia can include alcohol, caffeine, tobacco, cocaine, beta-blocker withdrawal, other stimulants, and medical conditions including anemia, dehydration, anxiety, pain, fever, pericarditis, and exercise to name a few (7).

In addition to the ECG, a 24-holter monitor will document elevated mean heart rates above normal for age, elevated daytime heart rates, and/or exaggerated elevation in sinus rate from supine to upright position (10). A diagnostic electrophysiology (EP) study should be considered if the etiology of the tachycardia is unclear (to rule out sinus node re-entry tachycardia). EP study consistent with IST would include slow warm up and cool down phases suggesting sinus node involvement, surface P-wave similar to that of normal sinus rhythm, and earliest activation arising near the sinus node area along the crista terminalis during mapping. IST is not initiated with programmed stimulation of the atria (11). In addition to electrophysiology testing, there is also a need for testing the autonomic nervous system. Neurologic, cardiovascular rehabilitation, and psychiatric consultations are often necessary because IST is a diagnosis of exclusion (10).

The primary method of treatment is a multidisciplinary approach. High dose beta-blockers are the first-line therapy and are often ineffective (7). Medications including beta-blockers, calcium channel blockers, class IC anti-arrhythmic agents and ivabradine are commonly used and decrease SA node automaticity (8). However, in patients with IST secondary to autonomic dysregulation, control of heart rate does not always lead to resolution of symptoms. In patients with no evidence of autonomic dysregulation, if biofeedback, meditation, and medical therapy fail, superolateral crista terminalis ablation should be considered (5, 10). Risks of RF ablation include SVC syndrome, diaphragmatic paralysis and persistent junctional rhythm. The prognosis of IST is benign over a mean follow-up of 6 years (9).

Sinus node re-entry tachycardia

Sino-atrial node re-entry tachycardia (SNRT) is a paroxysmal arrhythmia characterized by a focal re-entry circuit that is located entirely within the SA node or the peri-sinus atrial tissue (11). Incidence of SNRT is underestimated due to lack of symptoms in the majority. In patients undergoing electrophysiology study for supraventricular tachycardia, incidence ranges from 1.8%-16.9% (2). Incidence of SNRT is higher (10%) in those with underlying organic heart disease (12). A re-entry mechanism is present but it is not known whether the entire circuit is within the SA node or involves perisinus atrial tissue. Symptoms include palpitations, lightheadedness, presyncope, and rarely syncope (13). SNRT heart rate ranges from 80-200 beats/min. P-waves are similar to that of normal sinus rhythm. P-R interval is shorter than R-P interval. An atrio-ventricular (AV) nodal Wenkebach block may be present (14). Due to the similarity of SNRT to sinus tachycardia, it is underdiagnosed (15).

Criteria for diagnosis include: 1) paroxysmal tachycardia, 2) P-wave morphology and endocardial atrial activation similar to that of normal sinus rhythm, 3) inducibility with programmed premature atrial stimuli irrespective of the location of stimulation or the AV junction, 4) the ability to terminate the arrhythmia with atrial premature beat or atrial pacing, and 5) termination with vagal maneuvers or adenosine (2, 16). An electrophysiology study (EPS) is indicated in patients with frequent and poorly-tolerated episodes of tachycardia, unclear mechanism of tachycardia, and refractoriness to medications. Vagal maneuvers or adenosine may interrupt the tachycardia. Acutely, atrial pacing is effective. Beta blockers, calcium channel blockers, amiodarone, and digitalis can benefit patients with increased frequency of symptoms. However, prophylactic treatment of SNRT is not recommended. In patients undergoing an EPS, catheter ablation can be successfully performed at the same time (17).

Ectopic (focal) atrial tachycardia

Ectopic or focal atrial tachycardia (EAT) is a tachycardia mediated by inappropriate atrial impulse generation from a single atrial focus outside of the SA node (18). EAT is commonly found in children and teenagers and makes up approximately 15% of all newly diagnosed supraventricular tachycardias across all ages (18). Both genders are equally affected. Prevalence of EAT is 0.34% in asymptomatic male patients and 0.46% in symptomatic male patients (19). EAT can be due to three mechanisms: 1) enhanced automaticity, 2) triggered activity, and 3) microreentry (20). However, the exact mechanism is difficult to ascertain. In the majority of patients, the course is benign. Persistent incessant EAT can lead to ventricular dysfunction, leading to congestive heart failure and low cardiac output states, termed tachycardia-mediated cardiomyopathy. Termination of the rhythm can lead to improvement in ventricular function (21, 22). There is slowing of heart rate with time, with reversion to sinus rhythm or change in P-wave morphology (19).

Young patients are often asymptomatic until onset of left ventricular dysfunction. Patients may also have palpitations, lightheadedness, and exercise intolerance even with normal LV function (18). ECG shows a supraventricular tachycardia with rates within normal range to 300 beats per minute. ECG criteria for diagnosis include: 1) the P-wave morphology and axis different than that of normal sinus rhythm, 2) acceleration after initiation and deceleration before termination, 3) unaffected by presence of an atrio-ventricular block, and 4) an initial P-wave of the tachycardia similar to the subsequent P-waves (15). The QRS complex is similar to that of sinus rhythm. The location of the site of origin of the ectopic atrial tachycardia can be determined by noting P-wave frontal plane axis. "Warm-up" and "cool-down" patterns can be appreciated and are suggestive of an automatic mechanism. AV-block (Mobitz 1) can be appreciated episodically during sleep. Adenosine administration will demonstrate AV-block with continuous marching of P-waves (see Figure 1). Difficulty to terminate tachycardia with pacing maneuvers and external cardioversion are suggestive of an automatic EAT (18). Echocardiography at the time of diagnosis is important to document the baseline ventricular function (22). Electrophysiology testing is occasionally necessary to help differentiate between different types and mechanisms of tachycardia.

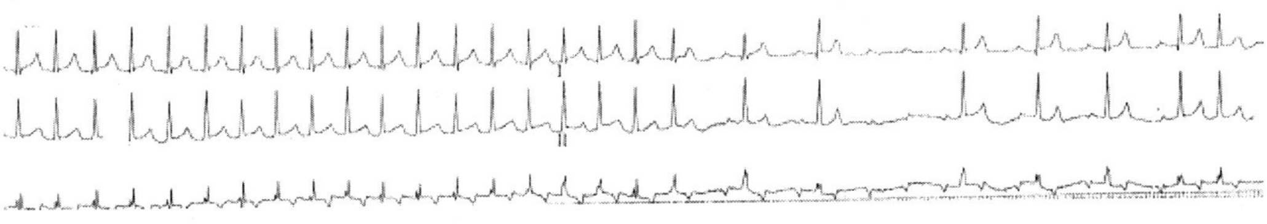

Figure 1. Ectopic atrial tachycardia with effect of adenosine.

Paroxysmal and incessant atrial tachycardia are difficult to treat medically (2). Acute therapy includes IV verapamil and IV beta blockers. There is no termination of tachycardia with atrial pacing, except for mild slowing of the heart rate. DC cardioversion may be effective only in those with micro-re-entry mechanism. Class IA (e.g., quinidine) and IC (e.g., flecainide, propafenone) antiarrhythmics are indicated for those without cardiac failure and Class III (amiodarone) is recommended in those with poor ventricular function (2). Chronic therapy includes calcium channel blockers, beta blockers, Classes IA, IC, and III anti-arrhythmics; Class IC is not indicated in those with coronary artery disease. Intravenous amiodarone or oral sotalol can reduce rates and restore sinus rhythm (23). Catheter ablation is successful in 86-90% with recurrence rate of 8% (18, 24). In children, 75% had restoration of normal sinus rhythm after medical therapy (22). In patients with medication refractory EAT or incessant EAT with tachycardia-induced cardiomyopathy, best therapy is ablation of the focus (2).

MULTIFOCAL (CHAOTIC) ATRIAL TACHYCARDIA

Multifocal (chaotic) atrial tachycardia (MAT) is a tachycardia characterized by electrocardiographic finding of multiple (at least three) distinct P-wave morphologies with irregular P-P intervals, isoelectric baseline between P-waves and ventricular rate >100 beats/min (2). MAT is a rare entity. In the pediatric age group, it is reported exclusively in neonates and infants, mostly associated with a normal heart (25). It is also associated with post-operative congenital heart disease, hypertrophic and dilated cardiomyopathies, and unrepaired atrial septal defects (18). Incidence is 0.2% among infants presenting with new onset arrhythmias (26). MAT is also associated with significant respiratory disease, hypoxemia, glucose intolerance, hypokalemia, digitalis, and chronic renal failure (27). Exact mechanism of MAT is unclear; however, automaticity versus triggered activity is postulated (18). Spontaneous resolution may occur in 50-80% of patients with MAT by 12-18 months of age (30). There is no recurrence of MAT in infants with normal cardiac structure (16, 29).

Most patients sent for cardiac evaluation are asymptomatic. If tachycardia is persistent, cardiomyopathy develops and symptoms consistent with cardiomyopathy arise. Diagnostic criteria include: 1) irregular atrial rates, 2) at least three different P-wave configurations, 3) isoelectric baseline between discrete P waves, 4) irregular P-P, P-R, and R-R intervals, and 5) absence of a dominant atrial pacemaker (30). Atrial rate may range from 150-500 beats/minute and ventricular rate is typically more than 100 bpm (see Figure 2) (30). MAT is usually not responsive to DC cardioversion, vagal maneuvers, or IV antiarrhythmics (29). However, digoxin, beta blockers, amiodarone, and flecainide are options to consider. Calcium channel blockers are not indicated in neonates and infants less than one year of age. When drug therapy is successful, it should be continued for 6-12 months. In rare cases with medication refractory MAT, multiple foci ablation may be required. In refractory cases, AV node ablation with ventricular pacemaker implantation may be necessary (18).

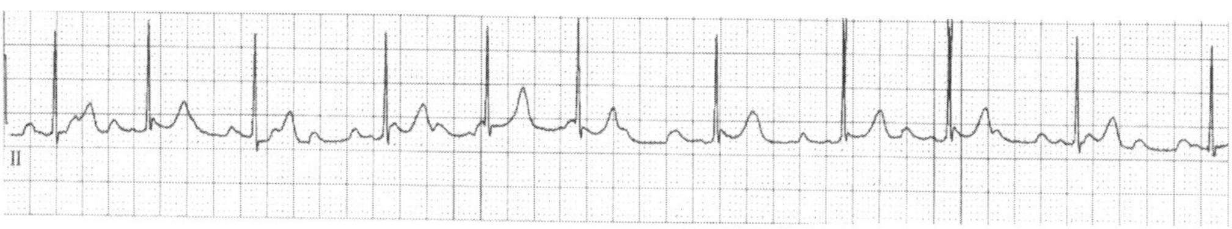

Figure 2. Multifocal atrial tachycardia.

ATRIAL FLUTTER

Atrial flutter is a regular atrial tachycardia due to a macro-reentrant rhythm confined to the atrium. There are two types of atrial flutter: 1) typical or Type I and 2) atypical or Type II. Typical atrial flutter is more common, dependent on the cavo-tricuspid isthmus, terminated by rapid atrial pacing and is further divided into counter-clockwise and clockwise circuits. Atypical atrial flutter may have a faster rate (>350 beats/minute) and is not cavo-tricuspid isthmus-dependent (31, 32). Left atrial flutter is also considered to be atypical (33). In a study of 380 patients with first flutter episode between 1 and 25 years of life, 81% had congenital heart disease, and 8% had normal hearts (34). Among adults, the incidence of atrial flutter overall was 88 per 100,000 person-years with male predominance (4:1) and is noted in patients with heart failure, pulmonary disease, thyrotoxicosis, post repair of congenital heart defects, and mitral valve disease (32, 35). The incidence of atypical atrial flutter is rare in patients without prior cardiac surgery. Atypical right atrial flutter occurs in 8% of patients with atrial flutter (36). Persistent or recurrent atrial flutter is common in patients post-cardiac surgery (32). The mechanism of atrial flutter is a re-entry mechanism with an excitable gap, within the atrium, right more than left (32). The flutter circuit requires an initially activated region to repolarize as the action potential travels through the slow conduction tissue and reactivates the initial part, thereby creating a re-entry circuit. The atrial activation along the circuit proceeds from the coronary sinus superiorly to the high right atrium area and craniocaudally along the free wall and medially to the isthmus between the tricuspid valve and the inferior vena cava in a counter-clockwise manner. There is an area of slow conduction in the posteroinferior aspect of the circuit. The clockwise or reverse typical circuit proceeds in the opposite direction (30).

In infants with no previous cardiac surgery, atrial flutter spontaneously converts in 26%. Congestive heart failure was more prevalent in those with atrial flutter of long duration. Of the infants with decreased ventricular function, all recovered normal function after conversion to sinus rhythm. If patients had additional arrhythmia, recurrence of atrial flutter was more likely (37). Atrial flutter persisting over a long period of time can evolve into atrial fibrillation (32). In neonates, 80% are asymptomatic and 20% may present with congestive heart failure (37). Patients can experience palpitations, dizziness, chest tightness, chest pain, shortness of breath, and fatigue. Hypotension, poor exercise tolerance, congestive heart failure and impaired cardiac output can also result from atrial flutter (2, 38).

On ECG, counterclockwise (typical) atrial flutter has negative flutter (F) waves in the inferior leads II, III, and aVF and positive F waves in Lead V1 (see Figure 3). Clockwise (reverse typical) atrial flutter shows positive F waves in the inferior leads II, III, and aVF and negative F waves in lead V1 (2). In typical atrial flutter, P waves are absent. The flutter rate can range from 240-340 beats/minute with no isoelectric interval between consecutive waves. Flutter rates in infants can be as high as 580 beats/minute with rapid ventricular response rates of 200 beats/minute with 2:1 AV conduction in 75% and variable block in the remainder (37). The QRS complexes appear normal unless there is rate-dependent aberrancy or block. Echocardiogram is indicated in those with congestive heart failure to evaluate ventricular function and structure.

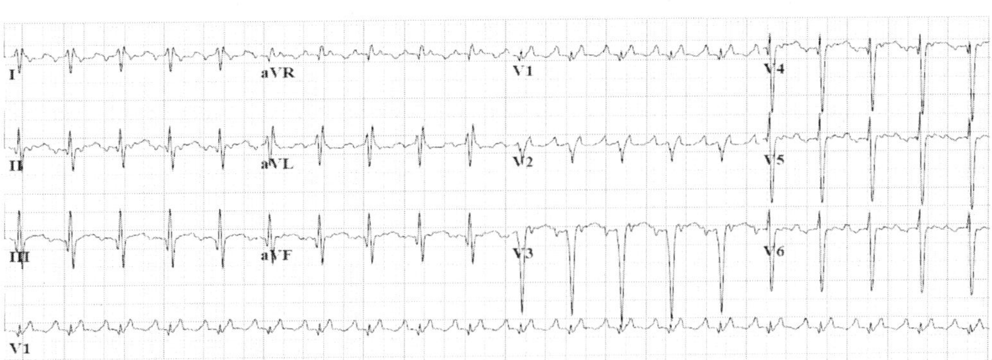

Figure 3. Atrial flutter.

The goal of flutter management is to decrease the ventricular rate and to restore normal sinus rhythm. The conversion to sinus rhythm is also dictated by the duration of the flutter. Management of atrial flutter is accomplished through electrical cardioversion, rapid atrial pacing, pharmacological therapy, and catheter ablation. Chronic anti-arrhythmic therapy may not be needed in those with uncomplicated, asymptomatic atrial flutter after conversion to sinus rhythm (23, 37). Drugs are successful in controlling atrial flutter in about 58% of young patients. Amiodarone, digoxin, and propranolol are found to be effective (34). Atrial flutter causing hemodynamic instability should be terminated acutely with electrical cardioversion (2J/Kg) (Class 1 level of evidence) (2, 37). Although cardioversion is successful acutely, atrial flutter recurs frequently. Recurrences of atrial flutter can be prevented by administering Classes IA, IC, and III anti-arrhythmic agents. Ventricular rate can be controlled with AV-nodal blockers such as digitalis and class II (beta blockers), III (amiodarone, sotalol), and IV (calcium channel blockers) anti-arrhythmic agents. Flecainide (Class 1C anti-arrhythmic) should not be administered alone; AV-node blocking agent as above should be used. As flecainide slows the atrial rate, it may facilitate 1:1 AV conduction, leading to clinical compromise (23). Calcium channel antagonists are contraindicated in children less than one year of age. Use of anticoagulation prior to conversion to sinus rhythm is warranted in patients with flutter for more than 48 hours and the duration is for at least six weeks.

When atrial flutter is refractory to medical management, transesophageal atrial overdrive pacing (TEAP) and catheter ablation are excellent options. In young adults with repaired congenital heart disease, 50-88% had successful ablation of recurrent atrial flutter (2). In a study by Ajisaka (1997), paroxysmal atrial flutter was terminated in greater than 50 percent of the adult subjects with low-output, short-duration TEAP (39). Catheter ablation is used to create a bidirectional conduction block across the cavo-tricuspid isthmus. In addition to palliating with catheter ablation, underlying causes of atrial flutter such as stimulants and sympathomimetic agents should also be eliminated.

INTRA-ATRIAL REENTRY TACHYCARDIA

Intra-atrial reentry tachycardia (IART) is a group of reentry tachycardias associated with repaired or unrepaired congenital heart disease (CHD). It is also known as slow atrial flutter, incisional atrial tachycardia, and macro-reentrant atrial tachycardia. IART is very often a late complication of cardiac surgery involving the atrium (40). IART is frequently associated with Fontan, Mustard, Senning, repaired tetralogy of Fallot, and TAPVR repairs. Prevalence of IART in early and intermediate term follow-up was 10 to 35%; however, with current management including a linear surgical incision and cryosurgical lesions at the time of Fontan completion, the occurrence is 3.5% (41). Risk factors for IART are older age of surgery and long-term follow-up. Incidence of IART often depends on the congenital heart disease and the surgery preceding the onset. Structural heart disease is present in about 89% of patients with IART (42). IART has a reentrant mechanism defined within the atrium and does not necessarily follow the atrial flutter circuit. Majority of the reentrant circuits are mainly confined to the right atrium (40). IART is intimately associated with atrial fibrillation and thromboembolic phenomena. Natural history is associated with increased frequency of recurrences, regardless of treatment with anti-arrhythmic medications or ablation (43). Intermediate follow-up post ablation of IART shows frequent recurrence with new IART configurations (44).

Symptoms in patients with IART can range from being asymptomatic to congestive heart failure to significant cardiovascular compromise, including sudden cardiac death (43). Sinus node dysfunction with symptomatic bradycardia is a common association with IART. Flutter morphology or uniform P waves are frequently noted with constant cycle length longer than typical atrial flutter (see Figure 4). Multiple ECG morphologies can be obtained from a single patient due to various activation circuits. There is often 1:1 AV conduction based on the cycle length. There is sudden onset and termination with pacing (40, 43). In refractory atrial reentry arrhythmias, an electrophysiology study must be conducted to further elucidate the nature of the substrate responsible for IART.

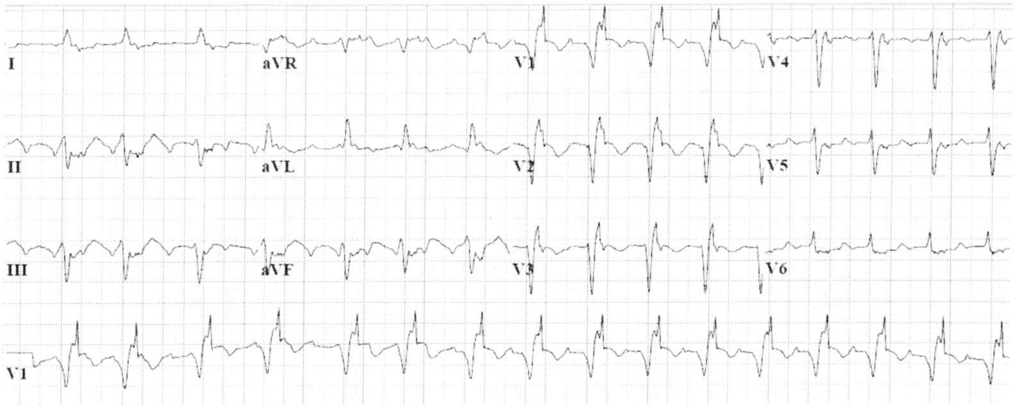

Figure 4. Intra-atrial re-entrant tachycardia.

Acute management in cardiovascular compromise consists of direct current (DC) cardioversion. Other options in clinically stable patients include anti-arrhythmic medications, atrial overdrive pacing, and anti-tachycardia pacing with pacemakers and transesophageal pacing. For chronic therapy, sotalol and amiodarone have been reported to be effective in approximately 60% (40). Implanted anti-tachycardia pacemakers provide relief from symptomatic tachycardia and bradycardia associated with sinus node dysfunction. In cases refractory to medical management, catheter ablation can be attempted. Intra-operative surgical Maze procedure (procedure which enables generation of scar lines within the atrium) is reserved for patients that have failed catheter ablation or are scheduled to undergo surgery for another indication. The need of anticoagulation is identical to patients with atrial flutter and atrial fibrillation.

ATRIO-VENTRICULAR RECIPROCATING TACHYCARDIA

Atrio-ventricular reciprocating tachycardia (AVRT) is a reentrant tachycardia with an accessory electrical connection between the atrial and ventricular myocardium in addition to the AV node (45). The accessory pathway (AP) can be "concealed" with only retrograde conduction, "manifest" with antegrade, or bidirectional conduction. The manifestation of antegrade conduction is presence of pre-excitation with short PR on the electrocardiogram during sinus rhythm suggestive of Wolff-Parkinson-White (WPW) syndrome. Orthodromic AVRT employs prograde conduction through the AV node and bundle of His with retrograde conduction through the AP. Antidromic AVRT employs AP for atrio-ventricular conduction with retrograde conduction through the bundle of His and AV node or another accessory connection.

AVRT is the most common cause of supraventricular tachycardia in children without prior cardiac surgery or neuromuscular disease, comprising 73 to 85 percent (46, 47). AVRT is more common in infancy compared to AVNRT, the incidence of which increases in older children and into adulthood (46). Accessory pathways are associated with congenital heart defects in 6-26% of the children. The common heart defects associated with accessory pathways are Ebstein's anomaly of the tricuspid valve, ventricular inversion (L-transposition of the great arteries), hypertrophic cardiomyopathy, and mitral valve prolapse (3). The reentrant mechanism of AVRT is characterized by an accessory pathway in the left or right atrio-ventricular grooves, i.e., extranodal pathway. Atriofascicular and nodofascicular (Mahaim), and atrionodal (James) AP are other variants. The left free wall is the most common site of the AP, followed by posteroseptal and right free wall AP (48). Even in patients with manifest AP, orthodromic narrow complex reciprocating tachycardia is still the most common manifestation.

In patients with WPW syndrome with onset less than two months of age, SVT disappeared in 93% and reappeared in 31% at an average age of eight years (49). In patients with onset after 5 years of age, seventy eight percent had persistence at seven years of follow-up. Multiple and right-sided AP were more frequent in patients with congenital heart disease (49). Congenital heart defects are present in 20-37% of patients with WPW (49, 50). Patients with WPW syndrome are also prone to develop atrial fibrillation with increased risk of sudden death (3). Symptoms are usually paroxysmal but may be persistent. Symptoms may occur with or without triggers, including activity and exertion. Location, rate, duration of tachycardia, and the type of AP very often determine the nature of symptoms. Infants tolerate higher rates of tachycardia compared to adolescents and adults. Infants tend to present with inconsolability and fussiness, decreased feeding, and are often asymptomatic. Older children perceive sensed tachycardia with or without associated symptoms including dizziness, lightheadedness, and mild chest discomfort. Heart failure symptoms with orthopnea, paroxysmal nocturnal dyspnea, fatigue, tachypnea, and/or diaphoresis are often present in those with persistent tachycardia (3). Sudden death is attributed to the presence of atrial fibrillation with rapid ventricular response across the accessory pathway (3). In orthodromic AVRT, shortness of breath, fatigue, and dizziness are common; syncope is less common (45). In antidromic AVRT, dizziness, syncope, and tendency towards unstable ventricular rhythm are more common than orthodromic AVRT (45).

ECG findings are determined by presence of tachycardia, normal sinus rhythm, and type of accessory pathway. In normal sinus rhythm, WPW syndrome is evident by the presence of pre-excitation (delta wave) with short PR interval. The pre-excited complex is a fusion complex resulting from initial pre-excitation of ventricular myocardium adjacent to the AP giving rise to the delta wave, followed by fusion of depolarization of the remainder of the ventricular myocardium by normal conduction. In orthodromic AVRT, the QRS complexes are narrow due to normal prograde conduction through the AV node and bundle of His and retrograde conduction via the AP (see Figure 5). Orthodromic AVRT have RP interval shorter than the PR interval with a P-wave on the upstroke of the T-wave during tachycardia, which differentiates it from AVNRT (3). In antidromic AVRT, the QRS complexes are wide due to antegrade conduction down the AP and retrograde conduction across the AV node or another AP. AV block terminates the tachycardia due to the role of AV node in the tachycardia. Mahaim AP has pre-excitation with widened QRS complexes but normal PR interval and usually manifest as a wide complex tachycardia with left bundle branch block pattern. Though the terminology is obsolete, Lown-Ganong-Levine (LGL) syndrome historically has been used to define normal QRS complexes with short PR interval and is now considered to be related to enhanced AV node conduction.

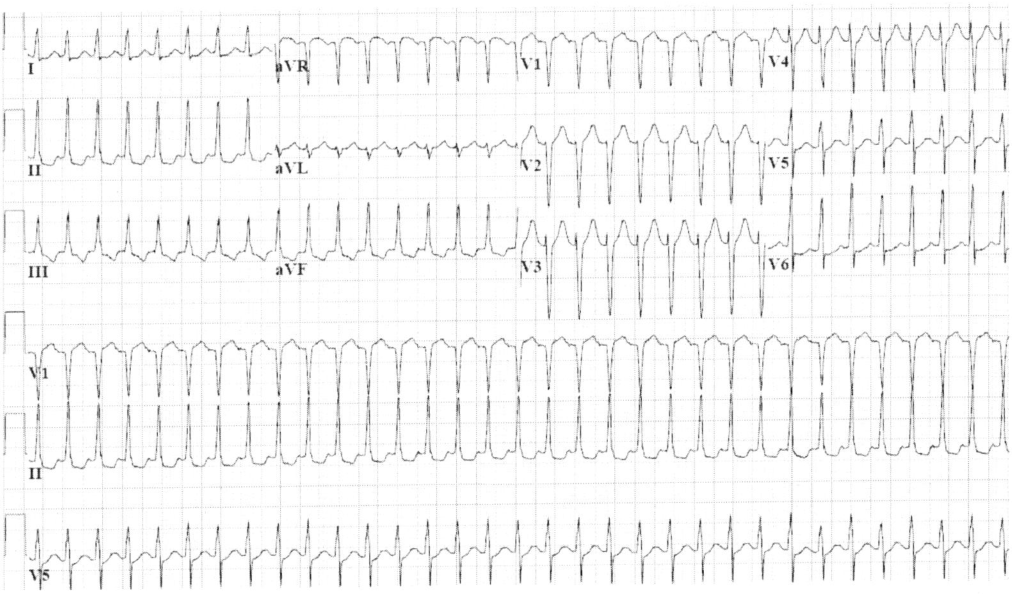

Figure 5. Orthodromic AV reciprocating tachycardia.

Baseline ECG during sinus rhythm may show preexcitation. Depending on the frequency of sensed tachycardia or other symptoms, a Holter monitor or a loop recorder can be used. Echocardiogram may be obtained to rule out structural heart defects. In patients with pre-excitation, exercise stress test to stratify the risk of sudden catastrophic event can be performed. Persistent pre-excitation at peak exercise may suggest a relatively short refractory period of the accessory fiber with a possible higher risk for sudden catastrophic event. Loss of preexcitation during exercise testing helps identify patients at low risk of sudden -arrhythmia related death (51). An electrophysiology study is recommended in patients requiring medical therapy other than beta blockers (45). To differentiate between narrow complex tachycardias, including concealed pathways, AVNRT, and atrial tachycardias, an EP study is required; an EP study will assist in differentiating antidromic AVRT from other wide-complex tachycardias.

Acute management in patients with significant hemodynamic compromise requires synchronized DC cardioversion. Adenosine administration is effective; verapamil, digoxin, and esmolol may be used. Flecainide and procainamide are recommended in pre-excited SVT (2). In stable patients, vagal maneuvers maybe effective in terminating the arrhythmia. Calcium channel blockers are contraindicated in infants. Catheter ablation is a Class I indication for managing AVRT (2). Left free wall AP was predictive of ablation success while right free wall, posteroseptal, septal, and multiple APs were predictive of recurrence (48). Medical therapy includes beta blockers to block AV node conduction and decrease premature ectopic beats, and class IA, IC, and III antiarrhythmics (40).

ATRIO-VENTRICULAR NODE REENTRY TACHYCARDIA

Atrio-ventricular node reentry tachycardia (AVNRT) is a reentry tachycardia that is dependent on existence of dual discrete pathways within or in proximity of the AV node, one with long conduction and short effective refractory period and the other with short conduction and long refractory period (52, 53). The typical ventricular rate in children ranges from 120 to 280 beats/minute (53). AVNRT is often associated with an accessory pathway. AVNRT is the most common SVT in adults but consists of 13% of SVT in children without underlying heart disease and rarely in children under two years of age (46). In infants, 15% of SVT was due to AVNRT (47). Dual AV node physiology is present in 33-35% of the children without clinical or inducible AVNRT in congenital or acquired heart disease (54). The "slow-fast" or typical form of the AVNRT is the most common form. A premature atrial or junctional beat blocks the fast pathway with subsequent antegrade conduction through the slow pathway. If the fast pathway recovers as the impulse conducts through the slow pathway, the substrate for reentry is present. In the less common "fast-slow" or atypical form of AVNRT, the premature ventricular impulse is blocked in the slow pathway and is conducted antegrade along the fast pathway. If the slow pathway recovers, a reentry substrate is present; antegrade conduction down the fast pathway and retrograde conduction up the slow pathway is present (53). The least common form is the "slow-slow" dual node physiology. There is retrograde atrial activation with early atrial activation in the low right atrium, followed by left and remaining right atrial activation (14).

AVNRT is not life-threatening and patients with minimal symptoms do well without therapy. Female patients are more symptomatic and tend to present with syncope (55). Symptoms include palpitations, chest pain, heart failure, and shock, and rarely syncope, dependent on the duration of the AVNRT. Tachycardia is paroxysmal. AVNRT is a regular narrow QRS complex tachycardia with abrupt onset and termination. The QRS complex may appear wider in case of baseline bundle branch block or rate dependent aberrant conduction. There is no preexcitation appreciated during normal sinus rhythm in sole AVNRT. In slow-fast AVNRT, retrograde P-waves are not appreciated and are located within the terminal part of the QRS complexes. In fast-slow AVNRT, the P waves have a superior axis with RP interval longer than PR interval. An electrophysiology study is indicated to definitively establish the diagnosis of AVNRT and dual AV node physiology.

Management of AVNRT is based on the frequency and the symptoms during the episodes. In those with infrequent, asymptomatic episodes, no treatment is necessary. Paroxysmal episodes may be terminated with Valsalva maneuver or carotid sinus massage. In acute decompensation, DC synchronized cardioversion, adenosine, IV beta blockers or digoxin can be employed (53). In patients with infrequent episodes desiring complete control, ablation is recommended. Patients with recurrent AVNRT refractory to beta blockers and calcium channel blockers, flecainide and sotalol are Class IIA recommendations. In recurrent, symptomatic patients with significant side effects of medications and those with poorly tolerated AVNRT with hemodynamic intolerance, catheter ablation of the slow AV nodal pathway is suggested (2).

JUNCTIONAL TACHY-ARRHYTHMIAS

Junctional ectopic tachycardia (JET), also called junctional automatic tachycardia, is an incessant tachycardia characterized by rapid heart rate with the focus of abnormal automaticity in the junction. Ventricular rates in patients with JET ranges from 140-370 beats/minute (56). Incidence of JET occurs in two cohorts: neonatal and post-operative patients. Congenital JET occurs in the first six months of life and a family history is usually present (57). Overall, JET occurs in 1% of congenital heart repairs (18). JET occurred in 22% of tetralogy of Fallot (TOF) repairs, 10% of atrio-ventricular canal defect repairs, and 3.7% of VSD repairs (58). Predictors of post-operative JET were younger age (59), lower body weight (60), resection of muscle bundles, higher bypass temperatures, and relief of right ventricular outflow tract obstruction through the right atrium (58). Although the mechanism of JET is unclear, abnormal (enhanced) automaticity of the junction has been put forth. In post-operative congenital heart disease patients, it is hypothesized that direct trauma or infiltrative hemorrhage of the conduction system leads to enhanced automaticity of the His bundle (58).

Congenital JET is associated with high mortality, most of which is attributed to sudden cardiac death (56). Concurrent arrhythmias may co-exist with JET, such as complete heart block, ventricular tachycardia, and persistent junctional reciprocating tachycardia. Post-operative JET is a transient state lasting on average 36 hours and is associated with higher mortality and longer intensive care unit (ICU) stay (18, 61). Congenital JET presents with cardiomegaly with concomitant heart failure in more than 50 percent, death in 35 percent (56), hydrops fetalis, and echocardiographic evidence of left ventricular dysfunction. In post-operative JET, the decreased ventricular filling time leads to cardiovascular compromise.

ECG criteria include 1) QRS morphology similar to that of sinus rhythm, 2) rapid ventricular rate, and 3) dissociated sinus rhythm with atrial rate often less than ventricular rate or retrograde 1:1 conduction (18). If variability exists in R-R interval, appropriately timed P-waves may conduct to the ventricular tissue (see Figure 6). An electrophysiology study is generally not necessary in patients with JET, unless ablation is being considered for medication-refractory symptoms (18). In cases of 1:1 retrograde conduction across the AV node, adenosine can clarify the underlying rhythm by blocking the AV node.

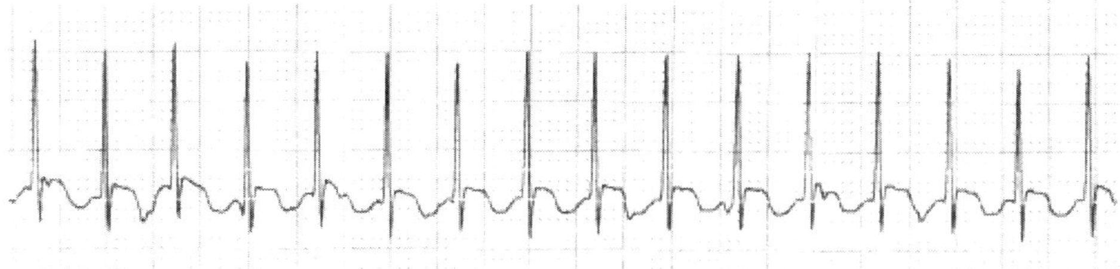

Figure 6. Junctional ectopic tachycardia.

Management of post-operative JET includes achievement of AV synchrony and rate control. Atrial pacing above the rate of JET may establish rate control (18). Post-operative JET is generally responsive to intravenous amiodarone, a class III antiarrhythmic (62). Mean length of time for termination of post-operative JET after loading and infusion of amiodarone was 4.5 hours with majority achieving control within 12 hours (63).Decreasing the body core temperature to 32-34°C, decreasing the sympathomimetic catecholamine levels, optimizing volume, electrolytes and hemoglobin contribute to decreased ventricular rate by decreasing the automaticity (64). Magnesium supplementation has been shown to be beneficial in prevention of post-operative JET (65). JET is unresponsive to DC cardioversion or overdrive pacing and programmed atrial or ventricular stimulation (66). Pharmacologic treatment of congenital JET with monotherapy is less successful than combined therapy with amiodarone, digoxin or class IA medication (57). Patients with drug-refractory congenital JET should undergo catheter ablation with maintenance of the normal atrio-ventricular conduction (18). A pacemaker is recommended in those children with evidence of impaired conduction with atrial stimulation, sinus dysfunction, or spontaneous AV block on ECG or Holter monitor (18).

PERSISTENT JUNCTIONAL RECIPROCATING TACHYCARDIA

Persistent or permanent junctional reciprocating tachycardia (PJRT) is a persistent tachycardia characterized by prograde conduction through the AV node and retrograde conduction through a slow accessory pathway located in the posteroseptal (74%) region with decremental conduction properties (67-69). PJRT is a narrow complex tachycardia with rates ranging from 120-250 beats/min and infants having higher tachycardia rates than children (70). PJRT consists of 1% to 6% of all supraventricular tachycardia (45, 70). It can present in infancy and into early childhood. PJRT has a reentrant mechanism with accessory pathways which are mostly isolated and in patients without congenital heart disease (67). In a recent study by Vaksmann et al. (2006), PJRT resolved spontaneously in 22 percent (67). Long term persistence of PJRT can lead to tachycardia-mediated cardiomyopathy, which resolves with appropriate rate control (69, 71). Uncontrolled PJRT may lead to death. Patients often are asymptomatic in childhood. Symptomatic patients present with intermittent palpitations, exercise intolerance, and syncope (70).

ECG shows retrograde P-wave in leads II, III, aVF, and left lateral leads, and R-P interval longer than P-R interval (70). The long R-P interval is attributed to the slow retrograde conduction. In sinus rhythm, there is no delta wave and P-R interval is normal, with narrow QRS complexes (68). PJRT is likely under-diagnosed in childhood and patients present with heart failure with associated ventricular dysfunction. An ECG and Holter monitor should be considered. An echocardiogram should be performed to assess the cardiac function and structure. An electrophysiology study and catheter ablation may be performed in refractory PJRT associated with decreased ventricular function (70).

Many patients with stable infrequent episodes and slow tachycardia may not require medical therapy (69). In pediatric patients, amiodarone and verapamil alone have success rates of 84-94% (67). Digoxin alone has a success rate of 50%. Hence, medical therapy with anti-arrhythmic drugs should be advocated prior to consideration of catheter ablation (72). Pediatric and adult patients with medication-refractory incessant PJRT should undergo catheter ablation, with good safety and efficacy (73).

VENTRICULAR TACHYCARDIA

Ventricular tachycardia (VT) is a tachycardia with rates greater than 120 beats per minute and originating within the ventricles or the lower conduction system with ventriculo-atrial dissociation. Non-sustained VT is defined as three or more consecutive beats of ventricular origin that terminate spontaneously with no hemodynamic compromise and lasting less than 30 seconds. Sustained VT persists longer than 30 seconds or requires medical or electrical intervention to terminate the tachycardia (74). In healthy teenage boys, short episodes of ventricular tachycardia were present in 3% (75). Incidence of VT is higher in patients with congenital heart disease. Approximately 30% of post-operative tetralogy of Fallot patients had sustained monomorphic VT and 4.4% had polymorphic VT, which contributes to 2% annual risk of sudden cardiac death (76, 77). VT originates in the RVOT in 60%-80% of structurally normal hearts (78). Idiopathic VT is also associated with aortic valve disease, corrected transposition of the great arteries, Ebstein's anomaly of the tricuspid valve, Eisenmenger's syndrome, long QT syndrome, unrepaired tetralogy of Fallot, arrhythmogenic right ventricular dysplasia, and myocardial infarction (77, 79, 80).

Ventricular tachycardia characterized by a reentry mechanism can be initiated and terminated with programmed stimuli (79). VT may also be secondary to automaticity or triggered activity. Post-operative congenital heart disease patients are at high risk of VT and sudden cardiac death. In patients with normal hearts, younger children (90%) and older populations (50%-70%) have resolution of VT within 2 to 10 years (81). However, symptomatic younger patients had worse prognosis (82). In patients with normal intracardiac anatomy, only 50% have an actual diagnosis such as hypertrophic cardiomyopathy, dilated cardiomyopathy, myocarditis, myocardial hamartoma, and metabolic disease (82). Ventricular tachycardia is present in 50%-60% of patients with dilated cardiomyopathy and is responsible for 8%-50% of deaths (83). Clinical presentation is variable (82). Symptoms may range from palpitations, light headedness, syncope, shortness of breath, neck fullness, and chest pain to death (84).

Monomorphic VT is a wide complex tachycardia with same QRS morphology, which suggests a single focus or re-entrant mechanism (see Figure 7). Polymorphic VT is a wide complex tachycardia with variable QRS morphology. Torsades de pointes is a form of polymorphic VT associated with long QT syndrome with variable electrical activation (Figure 8). Obtaining a thorough personal and family history including history of sudden cardiac death is important. An ECG of the arrhythmia is useful but very difficult to capture very often; however, a resting ECG is a Class 1 recommendation (85). Dyselectrolytemia, in particular, hypokalemia, hyperkalemia, and hypomagnesemia, should be ruled out. In patients with recurrent syncope, a holter monitor or event recorder is indicated. An echocardiogram is necessary to identify structural heart disease and evaluate cardiac function in those at risk for sudden cardiac death such as dilated, hypertrophic, and arrhythmogenic RV dysplasia, myocarditis, and inherited disorders (85). An exercise stress test is indicated in all individuals, regardless of age, known or suspected to have exercise-induced ventricular tachycardia. An electrophysiology study is warranted in patients with congenital/structural heart disease, those with unknown etiology of VT, and those with syncope of unknown etiology with LV dysfunction (85).

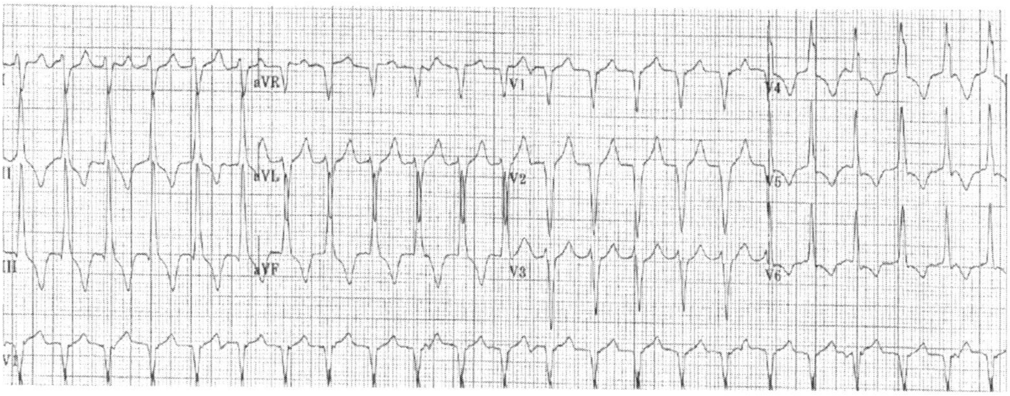

Figure 7. Ventricular tachycardia.

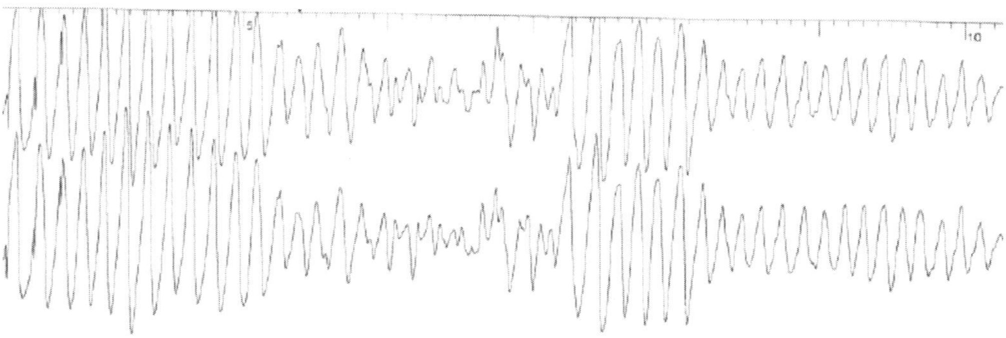

Figure 8. Torsades de pointes.

All wide complex tachycardias need to be treated like ventricular tachycardia unless proven otherwise. A-V dissociation, superior QRS axis and positive or negative concordance of QRS complexes in the precordial leads suggest ventricular origin. In patients with normal hearts, non-sustained VT has good prognosis. Avoid medications that prolong QT interval and correct electrolyte abnormalities. In patients with sustained VT with hemodynamic compromise, direct current (DC) cardioversion is indicated (85). In stable monomorphic VT, IV procainamide or amiodarone, and/or transvenous catheter pace termination may be employed. In patients with polymorphic VT, defibrillation, IV amiodarone and beta blockers may be employed. Internal cardiac defibrillator is indicated in patients with congenital heart disease who have survived cardiac arrest, patients with severely impaired ventricular function, and those on chronic optimal medical therapy with a life expectancy of at least one year (85).

CONCLUSION

Obtaining an ECG at the time of arrhythmia is of utmost importance in diagnosing and managing the tachy-arrhythmia. Assessing the atrial (P) and ventricular (QRS) activity on an ECG helps to narrow the differential diagnosis of tachyarrhythmia. If the atrial activity is more than the ventricular activity, the likely causes are atrial in origin. If the ventricular activity is more than the atrial activity, then the differential diagnosis includes junctional or ventricular origin of tachycardia. In case of 1:1 atrial and ventricular activity, the differential diagnosis would include AVRT, AVNRT, any atrial tachycardia with 1:1 AV conduction, junctional or ventricular tachycardia with 1:1 retrograde VA conduction. Physiologic sinus tachycardia is the sino-atrial node's response to endogenous and exogenous factors like fever, pain, dehydration, anxiety, hyperthyroidism, anemia and medications. Atrio-ventricular reciprocating tachycardia is the most common kind of SVT in children.

All wide complex tachycardias should be managed as ventricular tachycardia unless proven to be antidromic AV reciprocating tachycardia, SVT with aberration, SVT with baseline bundle branch block pattern or in patients with sodium channel blockers. DC cardioversion is the usually the primary method of treatment for acute hemodynamic decompensation due to tachy-arrhythmias. Referral to pediatric cardiology should be considered after obtaining hemodynamic stability for complex arrhythmias, when the etiology is unclear or further evaluation and/or intervention is required.

References

[1] Walsh E. Diagnosis and acute management of tachycardias. In: Walsh E, Saul J, Triedman J, eds. Cardiac arrhythmias in children and young adults with congenital heart disease. Philadelphia, PA: Lippincott Williams Wilkins, 2001:95-113.

[2] Blomstrom-Lundqvist Cea. ACC/AHA/ESC Guidelines for the managment of patients with supraventricular arrhythmias: Executive summary. J Am Coll Cardiol 2003;42(8):1493-1531.

[3] Van Hare G. Supraventricular tachycardia. In: Gillette P, Garson Jr. A, eds. Clinical pediatric arrhythmias. Philadelphia, PA: WB Saunders, 1999:97-120.

[4] Krahn A, Yee R, Klein G, Morillo C Inappropriate sinus tachycardia: evaluation and thearpy. J Cardiol Electrophysiol 1995;6(12):1124-8.

[5] Fogoros R. The electrophysiology study in the evaluation of the SA node, AV node, and His-Purkinje system, 4th ed. Malden, MA: Blackwell, 2006.

[6] Morillo C, Guzman J. Inappropriate sinus tachycardia: an update. Rev Esp Cardiol 2007; 60(Suppl 3):10-4.

[7] Olchansky B, Sullivan RM. Inappropriate sinus tachycardia. J Am Coll Cardiol 2013;61(8): 793-801.

[8] Chiale P, Garro H, Schmidberg J, Sanchez R, Acunzo R, Lago M, et al. Inappropriate sinus tachycardia may be related to an immunologic disorder involving cardiac beta adrenergic receptors. Heart Rhythm 2006;3(10):1182-6.

[9] Still A, Raatikainen P, Ylitalo A, Kauma H, Ikaheimo M, Kesaniemi Y, et al. Prevalence, characteristic and natural course of inappropriate sinus tachycardia. Europace 2005;7:104-12.

[10] Shen W. How to manage patients with inappropriate sinus tachycardia. Heart Rhythm 2005; 2(9):1015-9.

[11] Lin D, Callans D. Clinical arrhythmias: Mechanisms, features, and management. Supraventricular arrhythmias. In: Zipes D, Jaliffe J, eds. Cardiac electrophysiology from cell to bedside. Philadelphia, PA: Saunders, 2004:479-84.

[12] Garson Jr A, Gillette P. Electrophysiologic studies of supraventricular tachycardia in children. I. Clinical-electrophysiologic correlations. Am Heart J 1981;102(2):233-50.

[13] Gomes A, Hariman R, Kang P. Sustained symptomatic sinus node reentrant tachycardia: Incidence, clinical significance, electrophysiologic observations and the effects of antiarrhythmic agents. J Am Coll Cardiol 1985;5:45-7.

[14] Olgin J, Zipes D. Specific arrhythmias: Diagnosis and treatment. In: Zipes D, Libby P, Bonow R, Braunwald E, eds. Braunwald's heart disease. Philadelphia, PA: Elsevier Saunders, 2005:803-63.

[15] Hafeez Y, Grossman SA. Sinoatrial nodal reentrant tachycardia. Treasure Island, FL: StatPearls Publishing, 2019.
[16] Narula O. A mechanism for supraventricular tachycardia. Circulation 1974;50:1114-28.
[17] Goya M, Iesaka Y, Takahashi A, Mitsuhashi T, Yamane T, Soejima Y, et al. Radiofrequency catheter ablation for sinoatrial node reentrant tachycardia. Jap Circ J 1999;63:177-83.
[18] Walsh E. Automatic atrial and junctional tachycardias. In: Walsh E, Saul J, Triedman J, eds. Cardiac arrhythmias in children and young adults with congenital heart disease. Philadelphia, PA: Lippincott Williams Wilkins, 2001:115-35.
[19] Poutiainen A, Koistinen M, Airaksinen K, Hartikainen E, Kettunen R, Karjalainen J, et al. Prevalence and natural course of ectopic atrial tachycardia. Euro Heart J 1999;20(9):694-700.
[20] Roberts-Thomson K, Kistler P, Kalman J. Focal atrial tachycardia I: Clinical features, diagnosis, mechanisms, and anatomic location. Pac Clin Electrophysiol 2006;29(6):643-52.
[21] Packer D, Bardy G, Worley S, Smith M, Cobb F, Coleman R, et al. Tachycardia-induced cardiomyopathy: A reversible form of left ventricular dysfunction. Am J Cardiol 1986; 57(8):563-70.
[22] Naheed Z, Strasburger J, Benson Jr. D, Deal B. Natural history and management strategies of automatic atrial tachycardia in children. Am J Cardiol 1995;75(5-6):405-7.
[23] Skinner J, Sharland G. Detection and management of life threatening arrhythmias in the perinatal period. Early Hum Dev 2008;84(3):161-72.
[24] Hsieh M, Chen S. Catheter ablation in focal tachycardia. In: Zipes D, Haissaguerre M, eds. Catheter ablation of arrhythmias. Armonk, NY: Futura, 2002:185-204.
[25] Kastor J. Multifocal atrial tachycardia. New Eng J Med 1990;322:1713.
[26] Salim M, Case C, Gillette P. Chaotic atrial tachycardia in children. Am Heart J 1995; 129:831-3.
[27] Kones R, Phillips J, Hersh J. Mechanism and management of chaotic atrial mechanism. Cardiology 1974;59:92.
[28] Sokoloski M. Tachyarrhythmias confined to the atrium. In: Gillette P, Garson Jr. A, eds. Clinical pediatric arrhythmias, 2nd ed. Philadelphia, PA: WB Saunders, 1999.
[29] Bradley DJ, Fischback PS, Law IH, Serwer GA, Dick II M. The clinical course of multifocal atrial tachycardia in infants and children. J Am Coll Cardiol 2001;38(2):401-8.
[30] Shine KI, Kastor JA, Yurchak PM. Multifocal atrial tachycardia. Clinical and electrocardiographic features in 32 patients. N Engl J Med 1968;279:344-9.
[31] Saoudi N, Cosio F, Waldo A, Chen S, Lesaka Y, Lesh M, et al. A Classification of atrial flutter and regular atrial tachycardia according to electrophysiological mechanisms and anatomica bases. Euro Heart J 2001;22:1162-82.
[32] Waldo A. Atrial flutter: Mechanisms, clinical features, and management. In: Zipes D, Jaliffe J, eds. Cardiac electrophysiology from cell to bedside, 4th ed. Philadelphia, PA: Saunders, 2004:490-9.
[33] Garan H. Atypical atrial flutter. Heart Rhythm 2008;5:618-21.
[34] Garson Jr. A, Bink-Boelkens M, Hesslein P, Hordof A, Keane J, Neches W, et al. Atrial flutter in the young: A collaborative study of 380 cases. J Am Coll Cardiol 1985;6(4):871-8.
[35] Granada J, Uribe W, Chyou P, Maassen K, Vierkant R, Smith P, et al. Incidence and predictors of atrial flutter in the general population. J Am Coll Cardiol 2000;36(7):2242-6.
[36] Yang Y, Cheng J, bochoeycr A, Hamdan M, Kowal R, Page R, et al. Atypical right atrial flutters patterns. Circulation 2001;103(25):3092-8.
[37] Texter K, Kertesz N, Friedman R, Fenrich A. Atrial flutter in infants. J Am Coll Cardiol 2006;48(5):1040-6.
[38] Andrew P, Montenero A. Atrial flutter: A focus on treatment options for a common supraventricular tachyarrhythmia. J Cardiovasc Med 2007;8:558-67.
[39] Ajisaka H, Hiraki T, Ikeda H, Kubara I, Yoshida T, Ohga M, et al. Direct conversion of atrial flutter to sinus rhythm with low-output, short-duration transesophageal atrial pacing. Clin Cardiol 1997;20(9):762-6.
[40] Triedman J. Atrial reentrant tachycardias. In: Walsh E, Saul J, Triedman J, eds. Cardiac arrhythmias in children and young adults with congenital heart disease. Philadelphia, PA: Lippincott Williams Wilkins, 2001:137-59.

[41] Law IH, Alam O, Bove EL, Ohye RG, Bradley DJ, Yu S, et al. Follow-up of a prospective surgical strategy to prevent intra-atrial reentrant tachycardia following the Fontan operation. Circ Arrhythm Electrophysiol 2016;9(12):e004478.

[42] Haines D, DiMarco J. Sustained intraatrial reentrant tachycardia: Clinical, electrocardiographic and electrophysiologic characteristics and long-term follow-up. J Am Coll Cardiol 1990;15(6):1345-54.

[43] Triedman J. Atrial arrhythmias in congenital heart disease. In: Zipes D, Jaliffe J, eds. Cardiac electrophysiology from cell to bedside. Philadelphia, PA: Sanders, 2004:558-68.

[44] Triedman J, Bergau D, Saul J, Epstein M, Walsh E. Efficacy of radiofrequency ablation for control of intraatrial reentry tachycardia in patient with congenital heart disease. J Am Coll Cardiol 1997;30(4):1032-38.

[45] Blaufox A, Saul J. Accessory-pathway-mediated tachycardias. In: Walsh E, Saul J, Triedman J, eds. Cardiac arrhythmias in children and young adults with congenital heart disease. Philadelphia, PA: Lippincott Williams Wilkins, 2001:173-99.

[46] Ko J, Deal B, Strasburger J, Benson Jr. D. Supraventricular tachycardia mechanisms and their age distribution in pediatric patients. Am J Cardiol 1992;69(12):1028-32.

[47] Etheridge S, Judd V. Supraventricular tachycardia in infancy: Evaluation, management, and follow-up. Arch Pediatr Adolesc Med 1999;153(3):267-71.

[48] Calkins H, Yong P, Miller J, Olshansky B, Carlson M, Saul J, et al. Catheter ablation of accessory pathways, atrioventricular nodal reentrant tachycardia, and the atrioventricular junction: Final results of a prospective, multicenter clinical trial. Circulation 1999; 99(2):262-70.

[49] Perry J, Garson Jr. A. Supraventricular tachycardia due to Wolff-Parkinson-White syndrome in children: Early disappearance and late recurrence. J Am Coll Cardiol 1990;16(5):1215-20.

[50] Deal B, Keane J, Gillette P, Garson Jr. A. Wolff-Parkinson-White syndrome and supraventricular tachycardia during infancy: Management and follow-up. J Am Coll Cardiol 1985;5(1):130-5.

[51] Page RL, Joglar JA, Caldwell MA, Calkins H, Conti JB, Deal BJ, et al. ACC/AHA/HRS Guideline for the management of adult patients with supraventricular tachycardia. A report of the American College of Cardiology/American Heart Association tast force on clinical practice guidelines and the Heart Rhythm Society. J Am Coll Cardiol 2016;67(13):e27-e115.

[52] Lockwood D, Otomo K, Wang Z, Forresti S, Nakagawa H, Beckman K, et al. Electrophysiologic characteristics of atrioventricular nodal reentrant tachycardia: Implications for the reentrant circuits. In: Zipes D, Jaliffe J, eds. Cardiac electrophysiology from cell to bedside. Philadelphia, PA: Saunders, 2004:537-57.

[53] Zimmerman F. Atrioventricular node reentry tachycardia. In: Walsh E, Saul J, Triedman J, eds. Cardiac arrhythmias in children and young adults with congenital heart disease. Philadelphia, PA: Lippincott Williams Wilkins, 2001:161-72.

[54] Casta A, Wolff G, Mehta A, Tamer D, Garcia O, Pickoff A, et al. Dual atrioventricular nodal pathways: A benign finding in arrhythmia-free children with heart disease. Am J Cardiol 1980;46(6):1013-8.

[55] Drago F, Grutter G, Silvetti M, De Santis A, Di Ciommo V. Atrioventricular nodal reentrant tachycardia in children. Pediatr Cardiol 2006;27(4):454-9.

[56] Villain E, Vetter V, Garcia J, Herre J, Cifarelli A, Garson Jr. A. Evolving concepts in the management of congenital junctional ectopic tachycardia. A multicenter study. Circulation 1990;81(5):1544-9.

[57] Sarubbi B, Musto B, Ducceschi V, D'Onofrio A, Cavallaro C, Vecchione F, et al. Congenital junctional ectopic tachycardia in children and adolescents: A 20 year experience based study. Heart 2002;88:188-90.

[58] Dodge-Khatami A, Miller O, Anderson R, Goldman A, Gil-Jaurena J, Elliott M, et al. Surgical substrates of postoperative junctional ectopic tachycardia in congenital heart defects. J Thorac Cardiolvasc Surg 2002;123(4):624-30.

[59] Hoffman T, Bush D, Wernovsky G, Cohen M, Wieand T, Gaynor J, et al. Postoperative junctional ectopic tachycardia in children: Incidence, risk factors, and treatment. Ann Thorac Surg 2002;74(5):1607-11.

[60] Rekawek J, Kansy A, Miszczak-Knecht M, Manowska M, Bieganowska K, Brzezinska-Paszke M, et al. Risk factors for cardiac arrhythmias in children with congenital heart disease after surgical intervention in the early postoperative period. J Thorac Cardiolvasc Surg 2007; 133(4):900-4.

[61] Andreasen J, Johnsen S, Ravn H. Junctional ectopic tachycardia after surgery for congenital heart disease in children. Intensive Care Med 2008; 34(5):895-902.

[62] Shah M, Rhodes L. Management of postoperative arrhythmias and junctional ectopic tachycardia. Semin Thorac Cardiovasc Surg Pediatr Card Surg Annu 1998;1:91-102.

[63] Plumpton K, Justo R, Haas N. Amiodarone for post-operative junctional ectopic tachycardia. Cardiol Young 2005;15(1):13-8.

[64] Cabrera D, Rodrigo Carbonero D, Galdeano Miranda J, Martinez Corrales P, Pastor Menchaca E, Mucua Biurrun P, et al. [The treatment of post-operative junctional ectopic tachycardia]. An Esp Pediatr 2002;56(6):505-9. [Spanish]

[65] Dorman B, Sade R, Burnette J, Wiles H, Pinosky M, Reeves S, et al. Magnesium supplementation in the prevention of arrhythmias in pediatric patients undergoing surgery for congenital heart defects. Am Heart J 2000;139(3):522-8.

[66] Sarubbi B, Vergara P, D'Alto M, Calabro R. Congenital junctional ectopic tachycardia: Presentation and outcome. Ind Pac Electrophysiol J 2003;3(3):143-7.

[67] Vaksmann G, D'Hoinne C, Lucet V, Guillaumont S, Lupoglazoff J, Chantepie A, et al. Permanent junctional reciprocating tachycardia in children: A multicentre study on clinical profile and outcome. Heart 2006;92:101-4.

[68] Critelli G, Gallagher J, Monda V, Coltorti F, Scherillo M, Rossi L. Anatomic and electrophysiologic substrate of the permanent form of junctional reciprocating tachycardia. J Am Coll Cardiol 1984;4(3):601-10.

[69] Lindinger A, Heisel A, von Bernuth G, Paul T, Ulmer H, Kienast W, et al. Permanent junctional re-entry tachycardia. Eur Heart J 1998;19:936-42.

[70] Dorostkar P, Silka M, Morady F, Dick MI. Clinical course of persistent junctional reciprocating tachycardia. J Am Coll Cardiol 1999;33:366-75.

[71] Noe P, Van Driel V, Wittkampf F, Sreeram N. Rapid recovery of cardiac function after catheter ablation of persistent junctional reciprocating tachycardia in children. PACE 2002; 25(2):191-4.

[72] Drago F, Silvetti M, Mazza A, Anaclerio S, Pino A, Grutter G, et al. Permanent juncational reciprocating tachycardia in infants and children: Effectiveness of medical and non-medical treatment. Ital Heart J 2001;2(6):456-61.

[73] Aguinaga L, Primo J, Anguera I, Mont L, Valentino M, Brugada P, et al. Long-term follow-up in patients with the permanent form of junctional reciprocating tachycardia treated with radiofrequency ablation. PACE 1998;21(11):2073-8.

[74] Ventricular tachycardia. American Heart Association, 2007.

[75] Dickinson D, Scott O. Ambulatory electrographic monitoring in 100 healthy teenage boys. Br Heart J 1984;51(2):179-83.

[76] Khairy P, Landzberg M, Gatzoulis M, Lucron H, Lambert J, Marcon F, et al. Value of programmed ventricular stimulatino after tetralogy of Fallot repair: A multicenter study. Circulation 2004;109(16):1994-2000.

[77] Walsh E, Cecchin F. Arrhythmias in adult patients with congenital heart disease. Circulation 2007;115:534-45.

[78] Lerman B, Stein K, Markowitz S, Mittal S, Iwai S, eds. Ventricular tachycardia in patients with structurally normal hearts. Philadelphia, PA: Saunders, 2004.

[79] Callans D, Josephson M, eds. Ventricular tachycardia in patients with coronary artery disease. Philadelphia, PA: Saunders, 2004.

[80] Fontaine G, Fornes P, Hebert J, Prost-Squarcioni C, Fouven X, Hulot J, et al., eds. Ventricular tachycardia in arrhythmogenic right ventricular cardiomyopathies. Philadelphia, PA: Saunders, 2004.

[81] Alexander M. Ventricular arrhythmias in children and young adults. In: Walsh E, Saul J, Triedman J, eds. Cardiac arrhythmias in children and young adults with congenital heart disease. Philadelphia, PA: Lippincott Williams Wilkins, 2001:201-34.

[82] Davis A, Gow R, McCrindle B, Hamilton R. Clinical spectrum, Therapeutic management, and follow-up of ventricular tachycardia in infants and young children. Am Heart J 1996; 131:186-91.

[83] Galvin J, Ruskin J, eds. Ventricular tachycardia in patients with dilated cardiomyopathy. Philadelphia, PA: Saunders, 2004.

[84] Silka M, Garson Jr. A. Ventricular arrhythmias. In: Gillette P, Garson Jr A, eds. Clinical pediatric arrhythmias. Philadelphia, PA: WB Saunders, 1999:121-45.

[85] Zipes D, Camm A. ACC/AHA/ESC 2006 guidelines for management of patients with ventricular arrhythmias and the prevention of sudden cardiac death. J Am Coll Cardiol 2006; 48(5):e247-346.

In: Chronic Disease and Disability
Editors: DE Greydanus, P Anne, JD Rowlett et al.
ISBN: 978-1-53617-656-8

Chapter 7

MYOCARDITIS IN THE PEDIATRIC AND ADOLESCENT POPULATION

John D Rowlett*[*]*, MD, FAAP, FACP
St Joseph's/Candler Healthcare System, Savannah, Georgia,
Medical College of Georgia, Augusta, Georgia, United States of America
and Eastern Kentucky University, Richmond, Kentucky, United States of America

ABSTRACT

Myocarditis, an acute inflammatory condition of the heart that affects all age groups, is an increasingly recognized cause of morbidity and mortality in all age groups. Presenting symptoms can range from mild gastrointestinal complaints (i.e., vomiting, diarrhea) to overt cardiogenic shock with dysrhythmia and death. Most cases of myocarditis are either infectious or autoimmune in origin, though it also may be idiopathic in origin. The outcome can be improved in selected patients with prompt recognition of the clinical syndrome and when necessary, initiation of cardiovascular support including inotropic, ventilatory, and anti-arrhythmic measures; however, long-term morbidity and mortality are common. This discussion reviews the epidemiology, presentation, diagnosis, and management of myocarditis in children and adolescents.

INTRODUCTION

Myocarditis denotes an inflammatory condition of the myocardium which may be acute, sub-acute, or chronic (1). Though typically confined to the myocardium, the disease process may extend to the epicardium and less frequently to the pericardium (myopericarditis). There are many causative agents, and all can lead a dilated cardiomyopathy (DCM), overt heart failure, and death. This discussion now considers various features of pediatric myocarditis, including its incidence, etiologies, symptomatology, diagnostic evaluation, differential diagnosis, management, and clinical course (1).

[*] Corresponding Author's Email: drrowlett@gmail.com.

INCIDENCE AND ETIOLOGIES

The true incidence of myocarditis in children and young adults is unknown. Lipshultz et al. have estimated the incidence at 1.3 cases per 100,000 children per year (2). Clearly this underestimates the true burden of disease as many cases are sub-clinical and only the more severe cases typically seek medical attention. Further, of those who do seek medical care, the correct diagnosis may be difficult to establish. Durani and colleagues reported that less than 20% of pediatric patients were correctly diagnosed with myocarditis on initial presentation while Shu-Ling et al. reported that nearly 40% were initially diagnosed correctly (3, 4).

There is no sex difference in the occurrence of myocarditis until about age six at which point there is a marked progression to male predominance. By age eighteen years, 80% of the cases of clinical myocarditis are in male patients (5). This male predominance continues until the 5th decade when it becomes more evenly distributed. While it is postulated that estrogens are protective against myocarditis, other factors including genomic variations are likely contributory to this marked disparity (6).

The most common cause of myocarditis in children and young adults is an acute or sub-acute viral infection (see Table 1). Additional infectious etiologies include bacterial, protozoal, fungal, spirochetal, rickettsial, and parasitic organisms (Table 1). Non-infectious causes of acute and sub-acute myocarditis included autoimmune diseases, hypersensitivity reactions, and drugs. These causes are summarized in Table 1.

Table 1. Etiologies of myocarditis (1, 4, 12, 18, 32-34)

Infectious
Viral: Coxsackie B, Adenovirus, Cytomegalovirus, Echovirus, Epstein-Barr virus, Hepatis B, Hepatitis C, Human Herpes 6 virus, HIV, Influenza A and Influenza B, Mumps, Parvovirus, Poliomyelitis, Rubella, Varicella
Bacterial: Bartonella, Brucellosis, Chlamydia, Clostridia, Diphtheria, Gonococcal, Haemophilus, Legionella, Mycoplasma, Pneumococcal, Salmonella, Staphylococcus, Streptococcus,
Fungal: Histoplasmosis, Coccidiomycosis, Blastomycosis, Nocardia, Candida, Aspergillus
Protozoal: Toxoplasmosis, Leishmania, *Trypanasoma cruzi*
Other: Spirochetes (*Borrelia burgdorferi*, *Treponema pallidum*) Rickettsial, Parasitic
Autoimmune
Giant Cell myocarditis, Kawasaki disease, Systemic lupus, rheumatic disease (rheumatic fever, lupus, sarcoidosis, rheumatoid arthritis, dermatomyositis, scleroderma, polymyositis), celiac disease, myasthenia gravis, diabetes, Takayasu arteritis, thyrotoxicosis
Drugs
Chemotherapeutic agents (anthracyclines, cyclophosphamide, platinum-based drugs, check-point inhibitors), isoniazid, amphetamines, narcotics, cocaine, sulfonamides,
Other
Envenomation (snakes, scorpions, bees, spiders), radiation, heavy metals (copper, lead, iron), electrocution

PRESENTATION AND PHYSICAL FINDINGS

The initial presentation may be very benign; in one review fever and gastrointestinal complaints (i.e., abdominal pain, diarrhea, vomiting) were the presenting symptoms in approximately 80% of patients (7). Additional presenting symptoms may include typical viral/influenza syndrome features (i.e., cough, myalgias, fever), and tachycardia disproportionate to fever; typically, each degree of fever can be expected to raise resting heart rate 6-11 beats per minute. Severe cases of myocarditis may present with overt heart failure, dysrhythmias, heart blocks, and cardiogenic shock (8). Myocarditis is implicated in 12% of sudden cardiac death in children and 6% of adults (9, 10). In previously normal patients, myocarditis is the most common cause of acute heart failure.

Infants and young children may present with very vague symptoms and are more likely to progress to fulminant myocarditis requiring respiratory and/or cardiovascular support. In a review of 31 patients presenting to the emergency department with myocarditis, Freedman et al. reported the most common symptoms were respiratory distress (68%), lethargy (39%), and fever (30%); nearly three-fourths of children had a preceding viral prodromal illness (11).

Physical examination of the patient with myocarditis varies according to the severity of symptoms. Presenting vital signs may include some combination of tachycardia, tachypnea, hypotension, and in more severe cases, hypoxia. Depending on severity, mental status may range from irritable to moribund. In addition to tachycardia, the cardiac examination may reveal a gallop rhythm (S3 or S4, indicative of impaired ventricular function) and if there is significant pericardial disease, heart sounds may be muffled with or without a pericardial friction rub. Severe cases of pericardial disease may present with symptoms of cardiac tamponade including jugular venous distention, hypotension, muffled heart sounds, pulsus paradoxus, and a narrowed pulse pressure (4, 12). Additional physical findings may include hepatomegaly, poor perfusion, obtundation, peripheral edema and pulmonary rales.

DIAGNOSTIC EVALUATION

Diagnostic testing is guided by clinical presentation and suspicion of the underlying pathology. Patients presenting with fever and hypotension will likely get an extensive, non-specific workup including complete blood count, chemistry panel, lactic acid, procalcitonin, urinalysis, chest x-ray and an electrocardiogram. In the setting of hypotension, many of these results may be significantly altered but are individually non-specific.

The electrocardiogram (ECG) is rarely normal in myocarditis, but there are no pathognomonic ECG findings. Freedman et al. found that 93% of patients had an abnormal tracing, with abnormalities ranging from non-specific tachycardia, diminished voltage and inverted t-waves to overt heart blocks and ventricular dysrhythmias (11). Similarly, Durani and colleagues found the ECG to be abnormal in 100% of a cohort of 31 pediatric patients with myocarditis (12).

Chest radiography is routinely obtained on patients presenting with dyspnea, hypoxia, and/or unexplained tachypnea, with or without fever. Radiographic findings at presentation for patients with myocarditis range from normal to mild cardiomegaly, small pleural effusions and pulmonary venous congestion, to large pleural effusions and florid pulmonary edema. The most common abnormality is simple cardiomegaly, but the chest radiograph is neither sensitive nor specific in myocarditis (4).

Cardiac biomarkers are useful in the evaluation of suspected cases of myocarditis. Troponin is a complex of three regulatory proteins (Troponin C, I, and T) involved predominantly in muscle contraction. Troponin T and Troponin I are specific to cardiac muscle and are extensively used in evaluation for cardiac muscle ischemia and/or injury. Troponin is elevated in most but not all cases of myocarditis. Butto et al. reviewed 149 cases of myocarditis in pediatric as well as adolescent patients and found abnormal troponin (I or T) levels in 81% of patients at admission (13). The absolute level of elevation is not prognostic and this test lacks the necessary sensitivity or specificity to guide therapy (13). Brain natriuretic peptide (BNP) may help distinguish between cardiac and pulmonary causes of dyspnea. In cases of chronic dilated cardiomyopathies, the BNP may be persistently elevated, though the magnitude of elevation may trend volume status.

Echocardiography typically reveals global systolic dysfunction, but regional or segmental abnormalities may be detected. Echocardiography may exclude competing diagnoses such as pericarditis, valvular insufficiency, and anomalous left coronary artery (14).

Blood gases may reveal hypoxia and a metabolic acidosis in patients with hypoperfusion. Respiratory alkalosis may be seen early with tachypnea and transitions to respiratory acidosis in patients with progressive ventilatory failure. Inflammatory markers, such as sedimentation rate and C-reactive protein (CRP), may be abnormal but lack the sensitivity or specificity to aid in clinical diagnosis or disease management. It is important to obtain blood and urine cultures as well as viral respiratory polymerase chain reaction (PCR) panels on all critically ill patients presenting with hypotension. Again, these studies, though useful in competing diagnoses, have limited sensitivity and/or specificity in cases of myocarditis. Aspartate aminotransferase has been shown to be elevated in 92% of patients with probable myocarditis and 79% of patients with confirmed myocarditis (11).

Endomyocardial biopsy (EMB) has long been considered the gold standard for diagnosis of myocarditis but it too lacks sensitivity as the disease may be "patchy" resulting in frequent false-negative biopsies. Further, EMB requires invasive cardiac testing which is particularly risky in critically ill patients (15, 16). Cardiac magnetic resonance (CMR) is increasingly used to aid in the diagnosis of myocarditis in pediatric patients and is rapidly replacing EMB in many centers. CMR may demonstrate edema with the myocardium; enhanced scans may demonstrate myocardial necrosis and/or myocardial scar (17).

Absent a definitive diagnosis of myocarditis from EMB or CMR, most cases of myocarditis are diagnosed clinically. Myocarditis should be considered in cases where signs and symptoms of cardiac dysfunction (i.e., syncope, chest pain, dyspnea, tachycardia) are accompanied by elevated serum troponin and echocardiographic findings of ventricular abnormalities. Additional suggestive features include ECG changes and prodromal illness (18).

DIFFERENTIAL DIAGNOSIS

Differential diagnosis is governed by presenting symptoms but includes other causes of acute heart failure that include structural disease, cardiomyopathies (hypertrophic, ischemic, dilated), Kawasaki disease and sepsis. Patients presenting with hypotension and fever should be treated aggressively with broad-spectrum antibiotics until an etiology is determined. Myocardial dysfunction should be considered in all patients who fail to respond to large volume fluid resuscitation. Myocarditis should be considered in all cases of fever and hypotension which worsen in response to fluid challenges (suggesting cardiac dysfunction). Respiratory illnesses (i.e., asthma, bronchiolitis, pneumonia) can have similar presentations.

TREATMENT

The treatment of clinical myocarditis is largely supportive. As with all potentially critically ill patients, attention to the airway, ventilation, and circulation is paramount. When possible, children with suspected or confirmed myocarditis should be stabilized and transferred to a tertiary pediatric center. Initial fluid management may be difficult unless there is a clear diagnosis. Tachycardic, febrile, hypotensive patients are most commonly volume depleted and current recommendations call for the rapid infusion of up to 30 cc/kg of isotonic fluid for cases of suspected sepsis.

Unfortunately, in cases of myocarditis and congestive heart failure, such fluids may worsen the clinical scenario precipitously. Clinical management of more profound cases of myocarditis includes early judicious use of diuretics and inotropic agents (i.e., dobutamine, milrinone). Additional useful agents include norepinephrine, epinephrine, and dopamine (1, 19, 20). Dysrhythmias should be managed with amiodarone or lidocaine; electrical cardioversion may be necessary for unstable tachydysrhythmias.

Adequate tissue perfusion is a function of oxygenation, perfusion, and hemoglobin status. Packed red blood cells should be used judiciously to ensure adequate oxygen-carrying capacity. Supplemental oxygen should be provided to all patients with cardiac and/or respiratory dysfunction. Progressive respiratory symptoms, including hypoxia and respiratory fatigue, may necessitate endotracheal intubation. As in all cases, it is safer to do this in a controlled, anticipatory manner than in a crashing patient.

Extreme cases may require extracorporeal membrane oxygenation (ECMO), though even with the utilization of this technology, there is a high mortality. Nosaka and colleagues reviewed the clinical course and outcomes of 29 patients (median age 5 years) admitted to a Japanese children's hospital between 2002 and 2013; in this study, 16 patients required ECMO and 5 of these died (7). Of the surviving 24, favorable neurologic outcomes were noted in 23; also, of the five deaths, four were placed on ECMO *after* cardiopulmonary arrest while ten of the 11 patients electively were placed on ECMO survived (7).

Immunosuppressive agents (i.e., intravenous immune globulin [IVIG], corticosteroids) have been tried in adults and children with myocarditis with mixed results; at present, there is no consensus recommendation for the administration of IVIG or steroids in the acute phase for pediatric patients with suspected or proven myocarditis

Yen et al. reviewed 13 studies of pediatric patients with acute myocarditis in which 812 patients were treated with IVIG and 592 without IVIG treatment (21). Meta-analysis demonstrated no statistical difference in survival between the two treatment groups and the authors concluded that the routine use of IVIG in cases of myocarditis in children cannot be routinely recommended based on the currently available evidence (21).

Similarly, Li et al. reviewed nine databases and found 334 pediatric patients with myocarditis treated with either corticosteroids or IVIG (22). Follow-up ejection fractions (EF) on patients treated with corticosteroids failed to demonstrate improvement in EF, death rates, or heart transplantation (22). Contrary to the findings of Yen, Li found a statistically significant improvement for those patients treated with IVIG with increased EF, decreased death, and decreased heart transplantation (22). Li et al. concluded that IVIG therapy MIGHT be beneficial, but that there is no demonstrated role for corticosteroids in the treatment of pediatric myocarditis (22).

It is important to remember that this is a disparate population and clinically significant differences may be difficult to prove given age as well as etiology differences, advances in other forms of pediatric critical care, and other factors. Further, there may be a role for a combination of IVIG and steroids in restoring left ventricular function during the convalescent phase of myocarditis (23-25). Antivirals (i.e., acyclovir, ribarvirin) may be of benefit in selected cases of chronic viral myocardial disease but are not routinely recommended for acute myocarditis. Broad-spectrum antibiotics should initially be utilized in clinical settings consistent with unexplained hemodynamic compromise (1, 26).

Clinical Course

Myocarditis typically has ***three clinical phases:*** acute/viral, autoimmune/inflammatory, and potentially non-ischemic dilated cardiomyopathy in some. The acute or viral infection phase is characterized by vague viral symptoms including fever, malaise, and myalgias. This typically predates cardiac symptomatology by several days. Gastrointestinal symptoms are common that include diarrhea, vomiting, pain, and anorexia; respiratory symptoms are variable at this point.

This is soon followed by an autoimmunity and inflammatory stage caused by viral activation of the host immune system. This stage is associated with myocyte injury that can be seen on EMB. Myocyte injury manifests in a range of symptoms from mild fatigue to impaired left ventricular function as well as overt heart failure and myocardial necrosis; arrhythmias may develop during this period. Though controversial, it is in this recovery phase that there MAY be a role for immune modulators such as IVIG or corticosteroids.

A final phase of non-ischemic dilated cardiomyopathy develops in some patients. The majority of these patients can be managed with beta-blockers, diuretics, and ACE inhibitors, though some may progress to cardiac transplantation (18). Reported mortality for acute myocarditis ranges from 6% to 14%; late deaths occur in <5% of patients and typically involve persistent left ventricular dysfunction or complications from cardiac transplantation (18, 27, 28). Ventricular assist devices have been increasingly utilized as a bridge to cardiac transplantation (29). Despite advances in supportive care and the potential improvement of EF by immunosuppressive agents in the convalescent patient, from 5 to 20 percent of children with acute myocarditis will eventually require cardiac transplantation (28, 30, 31).

Conclusion

Myocarditis is the most common cause of acute heart failure in previously healthy children and adults. It is typically caused by an otherwise innocuous viral infection, though bacterial, fungal, protozoal, auto-immune, toxic, and idiopathic cases occur. Presenting symptoms range from mild gastrointestinal complaints and malaise to overt heart failure, respiratory distress, and sudden death. Diagnosis is largely clinical, though CMR may be useful. Prompt recognition of the clinical scenario and initiation of appropriate cardiovascular as well as respiratory support may improve outcome (32-34).

Currently there are no recommendation for immunosuppressive agents in the acute phase of myocarditis; these agents may be of limited utility in the convalescent phase. Myocarditis is associated with short-term mortality and long-term morbidity; many patients are left with a chronic dilated cardiomyopathy and up to 20% will eventually require cardiac transplantation.

REFERENCES

[1] Bergmann KR, Kharbanda A, Haveman L. Myocarditis and pericarditis in the pediatric patient: Validated management strategies. Pediatr Emerg Med Pract 2015;12(7):1-23.

[2] Lipshultz SE, Sleeper LA, Towbin JA, Lowe AM, Orav EJ, Cox GF, et al. The incidence of pediatric cardiomyopathy in two regions of the United States. N Engl J Med 2003;348(17):1647-55.

[3] Durani Y, Egan M, Baffa J, Selbst SM, Nager AL. Pediatric myocarditis: presenting clinical characteristics. Am J Emerg Med 2009;27(8):942-7.

[4] Shu-Ling C, Bautista D, Kit CC, Su-Yin AA. Diagnostic evaluation of pediatric myocarditis in the emergency department: a 10-year case series in the Asian population. Pediatr Emerg Care 2013; 29(3):346-51.

[5] Arola A, Pikkarainen E, Sipila JO, Pykari J, Rautava P, Kyto V. Occurrence and features of childhood myocarditis: A nationwide study in Finland. J Am Heart Assoc 2017;6(11). 6:e005306. doi: 10.1161/JAHA.116.005306.

[6] Fairweather D, Cooper LT Jr, Blauwet LA. Sex and gender differences in myocarditis and dilated cardiomyopathy. Curr Prob Cardiol 2013;38(1):7-46.

[7] Nosaka N, Muguruma T, Fujiwara T, Enomoto Y, Toida C, Morishima T. Effects of the elective introduction of extracorporeal membrane oxygenation on outcomes in pediatric myocarditis cases. Acute Med Surg 2015;2(2):92-7.

[8] Cooper LT Jr. Myocarditis. N Engl J Med 2009;360(15):1526-38.

[9] Levine MC, Klugman D, Teach SJ. Update on myocarditis in children. Curr Opin Pediatr 2010; 22(3):278-83.

[10] Lynge TH, Nielsen TS, Gregers Winkel B, Tfelt-Hansen J, Banner J. Sudden cardiac death caused by myocarditis in persons aged 1-49 years: a nationwide study of 14 294 deaths in Denmark. Forensic Sci Res 2019;4(3):247-56.

[11] Freedman SB, Haladyn JK, Floh A, Kirsh JA, Taylor G, Thull-Freedman J. Pediatric myocarditis: emergency department clinical findings and diagnostic evaluation. Pediatrics 2007;120(6):1278-85.

[12] Durani Y, Giordano K, Goudie BW. Myocarditis and pericarditis in children. Pediatr Clin North Am 2010;57(6):1281-303.

[13] Butto A, Rossano JW, Nandi D, Ravishankar C, Lin KY, O'Connor MJ, et al. Elevated troponin in the first 72 h of hospitalization for pediatric viral myocarditis is associated with ECMO: An analysis of the PHIS+ Database. Pediatr Card 2018;39(6):1139-43.

[14] Caforio AL, Pankuweit S, Arbustini E, Basso C, Gimeno-Blanes J, Felix SB, et al. Current state of knowledge on aetiology, diagnosis, management, and therapy of myocarditis: a position statement of the European Society of Cardiology Working Group on Myocardial and Pericardial Diseases. Eur Heart J 2013;34(33):2636-48.

[15] Brighenti M, Donti A, Giulia Gagliardi M, Maschietto N, Marini D, Lombardi M, et al. Endomyocardial biopsy safety and clinical yield in pediatric myocarditis: An Italian perspective. Catheterization and cardiovascular interventions. Catheter Cardiovasc Interv 2016;87(4):762-7.

[16] Canter CE, Simpson KE. Diagnosis and treatment of myocarditis in children in the current era. Circulation 2014;129(1):115-28.

[17] Banka P, Robinson JD, Uppu SC, Harris MA, Hasbani K, Lai WW, et al. Cardiovascular magnetic resonance techniques and findings in children with myocarditis: a multicenter retrospective study. J Cardiovasc Magn Reson 2015;17:96. doi:10.1186/s12968-015-0201-6.

[18] Allan CK Fulton DR. Clinical manifestations and diagnosis of myocarditis in children. UpToDate 2019. URL: https://www.uptodate.com.

[19] Blauwet LA, Cooper LT. Myocarditis. Prog Cardiov Dis 2010;52(4):274-88.

[20] Levi D, Alejos J. An approach to the treatment of pediatric myocarditis. Paediatr Drugs 2002; 4(10):637-47.

[21] Yen CY, Hung MC, Wong YC, Chang CY, Lai CC, Wu KG. Role of intravenous immunoglobulin therapy in the survival rate of pediatric patients with acute myocarditis: A systematic review and meta-analysis. Sci Rep 2019;9(1):10459. doi: 10.1038/s41598-019-46888-0.

[22] Li Y, Yu Y, Chen S, Liao Y, Du J. Corticosteroids and intravenous immunoglobulin in pediatric myocarditis: A meta-analysis. Front Pediatr 2019;7:342. doi. 10.3389/fped.2019.00342.

[23] Chen HS, Wang W, Wu SN, Liu JP. Corticosteroids for viral myocarditis. Cochrane Database Syst Rev 2013;10:Cd004471. doi: 10.1002/14651858.CD004471.pub3.

[24] Aziz KU, Patel N, Sadullah T, Tasneem H, Thawerani H, Talpur S. Acute viral myocarditis: role of immunosuppression: a prospective randomised study. Cardiol Young 2010;20(5):509-15.

[25] Camargo PR, Snitcowsky R, da Luz PL, Mazzieri R, Higuchi ML, Rati M, et al. Favorable effects of immunosuppressive therapy in children with dilated cardiomyopathy and active myocarditis. Pediatr Cardiol 1995;16(2):61-8.

[26] Simpson KE, Canter CE. Acute myocarditis in children. Expert Rev Cardiovasc Ther 2011;9(6):771-83.

[27] Wu MH, Wu ET, Wang CC, Lu F, Chen HC, Kao FY, et al. Contemporary postnatal incidence of acquiring acute myocarditis by age 15 years and the outcomes from a nationwide birth cohort. Pediatr Crit Care Med 2017;18(12):1153-8.

[28] Foerster SR, Canter CE, Cinar A, Sleeper LA, Webber SA, Pahl E, et al. Ventricular remodeling and survival are more favorable for myocarditis than for idiopathic dilated cardiomyopathy in childhood: an outcomes study from the Pediatric Cardiomyopathy Registry. Circ Heart Fail 2010; 3(6):689-97.

[29] Hetzer R, Loebe M, Potapov EV, Weng Y, Stiller B, Hennig E, et al. Circulatory support with pneumatic paracorporeal ventricular assist device in infants and children. Ann Thorac Surg 1998; 66(5):1498-506.

[30] Ghelani SJ, Spaeder MC, Pastor W, Spurney CF, Klugman D. Demographics, trends, and outcomes in pediatric acute myocarditis in the United States, 2006 to 2011. Circ Cardiovasc Qual Outcomes 2012;5(5):622-7.

[31] Butts RJ, Boyle GJ, Deshpande SR, Gambetta K, Knecht KR, Prada-Ruiz CA, et al. Characteristics of clinically diagnosed pediatric myocarditis in a contemporary multi-center cohort. Pediatr Cardiol 2017;38(6):1175-82.

[32] Schultz JC, Hilliard AA, Cooper LT, Jr., Rihal CS. Diagnosis and treatment of viral myocarditis. Mayo Clin Proc 2009;84(11):1001-9.

[33] Bajwa R, Cheema A, Khan T, Amirpour A, Paul A, Chaughtai S, et al. Adverse effects of immune checkpoint inhibitors (programmed death-1 inhibitors and cytotoxic T-lymphocyte-associated protein-4 inhibitors): Results of a retrospective study. J Clin Med Res 2019;11(4):225-36.

[34] Bejiqi R, Retkoceri R, Maloku A, Mustafa A, Bejiqi H, Bejiqi R. The diagnostic and clinical approach to pediatric myocarditis: A review of the current literature. Open Access Maced J Med Sci 2019; 7(1):162-73.

In: Chronic Disease and Disability
Editors: DE Greydanus, P Anne, JD Rowlett et al.
ISBN: 978-1-53617-656-8

Chapter 8

HYPERLIPIDEMIA IN CHILDREN

Manisha Ravi[1], BS and
Premchand Anne[2,*], MD, MPH, MBA, FAAP, FACP FACC
[1]Ohio State University College of Medicine, Columbus, Ohio, United States of America
[2]Pediatric Cardiology, Ascension St John Children's Hospital,
Detroit, Michigan, United States of America

ABSTRACT

Atherosclerotic cardiovascular disease (ASCVD) is the leading cause of mortality and morbidity in the United States, accounting for approximately 103 deaths per 100,000 people or 1 in 7 deaths yearly. Risk factors of atherosclerosis in the young include lipoprotein levels, cigarette smoking, body mass index, and systolic as well as diastolic blood pressures. Topics covered in this discussion include the physiology of lipid metabolism, pathophysiology of atherosclerosis, classification of hyperlipidemias, secondary causes of hyperlipidemias, and guidelines to evaluation of pediatric patients with hyperlipidemia. Finally, principles of management of hyperlipidemia are presented to aid the primary care clinician in managing this important condition in their pediatric patients.

INTRODUCTION

Atherosclerotic cardiovascular disease (ASCVD) is the leading cause of mortality and morbidity in the United States, accounting for approximately 103 deaths per 100,000 people or 1 in 7 deaths yearly (1). Although ASCVD manifests primarily in adulthood, early epidemiologic studies have shown that the onset and progression of atherosclerotic changes occur as early as the fetal period and is increased by elevated maternal cholesterol levels (2, 3). An autopsy study of coronary arteries on individuals from birth to 29 years of age who died showed that isolated macrophage foam cells in the intima of newborns was the earliest

* Correspondence: Premchand Anne, MD, MBA, MPH, FACC, FAAP, Pediatric Cardiology, Ascension St John Children's Hospital, Detroit, Michigan 48236, United States. Email: Premchand.Anne@ascension.org.

indication of the atherosclerotic process. Eight percent of children in this study developed advanced atheromas (4).

In children, adolescents and young adults, several epidemiologic studies demonstrated an association between age and atherosclerosis and lipoproteins and atherosclerotic changes. Earliest studies evaluated aortas and coronary arteries of young combat veterans of wars in Korea and Vietnam; these investigations demonstrated atherosclerotic changes and gross narrowing of the coronary arteries in 45-77.3% of the hearts (5, 6). Furthermore, evaluation of the aortas and coronary arteries during autopsies in persons between 15 and 19 years of age showed presence of fatty streaks and fibrous plaques and increased in number with age (7).

In an autopsy study of subjects between 6 and 30 years of age, antemortem low densisty lipoprotein cholesterol (LDL-C), very low density lipoprotein cholesterol (VLDL-C) and ponderal index strongly correlated with the aorta and coronary artery fatty streaks (8). This was further corroborated by identification of risk factors of atherosclerosis in the young, which included lipoprotein levels, cigarette smoking, body mass index, and systolic and diastolic blood pressures (9).

Noninvasive investigations using ultrasound technology demonstrated the presence of atherosclerotic changes in childhood and young adulthood. A strong association was shown between LDL-C and carotid intimal-medial thickness (indicator of subclinical atherosclerosis) and coronary artery calcification and childhood risk factors track into adulthood (10, 11). Using intravascular ultrasound in heart transplant patients, atherosclerotic changes, including coronary intimal thickness, were directly proportional to age and started in childhood (12).

WHY SCREEN, EVALUATE AND MANAGE PEDIATRIC HYPERLIPIDEMIA?

Appropriate cut points for lipoprotein levels led to identification of adolescents who develop hyperlipidemia in adulthood (13). Recent evidence has shown an association between risk reduction in childhood and delay in onset and progression of atherosclerotic heart disease. Risk reduction for ASCVD includes LDL-C reduction (14). The concept of cumulative LDL-C exposure relates age to a theoretical threshold at which ASCVD manifests; this threshold is determined by the level of LDL-C and the length of exposure to the LDL-C level (15). For example, a child with homozygous Familial Hypercholesterolemia (FH) may reach the threshold by mid-second decade of life whereas a child with heterozygous FH will reach the threshold by late-third decade to mid-fourth decade of life.

Therefore, lowering the LDL-C exposure earlier will delay reaching the threshold, which makes it imperative to reduce the significantly elevated LDL-C levels in children. This was further confirmed in a meta-analysis evaluating the polymorphisms manifesting in LDL-C reduction and comparing the benefits to statin-induced LDL-C reduction; the authors concluded that exposure to low LDL-C levels early in life is more beneficial than reducing the LDL-C level at a later age (16, 17). In order to reduce the LDL-C levels in childhood, it is necessary to screen children, identify those that will benefit from LDL-C reduction, evaluate, and manage them appropriately.

RISK FACTORS FOR ASCVD AND HYPERLIPIDEMIA

The National Cholesterol Education Program panel, first published in 1991 and later adapted by American Academy of Pediatrics in 1992, recommended that children reduce intake of saturated fat, total fat and cholesterol after 2 years of age (18). The American Heart Association (AHA) identified LDL-C, hypertension, unhealthy body weight, sedentary lifestyle, tobacco use and diabetes mellitus as significant risk factors that can present in childhood (19).

Various risk factors for hyperlipidemia have been investigated in children: high body mass index (BMI) (20-24), increased waist circumference (25,26), hypertension (27), short sleep durations (28), physical inactivity (29), excess adiposity (30), family history of premature coronary artery disease (31-33), poorly controlled Type I and Type II Diabetes Mellitus (DM) (34-36), presence of intellectual disabilities (37), antipsychotic drug treatment (38), and use of protease inhibitors (39).

In 1998, the American Academy of Pediatrics (AAP) recommended screening children with the risk factors identified by the AHA, with the addition of a low HDL-C level and family history of early ASCVD, at the discretion of the physician (40). With the progression of the obesity epidemic, the AAP included metabolic syndrome (a collection of risk factors for ASCVD) as a risk factor in the 2008 expert panel guidelines. The most recent expert panel guidelines published by the AAP (2011) expanded the risk factors to include age, gender, "predisposing conditions," inflammatory markers and perinatal factors (41).

PHYSIOLOGY OF LIPID METABOLISM

Hyperlipidemia, by definition, is an elevated level of fats in the blood. These fats include cholesterol and triglycerides. Cholesterol contains a tetracyclic ring structure with attached hydroxyl and hydrocarbon groups, providing both hydrophilic and hydrophobic properties to the molecule. Triglycerides are composed of three fatty acids with a glycerol backbone. Hyperlipidemia results from overproduction or impaired removal of these fats from the blood. These lipids are transported in the blood within lipoproteins. The apolipoproteins present on lipoproteins help direct metabolism of the particular lipoproteins. The five major lipoproteins involved in lipid metabolism are chylomicrons, low-density lipoprotein (LDL), intermediate-density lipoprotein (IDL), very low-density lipoprotein (VLDL), high-density lipoprotein (HDL) and chylomicrons. The lipoproteins deliver lipids to various organs and tissues through the exogenous, endogenous, and reverse transport mechanisms.

First, the exogenous pathway is involved in transporting dietary fat and cholesterol from the intestine to the tissues and the liver. The free fatty acids and monoglycerides, byproducts of emulsification of triglycerides by bile and pancreatic lipase, are absorbed into the enterocytes. Once inside the enterocyte, nascent chylomicrons are formed and transferred into the lymphatic system. As they enter the bloodstream, apolipoproteins (Apo CII and Apo E) attach to the nascent chylomicrons (mature-form). As these mature chylomicrons travel through the bloodstream, the-Apo CII activated lipoprotein lipase (LPL), present on blood vessels in various tissues, hydrolyzes the triglycerides to release fatty acids, which are taken up by the tissues. After triglyceride removal, chylomicrons are markedly reduced in size, forming cholesterol ester-rich chylomicron remnants. The majority of the chylomicron remnants are cleared by liver through binding of Apo E to hepatic receptors.

The second pathway of lipid metabolism is the endogenous pathway, which processes lipid synthesized within the liver. Nascent VLDL particles are synthesized by assembling triacylglycerols, cholesterol esters and ApoB-100, which are then released into the bloodstream via an ApoB 100-dependent mechanism mediated by microsomal triglyceride transfer protein (MTP). VLDL synthesis is determined by availability of triglycerides, which regulates ApoB 100 degradation versus secretion (42). In the bloodstream, the VLDL particles pick up Apo C-II and ApoE. The triglycerides are hydrolyzed once LPL is activated by Apo C-II, with release of fatty acids and glycerol to the peripheral tissues.

With the hydrolysis of triglycerides, the VLDLs are converted to IDLs, whose triglycerides are further hydrolyzed to form LDL molecules. The Apo B-100 on the LDL molecule interacts with the LDL-R, thereby facilitating removal of LDL molecules from the blood. The LDL particles are hydrolyzed in the hepatic cellular lysosomes. LDL molecules are also endocytosed by the peripheral cells, with release of cholesterol. The free cholesterol can regulate the rate of cholesterol synthesis within the peripheral cells as well the number of LDL-R on the cell surface. LDL-R expression subsequently significantly affects plasma LDL concentration.

Reduced hepatocyte cholesterol levels stimulate release and conversion of inactive sterol regulatory element binding proteins (SREBPs) to their active form. These activated transcription factors increase both LDL-R expression and HMG-CoA reductase-dependent cholesterol synthesis. Increased LDL-R expression allows for increased LDL uptake and subsequent cholesterol release (43). In states of cholesterol excess, lysosomal degradation of LDL-R is stimulated by binding of proprotein convertase subtilisin/kexin type 9 (PCSK9), which results in reduced hepatic LDL uptake (44).

The final pathway is the reverse cholesterol transport pathway, which is involved in mobilizing cholesterol from the peripheral tissues back to the liver. HDLs are the major lipoproteins involved in this pathway, with Apo A-1 being the major apolipoprotein associated with HDLs. As a sink for cholesterol in the form of cholesterol esters, the HDLs subtypes are involved in transferring cholesterol esters to LDL and VLDL particles in exchange for triglycerides, which can then be secreted into bile or converted into bile acids for excretion. Reduced triglyceride clearance and, therefore, elevated triglyceride levels are often linked to low HDL. The HDL molecules are also believed to have an antiatherogenic effect through inhibition of oxidation, inflammation, and apoptosis (45).

PATHOPHYSIOLOGY OF ATHEROSCLEROSIS

Atherosclerosis is a progressive disease process with its onset usually fetal life/early childhood and typical manifestation in adulthood. However, understanding the pathophysiology of atherosclerosis and its significant players will help appreciate the need to intervene for primary prevention starting in childhood. It is a multifactorial process that is initiated by damage to the endothelium, followed by accumulation of monocytes into the subendothelial space. The monocytes morph into macrophages and ingest oxidized LDL to form foam cells. Inflammatory processes, mediated by cytokine production, play an integral part in this disease progress.

With progressive accumulation of the foam cells and smooth muscle emigration into the subendothelial space, fatty streaks develop and mainly consist of live cells, triglycerides and cholesterol. Fatty streaks are the first visible evidence of an atherosclerotic process. This process leads to extracellular and intracellular lipid accumulation, formation of a fibrous cap, culminating in an atheroma formation. The associated luminal narrowing has the potential to cause peripheral claudication or angina depending on affected vessels. Additionally, the dead cells and extracellular matrix and lipid in the center of the plaque form a necrotic core. If the fibrous cap ruptures, this can lead to thrombosis and subsequent impedance of blood flow and ischemia. By decreasing the LDL-C level, the accumulation and oxidation of these particles is reduced, thereby inhibiting the early steps of atherosclerosis.

Table 1. Fredrickson classification of primary hyperlipidemia

Type		Elevated lipoprotein	Primary causes	Total cholesterol	Total triglyceride
I		Chylomicrons	Defective LPL Defective Apo CII	Normal	Markedly elevated
II	a	LDL-C	FH	Elevated	Normal
	b	LDL-C and VLDL	FCH	Elevated	Elevated
III		IDL	FD	Elevated	Elevated
IV		VLDL	FHTG	Normal to elevated	Elevated
V		VLDL and Chylomicrons	Familial Mixed Hypertriglyceridemia	Normal to elevated	Markedly elevated

CLASSIFICATION OF HYPERLIPIDEMIAS

Hyperlipidemias can result from the breakdown of underlying mechanisms in the three lipid metabolic pathways. Defective lipoproteins or apolipoproteins and their receptors can also manifest as hyperlipidemias, with three predominant phenotypes: hypercholesterolemia, hypertriglyceridemia, or a combination of both. The underlying mechanism can be of primary (inherited/genetic) or secondary (acquired) etiologies. The Frederickson classification of hyperlipidemias delineates the lipoprotein abnormalities associated with primary hyperlipidemias (see Table 1) (46). While hypercholesterolemia (LDL-C elevation) is the causal factor of ASCVD, marked elevation of triglycerides increases the patient's risk of pancreatitis. The age-appropriate levels for LDL-C and triglyceride levels and criteria for management will be discussed later.

PRIMARY CAUSES OF HYPERLIPIDEMIAS

The primary etiologies of hypercholesterolemia of interest are familial hypercholesterolemia (FH), familial combined hyperlipidemia (FCH), familial dysbetalipoproteinemia (FD), and polygenic hypercholesterolemia (PH). The underlying genetic causes and chief characteristics of each of these conditions are discussed below. Secondary causes must be eliminated before establishing the diagnosis of a primary hyperlipidemia. Understanding the pathophysiology will allow for proper management (non-pharmacologic and pharmacologic means) of these conditions.

Familial hypercholesterolemia is a monogenic disorder that is transmitted in an autosomal dominant manner and is primarily associated with decreased uptake of LDL from the blood. Although homozygous FH is uncommon (1 out of 1,000,000), the prevalence of FH is approximately 1 out of 500 to one out of 250 people (47, 48). The underlying causes of FH include mutations in genes involved in LDL-R and ApoB synthesis, or a gain of function mutation in PCSK9 enyzme. The defective LDL-R (>95% of the cases) is unable to recognize the LDL molecules, where as the defective Apo B (2-5% of the cases) prevents binding of LDL to LDL-R (49). The gain of function mutation in PCSK9 (<1% of cases) leads to increased destruction of LDL-R, thereby preventing recycling of the receptor back to the cell membrane (49). The autosomal recessive variant of FH is extremely rare.

Primary mode of diagnosis is clinical, with an emphasis on LDL-C levels (up to 1,100 mg/dL), tendon xanthomas (Achilles, patellar, and digital extensors), xanthalasma and corneal arcus in the young. Initial presentation for homozygous FH may be death due to a myocardial infarction (MI) within the early to mid second decade. Genetic testing confirming mutations in the LDL-R, ApoB, and PCSK9 genes can further help make the diagnosis. The lipoprotein phenotype is Type IIa.

Familial combined hyperlipidemia (FCH) is one of the most common causes of hyperlipidemia and is another monogenic disorder with an autosomal dominant transmission. Dyslipidemia associated with FCH can present as pure hypercholesterolemia, pure hypertriglyceridemia or a combination of both. The prevalence of FCH in the general population can be as high as two percent (50). Although there is difficulty with defining FCH to establish the diagnosis, the environmental factors play a significant role. With the environmental contribution from the obesity epidemic and metabolic syndrome, the prevalence of FCH is likely increasing.

The primary defect associated with FCH is the increased synthesis of Apo B-100 (VLDL-Apo B-100 and LDL-Apo B-100) due to decreased fatty acid oxidation and increased triglyceride synthesis. Other molecular defects have been implicated. This results in increased VLDL and small, dense LDL levels, often with elevated triglycerides (51, 52). There is premature ASCVD in individuals with FCH, although the incidence is beyond that of FH. The diagnosis of FCH is tricky but is consistent with an isolated LDL-C or triglyceride level or combined hyperlipidemia, first degree relative with early ASCVD, elevated Apo B-100 level and potential confirmation with genetic testing (52). The lipoprotein phenotype is Type IIb, IV, and V.

Familial dysbetalipoproteinemia (FD) is a primary hyperlipidemia that is predominantly inherited in an autosomal recessive manner, although other rare variants of FD follow autosomal dominant transmission. The frequency of FD is 1 out of 10,000 (53). The defect that is associated with FD is a mutation of the apolipoprotein E (Apo E), in particular the isoform E2. The prevalence of homozygosity for Apo E2 defect is commonly found in FD, although only 4 percent of those with homozygous E2 genotype develop FD. As with FCH, there is significant environmental influence, in addition to homozygous Apo E2 phenotype, that determines whether a child develops FD. These environmental cues include body mass index, nutrition, age and hormones.

Due to the Apo E defect, there is buildup of VLDL-remnants and chylomicron remnants due to impaired clearance (54). Clinical findings include tuberous or tuberoeruptive xanthomas on the elbows and knees, and palmar xanthomas (pathognomonic) and plantar streaks, premature ASCVD and recurrent pancreatitis. The lipid profile is remarkable for elevated total cholesterol that is slightly lower than the triglyceride level. This manifests as Type III lipoprotein phenotype.

Finally, polygenic hypercholesterolemia (PH) is the most common cause of hypercholesterolemia without a unique defect unlike the above three diagnoses. The prevalence of PH is 1 in 10 to 1 in 20 in the general population. The condition is due to a combination of multiple gene polymorphisms and environmental factors (i.e., dietary excess) that results in increased LDL levels; however, only those with an elevated Apo B-100 are at risk for ASCVD compared to those with normal Apo B-100. However, compared to FH, the elevation of LDL-C level in PH is milder. There is evidence of premature ASCVD, although the onset is delayed compared to FH. Family history is key to the diagnosis; less than ten percent of first degree relatives of those with PH have hyperlipidemia.

Hypertriglyceridemias

The primary causes of hypertriglyceridemia that are of interest are familial hyperchylomicronemia, familial hypertriglyceridemia (FHTG), and mixed hypertriglyceridemia. These etiologies can be monogenic or polygenic. Of the above three primary causes, familial hyperchylomicronemia is monogenic, follows autosomal recessive inheritance and occurs in 1 out of 1,000,000 with the heterozygotes mutation of LPL gene occurring 1 out of 600. Absence or defective lipoprotein lipase (LPL) is the primary cause. Other mutated genes for Apo C-II, Apo A-5, lipase maturation factor 1 (LMF1), and GPI-anchored HDL-binding protein 1 (GP1HBP1) also cause hyperchylomicronemia and associated hypertriglyceridemia in a Type I hyperlipoproteinemia (55, 56).

Lipemia retinalis is an important ocular sign of familial hyperchylomicronemia. It is a potentially reversible condition presenting with milky white retinal arteries and veins that result from elevated triglyceride levels. Ocular findings are caused by scattering of light by chylomicrons loaded with triglycerides. There is no observed reduction in visual acuity (57, 58). Common causes include autosomal recessive LPL or cofactor Apo C-II deficiency. Clinical grading is dependent on spread and correlates with severity of triglyceride elevation. Early stage involves milky whitening of peripheral retinal vessels at triglyceride levels 2500–3499 mg/dL. Progression to the posterior pole occurs at triglyceride levels between 3500–5000 mg/dL, characterizing the moderate stage. Finally, the fundus takes on a salmon colored appearance with diffuse whitening of retinal vessels at levels above 5000 mg/dL in the marked stage (57). The condition does not require direct treatment and is usually reversible with correction of serum triglyceride levels.

Next, familial hypertriglyceridemia (Type 4 hyperlipoproteinemia) is polygenic and is associated with elevated VLDL (55). FHTG is transmitted in an autosomal dominant manner. The frequency of FHTG is 1 out of 500 in the general population and is often associated with other comorbidities such as obesity and diabetes.

Table 2. Secondary causes of hyperlipidemia

Underlying condition	Mechanism	Resulting hyperlipidemia		
		LDL	TG	HDL
Overweight/obesity and nutrition	Overproduction of VLDL, decreased LPL activity	↑	↑	↓
Diabetes mellitus, type II	Decreased LPL activity, overproduction of VLDL	↑	↑	↓
Hypothyroidism	Down regulation of LDL-R, decreased hepatic lipase and LPL activity	↑	±↑	±↓
Anorexia nervosa	Decreased LDL-R, increased fat mobilization, decreased cholesterol and bile turnover	↑		
Medications	Varies	Varies		
Excess alcohol	Overproduction of VLDL	±↑	↑	↑
Cigarette smoking	Decreased LPL activity		↑	↓
Hyperglycerolemia	Glycerol kinase deficiency			

Mixed hypertriglyceridemia (Type 5 hyperlipoproteinemia) likely follows autosomal recessive inheritance and is associated with abdominal pain, hepatomegaly, and lipemia retinalis. The lipoprotein abnormalities include elevated VLDL and chylomicrons, with concomitant triglyceride elevation. In general, the main concern associated with hypertriglyceridemia, regardless of the cause, is the heightened risk of pancreatitis. Clinical presentation includes eruptive xanthomas, and abdominal pain.

SECONDARY CAUSES OF HYPERLIPIDEMIA

Secondary hyperlipidemias are dyslipidemias which are caused by underlying conditions, including unhealthy body weight, diabetes, hypothyroidism, and anorexia nervosa to mention a few. A comprehensive list of causes of secondary dyslipidemia is provided in the recent AAP Expert Panel guidelines (41). Table 2 summarizes the common causes of secondary hyperlipidemias, mechanism by which hyperlipidemia results and the lipid abnormality that results. In addition, secondary hyperlipidemias can compound the dyslipidemias due to the primary hyperlipidemias. The common comorbidities discussed below are relevant to the pediatric population and treating the comorbidity should produce an improvement in the dyslipidemia.

Overweight/obesity/nutrition

Unhealthy body weight, in the form of overweight or obesity, results when the intake of calories exceeds the expenditure of calories. Whether the intake of calories is in the form of refined carbohydrates, proteins, or fats, in addition to increased flux of free fatty acids, the liver overproduces Apo B-containing, triglyceride-rich lipoproteins, which manifest as increased small, dense LDL particles, diminished HDL-C levels, and increased triglyceride levels (59). The increased triglyceride levels lead to dense HDL particles due to transfer of triglycerides from VLDL to HDL via cholesterol-ester transfer protein (CETP) activity. There is also decreased LPL activity in skeletal muscle and decreased mRNA expression of LPL in adipose tissue, leading to increased remnant lipoproteins (59). The lipoprotein profile for nutrition rich in refined carbohydrates and fats is similar to that of individuals with an unhealthy body weight.

Diabetes mellitus

The dyslipidemia associated with diabetes depends on the activity of LPL. LPL requires adequate levels of insulin to function. In the case of type I diabetes mellitus, deficient insulin levels lead to deficient LPL activity. On the other hand, in type II diabetes with an insulin resistance state, LPL activity decreases and is often deficient, similar to that of obesity. The dyslipidemia of type 2 diabetes mellitus is similar to that of obesity due to similar underlying mechanisms (60). The increase in remnant lipoproteins can compound the effects of primary hyperlipoproteinemias discussed in the previous section.

Hypothyroidism

Hypothyroidism, whether overt or subclinical, is a well-known cause of secondary hyperlipidemia, in particular secondary hypercholesterolemia. This condition is primarily associated with an increase in LDL, IDL and Apo B levels (61). While hypothyroidism leads to decreased synthesis of cholesterol intracellularly by down-regulation of 3-Hydroxy-3-Methyl-Glutaryl Coenzyme A (HMGCoA) reductase, there is downregulation of the LDL-R expression, thereby decreasing clearance of LDL particles. The effect on triglycerides is dependent on LPL activity and is likely dependent on the levels of TSH. Due to diminished LPL activity, the Apo B-containing lipoproteins are triglyceride-rich and the lipoprotein profile is similar to and can contribute to type III hyperlipoproteinemias. Subclinical hypothyroidism (normal free thyroxine with elevated TSH) behaves similar to overt hypothyroidism as TSH levels increase (62).

Anorexia nervosa

Eating disorders are a common pathology seen in children and adolescents. Anorexia nervosa (AN), a condition resulting from starvation, is associated with hypercholesterolemia. The hypercholesterolemia associated with AN is counterintuitive given the hypocaloric, low-fat and hypocholesterolemic diet intake. The overall cholesterol synthesis in patients with AN is decreased. The hypercholesterolemia is attributed to reduced cholesterol and bile turnover and/or increased body fat mobilization, thereby leading to decreased cholesterol synthesis and decreased LDL-R activity. The decreased uptake of LDL-C due to LDL-R downregulation leads to elevated LDL-C levels (63). Furthermore, the hypothyroidism that is associated with AN also contributes to LDL-C elevation as described above.

Drugs

Medical therapies for various medical conditions and performance enhancement lead to secondary hyperlipidemias. The mechanisms vary by the class of drugs but they manifest as hypercholesterolemia, hypertriglyceridemia or a combination. Especially in adolescence and early adulthood, isotretinoin and oral contraceptives are commonly utilized. These two classes are associated with significant triglyceride elevations. Isotretinoin may promote exacerbation of a latent or predisposed hyperlipidemia, although the underlying mechanism is not well-known (64). The involvement of Apo E2 and Apo E4 may contribute to the hypertriglyceridemia with isotretinoin use.

Next, oral contraceptives, commonly used for polycystic ovarian syndrome, dysmenorrhea and prevention of pregnancy, lead to significant triglyceride and HDL-C elevations in those with higher estrogen components (65, 66). Another example of dyslipidemia associated with medical therapy is due to cyclosporine use in transplant patients. Cyclosporine is associated with increased VLDL and triglycerides due to increased Apo C-III which is an inhibitor of LPL and HL activity and decreased HDL-C levels. Cyclosporine is also associated with increase LDL levels due to decreased LDL-R on the hepatocytes and increased free cholesterol within the cytoplasm (67, 68).

Corticosteroids, whether used in asthma management, immunosuppression, or for other indications, are associated with a type IIb hyperlipoproteinemia. Corticosteroids contribute to hyperinsulinemia/insulin resistance, subsequently leading to decreased LPL activity and increased VLDL production and decreased triglyceride clearance. Anabolic steroids are associated with significant adverse lipid profiles. These agents are associated with a decrease in HDL-C and an increase in LDL-C (69). Compared to control subjects, those utilizing anabolic steroids had lower Apo A-1/B-100 ratios, which was congruent with the lipid changes. These changes are atherogenic (69, 70). Discussions with children/adolescents using anabolic steroids should include adverse effects of these agents, including the atherogenic effect.

Antipsychotic medications are indicated in patients with schizophrenia and certain mood disorders. Many of these medications are also approved for use in pediatric patients for similar indications (71). Second generation antipsychotic medications, while similar in efficacy to first generation antipsychotics, have a superior side effect profile with a reduction in extrapyramidal symptoms. Major drawbacks include weight gain and adverse metabolic effects of hyperglycemia and hypertriglyceridemia. The highest risk of hypertriglyceridemia is seen in the atypical antipsychotics clozapine, olanzapine, and quetiapine (72). Data suggests that the pediatric patient population may be at increased risk of weight gain and metabolic abnormalities compared to adults (71), suggesting that this population should be followed closely when placed on these medications. While the underlying mechanism of hyperlipidemia associated with atypical antipsychotic use is unclear, the resulting enhanced lipogenesis and inhibited lipolysis, as well as the promotion of insulin-mediated reduced adipocyte lipolysis may contribute to this dyslipidemia (73).

Beta blockers act as competitive antagonists at the beta adrenergic receptor, preventing the binding and action of the catecholamines, epinephrine and norepinephrine. This class of medications is commonly used to treat arrhythmias and hypertension. Older generation beta blockers do not contain the vasodilating characteristics that are present in the newer generation medications. These older generation beta blockers (atenolol, metoprolol, and propranolol) are found to raise triglyceride levels and reduce HDL-C (74, 75). A proposed mechanism for the associated dyslipidemia is due to the promotion of insulin resistance by beta blockers. First, insulin clearance is decreased with beta blockers, which results in elevated plasma insulin levels (74). Second, the reduction in cardiac output associated with non-vasodilating beta blockers, which may be a result of unopposed alpha-1 adrenergic activity, reduces glucose uptake by skeletal muscles (74, 75). Both mechanisms contribute to subsequent development of insulin resistance.

Diuretics are used to increase urine production in the treatment of hypertension and heart failure. Thiazide diuretics act on the Na^+/Cl^- cotransporter in the distal convoluted tubule of the kidney nephron to inhibit sodium and chloride reabsorption. Loop diuretics act on $Na^+/K^+/2Cl^-$ symporter in the thick ascending limb of the Loop of Henle to inhibit sodium reabsorption. As a result of diuretic use, water is retained in the tubule for excretion in the urine. Diuretics have been shown to cause increases in cholesterol and triglyceride levels in a dose-dependent fashion and exert the greatest effect on black populations (76). Therefore, high doses of these medications should be used with caution.

Excess alcohol use

Although limited alcohol use is associated with beneficial effects (increase in HDL-C), excess alcohol use is associated with an adverse lipid profile. The lipid profile is characteristic of a type IV or type V lipoproteinemia with VLDL excess and rarely but additional chylomicron excess, respectively (77). There was no significant change in the LDL-C in those with moderate alcohol consumption but a dose-response relationship with HDL-C and triglyceride levels (78).

Cigarette smoking

Cigarette smoking has a lipid profile that is atherogenic; however, the tobacco use is also a risk factor that is independent of lipoprotein levels (79). Epidemiologic studies have noted a higher levels of triglycerides due to elevated VLDL levels and Apo B levels in smokers. They also showed an increase in LDL-C and a decrease in HDL-C and its predominant apolipoprotein (Apo A-1) independent of the triglyceride level (80,81). The benefit of smoking cessation is that the lipid profiles of former smokers were comparable to those in nonsmokers.

Hyperglycerolemia

Hyperglycerolemia is a cause of pseudohypertriglyceridemia. The enzymatic defect associated with the diagnosis is mutation in the gene encoding glycerol kinase, which phosphorylates glycerol to form glycerol-3-phosphate. This is an X-linked recessive defect (82). Deficiency of this enzyme leads to accumulation of glycerol and inability to synthesize triglycerides. Routine testing of a fasting lipid profile will reveal an elevated triglyceride level. Initiation of treatment with dietary measures including refined carbohydrate restriction, and initiation of omega-3-acid ethyl esters and triglyceride-lowering pharmacotherapies do not reduce or resolve the hypertriglyceridemia. In such a case, performing a glycerol-blanked (glycerol-corrected) triglyceride level will demonstrate the discrepancy between triglyceride level and a markedly elevated glycerol level.

EVALUATION OF A HYPERLIPIDEMIA

A practical and systematic approach to evaluation of a hyperlipidemia is the key to establishing a clinical diagnosis. Initial hyperlipidemia evaluation must include a thorough evaluation of the patient's medical history, family history, clinical chemistry assessment including lipoprotein and physical exam. The purpose of the evaluation is to determine whether the hyperlipidemia is of primary etiology, secondary etiology, or a primary etiology with secondary contributions from comorbidities.

Medical history

When questioning about the medical history, it is important to establish when the initial diagnosis of a hyperlipidemia was established and whether the hyperlipidemia is a hypercholesterolemia, hypertriglyceridemia or a combination of both. While obtaining the medical history, it is important to consider secondary causes that may affect the lipid profile, whether fasting or non-fasting. Non-fasting profile may be more practical in children for an initial assessment and confirmed, if needed, with a fasting lipid profile.

Lipid profile assessment

The timing of the initial screen maybe relevant if pubertal time is of value. It is well recognized that the total cholesterol and LDL-C levels decrease by 10 to 20 percent during puberty. Therefore, the AAP Expert Panel recommended universal screening of children between 9 and 11 years of age, a period which is pre-pubertal for most children (41). A non-fasting lipid profile followed by an average of two fasting lipid profiles is recommended if a hyperlipidemia is noted on the nonfasting lipid profile or an average of two fasting lipid profiles to confirm the diagnosis of hyperlipidemia. In addition, it is recommended that children 2 to 8 years of age and 12 to 16 years of age be screened if there are significant risk factors.

These risk factors include: 1) parent with total cholesterol ≥240 mg/dL or known dyslipidemia, 2) child with diabetes, hypertension, BMI ≥95th percentile, or cigarette smoking, 3) child with at least one family member with early manifestation of ASCVD (<55 years in males and <65 years in females), and 4) child with a moderate- or high-risk medical condition (41). For children in these two age groups, two fasting lipid profiles performed two to twelve weeks apart should be averaged. It is also important to note whether the lipid profile was obtained while fasting or at a random time. If done in a non-fasting state, then the non-HDL-C level must be used. The recommended lipid and lipoprotein level cut points are different for children and adolescents and those in the young adult category. Tables 3 and 4 present the cutoffs as acceptable, borderline-high and high for the two groups.

Table 3. Lipid and lipoprotein cut points for children and adolescents (adapted from the Expert Panel Guidelines) (41)

Category	Acceptable (mg/dL)	Borderline-High (mg/dL)-75%	High (mg/dL)-95%
Total cholesterol	<170	170-199	≥200
LDL cholesterol	<110	110-129	≥130
Non-HDL cholesterol	<120	120-144	≥145
HDL cholesterol	>45	40-45	
Triglycerides			
0-9 years	<75	75-99	≥100
10-19 years	<90	90-129	≥130

Table 4. Lipid and lipoprotein cut points for young adults (adapted from the Expert Panel Guidelines) (41)

Category	Acceptable (mg/dL)	Borderline-High (mg/dL)	High (mg/dL)
Total cholesterol*	<190	190-224	≥225
LDL cholesterol*	<120	120-159	≥160
Non-HDL cholesterol*	<150	150-189	≥190
Triglycerides#	<115	115-149	≥150
HDL cholesterol@	>45		

*Borderline: 75-94%; #Borderline-High: 75-89%; @Acceptable: >50%.

Family history

After the medical history, a detailed family history must be delineated. It is important to identify any first degree relatives, including siblings, with hyperlipidemia and/or early manifestation of ASCVD (cerebrovascular accident (CVA), myocardial infarction (MI), peripheral vascular disease or other coronary equivalents). In addition to early ASCVD, other significant comorbidities, such as diabetes mellitus, chronic kidney disease, autoimmune diseases, must be documented in the family history. The family history should extend to paternal and maternal grandparents to document early onset ASCVD to overcome undiagnosed, subclinical ASCVD in first degree relatives. Preparing a pedigree will help establish patterns of inheritance, if any exist. Determining the presence or absence of the mode of inheritance can help establish the diagnosis for the hyperlipidemia.

Laboratory assessment

Next, laboratory assessment will contribute to confirmation of the diagnosis responsible for the hyperlipidemia. The clinical chemistry assessment must include thyroid function tests, glycemic indices, liver enzymes, renal indices to exclude thyroid disease, diabetes mellitus/insulin resistance, hepatic disease, and renal disease. Lipoprotein(a), Lp(a), must be assessed in children with hemorrhagic or ischemic stroke. Lipoprotein(a) is an independent risk factor for ASCVD (83). Although Lp(a) is associated with ASCVD in adulthood, identification of an elevated Lp(a) may prompt more aggressive therapy for LDL-C reduction. If dysbetalipoproteinemia is under consideration, an Apo E genotype is warranted to see if the Apo E genotype is E2/E2. A lipoprotein electrophoresis is often indicated to determine whether hypertriglyceridemia is due to triglycerides or due to chylomicrons or secondary to elevated VLDL and IDL levels.

Physical exam (lipid deposition) findings

Finally, a thorough physical exam is critical in establishing a diagnosis as a cause of a particular hyperlipidemia. Findings of particular interest include obesity, corneal arcus and xanthalasma, xanthomata (tendon, tuberous, eruptive, and planar), and bruits and diminished pulses. As mentioned above, obesity is associated with increased triglycerides and LDL-C levels and a decreased HDL-C level. Assessing height percentile, weight percentile, and body mass index percentile for age and gender is important to characterize the unhealthy weight as overweight or obesity. Corneal arcus is lipid deposition consisting of cholesterol and triglycerides in the periphery of the cornea and is usually a benign finding. Xanthalasma palpebrarum are yellow lesions in the dermis and localized to the medial aspects of the upper and lower eyelids and consist of cholesterol in xanthoma cells (84).

Xanthomas are categorized into tendinous, tuberoeruptive, tuberous, and planar types (85). Tendinous xanthomas are pathognomonic of FH and contain free and esterified cholesterol; they are also often seen in sitosterolemia and cerebrotendinous xanthomatosis. The most common location for tendinous xanthomas are the Achilles tendons but are also found on digits, elbows, and knees; tendinous xanthomas are either persistent or resolve after prolonged period of time. Tuberous and tuberoeruptive xanthomas are characteristic of FD; these are nontender, yellow-orange, firm nodules on extensor surfaces (elbows and knees) which usually resolve in a few months post initiation of treatment.

Eruptive xanthomas are non-tender, yellowish raised lesions present on the elbows, shoulders and buttocks. These are present in conditions with markedly elevated triglyceride levels as in uncontrolled diabetes mellitus and usually resolve within weeks upon treating the underlying condition. Finally, planar xanthomas are yellowish deposits on palmar surfaces and are specifically associated with FD.

Finally, bruits and diminished pulses are rare findings in children, adolescents and young adults. Bruits and diminished pulses manifest as a result of obstructive disease; in the setting of hyperlipidemia, this is due to obstruction resulting from plaque and atheroma formation. If the hyperlipidemia is managed effectively, the atherosclerotic changes may stabilize.

MANAGEMENT OF HYPERLIPIDEMIA

Management of hyperlipidemia is two-fold once the hyperlipidemia and its etiology is clear. The primary intervention is lifestyle change involving nutrition and physical activity, before initiating pharmacotherapy suitable for the hyperlipidemia.

Nutrition

From the NCEP Pediatric Panel, the recommended diet restricts total fat to <30% of total calories, saturated fat to <10% of total calories and dietary cholesterol to <300 mg/day (86). In children with an identified hypercholesterolemia, further restriction of saturated fat and cholesterol is required (<7% of calories due to fat and cholesterol to <200 mg/day, respectively). Besides restricting dietary fat, saturated fat and cholesterol intake, addition of plant stanols/sterols of approximately 2 grams/day decreases LDL-C by an additional 9-20% in children (87). Another dietary supplement is soluble fiber, in particular psyllium husk. In children, psyllium use of 6 grams/day in 2-12 year olds and 12 grams/day in >12 year old children had multiple benefits: 1) decrease in postprandial glucose level of 20%, 2) decrease in serum LDL-C of 22%, 3) decrease in triglyceride levels of 20%, and 4) increase in HDL-C of 3% (41, 88, 89).

Children with diabetes and/or obesity can benefit from psyllium supplementation. In those with hypertriglyceridemia, refined carbohydrate restriction and caloric restriction are required to achieve some nonpharmacological benefit and control. If further control is needed, Cardiovascular Health Integrated Lifestyle Diet (CHILD-1 and CHILD-2) diets are recommended per the 2011 Expert panel guidelines (41). A consultation with a registered dietician should be encouraged to bring about an informed lifestyle change.

Activity

A companion of dietary modification under nonpharmacologic intervention and lifestyle change is physical activity. The benefits of moderate to vigorous physical activity are: 1) decreased body fat and BMI, 2) improved lipid profile, and 3) decreased insulin resistance. The Expert Panel guidelines recommend one hour of activity per day, at least three times a week, for children over 5 years of age (41). A pedometer should be obtained for the child, with the goal of taking 10,000 steps per day. Reduction of "tube time" to less than two hours per day is also warranted.

Pharmacotherapy

Pharmacotherapy is an option available to the physician to control the dyslipidemia that is suboptimally controlled with nutrition and activity interventions. The purpose of pharmacotherapy in hypercholesterolemia is to reduce the LDL-C burden within the vasculature to mitigate the atherosclerotic changes and delay their onset in children. The criteria for medical therapy to achieve the LDL-C goal include: 1) LDL-C ≥190 mg/dL after dietary intervention in a child 10 years or older, or 2) LDL-C between 160 and 189 mg/dL after dietary intervention in a child 10 years or older and either a positive family history in first degree relatives, one high-level risk factor or two moderate level risk factors/conditions.

LDL-C reduction

There are three drug classes that are currently utilized for decreasing the LDL-C levels to achieve the goal of ≤130 mg/dL (<95%). These include bile acid-binding resins/sequestrants (BAS), statins, and an intestinal cholesterol absorption inhibitor (ezetimibe). An upcoming class of therapy for LDL-C reduction in children are proprotein convertase subtilisin kexin 9 (PCSK9) inhibitors.

First, the mechanism by which BAS work is to prevent reuptake of bile acids in the intestine, which leads to depletion of intracellular cholesterol during the synthesis of bile acids de novo. Consequently, the LDL-R are upregulated which leads to uptake of LDL-C from the blood and lowering of the LDL-C in the blood. BAS are poorly tolerated for the quantity of medication that needs to be ingested and gastrointestinal side effects that are frequently reported. The side effect profile leads to poor compliance which further compounds the relative inefficacy compared to the statins and ezetimibe. In those with a mixed hyperlipidemia, BAS can increase the triglyceride further, which may necessitate a second medication to lower triglycerides where diet may have controlled the triglyceride elevation.

Next class of medications is the statins. Statins inhibit HMGCoA reductase, thereby decreasing intracellular cholesterol, which leads to upregulation of LDL-R and uptake of LDL-C in the blood. The statins, in general, are more effective when taken at bed time due to their half-lives. Two classes of statins are available: lipophilic and hydrophilic statins. Lipophilic statins are lovastatin, simvastatin, and atorvastatin whereas the hydrophilic statins are pravastatin and rosuvastatin. The lipophilic statins are known to cross the blood-brain barrier, which is a concern in a growing child. Side effects (although rare) of statins include myopathy, hepatic transaminase elevations, and rhabdomyolysis. The side effects tend to be less pronounced in the pediatric population when using hydrophilic statins (rosuvastatin and pravastatin).

When prescribing a statin at a certain dose, it is important to consider the age of the patient, the weight of the patient, and the degree of LDL-C elevation. It is common practice to start below the prescribed starting doses which are commonly used in adults and titrate up as necessary. The starting (adult) dose determines the efficacy of the medication; beyond the starting dose, doubling the dose will provide a diminishing LDL-C reduction. For example, if the starting dose of pravastatin (20 mg) provides a 33% reduction in LDL-C levels, doubling the dose to 40mg may only add another 6-7% reduction in LDL-C levels. In the case of lipophilic statins, increasing the dose can lead to a small reduction of LDL-C at the expense of higher number of side effects described above. For the children seen in the Pediatric Lipid Clinic at our institution and started on statins, no side effects have been reported over the past six years; this is in part due to the preferential use of pravastatin and rosuvastatin.

The other alternative for LDL-C reduction in children is ezetimibe, which is a second line therapy. The mechanism of action for ezetimibe is inhibition of the Niemann-Pick C1-like1(NPC1L1) protein in the intesting brush border (enterocytes). Inihibition of NPC1L1 protein leads to decreased absorption of cholesterol, which consequently leads to upregulation of LDL-R and a decrease in LDL-C in the blood. The degree of LDL-C reduction is expected to be around 25 to 30%. Only one dose (10mg) exists.

Finally, investigations are being conducted on PCSK9 inhibitor use in children. To start, proprotein convertase subtilisin kexin 9 (PCSK9) is produced by the PCSK9 gene located on chromosome 1p32 and exerts its effects by binding to the LDL-R. Enzymatic activity of PCSK9 leads to a reduction in LDL-R activity through enhancement of lysosomal degradation (90-92). Targets for LDL-R degradation are in the liver and to a lesser extent in the brain, kidney, and small intestines (93). These effects result in elevated plasma LDL-C levels. A deficiency in enzyme activity due to loss of function mutations has been shown to inhibit LDL-R degradation and reduce LDL-C levels. Conversely, gain of function mutations in the gene lead to familial autosomal dominant hypercholesterolemia (ADH), which is characterized by elevated LDL-C levels (90,94).

PCSK9 inhibitors are monoclonal antibodies that function to inhibit PCSK9 activity and ultimately reduce LDL-C levels. Two antibodies are currently available: alirocumab, evolocumab. These IgG antibodies attach to PCSK9 and cause a functional deficiency of the enzyme by preventing its binding with LDL-R. The inhibition of PCSK9-facilitated LDL-R degradation results in a buildup of LDL-R and greater clearance of plasma LDL-C (95). Clinical trials performed in adults have confirmed a reduction in risk with these monoclonal antibodies (91). Their use is currently indicated to supplement statin therapy in high-risk populations, such as those with familial hypercholesterolemia (FH) and ASCVD (96, 97), with cost as the major limitation to their use.

PCSK9 inhibitor use in pediatric patients is not as well established as in adults. Studies including pediatric patients are currently investigating the efficacy and safety of evolocumab in the high-risk population of patients with FH. The Trial Evaluating PCSK9 Antibody in Subjects with LDL Receptor Abnormalities (TESLA) Part B study found that 420 mg evolocumab dosed every 4 weeks resulted in reduction of LDL-C levels and was relatively well-tolerated amongst subjects with homozygous FH between the ages of 12 and 80 years (98). Of the 11 patients enrolled in the study under the age of 18, 8 patients received evolocumab (98, 99). Similarly, the Trial Assessing Long-Term Use of PCSK9 Inhibition in Patients with Genetic LDL Disorders (TAUSSIG) is an ongoing trial studying homozygous FH patients aged 12-80 years who are receiving lipid apheresis. Preliminary data suggests that PCSK9 inhibitors may be beneficial in this patient population (100). The current HAUSER-RCT study is specifically investigating pediatric patients (age 11-17) with heterozygous FH and the utility of evolocumab as an adjunct to diet and other therapies in this population (99). The role of the PCSK9 inhibitor evolocumab in pediatric patients is promising; yet, continued investigation is necessary to establish indications for its use.

Triglyceride reduction

In the case of triglycerides, the intent of pharmacotherapy is to minimize the risk of pancreatitis by lowering the triglyceride level aggressively. Per the Expert Panel guidelines (41), children with average triglyceride level ≥500 mg/dL or a single elevation of ≥1000 mg/dL should be started on omega-3 fatty acids, fibrate or Niacin. Three primary classes of medications prescribed for triglyceride reduction are the omega-3-acid ethyl esters, fibrates, and Niacin. Due to the decreased use of niacin due to side effects, it will not be discussed. Omega-3-acid ethyl esters reduce triglyceride levels by decreasing hepatic triglyceride synthesis, decrease VLDL synthesis and secretion, increase VLDL metabolism, and increase LPL activity (101). Omega-3 fatty acids are expected to reduce the triglyceride level by 20 to 50%. Full prescription dose of omega-3-acid ethyl ester is two grams orally, twice a day.

Fibrates are useful in reducing the triglyceride levels if omega-3 fatty acids are not an option. The mechanism by which fibrates operate is to activate peroxisome proliferator-activated receptors (PPARs). There also increase LPL activity and inhibit Apo CIII which is a potent inhibitor of LPL. Fibrates also reduce VLDL production but induce synthesis of HDL apolipoproteins to increase HDL levels (102). Fibrates are expected to reduce triglyceride levels by 20 to 50 percent and increase HDL-C by 6-20 percent (101). Although six fibrates are available (bezafibrate, ciprofibrate, clofibrate, clinifibrate, gemfibrozil, and fenofibrate), only two are commonly used due to the efficacy and lower side effects: gemfibrozil and fenofibrate (less drug interactions of the two).

Safety labs

The initiation and maintenance of lipid-lowering drug therapies warrant careful follow up to monitor for organ damage. Therefore, 6-8 weeks post-initiation of pharmacotherapies, a laboratory assessment including a fasting lipid profile, AST, ALT, fasting glucose, creatine kinase levels should be checked routinely. If a fibrate is initiated for hypertriglyceridemia management, an alkaline phosphatase, and a total bilirubin should also be checked. Once the laboratory values have reached a steady state, including resolution of the dyslipidemia, the frequency of the safety lab assessments can be less frequent.

AAP Recommendations for preventive pediatric health care (risk assessment and screening)

2015 (103):
Dyslipidemia risk assessment at ages: 24 months, 4, 6, 8, 12-17 years
Dyslipidemia screening between ages: 9-11 years and 18-21 years

2017 (104):
Dyslipidemia screening between ages: 9-11 years and 17-21 years

Conclusion

Identification of hyperlipidemia in children is increasing in frequency, partly due to the growing obesity epidemic and the most recent Expert Panel guidelines from the AAP in 2011. Evaluating the patient in a systematic manner will help avoid unnecessary testing for the patient and unnecessary anxiety for the parent-child unit. Understanding the current guidelines and the rationale for therapy will benefit those under a physician's care, by mitigating the effects of the dyslipidemia. Conducting a thorough evaluation and prescribing appropriate non-pharmacologic and pharmacologic therapies will lead to primary prevention of ASCVD at a young age. Primum non nocere (first do no harm)!

REFERENCES

[1] Kochanek KD, Murphy SL, Xu J, Arias E. Mortality in the United States, 2013. NCHS data brief, no 178. Hyattsville, MD: National Center for Health Statistics, Centers for Disease Control and Prevention, US Department of Health and Human Services, 2014.

[2] Napoli C, D'Armiento FP, Mancini FP, Postiglione A, Witztum JL, Palumbo G, et al. Fatty streak formation occurs in human fetal aortas and is greatly enhanced by maternal hypercholesterolemia: intimal accumulation of LDL and its oxidation precede monocyte recruitment into early atherosclerotic lesions. J Clin Invest 1997;100(11):2680-90.

[3] Palinski W, Napoli C. The fetal origins of atherosclerosis: maternal hypercholesterolemia, and cholesterol-lowering or antioxidant treatment during pregnancy influence in utero programming and postnatal susceptibility to atherogenesis. FASEB J 2002;16(11):1348-60.

[4] Stacy HC. Evolution and progression of atherosclerotic lesions in coronary arteries of children and young adults. Arteriosclerosis 1989; 9(1 Suppl):I19-32.

[5] Enos WF, Holmes RH, Beyer J. Coronary disease among United States soldiers killed in action in Korea: Preliminary report. JAMA 1953;152(12):1090-3.

[6] McNamara JJ, Molot MA, Stremple JF, Cutting RJ. Coronary artery disease in combat casualities in Vietnam. JAMA 1971;216(7):1185-7.

[7] Natural history of aortic and coronary atherosclerotic lesions in youth. Findings from the PDAY study. Pathobiological determinant of Atherosclerosis in Youth (PDAY) Research Group. ATVB 1993;13:1291-8.

[8] Berenson GS, Wattigney WA, Tracy RE, Newman WP 3rd, Srinivasan SR, Webber LS, et al. Atherosclerosis of the aorta and coronary arteries and cardiovascular risk factors in persons aged 6 to 30 years and studied at necropsy (The Bogalusa Heart Study). Am J Cardiol 1992;70(9):851-8.

[9] Berenson GS, Srinivasan SR, Bao W, Newman WP 3rd, Tracy RE, Wattigney WA. Association between multiple cardiovascular risk factors and atherosclerosis in children and young adults. N Engl J Med 1998; 338(23):1650-6.

[10] Jarvisalo MJ, Jartti L, Nanto-Salonen K, Irjala K, Ronnemaa T, Hartiala JJ, et al. Increased aortic intima-media thickness: a marker of preclinical atherosclerosis in high-risk children. Circulation 2001; 104:2943–7.

[11] Davis PH, Dawson JD, Riley WA, Lauer RM. Carotid intimal-medial thickness is related to cardiovascular risk factors from childhood through middle age. Circulation 2001;104;2815-9.

[12] Tuzcu EM, Kapadia SR, Tutar E, Ziada KM, Hobbs RE, McCarthy PM et al. High prevalence of coronary atherosclerosis in asymptomatic teenagers and young adults: evidence from intravascular ultrasound. Circulation 2001;103(22):2705-10.

[13] Magnussen CG, Raitakari OT, Thomson R, Juonala M, Patel DA, Viikari JS, et al. Utility of currently recommended pediatric dyslipidemia classifications in predicting dyslipidemia in adulthood: evidence from the Childhood Determinants of Adult Health (CDAH) study, Cardiovascular Risk in Young Finns Study, and Bogalusa Heart Study. Circulation 2008;117(1):32-42.

[14] Cholesterol Treatment Trialists' (CTT) Collaboration, Baigent C, Blackwell L, Emberson J, Holland LE, Reith C, Bhala N, et al. Efficacy and safety of more intensive lowering of LDL cholesterol: a meta-analysis of data from 170,000 participants in 26 randomised trials. Lancet 2010;376 (9753):1670-81.

[15] Horton JD, Cohen JC, Hobbs HH. PCSK9: a convertase that coordinates LDL catabolism. J Lipid Res 2009;50(Suppl):S172-7.

[16] Ference BA, Yoo W, Alesh I, Mahajan N, Mirowska KK, Mewada A, et al. Effect of long-term exposure to lower low-density lipoprotein cholesterol beginning early in life on the risk of coronary heart disease: a Mendelian randomization analysis. J Am Coll Card 2012; 60(25):2631-9.

[17] Ference BA, Mahajan N. The Role of Early LDL Lowering to prevent the onset of Curr Atheroscler Rep 2013;15(4):312.

[18] Cholesterol Education Program. Report of the Expert Panel on Blood Cholesterol in Children and Adolescents. Bethesda, MD: National Cholesterol Education Program, 1991.

[19] Strong WB, Deckelbaum RJ, Gidding SS, Kavey RE, Washington R, Wilmore JH, et al. Integrated cardiovascular health promotion in childhood: a statement for health professionals from the

Subcommittee on Atherosclerosis and Hypertension in Childhood of the Council on Cardiovascular Disease in the Young, American Heart Association. Circulation 1992;85:1638-50.

[20] Raman A, Sharma S, Fitch MD, Fleming SE. Anthropometric correlates of lipoprotein profile and blood pressure in high BMI African American children. Acta Paediatrica 2010;99(6):912-9.

[21] Costa GB, Horta N, Resende ZF, Souza G, Barreto LM, Correia LH, et al. Body mass index has a good correlation with proatherosclerotic profile in children and adolescents. Arq Bras Cardiol 2009;93(3):261-7.

[22] Azita F, Asghar Z, Gholam-Reza S. Relationship of body mass index with serum lipids in elementary school students. Ind J Pediatr 2009; 76(7):729-31.

[23] Eissa MA, Wen E, Mihalopoulos NL, Grunbaum JA, Labarthe DR. Evaluation of AAP guidelines for cholesterol screening in youth: Project HeartBeat! Am J Prev Med 2009;37(1 Suppl):S71-7.

[24] Quijada Z, Paoli M, Zerpa Y, Camacho N, Cichetti R, Villarroel V, et al. The triglceride/HDL-cholesterol ratio as maker of cardiovascular risk in obese children; association with traditional and emergent risk factors. Pediatr Diabetes 2008;9(5):464-71.

[25] Korsten-Reck U, Kromeyer-Hauschild K, Korsten K, Baumstark, MW, Dickhuth HH, Berg A. Frequency of secondary dyslipidemia in obese children. Vasc Health Risk Manag 2008;4(5):1089-94.

[26] Plachta-Danielzik S, Landsberg B, Johannsen M, Lange D, Müller MJ. Association of different obesity indices with blood pressure and blood lipids in children and adolescents. Br J Nutr 2008;100(1):208-18.

[27] Liao CC, Su TC, Chien KL, Wang JK, Chiang CC, Lin CC, et al. Elevated blood pressure, obesity, and hyperlipidemia. J Pediatr 2009; 155(1):79-83e1.

[28] Gangwisch JE, Malaspina D, Babiss LA, Opler MG, Posner K, Shen S, et al. Short sleep duration as a risk factor for hypercholesterolemia: analysis of the National Longitudinal Study of Adolescent Health. Sleep 2010;33(7):956-61.

[29] Leblanc AG, Janssen I. Dose-responsive relationship between physical activity and dyslipidemia in youth. Can J Cardiol 2010;22(6):201-5.

[30] McFarlin BK, Johnston CA, Tyler C, O'Connor DP, Strohacker KA, Reeves R, et al. Relation between adiposity and disease risk factors in Mexican American children. J Pediatr Gastroenterol Nutr 2009; 49(4):450-5.

[31] van der Graaf A, Kalstelein JJ, Wiegman A. Heterozygous familial hypercholesterolemia in childhood: cardiovascular risk prevention. J Inherit Metabol Dis 2009;32(6):699-705.

[32] Lapinleimu J, Lapinleimu H, Nuotio IO, Rönnemaa T, Simell OG, Viikari JS, et al. Expression of common familial dyslipidemia in early childhood. Atherosclerosis 2009;204(2:)573-9.

[33] Kelishadi R, Ardalan G, Adeli K, Motaghian M, Majdzadeh R, Mahmood-Arabi MS, et al. Factor analysis of cardiovascular risk clustering in pediatric metabolic syndrome: CASPIAN study. Ann Nutr Metab 2007;51 (3):208-15.

[34] Edge JA, James T, Shine B. Longitudinal screening of serum lipids in children and adolescents with Type I diabetes in a UK clinic population. Diab Med 2008;25(8):942-8.

[35] Newfield RS, Dewan AK, Jain S. Dyslipidemia in children with type 2 diabetes vs. obesity. Pediatr Diabetes 2008;9(2):115-21.

[36] Maahs DM, Wadwa RP, McFann K, Nadeau K. Longitudinal lipid screening and use of lipid-lowering medications in pediatric type 1 diabetes. J Pediatr 2007;150(2):146-50.

[37] Wallen EF, Mullersdorf M, Christensson K, Malm G. High prevalence of cardio-metabolic risk factors among adolescents with intellectual disability. Acta Paediatrica 2009;98(5)853-9.

[38] Morrato EH, Nicol GE, Maahs D, Druss BG, Hartung DM, Valuck RJ, et al. Metabolic screening in children receiving antipsychotic drug treatment. Arch Pediatr Adolesc Med 2010; 164(4)344-51.

[39] Tassiopoulos K, Williams PL, Seage GR 3rd, Crain M, Oleske J, Farley J, et al. Association of hypercholesterolemia incidence with antiretroviral treatment, including protease inhibitors, among perinatally HIV-infected children. J Acquir Immune Defic Syndr 2008; 47(5):607-14.

[40] Committee on Nutrition. Cholesterol in children. American Academy of Pediatrics. Pediatrics 1998;101(1 pt 1):141-7.

[41] Expert Panel on Integrated Guidelines for Cardiovascular Health and Risk Reduction in Children and Adolescents: Summary Report. Pediatrics 2011;128(Suppl 5):S213-56.

[42] Tiwari S, Siddiqi SA. Intracellular trafficking and secretion of VLDL. ATVB 2012;32(5):1079-86.

[43] Goldstein JL, Brown MS. The LDL receptor. ATVB 2009;29(4):431-438.

[44] Lagace TA. PCSK9 and LDLR degradation: regulatory mechanisms in circulation and in cells. Curr Opin Lipid 2014;25(5):387.

[45] Kontush A, Chapman MJ. Antiatherogenic small, dense HDL—guardian angel of the arterial wall? Nature Rev Cardiology 2006;3(3): 144.

[46] Fredrickson DS, Lees RS. A system for phenotyping hyperlipoproteinemias. Circulation 1965;31(3):321–7.

[47] Goldstein JL, Brown MS. Molecular medicine. The cholesterol quartet. Science 2001;292(5520):1310-2.

[48] Benn M, Watts GF, Tybjaerg-Hansen A, Nordestgaard BG. Familial hypercholesterolemia in the Danish general population: prevalence, coronary artery disease, and cholesterol-lowering medication. J Clin Endocrinol Metab 2012; 97(11):3956–64.

[49] Cuchel M, Bruckert E, Ginsberg HN, Raal FJ, Santos RD, Hegele RA, et al; for the European Atherosclerosis Society Consensus Panel on Familial Hypercholesterolaemia. Homozygous familial hypercholesterolaemia: new insights and guidance for clinicians to improve detection and clinical management. A position paper from the Consensus Panel on Familial Hypercholesterolaemia of the European Atherosclerosis Society. Eur Heart J 2014;35(32):2146-57.

[50] Iwata F, Okada T, Kuromori Y, Hara M, Harada K. Screening for familial combined hyperlipidemia in children using lipid phenotypes. J Atherosclerosis Thromb 2003;10(5):299-303.

[51] Sniderman AD, Ribalta J, Castro Cabezas M. How should FCH be defined and how should we think about its metabolic bases? Nutr Metab Cardiovasc Dis 2001;11:259-73.

[52] Gaddi A, Cicero AFG, Odoo FO, Poli A, Paoletti R. Practice guidelines for familial combined hyperlipidemia: an update. Vasc Health Risk Manag 2007;3(6):877-86.

[53] Fung M, Hill J, Cook D, Frohlich J. Case series of type III hyperlipoproteinemias in children. Br Med J Case Rep 2011. doi:10.1136/bcr.02.2011.3895.

[54] Vermeer BJ, Frants RR, Havekes LM. Familial Dysbetalipoproteinemia: A genetically heterogenous disease caused by mutations of the ligand Apolipoprotein E. J Invest Derm 1992;98:57S-60S.

[55] Hegele R. Plasma lipoproteins: genetic influences and clinical implications. Nat Rev Genet 2009;10(2):109-21.

[56] Surendran RP, Visser ME, Heemelaar S, Wang J, Peter J, Defesche JC, et al. Mutations in LPL, APOC2, APOA5, GP1HBP1 and LMF1 in patients with severe hypertriglyceridaemia. J Int Med 2012; 272(2):185-96.

[57] Zahavi A, Snir M, Kella YR. Lipemia retinalis: case report and review of the literature. J Amer Asson Ped Ophth Strab 2013;17(1):110-1.

[58] Jain NC, Vanteri J, Shah PK, Narendran V. Lipemia retinalis in 1-month-old infant. Oman J Ophth 2017;10(1).

[59] Klop B, Elte JWF, Cabezas MC. Dyslipidemia in obesity: mechanisms and potential targets. Nutrients 2013;5:1218-40.

[60] Mooradian AD. Dyslipidemia in type 2 diabetes mellitus. Nat Clin Pract Endocrinol Metab 2009;5(3):150-9.

[61] Jin T, Teng X. Update on lipid metabolism and thyroid disorders. J Endocrinol Diab Obes 2014;2(3):1043.

[62] Rizos CV, Elisaf MS, Liberopoulos EN. Effects of thyroid dysfunction on lipid profile. Open Cardiovasc Med J 2011;5:76-84.

[63] Weinbrenner T, Züger M, Jacoby GE, Herpertz S, Liedtke R, Sudhop T, et al. Lipoprotein metabolism in patients with anorexia nervosa: a case-control study investigating the mechanisms leading to hypercholesterolemia. Br J Nutr 2004;91:959-69.

[64] Radondi N, Darioli R, Ramelet A, Hohl D, Lenain V, Perdrix J, et al. High risk for hyperlipidemia and the metabolic syndrome after an episode of hypertriglyceridemia during 13-cis retinoic acid therapy for acne: a pharmacogenetics study. Ann Intern Med 2002;136(8):582-9.

[65] Shufelt CL, Merz CNB. Contraceptive hormone use and cardiovascular disease. J Am Coll Cardiol 2009;53(3):221-31.

[66] Halperin IJ, Kumar SS, Stroup DF, Laredo SE. The association between the combined oral contraceptive pill and insulin resistance, dysglycemia, and dyslipidemia in women with polycystic ovary syndrome: a systemic review and meta-analysis of observational studies. Hum Reprod 2011;26(1):191-201.

[67] Kuster GM, Drexel H, Bleisch JA, Rentsch K, Pei P, Binswanger U, et al. Relation of cyclosporine blood levels to adverse effects on lipoproteins. Transplantation 1994;57(10):1479-83.

[68] Kockx M, Kritharides L. Cyclosporin A-induced hyperlipidemia. In: Frank S, Kostner G, eds. Lipoproteins: Role in health and diseases. London: IntechOpen, 2012:337-54.

[69] Lenders JW, Demacker PN, Vos JA, Jansen Pl, Joitsma J, van't Laar A, et al. Deleterious effects of anabolic steroids on serum lipoproteins, blood pressure, and liver function in amateur body builders. Int J Sports Med 1988;9(1):19-23.

[70] Gheshlaghi F, Piri-Ardakani M, Masoumi GR, Behjati M, Paydar P. Cardiovascular manifestations of anabolic steroids in association with demographic variables in body building athletes. J Res Med Sci 2015; 20(2):165-8.

[71] De Hert M, Dobbelaere M, Sheridan EM, Cohen D, Correll CU. Metabolic and endocrine adverse effects of second-generation antipsychotics in children and adolescents: a systematic review of randomized, placebo controlled trials and guidelines for clinical practice. Euro Psych 2011;26(3):144-58.

[72] Meyer JM, Koro CE. The effects of antipsychotic therapy on serum lipids: a comprehensive review. Schizo Res 2004;70(1):1-17.

[73] Chaggar PS, Shaw SM, Williams SG. Effect of antipsychotic medications on glucose and lipid levels. J Clin Pharm 2011;51(5): 631-8.

[74] Deano R, Sorrentino M. Lipid effects of antihypertensive medications. Curr Athero Rep, 2012;14(1):70-7.

[75] Fonseca VA. Effects of β-blockers on glucose and lipid metabolism. Curr Med Res Opin, 2010;26(3):615-29.

[76] Kasiske BL, Ma JZ, Kalil RS, Louis TA. Effects of antihypertensive therapy on serum lipids. Ann Int Med 1995;122(2):133-41.

[77] Lakshmipathy A, Krishnamani R, DeSio FJ. Unusual lipid and metabolic abnormalities secondary to alcohol abuse. Hosp Physician 2004;40(8):43-6.

[78] Brien SE, Ronksley PE, Turner BJ, Mukamal KJ, Ghali WA. Effect of alcohol consumption on biological markers associated with risk of coronary heart disease: systematic review and meta-analysis of interventional studies. BMJ 2011;342:d636. doi:10.1136/bmj.d636.

[79] How tobacco smoke causes disease. The biology and behavioral basis for smoking-attributable disease. A report of the surgeon general. Atlanta, GA: CDC, 2010.

[80] Mero N, Syvanne M, Eliasson B, Smith U, Taskinen MR. Postprandial elevation of ApoB-48-containing triglyceride-rish particles and retinyl esters in normolipemic males who smoke. Arterioscler Thromb Vasc Biol 1997;17(10):2096-102.

[81] Mero N, Van Tol A, Scheek LM, Van Gent T, Labeur C, Rosseneu M, et al. Decreased postprandial high density lipoprotein cholesterol and apolipoproteins A-I and E in normolipemic smoking men: relations with lipid transfer proteins and LCAT activities. J Lipid Res 1998; 39(7):1493-502.

[82] Glycerol kinase deficiency. Online Mendelian Inheritance in Man. URL: http://www.omim.org/entry/307030.

[83] Nordestgaard BG, Chapman MJ, Ray K, Boren J, Andreotti F, Watts GF, et al. Lipoprotein(a) as a cardiovascular risk factor: current status. Eur Heart J 2010;31(23):2844-53.

[84] Urbano F. Ocular signs of hyperlipidemia. Hospital Physician 2001; 37(11):51-3.

[85] Miller M, Vogel RA. Clinical signs and syndromes associated with premature coronary artery disease. In: Miller M, Vogel RA, eds. The practice of coronary disease prevention. Baltimore, MD: Williams Wilkins, 1996:24-35.

[86] NCEP Expert Panel of Blood Cholesterol Levels in Children and Adolescents. National Cholesterol Education Program (NCEP): highlights of the report of the Expert Panel on Blood Cholesterol Levels in Children and Adolescents. Pediatrics 1992;89(3):495–501.

[87] Gylling H, Siimes MA, Miettinen TA. Sitostanol ester margarine in dietary treatment of children with familial hypercholesterolemia. J Lipid Res 1995;36:1807-12.

[88] Moreno LA, Tresaco B, Bueno G, Fleta J, Rodriquez G, Garagorri JM, et al. Psyllium fibre and the metabolic control of obese children and adolescents. J Physiol Biochem 2003;59(3):235-42.

[89] Ribas SA, Cunha DB, Sichieri R, da Silva LC. Effects of psyllium on LDL-cholesterol concentrations in Brazilian children and adolescent: a randomized, placebo-controlled, parallel clinical trial. Br J Nutr 2014; 13:1-8.

[90] Chaudhary R, Garg J, Shah N, & Sumner A. PCSK9 inhibitors: A new era of lipid lowering therapy. World journal of cardiology, 2017;9(2): 76.

[91] Wilson PW, Polonsky TS, Miedema MD, Khera A, Kosinski AS, Kuvin JT. Systematic Review for the 2018 AHA/ACC/AACVPR/AAPA/ABC/ACPM/ADA/AGS/APhA/ASPC/NLA/PCNA Guideline on the Management of Blood Cholesterol: A Report of the American College of Cardiology/ American Heart Association Task Force on Clinical Practice Guidelines. Circulation 2018; doi: 10.1161/ CIR.0000000000000626.

[92] Seidah NG, Awan Z, Chrétien M, Mbikay M PCSK9: A key modulator of cardiovascular health. Circ Res 2014;114(6):1022-36.

[93] Schulz R, Schlüter KD. PCSK9 targets important for lipid metabolism. Clin Res Card Supp 2017;12(1):2-11.

[94] Cohen JC, Boerwinkle E, Mosley Jr TH, Hobbs HH. Sequence variations in PCSK9, low LDL, and protection against coronary heart disease. New Engl J Med, 2006;354(12):1264-72.

[95] Rosenson RS, Hegele RA, Fazio S, Cannon CP. The evolving future of PCSK9 inhibitors. J Amer Coll Card, 2018;72(3):314-29.

[96] Lloyd-Jones DM, Morris PB, Ballantyne CM, Birtcher KK, Daly DD, DePalma SM et al. 2016 ACC expert consensus decision pathway on the role of non-statin therapies for LDL-cholesterol lowering in the management of atherosclerotic cardiovascular disease risk: a report of the American College of Cardiology Task Force on Clinical Expert Consensus Documents. J Amer Coll Card 2016;68(1):92-125.

[97] Knickelbine T, Garberich R, White S, Oberembt S, Wills S, Miedema M, et al. PCSK9 inhibitors in patients with familial hypercholesterolemia and/or CVD: The impact of a systematic, team-based approach to prescription on rates of insurance approval and lipid lowering. J Amer Coll Card 2018;71(11):A1728.

[98] Raal FJ, Honarpour N, Blom DJ, Hovingh GK, Xu F, Scott, R, et al. Inhibition of PCSK9 with evolocumab in homozygous familial hypercholesterolaemia (TESLA Part B): a randomised, double-blind, placebo-controlled trial. Lancet 2015;385(9965):341-50.

[99] Gaudet D, Langslet G, Gidding SS, Luirink IK, Ruzza A, Kurtz C, et al. Efficacy, safety, and tolerability of evolocumab in pediatric patients with heterozygous familial hypercholesterolemia: Rationale and design of the HAUSER-RCT study. J Clin Lipid 2018;12(5):1199-1207.

[100] Bruckert E, Blaha V, Stein EA, Raal FJ, Kurtz CE, Honarpour N, et al. Trial assessing long-term use of PCSK9 inhibition in patients with genetic LDL disorders (TAUSSIG): efficacy and safety in patients with homozygous familial hypercholesterolemia receiving lipid apheresis. Circulation 2014;130:A17016.

[101] Bays HE, Tighe AP, Sadovsky R, Davidson MH. Prescription omega-3 fatty acids and their lipid effects: physiologic mechanisms of action and clinical implications. Expert Rev Cardiovasc Ther 2008;6(3):391-409.

[102] Staels B, Dallongeville J, Auwerx J, Schoonjans K, Leitersdorf E, Fruchart J. Mechanism of action of fibrates on lipid and lipoprotein metabolism. Circulation 1998;98:2088-93.

[103] Committee on Practice and Ambulatory Medicine and Bright Futures Periodicity Schedule Workgroup. 2015 recommendations for preventive pediatric health care. Pediatrics 2015;136(3):e727-9.

[104] Committee on Practice and Ambulatory Medicine. 2017 recommendations for preventive pediatric health care. Pediatrics 2017;139(4):e20170254.

In: Chronic Disease and Disability
Editors: DE Greydanus, P Anne, JD Rowlett et al.
ISBN: 978-1-53617-656-8

Chapter 9

CARDIOVASCULAR COMPLICATIONS OF OBESITY

Stuart Covi, MD and
Premchand Anne*, MD, MPH, MBA, FAAP, FACP, FACC
Pediatric Cardiology, Ascension St John Children's Hospital,
Detroit, Michigan, United States of America

ABSTRACT

Cardiovascular complications of obesity are numerous and considered critical aspects of human health. A number of these complications are considered in this discussion including obesity cardiomyopathy, pulmonary hypertension and sleep apnea, hypertension and dyslipidemia associated with obesity. Primary care clinicians caring for overweight and/or obese pediatric patients much be cognizant of such potential complications and work to effectively manage the state of obesity to minimize cardiovascular complications, thereby allowing healthier childhood/later adulthood.

INTRODUCTION

Childhood obesity is a worldwide epidemic in many countries, with prevalence sharply rising in recent decades. Since 1980, the prevalence of obesity has doubled in more than 70 countries and continuously increasing in many others (1). Global obesity estimates for 5-17-year olds based upon International Obesity Task Force (IOTF) standards from 2010-2013 were at 3-4%, with overweight/obesity at 12-14%; however, significant variation exists between countries. Whereas children in Africa and Asia have overweight/obesity levels as low as 4-8%, others like the America's and Europe are as high as 20-28% (2).

Even within certain countries, geographical differences have emerged. In Europe, a North-South gradient has been found with overweight/obesity as low as 15% in Norway vs. 36% in Italy from 2009-2010 (7-8 yo) [IOTF definition] (3). Although genetic factors may have an

* Correspondence: Premchand Anne, MD, Pediatric Cardiology, Ascension St John Children's Hospital, 22201 Moross, Suite 275, PB II, Detroit, MI 48236, United States. Email: Premchand.anne@ascension.org.

impact, surveys found that all countries in the various regions of Europe had a marked increase in prevalence indicating other factors at play (4). In particular, certain developed countries such as the United States (US) have seen prevalence of obese children (ages 2-19) more than triple from 1971 to 2008, reaching nearly 17% for both children and adolescents (5). In addition, obesity prevalence was 8.9% among 2- to 5-year-old children between 2011 and 2014 (6). In addition to age and gender, the prevalence of unhealthy body weight (overweight and obesity) also varies by ethnicity and race.

DEFINITIONS

Definitions of overweight and obesity currently use two international references, the World Health Organization (WHO) and the International Obesity Task Force (IOTF) [now the World Obesity Federation (WOF)]. The WHO reference points were originally based on United States reference data using body mass index (BMI) range of 85th percentile up to 95th percentile to define overweight and 95th percentile and greater as obese for age and gender (7). Due to difficulties in comparing surveys with differing national reference curves, the IOTF expert panel was established in 1995 based upon pooled international data (4, 8). The IOTF defines overweight and obesity as BMI percentile curves that pass through cut-off points of 25 and 30 kg/m^2 at age 18, respectively, and are age and gender specific (9, 10).

PARENTAL ASSOCIATIONS

Overweight and obesity, regardless of how they are defined, are chronic problems that are associated with chronic comorbidities. However, these chronic problems and CVD risk factors in children are associated with their parental childhood BMI and low density lipoprotein cholesterol (LDL-C) rather than the parental BMI and LDL-C levels (11). These comorbidities can range from metabolic syndrome and sleep apnea to cardiovascular conditions. Many of the comorbidities associated with overweight and obesity manifest in adulthood.

Adults with obesity have been found to have a higher likelihood of children with obesity, implying a potential "passing on" effect (12, 13). Maternal obesity has been shown to affect offspring phenotype, predisposing children to diseases such as obesity, dyslipidemia, type 2 diabetes, and hypertension later in life (14). Proposed epigenetic mechanisms for such changes include programming of the hypothalamic appetite regulating centers and methylation/histone modification (15, 16). Epigenetic changes as early as in utero could result in a perpetuating cycle of obesity, and may be inherited trans-generationally (14).

Cardiovascular complications of pediatric obesity include hypertension, hyperlipidemia, increased left ventricular mass, premature cardiovascular morbidity and mortality (due to coronary artery disease, cerebrovascular accidents, and renovascular disease) in adulthood (17). In this discussion, we will focus on the impact of unhealthy body weight on cardiac changes, pulmonary hypertension, elevated blood pressure, dyslipidemia and sudden death.

CHANGES IN CARDIAC-VASCULAR STRUCTURE AND HEMODYNAMICS

Obesity cardiomyopathy is a diagnosis, the onset of which occurs in children and adolescents (18). It is characterized by hypertrophy of the myocardium, increased cardiac mass (15-20% higher than normal weight subject) and enlargement of the cardiac chambers (19-22). There is a direct correlation of 0.6 between the degree of obesity and left ventricular mass and left ventricular size (left ventricular end-diastolic dimension) in pediatric subjects (23, 24). Jing et al. (25) compared obese/overweight and healthy-weight subjects using cardiac magnetic resonance imaging; the study revealed 23 percent greater indexed left ventricular mass ($g/m^{2.7}$) and 10 percent thicker left ventricular myocardium (25).

Furthermore, obese children as young as eight years had evidence of cardiac remodeling in the form of concentric or eccentric hypertrophy; longitudinal and circumferential strains were most impaired in obese children with concentric hypertrophy, indicating cardiac contractile dysfunction (25). However, the increase in cardiac mass and chamber sizes are not necessarily associated with the excess adipose tissue, i.e., non-lean body mass. They are correlated with the higher lean body mass that is characteristic of the overweight and obese children (26, 27).

Besides cardiac structural changes, hemodynamic changes occur among the children with unhealthy body weight. The hemodynamic changes associated with obesity among the youth are increased resting stroke volume and resultant increased cardiac output. Main contributing factors associated with these physiological adaptation/pathophysiological changes are increased lean body mass leading to increase oxygen delivery requirement and uptake, and increased blood volume necessitated by the need for increased oxygen delivery (24, 28).

In addition to the structural cardiac changes resulting from obesity cardiomyopathy, there are changes in cardiac systolic and diastolic function. The depression in systolic function is evident in childhood, based on the duration of the obesity. Multiple studies have reported decreased systolic function in the obese youth (27, 29-31). Mehta et al. (20) reported echocardiographic presence of diastolic dysfunction among obese and overweight children. The etiology of systolic and diastolic dysfunction was speculated to be due to "myocardial fatigue" due to chronic volume overload with subsequent asymptomatic high output congestive heart failure (18).

Epicardial fat (adipose tissue present between the pericardium and the outer wall of the myocardium) has been previously identified as a cardiovascular disease risk predictor in adults (32). Recent studies have noted larger deposits of epicardial fat in obese children compared to sex- and age-matched children, which has significant implications as these children go into adulthood (33-36). In addition, the epicardial fat deposition tracks directly with indexed LV mass and carotid intimal medial thickness (CIMT) (35). Increased CIMT, along with arterial stiffness and endothelial dysfunction, indicate evidence of arterial wall damage, which can accentuate and promote accelerated atherosclerosis (36, 37). Obesity/overweight is also associated with advanced vascular age (38). Summarily, unhealthy body weight can accelerate atherosclerosis from early childhood and increase risk of cardiovascular disease.

The impact of obesity in childhood is real. Although symptoms of congestive heart failure, lower extremity edema and oxygen dependence are not common in childhood and adolescence, the effect of "excess baggage" that is carried during physical activity can influence activity time (18). There is a negative correlation between distance walked/ran on a 12-minute walk/run and the child's body mass index (BMI) (39). Several studies have also demonstrated that the maximal aerobic capacity (expressed as VO_2 max per kilogram) is related directly to the lean body mass. The maximal aerobic capacity maybe lower in obese children due to the higher fat mass which will decrease VO_2 max after normalization by weight although there is no decrease in cardiac functional reserve capacity (18, 40).

Pediatric obesity is associated with increased cardiac mass in adulthood (41). The increased cardiac mass, eccentric left ventricular hypertrophy, and biventricular enlargement are associated with congestive heart failure. These changes are independent of coronary artery disease, sleep apnea, and systemic hypertension (42). One benefit of weight loss (whether lifestyle changes, or medical and/or surgical weight loss) is the reversal of the pathophysiological changes (43, 44). Weight loss, whether with diet alone, exercise alone, or a combination, have shown reversibility of cardiovascular risk markers in children (45). By establishing and promoting healthy(ier) body weight childhood, the early and late clinical manifestations of obesity cardiomyopathy can be prevented and/or ameliorated before adulthood.

PULMONARY HYPERTENSION AND SLEEP APNEA

Pulmonary arterial hypertension is defined as a mean pulmonary artery pressure (PAP) of 25 mmHg or greater in the setting of pulmonary capillary wedge pressure $\leq$ 15 mmHg and pulmonary vascular resistance $\geq$3 (46). Per the World Health Organization Symposium on Pulmonary Hypertension, there are now five recognized categories of pulmonary arterial hypertension (PH) (47, 48). These categories are: 1) pulmonary arterial hypertension, 2) PH due to left heart disease, 3) PH due to lung disease and/or hypoxia, 4) chronic thromboembolic PH, and 5) PH with unclear multifactorial mechanisms (47, 48). Up to 46% of patients with pulmonary arterial hypertension have no clear etiology, and are therefore classified as idiopathic PH (49). Sleep-disordered breathing is categorized under category 3; sleep-disordered breathing is a spectrum ranging from normal breathing to severe obstructive sleep apnea.

Obstructive sleep apnea (OSA) is a significant etiology of PH. It is estimated that approximately 20% of individuals with OSA have pulmonary hypertension (50). The World Health Organization has maintained BMI an unlikely risk factor for PH, and available data has conflicting results (50). Pulmonary hypertension was more prevalent in patients with sleep apnea syndrome (SAS), and was related to severity of obesity (51). Others did not find a difference in weight between pulmonary hypertension and normal groups in patients with obstructive sleep apnea (52). Using the much larger primarily adult based Registry to Evaluate Early and Long-Term PAH Disease Management (REVEAL), mean BMI was no different for patients with category 1 PH than the normal comparison group (53). However, subgroup analysis demonstrated higher percentages of obese patients (IPAH and PH from drugs) and mean BMI (PH from drugs) compared to controls. Hence, it appears obesity may be a risk factor within certain categories of pulmonary hypertension.

Obstructive sleep apnea syndrome (OSAS), as defined by the American Thoracic Society, is characterized by snoring, labored breathing during sleep, nocturnal enuresis, hyperactivity, and attention deficit (54). It is associated with recurrent episodes of upper airway obstruction (partial or complete) with snoring, with associated hypoxemia and sleep disturbance as well as fragmentation (55, 56). It is estimated that ten percent of children with OSAS are obese (57). On the other hand, 55-59% of obese children are reported to have OSAS (58, 59).

Besides its association with obesity and pulmonary hypertension, OSA is associated with endothelial dysfunction in children, which is a precursor to atherosclerosis (60). The severity of endothelial dysfunction is positively correlated with the degree and duration of obesity and the severity of OSA. Obstructive sleep apnea has been shown to be independently associated with systemic and pulmonary vascular hypertension (61, 62).

OSA is associated with increased sympathetic tone, which leads to vasoconstriction and subsequent systemic hypertension. Systemic hypertension, however, is believed to be a possible risk factor for development of pulmonary arterial hypertension with BMI as a strong determinant (50). As a more speculative theory, PH patients have diminished exercise capacity and may therefore be more prone to obesity; however, further research is needed to establish this relationship (53).

Furthermore, OSA is associated with atrial as well as ventricular ectopy and arrhythmias and episodic bradycardia as well as tachycardia due to hypoxia-stimulated vagal output with associated bradycardia and post-episodic sympathetic output leading to tachycardia. Hypoxia associated with OSA may cause atrioventricular blocks and sinus pauses, transiently prolong QT interval primarily in Long QT syndromes, with potential for sudden cardiac death, albeit rare. Finally, the disrupted sleep pattern may contribute to further weight gain, thereby increasing the BMI.

OSAS management

In children with OSAS, the primary treatment is adenotonsillectomy and this procedure improves the nadir oxygenation level significantly in the obese population with concomitant adenotonsillar hypertrophy. Long term effects of adenotonsillectomy have indicated a decrease in diastolic blood pressure (63, 64). However, presence of residual or recurrent OSAS demonstrated an increase in systolic and diastolic blood pressures (63). A secondary option if adenotonsillectomy does not relieve OSA, is continuous positive airway pressure (CPAP). In order to reduce the likelihood of recurrence of OSAS, achieving a healthier body weight can be beneficial. Bariatric surgery in morbidly obese children with skeletal and psychological maturity should be considered if the child has failed multiple attempts at weight loss (65). A referral to an otorhinolaryngologist may be helpful in identifying additional treatments if weight loss after adenotonsillectomy is insufficient to treat OSAS.

In 2012, the American Academy of Pediatrics published clinical practice guidelines for the diagnosis and management of OSAS. The recommendations were to: 1) screen all children and adolescents for snoring; 2) test children with snoring; 3) establish that adenotonsillectomy is the primary treatment for adenotonsillar hypertrophy; 4) monitor high-risk post-operative patients in the inpatient setting; 5) perform objective testing on post-operative patients to determine recurrence or residual OSAS; 6) use continuous positive airway pressure, if needed; 7) recommend weight loss for those children with unhealthy body weight (overweight/obese); and 8) consider intranasal steroids for those with mild OSAS for mild post-operative OSAS or if adenotonsillectomy is contraindicated (66).

HYPERTENSION

Hypertension in children and adolescents is defined as systolic (SBP) or diastolic blood pressures (DBP) ≥ 95th percentile for age, sex and height percentile (67). Normative and abnormal systolic as well as diastolic blood pressure percentiles are available for age, sex and height percentile (67, 68). Hypertension is divided into primary (essential) and secondary groups. The predominant cause of secondary pediatric hypertension was due to renal etiologies, which have become rare; however, hypertension associated with obesity, is now commonplace due to the current obesity epidemic (69). BMI is a strong determinant of hypertension, even more so than family history and activity level (70, 71).

Obese adolescents have an average systolic blood pressure 7.6 mmHg than normal weight peers, and for every unit increase in BMI z-scores, there is an associated increase in SBP (71). An estimated 37% of childhood hypertension could be attributed to unhealthy body weight, and the odds of systolic hypertension are 2.5-3.7 times higher in obese children compared to non-obese children (72, 73). Overweight children in the Bogalusa Heart Study were more likely to have elevated systolic and diastolic blood pressures compared to normal weight adolescents (74). In fact, the prevalence of isolated systolic hypertension among children and adolescents who were both obese and had a blood pressure greater than the 95 percentile was 94 percent (75).

Mechanisms of obesity-induced hypertension include a hyperactive sympathetic nervous system, leading to increased sodium retention and elevated systemic vascular resistance (76, 77). Aside from the sympathetic nervous system, direct deposition of lipids and vascular fibrosis have been associated with increased systemic vascular resistance as well (76).

Obese children and adolescents have been shown to have diminished baroreceptor sensitivity, an important component in the regulation of blood pressure (78). Moreover, severity of obesity correlates with the activation of the Renin-Angiotensin-Aldosterone System (RAAS), with elevated levels of aldosterone found in obese children, and may be important in regulation of their blood pressure (79). Weight appears to be one of the most important factors related to hypertension in children and adolescents worldwide (80).

In overweight and obese children, there is significant adipose tissue dysfunction leading to an imbalance of pro- and anti-inflammatory activity within the adipose tissue and the individual adipocyte (77). In addition, increased oxidative stress contributes to hypertension by activating the sympathetic nervous system, with subsequent involvement of the hypothalamus and its downstream functions (81). Importantly, an increase in arterial blood pressure in youth predicts hypertension in adulthood (80). Cardiovascular diseases are thought to develop over the course of life, beginning as young as the fetal period, with hypertension as a major risk factor (82).

A primary challenge facing obese and overweight children is screening them for hypertension. This challenge arises from the inability to use standard pediatric cuffs that would be appropriate for normal weight children. Using a cuff that is too small will inaccurately provide elevated blood pressure whereas a larger cuff may provide lower blood pressures. Increased arm circumference (and relatively short arm length with respect to the arm circumference) and the shape of the arm further contribute to this difficulty in assessing an accurate blood pressure (77).

The Expert Panel from the American Academy of Pediatrics (AAP) has recommended yearly blood pressures and more frequent analysis if blood pressure is elevated on routine clinic visits (68). Besides checking and establishing elevated blood pressure, secondary etiologies must be assessed and treated. Obstructive sleep apnea (OSA) as mentioned above, toxicology screens, hyperparathyroidism and hyperthyroidism should also be evaluated.

When obesity or overweight is the most likely etiology of hypertension in children, weight loss is the primary treatment in the obese category for children over six years of age and weight maintenance for those in the overweight category (68, 83). Dietary modifications with caloric restriction via refined carbohydrate and saturated fat restrictions ought to be considered. Various paradigms are available for dietary and lifestyle interventions (68). Secondary causes of hypertension, besides unhealthy body weight, should be identified and cardiology and/or nephrology consultations may be warranted for further evaluation. Such evaluation must include workup for potential early end-organ damage in children based on the duration of obesity, hypertension and other cardiovascular risk factors (67, 84).

DYSLIPIDEMIA

Dyslipidemia and hypertension are common comorbidities in individuals with obesity (84). Metabolic syndrome, a cluster of the aforementioned conditions along with obesity, is a major risk factor for development of cardiovascular diseases throughout life (85). As an important factor involved in cardiovascular disease development, significantly elevated hazard ratios (HR) for coronary heart disease [4.9], death from stroke [2.1], sudden death [3.5], and death from total cardiovascular causes [3.5] have been found in large longitudinal studies of obese vs. non-obese groups (82, 86). Even those with a BMI at the 50-74th percentile in adolescence have been shown to have increase in the risk of cardiovascular and all-cause death during a 40 year follow up period (86). The Global Burden of Disease Collaborators assessed 195 countries and found that 70 percent of adult deaths related to high BMI were due to cardiovascular disease (1).

The dyslipidemia associated with overweight and obesity is characterized by overproduction of apolipoprotein B containing triglyceride-rich lipoproteins and free fatty acid (FFA), small, dense low density lipoprotein (LDL) particles, decreased high density lipoprotein (HDL) cholesterol levels with HDL dysfunction (87). The lipid profile in obese/overweight children is similar to that of individuals with diets that are rich in refined carbohydrates and saturated fats. Postprandial triglyceride levels are elevated in obese and overweight patients. In obese children, triglyceride-rich lipoprotein lipolysis is impaired due to decreased lipoprotein lipase (LPL) levels in adipose tissue and LPL activity in skeletal muscle (88, 89). LPL is essential in the breakdown of triglycerides.

In the presence of hypertriglyceridemia, there is exchange of cholesterol esters for triglycerides between HDL and very low density lipoprotein (VLDL) as well as LDL molecules through the activity of cholesterol ester transfer protein (CETP); this action leads to denser, small, dysfunctional HDL (reduced affinity for apolipoprotein A-1) and triglyceride-depleted, small, dense LDL molecules (89). The small, dense LDL particles are considered to be atherogenic. The role of elevated triglyceride levels in atherosclerotic cardiovascular disease (ASCVD) is under investigation.

Addition of eicosapentanoic acid (EPA) via prescriptions or over-the-counter fish oil therapy has been shown to reduce triglyceride levels. In addition, addition of EPA to a statin reduced primary cardiovascular endpoints in adult patients with acute coronary syndromes (90). As is the case with many childhood conditions, obesity-related dyslipidemias can manifest in childhood and more significant cardiovascular complications track into adulthood.

Conclusion

The effects of obesity on the heart are acute and chronic while ranging from cellular to gross structural changes. The duration of obesity is a significant predictor and prognosticator of various cardiac abnormalities. As mentioned above, achieving a healthier body weight has been shown to reverse some changes that manifest in childhood while other changes may be chronic and track into adulthood.

It is imperative to address the overweight and obesity conditions early on in childhood to minimize their impact on significant morbidity and mortality. Although numerous cardiovascular and non-cardiovascular comorbidities arise secondary to unhealthy bodyweight, the impact of achieving sustained weight loss, whether small or large, can resolve or mitigate progression of the cardiovascular comorbidities.

References

[1] Afshin A, Forouzanfar M, Reitsma M, Sur P, Estep K, Lee, A, et al. Health effects of overweight and obesity in 195 countries over 2 years. The GBD 2015 Obesity Collaborators. N Engl J Med 2017;377(1):13-27.

[2] International Association for the Study of Obesity. Online database of national prevalence data from published national surveys. London: IASO, 2014.

[3] Wijnhoven TM, van Raaij JM, Spinelli A, Rito AI, Hovengen R, Kunesova M, et al. WHO European Childhood Obesity Surveillance Initiative 2008: weight, height and body mass index in 6-9-year-old children. Pediatr Obes 2013;8(2):79-97.

[4] Lobstein T. Prevalence and trends across the world. In: Frelut ML, ed. The ECOG's eBook on child and adolescent obesity, 2015. URL: www.coursehero.com.EAES.

[5] Ogden C, Carroll M. Prevalence of obesity among children and adolescents: United States, Trends 1963-1965 Through 2007-2008. NCHS Health E-Stat. Hyattsville, MD: NCHS, 2014.

[6] Ogden CL, Carroll M, Fryar CD, Flegal KM. Prevalence of obesity among adults and youth: United States, 2011-2014. NCHS data brief. 20 219. Hyattsville, MD: NCHS, 2015.

[7] World Health Organization. Physical status, the use and interpretation of anthropometry. WHO Technical Report Series No. 854. Geneva: WHO, 1995. World Obesity (formerly IASO) History. 2015. URL: https://www.worldobesity.org/who-we-are/history/.

[8] Cole TJ, Belizzi MC, Felgal KM, Dietz AH. Establishing a standard definition for child overweight and obesity worldwide: international survey. BMJ 2000;320(7244):1240-5.

[9] Cole TJ, Lobstein T. Extended international (IOTF) body mass index cut-offs for thinness, overweight and obesity. Pediatr Obes 2012;7:284-94.

[10] Chen W, Srinivasan SR, Bao W, Berenson GS: The magnitude of familial associations of cardiovascular risk factor variables between parents and offspring are influenced by age: the Bogalusa Heart Study. Ann Epidemiol 2001;11:522–8.

[11] Carolan-Olah M, Duarte-Gardea M, Lechuga J. A critical review: early life nutrition and prenatal programming for adult disease. J Clin Nurs 2005;24:3716-29.

[12] Chang L, Neu J. Early factors leading to later obesity: interactions of the microbiome, epigenome, and nutrition. Curr Probl Pediatr Adolesc Health Care 2015;45(5):134-42.

[13] Zambrano E, Ibáñez C, Martinez-Samayoa PM, Lomas-Soria C, Durand-Carbajal M, Rodríquez-González GL. Maternal obesity: lifelong metabolic outcomes for offspring from poor developmental trajectories during the perinatal period. Arch Med Res 2016;47(1):1-12.

[14] Roth C, Sathyanarayana S. Mechanisms affecting neuroendocrine and epigenetic regulation of body weight and onset of puberty: potential implications in the child born small for gestational age (SGA). Rev Endocr Metab Disord 2012:13;129-40.

[15] Franks PW, Ling C. Epigenetics and obesity: the devil is in the details. BMC Med 2010;8:88. doi: 10.1186/1741-7015-8-88.

[16] Hambdy RC. Obesity: An epidemic. South Med J 2003;96:531-2.

[17] Rowland TW. Effect of obesity on cardiac function in children and adolescents: A review. J Sports Science Med 2007;6:319-26

[18] Koehler B, Malecka-Tendera E, Drzewiecka B. Function of the cardiovascular system in children with simple obesity. Part II. Echocardiographic assessment. Matera Medica Polonica 1997;70:131-3.

[19] Mehta SK, Holliday C, Hayduk L, Wiersma L, Richards N, Younoszai A. Comparison of myocardial function in children with body mass indexes >25 versus those <25 kg/m2. Am J Cardiol 2004;93(3):1567-9.

[20] Di Salvo G, Pacileo G, Del Giudice EM, Natale F, Limongelli G, Verrengia M, et al. Abnormal myocardial deformation properties in obese, non-hypertensive children: an ambulatory blood pressure monitoring, standard echocardiographic, and strain rate imaging study. Eur Heart J 2006;27(2):2689–95.

[21] Friberg P, Allansdotter-Johnsson A, Ambring A, Ahl R, Arheden H, Framme J, et al. Increased left ventricular mass in obese adolescents. Eur Heart J 2004;25(11):987-92.

[22] Kono Y, Yoshinaga M, Oku S, Nomura Y, Nakamura M, Aihoshi S. Effect of obesity on echocardiographic parameters in children. Int J Cardiol 1994;46(1):7-13.

[23] Rowland T, Dunbar NS. Effects of obesity on cardiac function in adolescent females. Am J Lifestyle Med 2007;1(4):282-5.

[24] Jing L, Binkley CM, Suever JD, Umasankar N, Haggerty CM, Rich J, et al. Cardiac remodeling and dysfunction in childhood obesity: a cardiovascular magnetic resonance study. J Cardiovasc Magn Reson 2016;18(1):28. doi: 10.1186/s12968-016-0247-0.

[25] Janz KF, Burns TL, Mahoney LT. Predictors of left ventricular mass and resting blood pressure in children: the Muscatine Study. Med Sci Sports Exer 1995;27:818-25.

[26] Gutin B, Treiber F, Owens S, Mensah GA. Relations of body composition to left ventricular geometry and function in children. J Pediatr 1998;132:1023-7.

[27] Giordano U, Ciampalini P, Turchetta A, Santilli IA, Calzolari F, Crinò A, et al. Cardiovascular hemodynamics: relationships with insulin resistance in obese children. Pediatr Cardiol 2003;24(6):548-52.

[28] Lauer MS, Anderson, KM, Levy D. Separate and joint influences of obesity and mild hypertension on left ventricular mass and geometry: The Framingham Heart Study. J Am Coll Cardiol, 2006;19:130-4.

[29] Chinali,M, de Simone G, Roman MJ, MJ, Lee ET, Best LG, Howard BV, et al. Impact of obesity on cardiac geometry and function in a population of adolescents: the Strong Heart Study. J Am Coll Cardiol 2006;47(11) 2267-73.

[30] Mensah GA, Treiber FA, Kapuku GK. Patterns of body fat deposition in youth and their relation to left ventricular markers of adverse cardiovascular prognosis. Am J Cardiol 1999;84:583-8.

[31] Iacobellis G, Ribaudo MC, Assael F, Vecci E, Tiberti C, Zappaterreno A, et al. Echocardiographic epicardial adipose tissue is related to anthropometric and clinical parameters of metabolic syndrome: a new indicator of cardiovascular risk. J Clin Endocrinol Metab 2003;88:5163–8.

[32] Ozdemir O, Hizli S, Abaci A, Agladioglu K, Aksoy S. Echocardiographic measurement of epicardial adipose tissue in obese children. Pediatr Cardiol 2010;31:853–60.

[33] Manco M, Morandi A, Marigliano M, Rigotti F, Manfredi R, Maffeis C. Epicardial fat, abdominal adiposity and insulin resistance in obese pre-pubertal and early pubertal children. Atherosclerosis 2013;226:490–5.

[34] Abaci A, Tascilar ME, Saritas T, Yozgat Y, Yesilkaya E, Kilic A, et al. Threshold value of subepicardial adipose tissue to detect insulin resistance in obese children. Int J Obes (Lond) 2009;33:440–6.

[35] Cote AT, Harris KC, Panagiotopoulos C, Sandor GGS, Devlin AM. Childhood obesity and cardiovascular dysfunction. J Am Coll Cardiol 2013;62(15):1309-19.

[36] Urbina EM, Kimball TR, Khoury PR, Daniels SR, Dolan LM. Increased arterial stiffness is found in adolescents with obesity or obesity-related type 2 diabetes mellitus. J Hypertens 2010;28:1692–8.

[37] Le J, Zhang D, Menees S, Chen J, Raghuveer G. "Vascular age" is advanced in children with atherosclerosis-promoting risk factors. Circ Cardiovasc Imaging 2010;3:8–14.

[38] Drinkard B, McDuffie J, McCann S, Uwaifo GI, Nichlson J, Yanovsky JA. Relationships between walk/run performance and cardiorespiratory fitness in adolescents who are overweight. Phys Ther 2001;81:1889-96.

[39] Goran M, Fields DA, Hunter GR, Herd SL, Weinsler RL. Total body fat does not influence maximal aerobic capacity. Int J Obes 2000;24:841-8.

[40] Li X, Li S, Ulusoy E, Chen W, Srinivasan SR, Berenson GS. Childhood adiposity as a predictor of cardiac mass in adulthood: the Bogalusa Heart Study. Circulation 2004;110(22):3488-92.

[41] Alpert MA, Alexander K. Cardiac morphology and obesity in man. In: The Heart and Lung in Obesity. Eds: MA Alpert and JK Alexander. Armonk, NY: Futura, 1998:25-44.

[42] Alpert MA, Lambert CR. Terry BE, Kelly DL, Panayiotou H, Mukerji V, et al. Effect of weight loss on left ventricular mass in nonhypertensive morbidly obese patients. Am J Cardiol 1994;73(12):918-21.

[43] MacMahon SW, Wilcken DE, MacDonald GJ. The effect of weight reduction on left ventricular mass. A randomized, controlled trial in young overweight hypertensive patients. N Engl J Med 1986;314(6):334-9.

[44] Ayer J, Charakida M, Deanfield JE, Celermajer DS. Lifetime risk: childhood obesity and cardiovascular risk. Eur Heart J 2015;36:1371-6.

[45] Abman S, Hansmann G, Archer S, Ivy DD, Adatia I. Pediatric pulmonary hypertension guidelines from the American Heart Association and American Thoracic Society. Circulation 2015;132:2037-99.

[46] Galiè N, Simonneau G. The fifth world symposium on pulmonary hypertension. J Am Coll Cardiol 2013;62(25):D1-3.

[47] Simmoneau G, Gatzoulis MA, Adatia I, Celermajer D, Denton C, Ghofrani A, et al. Updated clinical classification of pulmonary hypertension. J Am Coll Cardiol 2013;62(25 Suppl):D34-41.

[48] Badesch D, Raskob G, Elliott G, Krichman AM, Farber HW, Frost AE, et al. Pulmonary arterial hypertension: baseline characteristics from the REVEAL registry. Chest 2010;137(2):376-87.

[49] Taichman D, Mandel J. Epidemiology of pulmonary arterial hypertension. Clin Chest Med 2007;28:1-22.

[50] Bady E, Achkar A, Pascal S, Orvoen-Frija E, Laaban J-P. Pulmonary arterial hypertension in patients with sleep apnoea syndrome. Thorax 2000;55:934-9.

[51] Weitzenblum E, Krieger J, Apprill M, Vallee E, Herhart M, Ratomahharo J, et al. Daytime pulmonary hypertension in patients with obstructive sleep apnea syndrome. Am Rev Respir Dis 1988;138:345-9.

[52] Burger C, Foreman A, Miller D. Comparison of body habitus in patients with pulmonary arterial hypertension enrolled in the registry to evaluate early and long term-PH disease management with normative values from the National Health and Nutrition Examination Survey. Mayo Clin Proc 2011;86(2):105-12.

[53] No authors listed. American Thoracic Society. Cardiorespiratory sleep studies in children. Establishment of normative data and polysomnographic predictors of morbidity. Am J Respir Crit Care Med 1999;160(4):1381–7.

[54] Arens R, Muzumdar H. Childhood obesity and obstructive sleep apnea syndrome. J Appl Physiol 2010;108(2):436-44.

[55] Narang I, Mathew JL. Childhood Obesity and obstructive sleep apnea. J Nutr Metab 2012;2012:134202. doi:10.1155/2012/134202.

[56] Guilleminault C, Korobkin R, Winkle R. A review of 50 children with obstructive sleep apnea syndrome. Lung 1981;159(5):275–87.

[57] Kalra M, Inge T, Garcia V, Daniels S, Lawson L, Curti R, et al. Obstructive sleep apnea in extremely overweight adolescents undergoing bariatric surgery. Obes Res 2005;13:1175–9.

[58] Silvestri JM, Weese-Mayer DE, Bass MT, Kenny AS, Hauptman SA, Pearsall SM. Polysomnography in obese children with a history of sleep-associated breathing disorders. Pediatr Pulmonol 1993;16:124–9.

[59] Bhattacharjee R, Kim J, Alotaibi WH, Kheirandish-Gozal L, Capdevila OS, Gozal D. Endothelial dysfunction in children without hypertension: potential contributions of obesity and obstructive sleep apnea. Chest 2012;141:682–91.

[60] Bhattacharjee R, Kheirandish-Gozal L, Pillar G, Gozal D. Cardiovascular complications of obstructive sleep apnea: evidence from children. Prog Cardiovasc Dis 2009;51:416-33.

[61] Gozal D, Kheirandish-Gozal L. Childhood obesity and sleep: relatives, partners, or both? Ann NY Acad Sci 2012;1264:135–41.

[62] Amin R, Anthony L, Somers V, Fenchel M, McConnell K, Jefferies J, et. al. Growth velocity predicts recurrence of sleep-disordered breathing 1 year after adenotonsillectomy. Am J Respir Crit Care Med 2008;177(6):654–9.

[63] Kaditis A. Blood pressure after adenotonsillectomy in children with obstructive sleep-disordered breathing. Am J Respir Crit Care Med 2008;178(8):882.

[64] Watson SE, Zhoukai BS, Wanzhu T, Hasnaa Jalou, Brubaker JL, Gupta S, et al. Obstructive sleep apnea in obese adolescents and cardiometabolic risk markers. Pediatr Obes 2014;9 (6):471-7.

[65] Marcus CL, Brooks LJ, Draper KA, Gozal D, Halbower AC, Jones J, et al. Diagnosis and management of childhood obstructive sleep apnea syndrome. Pediatrics 2012;130(3):e714-55.

[66] National High Blood Pressure Education Program. Working Group on High Blood Pressure in Children and Adolescents. The fourth report on the diagnosis, evaluation, and treatment of high blood pressure in children and adolescents. Pediatrics 2004;114(2 Suppl 4th Rep):555-76.

[67] Expert panel on integrated guidelines for cardiovascular health and risk reduction in children and adolescent; National Heart, Lung, and Blood Institute. summary report. Pediatrics 2011;128(Suppl 5):S213-56.

[68] Sorof J, Daniels S. Obesity hypertension in children: A problem of epidemic proportions. Hypertension 2002;40:441-7.

[69] Sorof J, Lai D, Turner J, Poffenbarger T, Portman RJ. Overweight, ethnicity, and the prevalence of hypertension in school-aged children. Pediatrics 2004;113(3 Pt 1):475-82.

[70] Shi Y, de Groh M, Morrison H. Increasing blood pressure and its associated factors in Canadian children and adolescents from the Canadian Health Measure Survey. BMC Public Health 2012;12:388. doi: 10.1186/1471-2458-12-388.

[71] Chiolero A, Cachat F, Burnier M, Paccaud F, Bovet P. Prevalence of hypertension in school schildren based on repeated measurements and association with overweight. J Hypertens 2007;25(11):2209-17.

[72] Rosner B, Prineas R, Daniels SR, Loggie J. Blood pressure differences between blacks and whites in relation to body size among US children and adolescents. Am J Epidemiol 2000;151:1007-19.

[73] Friedman DS, Dietz WH, Srinivasan SR, Berenson GS. The relation of overweight to cardiovascular risk factors among children and adolescents: the Bogalusa Heart Study. Pediatrics1999;103:1175–82.

[74] Sorof JM, Poffenbarger T, Franco K, Bernard L, Portman RJ. Isolated systolic hypertension, obesity, and hyperkinetic hemodynamic states in children. J Pediatr 2002;140:660–6.

[75] Bogaert YE, Linas S.: The role of obesity in the pathogenesis of hypertension. Nat Clin Pract Nephrol 2009;5:101-11

[76] Brady TM. Obesity-related hypertension in children. Front Pediatr 2017;5:197; doi:10.3389/fped.2017.00197.

[77] Dangardt F, Volkmann R, Chen Y, Osika W, Marild S, Friberg P. Reduced cardiac vagal activity in obese children and adolescents. Clin Physiol Funct Imaging 2011;31(2):108-13.

[78] Rocchini A, Katch V, Grekin R, Moorehead C, Anderson J. Role for aldosterone in blood pressure regulation of obese adolescents. Am J Cardiol 1986;57(8):613-8.

[79] Rodriques AN, Abreu GR, Resende RS, Goncalves WL, Gouvea SA. Cardiovascular risk factor investigation: A pediatric issue. Int J. Gen Med 2013;6:57-66.

[80] Dorresteijn JA, Visseren FL, Spiering W. Mechanisms linking obesity to hypertension. Obes Rev 2012;13:17–26.

[81] Zachurzok A, Malecka-Tendera E. Cardiovascular complications of obesity. In: Frelut ML, ed. The ECOG's eBook on child and adolesent obesity, 2015. URL: http://ebook.ecog-obesity.eu/chapter-clinics-complications/cardiovascular-complications-obesity/?utm_source=text&utm_medium=article-link&utm_campaign=ebook-en.

[82] Spear BA, Barlow SE, Ervin C, Ludwig DS, Saelens BE, Schetzina KE, et al. Recommendations for treatment of child and adolescent overweight and obesity. Pediatrics 2007;120(Suppl 4):S254–88.

[83] Reaven GM. Insulin resistance and compensatory hyperinsulinemia: role in hypertension, dyslipidemia, and coronary heart disease. Am Heart J 1991;121:1283-8.

[84] Isomaa B, Almgren P, Tuomi T, Forsén B, Lahti K, Nissén M, et al. Cardiovascular morbidity and mortality associated with the metabolic syndrome. Diabetes Care 2001;24(4):683-9.

[85] Twig G, Yaniv G, Levin H, Leiba A, Goldberger N, Derazne E, et al. Body-mass index in 2.3 million adolescents and cardiovascular death in adulthood. N Engl J Med 2016;374(25):2430-40.

[86] Klop B, Elte JWF, Cabezas MC. Dyslipidemia in obesity: mechanisms and potential targets. Nutrients 2013;5:1218-40.

[87] Klop B. Jukema JW, Rabelink TJ, Castro Cabezas M. A physician's guide for the management of hypertriglyceridemia: The etiology of hypertriglyceridemia determines treatment strategy. Panminerva Med 2012;54:91–103.

[88] Clemente-Postigo M, Queipo-Ortuno MI, Fernandez-Garcia D, Gomez-Huelgas R, Tinahones FJ, Cardona F. Adipose tissue gene expression of factors related to lipid processing in obesity. PLoS One 2011;6:e24783; doi:10.1371/journal.pone.0024783.

[89] Subramanian S, Chait A. Hypertriglyceridemia secondary to obesity and diabetes. Biochim Biophys Acta 2012;1821:819–25.

[90] Nosaka K, Miyoshi T, Iwamoto M, Kajiya M, Okawa K, Tsukuda S, et al. Early initiation of eicosapentanoic acid and statin treatment is associated with better clinical outcomes than statin alone in patients with acute coronary syndromes: 1-year outcomes of a randomized controlled study. Int J Cardiol 2017;228:173-9.

In: Chronic Disease and Disability
Editors: DE Greydanus, P Anne, JD Rowlett et al.
ISBN: 978-1-53617-656-8

Chapter 10

PEDIATRIC PULMONARY THROMBOEMBOLIC DISEASE

John D Rowlett*, MD, FAAP, FACP
Pediatric Emergency Medicine and Pediatric Hospital Medicine,
St Joseph's/Candler Healthcare System, Savannah, Georgia,
Medical College of Georgia, Augusta, Georgia
and Eastern Kentucky University, Richmond, Kentucky, United States

ABSTRACT

Pulmonary embolism occurs when thrombus forms in the venous vasculature and propagates to the pulmonary vasculature. These clots, often asymptomatic prior to migration, are an increasing problem in the adult and pediatric population. Mortality and morbidity from acute pulmonary embolism is high. After a review of the historical context of venous thromboembolism (VTE), this discussion details the recent increase, risk factors and other contributing causes of VTE in children. Presenting symptoms, physical examination, and diagnostic strategies are also reviewed. In addition, VTE management is presented that includes unfractionated heparin (UFH), low molecular weight heparins (LMWH: enoxaparin, dalteparin, fondaparinux), warfarin and the potential impact of the novel anti-coagulants (i.e., rivaroxaban, dabigatran, apixaban, edoxaban). This discussion concludes with a review of the applicable inherited thrombophilias and their impact on both the presentation and long-term management of venous thromboembolism in children.

INTRODUCTION

Pulmonary embolism occurs when a thrombus forms in the venous vasculature and propagates to the pulmonary vasculature. These clots, often asymptomatic prior to migration, are an increasing problem in the adult and pediatric population. Though he never actually defined the triad attributed to his name, the German pathologist Rudolph Virchow (1821-1902) described

* Corresponding Author's Email: drrowlett@gmail.com.

the combination of "interrupted blood flow" (stasis), "alterations in the blood" (hypercoagulability), and "irritation of the vessel and its vicinity" (endothelial injury) (1, 2). He wrote about "the detachment of larger or smaller fragments from the end of the softening thrombus which are carried along by the current of blood and driven into remote (pulmonary) vessels. This gives rise to the very frequent process on which I have bestowed the name of Embolia" (3). The Italian anatomist, Giovanni Morgagni (1682-1771), was the first to describe a case of fatal pulmonary embolism (PE) in 1740; he noted:

> A man was admitted to the hospital with a broken leg. Soon after, physicians found he was "without a pulse and then he died." The autopsy revealed "the heart and the major vessels were full of clots." Where is the disease?

While correctly determining the cause of death, Morgagni did not realize that the source of the clot was the fractured leg (4, 5). The first reported case of pulmonary embolism in a child was in 1953, when Cashman reported the case of a 9-year-old boy who was five days removed from an appendectomy (6). The patient developed sudden left-sided chest pain, tachycardia, hypoxia, shock, and characteristic electrocardiogram changes; he was treated with fluids, heparin, and oxygen and survived (6).

EPIDEMIOLOGY

Venous thromboembolism (VTE) and pulmonary embolism (PE) affect up to one million persons in the United States annually. As many as 100,000 persons in the United States die each year from pulmonary embolisms; in 25% of the cases, sudden death is the initial and only presenting symptom (7). Clearly many cases of "sudden death" are secondary to massive pulmonary embolism but absent an autopsy, the diagnosis is not made. The incidence of VTE/PE in children is markedly lower than in adults but has increased more than 70% in recent years.

RISK FACTORS

One institution reported 58 cases of VTE per 10,000 hospital admissions which was increased from 35 cases per 10,000 admissions just 7 years prior (8). Most children in this series had co-morbidities that are identified risk factors for VTE (see Table 1); these included having a malignancy, trauma, central venous catheter, sepsis, or an inherited thrombophilia (8). There was also an absolute increase in other children for VTE (8). The cause (s) of this increase are incompletely understood but are probably multi-factorial; these include increased use of central venous and peripheral catheters, obesity, sicker patients, and increased survival of patients who might have previously succumbed to their illness/injury.

Hume reported that, among pediatric patients admitted for elective general surgery, there was an increased risk (9-fold) of VTE; however, the absolute risk is quite small (0.4 per 1000-person years) (9). Children undergoing abdominal surgeries were at higher risk and no cases were reported among those undergoing outpatient surgery. Significantly, the majority of clots were identified after hospital discharge (9). The incidence of post-operative DVT in healthy adolescents is low. For example, Lau reported an overall incidence of confirmed symptomatic VTE after elective arthroscopic knee procedures of 0.27% (10).

Table 1. Risk factors for VTE in children (12, 24, 27, 45-49)

1. Indwelling central venous catheter (#1 cause)
2. Infection
    a. General (sepsis, pro-inflammatory state)
    b. Local
        i. Otitis media and mastoiditis associated with cerebral sinus venous thrombosis
        ii. Osteomyelitis associated with neighboring vein thrombosis
3. Lower extremity injury
4. Trauma
5. General surgery
6. Immobility (3 or more days)
7. Malignancy, especially Acute lymphocytic leukemia
8. Critical Illness
    c. Ventilator more than 4 days
    d. Hypovolemia
    e. Sepsis
    f. Indwelling lines
9. Certain Disease States
    g. Sickle Cell Anemia
    h. Nephrotic Syndrome
    i. Systemic lupus
    j. Cystic fibrosis
    k. Inflammatory Bowel Disease
    l. Congenital Heart disease
        i. Native shunts
        ii. Surgical shunts
    m. Liver Failure
10. Prolonged total parenteral nutrition
11. Inherited Thrombophilias
    n. Factor V Leiden deficiency
    o. Protein C, Protein S Deficiency
    p. Anti-phospholipid antibody syndrome
    q. Prothrombin 20210 gene mutation
    r. Anti-thrombin III deficiency
12. Obesity (low grade inflammatory state, increased endothelial dysfunction; increased platelet activation
13. Idiopathic

Patients with cystic fibrosis are at increased risk for VTE due to increased use of central catheters, acquired thrombophilia secondary to vitamin deficiencies, malnutrition, hepatic dysfunction, and chronic inflammation. Because of often severe underlying lung disease, the morbidity and mortality is increased. Further, the long-term risk of increased pulmonary hypertension is potentially more serious in this setting (11).

Obesity

Obesity is a well-recognized risk factor for VTE in both children (odds ratio 2.1) and adults; in some pediatric series, it the most commonly identified risk (12). The increased incidence of childhood obesity in the United States is well documented (13). Concurrent with the increase in childhood obesity has been a well-documented increase in pediatric VTE events. The increased risk is associated with obesity (BMI >30) but not overweight (BMI-25-30) (12). In Denmark, where there has been no increase in childhood obesity, there was no clinically significant increase in VTE in children between 1994 and 2006 (8, 14).

Multiple mechanisms have been proposed for the increased incidence of VTE in obese patients. Interesting, all of three components of Virchow's triad are adversely impacted by obesity. Increased abdominal pressure may decrease intra-abdominal flow (stasis), while obesity is a low-grade inflammatory state associated with vessel changes (endothelial); also, pro-thrombotic changes (blood) occur that include increased platelet activation, increased levels of plasminogen activator inhibitor and other pro-coagulants (Factor Vii, VIII, fibrinogen, von Willebrand factor) (15).

Critical illness

Critically ill children are at increased risk for VTE because of both the disease and its treatment. VTE risk factors include sepsis, mechanical ventilation (more than 4 days), hypovolemia, immobility and the use of central venous catheters. Of these, the presence of a central venous catheter is the most important risk factor for VTE; 85% of cases of VTE in critically ill children are related to central venous catheters. Asymptomatic DVTs were detected in 16% of all pediatric ICU patients with central lines (16-19). Recognition and treatment of asymptomatic DVT is crucial as nearly 50% of pulmonary embolisms in children arise from unrecognized DVT (20). The introduction of heparin-bonded central venous catheters has been shown to dramatically decrease the rate of both thrombosis and infection (21).

Oral contraception

The use of oral contraception and hormone supplementation is a well-described risk factor for VTE. It is important to note that for women with VTE attributed to hormonal supplementation, 96% had additional risk factors for VTE, including 27% with an inherited thrombophilia. Of those identified with an inherited thrombophilia two out of three had no family history of VTE (22).

Mortality rates

Mortality rates in pediatric PE are as high as 20%. Children are less likely to die from acute VTE than adults because of the absence (frequently) of co-morbidities including cardiac, renal, and pulmonary disease (20, 23-25).

DIAGNOSIS

The presentation of pulmonary embolism in children ranges from dramatic to subtle. Physical findings may range from profound (i.e., cardiac arrest, syncope, right heart failure, cyanosis, hypotension, dysrhythmia, pallor) to a near normal exam (25). The most common presenting signs of VTE in children are chest pain, shortness of breath, dyspnea, tachycardia, and cough (20). Symptoms may be vague (pain, dyspnea) and frequently overlap with more common diseases. Given large pulmonary reserves, small peripheral emboli may have minimal symptoms; some children with pulmonary emboli have normal vital signs on presentation.

The diagnosis of VTE in children is frequently delayed; in one retrospective, only 40% of pediatric patients with pulmonary embolism were diagnosed in the emergency department (26). The remaining 60%, were admitted with other diagnoses (i.e., pneumonia, respiratory distress, deep venous thrombosis) before subsequently being diagnosed with a pulmonary embolism. The median time to diagnosis for this group was 2 days after admission. Eighty percent of these patients had identifiable risk factors (obesity was most common); 45% had two or more risk factors for thromboembolic disease (26).

A high index of suspicion for pulmonary embolism is required in patients presenting with shortness of breath, tachypnea, cough, tachycardia, syncope, pleuritic chest pain or signs of a deep venous thrombosis. Patients with sickle cell disease are both prone to VTE and delayed diagnosis as the symptoms of pulmonary embolism and sickle chest syndrome overlap (27, 28).

Many well established clinical prediction rules for the likelihood of pulmonary embolism in adult populations have been proposed. The two most common (i.e., Wells criteria and PERC (Pulmonary Embolism Rule-out Criteria) have not been shown to be effective predictors in pediatric population. The Wells sensitivity is 86% vs a specificity of 60%; in the PERC, it is 100% and 24% respectively. Even when adding in clinical criteria (i.e., contraception, tachycardia, hypoxia), sensitivity and specificity were unacceptably low (90% and 56%).

Laboratory testing

Laboratory testing is of limited utility in the diagnosis of pulmonary embolism in children. For example, d-dimer, a degradation product of cross-linked fibrin, has been shown to be very sensitive (but not specific) for the detection of pulmonary embolism in adult patients. Pediatric specific data on the utility of the d-dimer test are lacking. Further, the d-dimer is frequently elevated in children by concomitant diseases (e.g., infectious, neoplastic, and inflammatory). Unfortunately, the addition of the d-dimer test to Wells or PERC decision rules has failed to significantly improve the utility of these strategies for children. Given the very low incidence of pulmonary embolism in children, further studies to delineate this will be difficult and a high index of suspicion is necessary in the appropriate clinical setting (29, 30). As discussed, the utilization of the d-dimer test is limited by the high false-positive rate.

Complete blood count, chemistries, and coagulation studies are typically normal, though may be affected by underlying or concomitant processes and are therefore not discriminatory. Arterial blood gases may be helpful if significant hypoxia is present; pC02 may be decreased secondary to tachypnea from underlying disease process, anxiety, or the simple pain of an arterial puncture. The non-invasive combination of pulse oximetry and end-tidal pC02 monitoring can give an accurate picture of both oxygenation and ventilation but is not enough to either diagnose or exclude pulmonary embolism. Cardiac biomarkers (i.e., troponin, brain natriuretic peptide [BNP]) are normal in patients with small (low-risk) PEs but are elevated in sub-massive and massive embolic events.

Electrocardiography

Electrocardiogram (ECG) changes are non-specific in both pediatric and adult patients with demonstrated pulmonary embolisms. The most common ECG abnormality in children with proven pulmonary embolism is tachycardia. Additional findings reflect right heart changes secondary to increased pulmonary pressures and include right axis deviation, incomplete right bundle branch block, and complete right heart block. The pathognomonic adult ECG finding in pulmonary embolism (s1q3t3), predictive of cor pulmonale/right heart strain, has not been validated in children.

Echocardiography

Similarly, echocardiography may demonstrate elevated right sided pressures with a dilated right ventricle, abnormal interventricular septal motion, tricuspid regurgitation, hypokinesis, and failure of the inferior vena cava to collapse during inspiration. These findings have been associated with increased morbidity and mortality in adults. However, patients with clinically significant smaller pulmonary emboli may have essentially normal echocardiograms (31).

Computed tomography angiography

Multi-detector computed tomography angiography (CTA) of the pulmonary vasculature has become the standard modality for diagnosing pulmonary embolism in children and adolescents. CTA has greater sensitivity and specificity than ventilation-perfusion scans (32). CTA can be used to estimate right ventricular volume overload in adult studies. An abnormally increased right ventricle/left ventricle diameter ratio on CT has been associated with a 2.5 increase in all-cause mortality and a 5x increase in PE mortality in adults; applicability of this to children and adolescents is unclear (33). CTA can define clot burden and provide information which may alter therapy (utilization of thrombolysis, thrombectomy).

CTA of the chest has the added benefit of finding alternative diagnoses in patients suspected of having PE but who had a normal CT angiogram. In a recent series of 96 pediatric patients, 57 patients without evidence of PE (59%) were found to have an alternative diagnosis;

these included pneumonia, atelectasis, malignancy, congenital heart disease, pulmonary hypertension, pulmonary nodules, pericardial effusion, fat embolism, right atrial thrombus, and rib fractures (34). CTA may miss very small peripheral pulmonary emboli but this is less likely with newer protocols. CT imaging does have significant radiation exposure and uses contrast dye which has been associated with both allergic and nephrotoxic complications.

Magnetic resonance angiography

Contrast-enhance pulmonary magnetic resonance angiography (MRA) is an alternative to CT angiogram. In addition to avoiding the significant amount of radiation associated with CTA, MRA defines cardiac anatomy and can be used in persons who cannot tolerate CT radiocontrast dye (35, 36). Sedation may be required for this procedure, though scanning times are decreasing with faster magnets and protocols. The contrast used with MRA has fewer side effects than the contrast used with CT angiography. Similar to CTA, MRA may miss small peripheral emboli.

Medical imaging conclusion

Nuclear medicine ventilation-perfusion scanning was long the standard for diagnosing pulmonary emboli and is still occasionally useful. Patients are exposed to less radiation than with CTA; however, the test is technically difficult to complete in younger patients and the comparably lower sensitivity and specificity (to CTA or MRA) limit its use. Ventilation-perfusion scanning remains the imaging procedure of choice for diagnosing chronic thromboembolic pulmonary hypertension (CTEPH), a sequelae in up to 10% of adult patients with pulmonary embolism.

Management

Patients with pulmonary emboli are stratified into one of three categories: minor, sub-massive and massive. Minor pulmonary emboli are associated with normal vital signs and normal bio-markers. Sub-massive pulmonary embolisms are characterized by elevated bio-markers and normal vital signs. Massive pulmonary embolisms are characterized by cardiovascular or respiratory compromise.

The initial management of acute pulmonary embolism is guided by the patient's overall hemodynamic status. Patients with minor pulmonary embolisms may only need pain control; others may need intravenous fluids, supplemental oxygen, and cardio-pulmonary monitoring with continuous pulse oximetry as well as end-tidal CO_2 monitoring if available. These patients will require immediate anti-coagulation with either unfractionated heparin (UFH) or low molecular weight heparin (LMWH).

Anti-coagulation

Unfractionated heparin (UFH) has been used for more than 50 years to treat thrombosis. UFH requires hospitalization and frequent blood draws; side effects include thrombocytopenia (HIT: heparin-induced thrombocytopenia), bleeding, and osteoporosis. In recent years, low molecular weight heparin (LMWHs) have become the initial drug of choice for anti-coagulation in children; LMWH include enoxaparin, dalteparin, fondaparinux. LMWH can be administered subcutaneously and unlike UFH does not require hospitalization. The use of LMWH requires minimal monitoring and the risk of drug-induced thrombocytopenia is negligible. Limited monitoring is necessary and unlike UFH, the incidence of drug-induced thrombocytopenia is negligible. The effectiveness of LMWH is less reliable in very young and obese patients. Fondaparinux, a selective Xa inhibitor LMWH, can be given once daily in children (37). The anti-coagulation effects of UFH and LMWHs can be reversed with protamine.

Sub-massive PE

Sub-massive pulmonary embolism presents with elevated biomarkers (i.e., troponin, BNP) and stable hemodynamics. EKG changes may include changes of right heart strain/cor pulmonale; this can include right axis deviation, incomplete or complete right bundle branch block, s1q3t3, and anterolateral t wave inversion. In addition to monitoring, pain control, and intravenous fluids, patients may need supplemental oxygen. It is important to remember that patients with low risk or sub-massive pulmonary emboli may quickly evolve in to more complicated scenarios (i.e., massive pulmonary embolus) should additional venous thrombus migrate to the pulmonary circulation.

Patients with sub-massive pulmonary embolism require full anti-coagulation with either UFH or LMWH. To date there is no consensus among the major adult guidelines (i.e., American Heart Association, American College of Chest Physicians, American College of Emergency Physicians, European Society of Cardiology) about the use of thrombolytic therapy (peripheral or catheter-directed) for patients with sub-massive pulmonary emboli.

Massive PE

Massive pulmonary emboli present with hypotension, arrhythmias, hypovolemic shock, left ventricular dysfunction, bradycardia, and sudden death. About 5% of adult pulmonary embolisms are massive; however, the real incidence is unknown as some cases of sudden death are undoubtedly attributable to massive pulmonary embolism. The incidence of massive pulmonary embolism in children is less in part because of increased cardiopulmonary reserve and the absence of co-morbidities (i.e., diabetes, heart disease, lung disease).

Initial therapy is aimed at cardiovascular support including use of inotropes and mechanical ventilation. Unfortunately, large saddle-type pulmonary emboli may be refractory to these therapies as there is essentially no pulmonary flow and oxygenation, even with mechanical ventilation, is impossible. In these scenarios, practitioners should consider thrombolytic therapy with recombinant tissue plasminogen activator. Full dose thrombolytics may restore partial pulmonary arterial flow allowing for improved oxygenation and resuscitation. Full dose thrombolytics, particularly if delivered peripherally, have been associated with intra-cerebral bleeding and death (38). Full dose thrombolytics are effective but carry a higher rate of serious and sometimes fatal bleeding complications including intracerebral hemorrhage.

Table 2. Virchow revisited: Risk factors for pediatric thromboembolism (31)

1. Damage to Endothelium
    a. Trauma
    b. Surgery
    c. Central venous catheter
    d. Chronic inflammatory state
        i. Inflammatory bowel disease
        ii. Sickle cell anemia
        iii. Obesity
        iv. Cystic Fibrosis
    e. Infection/Sepsis
    f. Anti-phospholipid antibodies
2. Thrombophilia (alterations in blood)
    a. Acquired
        i. Cancers
        ii. Medications (including hormones)
        iii. Obesity
        iv. Pregnancy
        v. Nephrotic Syndrome
    b. Inherited
        i. Factor V Leiden syndrome
        ii. Prothrombin 20210 gene mutation
        iii. Protein C/Protein S deficiency
        iv. Anti-thrombin III deficiency
3. Stasis
    a. Sepsis/shock
    b. Hypovolemia
    c. Immobility
    d. Heart disease
        i. Congenital heart disease
        ii. Cardiomyopathies
        iii. Shunts
    e. Total parenteral nutrition

Long-term anti-coagulation

All patients with acute pulmonary embolism require long-term anti-coagulation. Current options for long-term anticoagulation in patients under age 18 years include warfarin and LMWH. Historically the vitamin K antagonist warfarin has been used for long-term anti-coagulation in children. Warfarin (Coumadin) is inexpensive and administered orally, but has many problems. Dosing is unreliable and requires frequent monitoring; therapeutic levels are difficult to maintain and are affected by diet and other medications. Home monitoring is now available and this is a viable option for older patients requiring long-term anti-coagulation.

Bleeding risks are real but can generally be managed with vitamin K (oral, intramuscular, or intravenous), fresh frozen plasma, and in severe cases, prothrombin complex concentrate.

Novel anti-coagulants (NOACs) (rivaroxaban, dabigatran, apixaban, edoxaban) are widely used for maintenance anti-coagulation in adults. Though expensive, these drugs do not have significant interactions and are not affected by diet. There is no need for routine laboratory monitoring of NOACS. Multiple clinical trials are ongoing, but currently none of the novel anticoagulants are approved for use in children (39-41).

The duration of anti-coagulation therapy depends on multiple factors. All patients require anti-coagulation for a minimum of three months. For selected patients with "provoked" thrombosis (e.g., surgery, trauma, central venous catheter), three months may be sufficient. For patients with an "unprovoked" thrombosis, anti-coagulation for a minimum of six months is recommended (16).

Up to 8% of the US population has an inherited thrombophilia (7). Patients with inherited thrombophilia may present with what appears to be a provoked thrombosis, and for this reason more extensive testing may be considered, especially if there is a family history of venous thromboembolic disease; up to 35% of pediatric patients may have an unrecognized inherited thrombophilia (7, 42, 43). All patients with a second thrombosis, even in the presence of central venous catheters, require further evaluation (see Table 3).

Table 3. Recommended testing for inherited thrombophilia (16, 50, 51)

1. Prothrombin 20210 gene mutation
2. Anti-phospholipid antibodies
3. Protein C activity level
4. Protein S activity level
5. Anti-thrombin III activity level
6. Factor V Leiden assay
7. Fasting homocysteine

CONCLUSION

Pulmonary embolism occurs when a thrombus forms in the venous vasculature and propagates to the pulmonary vasculature. Venous thromboembolism (VTE) and pulmonary embolism (PE) affect up to 1 million persons in the United States annually. Risk factors, diagnostic considerations, and management options for adults and children are presented in this discussion.

The long-term prognosis for children surviving pulmonary embolism is excellent. Less than 10% of adult patients with pulmonary embolism (study range 0.1% to 10%) develop chronic thromboembolic pulmonary hypertension (CTEPH). The risk of CTEPH in children is unknown; most children who develop this syndrome (66%) have an underlying thrombophilia. Patients with CTEPH may have a normal CTA and are best diagnosed with VQ scanning. Selected children with CTEPH may benefit from surgical pulmonary thrombo-endarterectomy (44).

REFERENCES

[1] Lowe GD. Virchow's triad revisited: abnormal flow. Pathophysiol Haemost Thromb 2003;33(5-6):455-7.

[2] Chung I, Lip GY. Virchow's triad revisited: blood constituents. Pathophysiol Haemost Thromb 2003;33(5-6):449-54.

[3] Huth E, Murray TJ. Medicine in quotations: Views of health and diseases through the ages, Second ed. Philadelphia, PA: American College of Physicians, 2006.

[4] Zampieri F, Zanatta A, Basso C, Thiene G. Cardiovascular medicine in Morgagni's De sedibus: dawn of cardiovascular pathology. Cardiovasc Pathol 2016;25(6):443-52.

[5] McFadden PM, Ochsner JL. A history of the diagnosis and treatment of venous thrombosis and pulmonary embolism. Ochsner J 2002;4(1):9-13.

[6] Cashman M. Massive Pulmonary embolism in a boy aged 9 years. Arch Dis Child 1956;160:474-6.

[7] Beckman MG, Hooper WC, Critchley SE, Ortel TL. Venous thromboembolism: a public health concern. Am J Prev Med 2010;38(4 Suppl):S495-501.

[8] Raffini L, Huang YS, Witmer C, Feudtner C. Dramatic increase in venous thromboembolism in children's hospitals in the United States from 2001 to 2007. Pediatrics 2009;124(4):1001-8.

[9] Humes DJ, Nordenskjold A, Walker AJ, West J, Ludvigsson JF. Risk of venous thromboembolism in children after general surgery. J Pediatr Surg 2015;50(11):1870-3.

[10] Lau BC, Jagodzinski J, Pandya NK. Incidence of symptomatic pulmonary embolus and deep vein thrombosis after knee arthroscopy in the pediatric and adolescent population. Clin J Sport Med 2017 Oct 10. doi: 10.1097/JSM.0000000000000519.

[11] Takemoto CM, Sohi S, Desai K, Bharaj R, Khanna A, McFarland S, et al. Hospital-associated venous thromboembolism in children: incidence and clinical characteristics. J Pediatr 2014;164(2):332-8.

[12] Stokes S, Breheny P, Radulescu A, Radulescu VC. Impact of obesity on the risk of venous thromboembolism in an inpatient pediatric population. Pediatr Hematol Oncol 2014;31(5):475-80.

[13] Dietz WH. Overweight in childhood and adolescence. New Engl J Med 2004;350(9):855-7.

[14] Tuckuviene R, Christensen AL, Helgestad J, Johnsen SP, Kristensen SR. Paediatric arterial ischaemic stroke and cerebral sinovenous thrombosis in Denmark 1994-2006: A nationwide population-based study. Acta Paediatrica 2011;100(4):543-9.

[15] Steffen LM, Cushman M, Peacock JM, Heckbert SR, Jacobs DR, Jr., Rosamond WD, et al. Metabolic syndrome and risk of venous thromboembolism: longitudinal Investigation of thromboembolism etiology. J Thromb Haemost 2009;7(5):746-51.

[16] Monagle P, Chan AKC, Goldenberg NA, Ichord RN, Journeycake JM, Nowak-Göttl U, et al. Antithrombotic therapy in neonates and children: Antithrombotic therapy and prevention of thrombosis, 9th ed: American College of Chest Physicians Evidence-Based Clinical Practice Guidelines. Chest 2012;141(2 Suppl): e737S-e801S.

[17] Faustino EVS, Spinella PC, Li S, Pinto MG, Stoltz P, Tala J, et al. Incidence and acute complications of asymptomatic central venous catheter-related deep venous thrombosis in critically ill children. J Pediatrics 2013;162(2):387-91.

[18] Polikoff LA, Faustino EVS. Venous thromboembolism in critically ill children. Curr Opin Pediatr 2014;26(3):286-91.

[19] Higgerson RA, Lawson KA, Christie LM, Brown AM, McArthur JA, Totapally BR, et al. Incidence and risk factors associated with venous thrombotic events in pediatric intensive care unit patients. Pediatr Crit Care Med 2011;12(6):628-34.

[20] Biss TT, Brandao LR, Kahr WH, Chan AK, Williams S. Clinical features and outcome of pulmonary embolism in children. Br J Haematol 2008;142(5):808-18

[21] Pierce CM, Wade A, Mok Q. Heparin-bonded central venous lines reduce thrombotic and infective complications in critically ill children. Intensive Care Med 2000;26(7):967-72.

[22] Pillai P, Bonny AE, O'Brien SH. Contraception-related venous thromboembolism in a pediatric institution. J Pediatr Adolesc Gynecol 2013;26(3):186-8.

[23] Spentzouris G, Scriven RJ, Lee TK, Labropoulos N. Pediatric venous thromboembolism in relation to adults. J Vasc Surg 2012;55(6):1785-93.

[24] Andrew M, David M, Adams M, Ali K, Anderson R, Barnard D, et al. Venous thromboembolic complications (VTE) in children: first analyses of the Canadian Registry of VTE. Blood 1994;83(5):1251-7.
[25] van Ommen CH, Peters M. Venous thromboembolic disease in childhood. Semin Thromb Hemost 2003;29(4):391-404.
[26] Agha BS, Sturm JJ, Simon HK, Hirsh DA. Pulmonary embolism in the pediatric emergency department. Pediatrics 2013;132(4):663-7.
[27] Burnham JM, Broussard M, Milbrandt T. Bilateral pulmonary embolism in an adolescent with sickle cell disease and a recent total hip arthroplasty: a case report and review of the literature. Iowa Orthop J 2014;34:107-10.
[28] Mornand P, Chalard F, Romain AS, Rohr M, Paluel-Marmont C, Niakate A, et al. Bilateral pulmonary embolism mimicking acute chest syndrome in an adolescent with sickle cell disease. Arch Pediatr 2017;24(7):625-9. [French]
[29] Hennelly KE, Baskin MN, Monuteuax MC, Hudgins J, Kua E, Commeree A, et al. Detection of pulmonary embolism in high-risk children. J Pediatr 2016;178:214-8.e3.
[30] Biss TT, Brandao LR, Kahr WHA, Chan AKC, Williams S. Clinical probability score and D-dimer estimation lack utility in the diagnosis of childhood pulmonary embolism. J Thromb Haemost 2009;7(10):1633-8.
[31] Zaidi AU, Hutchins KK, Rajpurkar M. Pulmonary embolism in children. Front Pediatr 2017;5:170. doi: 10.3389/fped.2017.00170.
[32] Tang CX, Schoepf UJ, Chowdhury SM, Fox MA, Zhang LJ, Lu GM. Multidetector computed tomography pulmonary angiography in childhood acute pulmonary embolism. Pediatr Radiol 2015;45(10):1431-9.
[33] Meinel FG, Nance JW, Jr., Schoepf UJ, Hoffmann VS, Thierfelder KM, Costello P, et al. Predictive value of computed tomography in acute pulmonary embolism: Systematic review and meta-analysis. Am J Med 2015;128(7):747-59.
[34] Lee EY, Kritsaneepaiboon S, Zurakowski D, Arellano CM, Strauss KJ, Boiselle PM. Beyond the pulmonary arteries: alternative diagnoses in children with MDCT pulmonary angiography negative for pulmonary embolism. AJR Am J Roentgenol 2009;193(3):888-94.
[35] Benson DG, Schiebler ML, Repplinger MD, Francois CJ, Grist TM, Reeder SB, et al. Contrast-enhanced pulmonary MRA for the primary diagnosis of pulmonary embolism: current state of the art and future directions. Br J Radiol 2017;90(1074):20160901. doi: 10.1259/bjr.20160901.
[36] Benson DG, Schiebler ML, Nagle SK, Francois CJ. Magnetic resonance imaging for the evaluation of pulmonary embolism. Top Magn Reson Imaging 2017;26(4):145-51.
[37] Young G, Yee DL, O'Brien SH, Khanna R, Barbour A, Nugent DJ. FondaKIDS: a prospective pharmacokinetic and safety study of fondaparinux in children between 1 and 18 years of age. Pediatric Blood Cancer 2011;57(6):1049-54.
[38] Jaff MR, McMurtry MS, Archer SL, Cushman M, Goldenberg N, Goldhaber SZ, et al. Management of massive and submassive pulmonary embolism, iliofemoral deep vein thrombosis, and chronic thromboembolic pulmonary hypertension: a scientific statement from the American Heart Association. Circulation 2011;123(16):1788-830.
[39] Law C, Raffini L. A guide to the use of anticoagulant drugs in children. Paediatr Drugs 2015;17(2):105-14.
[40] Mitchell LG, Goldenberg NA, Male C, Kenet G, Monagle P, Nowak-Göttl U, et al. Definition of clinical efficacy and safety outcomes for clinical trials in deep venous thrombosis and pulmonary embolism in children. J Thromb Haemost 2011;9(9):1856-8.
[41] Antoniou S. Rivaroxaban for the treatment and prevention of thromboembolic disease. J Pharm Pharmacol 2015;67(8):1119-32.
[42] Biss TT, Rajpurkar M, Williams S, van Ommen CH, Chan AKC, Goldenberg NA. Recommendations for future research in relation to pediatric pulmonary embolism: communication from the SSC of the ISTH. J Thromb Haemost 2018;16(2):405-408.
[43] Laygo RJ, Rowlett JD. Anticardiolipin antibody syndrome in an adolescent with recurrent deep vein thrombosis. South Med J 1994;87:S97.

[44] Madani MM, Wittine LM, Auger WR, Fedullo PF, Kerr KM, Kim NH, et al. Chronic thromboembolic pulmonary hypertension in pediatric patients. J Thorac Cardiovasc Surg 2011;141(3):624-30.

[45] Mahajerin A, Branchford BR, Amankwah EK, Raffini L, Chalmers E, van Ommen CH, et al. Hospital-associated venous thromboembolism in pediatrics: a systematic review and meta-analysis of risk factors and risk-assessment models. Haematologica 2015;100(8):1045-50.

[46] Gerotziafas GT. Risk factors for venous thromboembolism in children. Int Angiol 2004;23(3):195-205.

[47] Nylund CM, Goudie A, Garza JM, Crouch G, Denson LA. Venous thrombotic events in hospitalized children and adolescents with inflammatory bowel disease. J Pediatr Gastroenterol Nutr 2013;56(5):485-91.

[48] Kim SJ, Sabharwal S. Risk factors for venous thromboembolism in hospitalized children and adolescents: A systemic review and pooled analysis. J Pediatr Ortho B 2014;23(4):389-93.

[49] Mahajerin A, Croteau SE. Epidemiology and risk assessment of pediatric venous thromboembolism. Front Pediatr 2017;5:68. doi: 10.3389/fped.2017.00068.

[50] Young G. Anticoagulants in children and adolescents. Hematology Am Soc Hematol Educ Program 2015;2015:111-6.

[51] Young G. How I treat pediatric venous thromboembolism. Blood 2017;130(12):1402-8.

In: Chronic Disease and Disability
Editors: DE Greydanus, P Anne, JD Rowlett et al.
ISBN: 978-1-53617-656-8

Chapter 11

EMERGING THERAPIES FOR PEDIATRIC THROMBOEMBOLIC DISEASE

John D Rowlett*[1-3,*]*, MD, FAAP, FACP and Carson S Villa*[4]*, BS

[1]Pediatric Emergency Medicine and Pediatric Hospital Medicine,
St Joseph's/Candler Healthcare System, Savannah, Georgia, United States of America
[2]Medical College of Georgia, Augusta, Georgia, United States of America
[3]Eastern Kentucky University, Richmond, Kentucky, United States of America
[4]College of Pharmacy, Lipscomb University, Nashville, Tennesee,
United States of America

ABSTRACT

Pediatric thromboembolism is an uncommon, but potentially life-threatening and occasionally fatal event in pediatric individuals. This discussion reflects on recent advances in thrombolytic therapy that have been in the adult populations and are applied to the pediatric population. After a historical refection, this discussion reviews various thrombolytics with the main emphasis on tissue plasminogen activator (tpa). Absolute and relative contraindications to thrombolysis are considered as well as general precautions for patients undergoing thrombolysis. Various medications used for the management of adult thromboembolic disease are noted that include rivaroxaban, dabigatran, apixaban, and edoxaban.

INTRODUCTION

Pediatric thromboembolism is an uncommon but potentially life-threatening and occasionally fatal clinical event. A high index of suspicion, rapid clinical diagnosis, and aggressive supportive care are necessary to support the pediatric patient with an acute pulmonary embolism. Recent advances in thrombolytic therapy in adult patients with multiple conditions, including pulmonary embolism, have shown significant improvements in both morbidity and

---

* Corresponding Author's Email: drrowlett@gmail.com.

mortality. Little data exists regarding the use of similar strategies in pediatric patients; however, given the success of the adult trials and the disease burden associated with pediatric pulmonary thromboembolism, aggressive therapy with thrombolytics is becoming increasingly common.

Surgical and catheter-based therapies (thrombectomy, thrombolysis) developed in adult populations are becoming more widely used in pediatric practice. Finally, the introduction of novel anticoagulants has fundamentally changed the treatment of venous thromboembolic disease and pulmonary embolism in adults. Also, the eventual inclusion of these drugs in pediatric protocols will profoundly change management of pulmonary embolisms in children and adolescents.

HISTORICAL CONSIDERATIONS

Direct thrombectomy is a well-established albeit invasive procedure for the removal of large clot volumes. In 1872 the German surgeon Friedrich Trendelenburg (1844-1924) performed embolectomies on two patients with pulmonary embolism; unfortunately, neither survived more than two days. A pupil of Trendelenburg, Martin Kirschner (1879-1924) successfully performed in 1924 a pulmonary embolectomy, which complicated the post-operative course of a routine hernia repair (1, 2).

Eini (3) reviewed the literature on massive pulmonary embolism in children in he found a total of 39 cases reported between 1953 and 2011. Nearly 50% of these patients died without any treatment; 15 were treated with embolectomy (with cardiac bypass) in which 12 of these survived. Five patients in this series received either native or recombinant tissue plasminogen activator (tpa); this study noted that one survived, two died, and two failed use of tPA and underwent embolectomy (one survived) (3). This was a very diverse patient group with risk factors ranging from simple immobilization to major diseases (e.g., congenital heart disease, malignancy, cardiomyopathy, sepsis).

Given the success of prior embolectomies, Eini successfully performed fiber-optic guided embolectomy on two small children (an 11-day-old infant and a 2-year-old boy) with massive pulmonary embolism (3). Badheka (4) recently reported a successful surgical thrombo-embolectomy; this was accomplished in a chronically ill patient who had a tracheostomy, developed obstructive shock secondary to a massive pulmonary embolism, and received extracorporeal membrane oxygenation (ECMO) (4).

TISSUE PLASMINOGEN ACTIVATOR (TPA)

In 1947, researchers discovered a substance (initially named "fibrinokinase") in animal tissue which could activate plasminogen; this was later isolated and renamed "tissue plasminogen activator" (tPA) (2). In 1981, two patients with post-renal transplant renal vein thrombosis were successfully treated (recanalization of the thrombosed renal vein) with intravenous infusion of tPA. In 1983, tPA was successfully used to treat acute myocardial infarction; 6 of 7 patients recanalized previously occluded arteries within 60 minutes of the infusion (2). A recombinant form (rtpa) was developed and used in 1984 to successfully treat acute myocardial infarctions.

Currently available agents for thrombolysis include streptokinase, urokinase, and recombinant tissue plasminogen activator. Recombinant tissue plasminogen activator (rtPA) has become the most commonly utilized drug because of a superior safety profile (less immunogenic), improved in vitro clot lysis, and wide-spread availability (5). Recombinant tissue plasminogen activator (rtPA) has found widespread use in adults for the treatment of heart attacks, pulmonary embolism, peripheral arterial thrombosis, and most recently, cerebrovascular occlusions. Though percutaneous catheter based treatments have largely supplanted the use of rtPA in acute coronary disease, thrombolysis is still a crucial component of acute therapy for massive pulmonary embolism, selected cases of sub-massive pulmonary embolism, selected strokes, occluded catheters, and acute arterial and venous occlusions (6).

Thrombolytics (essentially rtPA but occasionally heparin) can be delivered through a peripheral intravenous (IV) route or through an endovascular catheter (catheter-directed thrombolysis, (CDT). Additionally, some catheters may be utilized via aspiration or rotational thrombectomy for removal of some or all of the clot burden, in addition to delivering thrombolytic drugs (heparin or rtPA) at the site of the clot.

THROMBOLYSIS IN PEDIATRICS

Thrombolysis has been utilized in pediatrics for a variety of conditions including those listed in Table 1 (7-10). A combination of pharmaco-mechanical thrombectomy (PMT) and catheter-directed thrombolysis with rtPA infusion was successfully used to treat extensive iliofemoral deep vein thrombosis (DVT) in a 9-year-old boy (11). Patients with congenital heart disease are at increased risk for thrombosis (implanted/created shunts, cardiomyopathy); tpa has been successfully used to treat native and surgical vessel shunts in this population (12). The ventricular assist device (VAD) has become an important bridge between surgeries and potential orthotopic heart transplant in children and adults. Unfortunately, such devices are known to increase the risk of thrombosis. Thrombolysis with rtPA has been successfully used to treat bilateral pulmonary emboli in a child on Bi-VAD (bi-ventricular assist device) who was then successfully bridged to heart transplantation (13).

Table 1. Pediatric uses of thrombolysis (7-10)

1.	Salvage of occluded central venous access
2.	Shunt thrombosis in the setting of congenital heart disease
3.	Arterial thrombosis with tissue ischemia
4.	Coronary artery thrombosis in the setting of Kawasaki disease
5.	Superior vena cava syndrome
6.	Pulmonary embolism (PE) with hypotension
7.	Shock with resultant right heart strain/failure and PE

Multi-disciplinary institutional protocols have been developed for percutaneous endovascular thrombolysis for children with deep vein thrombosis (DVT) and have been modified for catheter-directed thrombolysis (CDT) for pulmonary embolism (PE) (12, 14, 15). Catheter directed thrombolysis with rtPA infusion has been used successfully in adults with thrombosis using a multi-side hole catheter rotational embolectomy, suction embolectomy and rheolytic as well as aspiration thrombectomy; data are limited in children but these appears to be emerging and safe therapies (16).

Bavare reported a series of five pediatric patients (median age 16.5 years, each having multiple risk factors) with massive pulmonary embolism who were treated with augmented (ultrasound) catheter directed infusion of rtPA with the EKOS™ system. The EKOS™ uses targeted ultrasonic waves with rtPA to effectively target the entire clot; this system has a higher success rate, uses less thrombolytic drug, and has fewer bleeding complications than traditional CDT (17,18). Four patients had complete resolution at 24 hours; all five survived with no mortality or treatment-related complications (19). Morgan reported a series of five adolescents with cardiac arrest secondary to PE; during the study period, this represented 6% of all pediatric arrests and 25% of all adolescent in hospital arrests (20), All of the patients has multiple risk factors for venous thromboembolism (VTE), all five patients were treated with intravenous tPA, and four (80%) survived to hospital discharge (20).

Thrombolysis has been shown to be effective for established clots less than 14 days old (83% response rate to tPA). If delivered directly to the embolus (CDT), rtPA has been shown to be safe and effective for clots up to 60 days old (21). Thrombolysis, whether systemic or catheter directed, is not without significant risks including intracranial bleeding, epidural hematoma (in a patient with underlying malignancy), and death (22). Accordingly, well-established absolute exclusion criteria (see Table 2) have been established in adult populations and are applicable to pediatric patients. Further, relative contraindications (Table 3) and general precautions (Table 4) have been established (5, 7, 15, 22).

Table 2. Absolute contraindications to thrombolysis

1.	Active bleeding
2.	Thrombocytopenia (<100,000)
3.	Recent (10 days or less) major trauma, surgery, puncture of a non-compressible vessel, or organ biopsy.
4.	Intracranial hemorrhage, intracranial infarction, or intra-spinal surgery within past 60 days.
5.	CPR or prolonged asphyxia in the past 7 days
6.	Know significant right-to-left intra-cardiac shunt
7.	Extreme prematurity

Table 3. Relative contraindications to thrombolysis

1.	Pregnancy
2.	Puerperium
3.	Arteriovenous malformations
4.	Neoplasms
5.	Uncontrolled hypertension
6.	Infective Endocarditis
7.	Contraindication to imaging (contrast allergy, renal failure)

Table 4. General precautions for patients undergoing thrombolysis

1.	No arterial punctures
2.	Avoid new line placements if possible
3.	Limit patient movement/manipulation (physiotherapy)
4.	Avoid ng tubes and urinary catheters if possible
5.	Avoid non-steroidal anti-inflammatory drugs, anti-platelet medications
6.	If less than 3 months of age, intracranial imaging before and after thrombolysis if feasible

The optimal dose for tPA infusion in CDT in children is unknown. Low dose tPA (0.01-0.06 mg/kg/hour) has been shown in some studies to be as effective as higher dose (0.1-0.5 mg/kg/hr) (15, 23). Once stable, patients can be started on unfractionated heparin (UFH) or low-molecular weight heparin (LMWH) and transitioned to outpatient treatment with either LMWH or vitamin K antagonist (warfarin). The eventual approval of novel anticoagulants will change the long-term management. Duration of therapy is dependent on multiple factors including status (provoked or unprovoked) and possible genetic predisposition. A minimum of three months is recommended for provoked events; unprovoked events require a minimum of six-months of anticoagulation. However, in some cases (i.e., inherited thrombophilia) the recommendation may be life-long (24).

CONCLUSION

Pediatric thromboembolism is a serious event, but current management options can be beneficial with reduced morbidity and mortality. Surgical and catheter-based therapies (thrombectomy, thrombolysis) developed in adult populations are becoming more widely used in pediatric practice. The use of tissue plasminogen activator (tPA) has been an exciting development that began in the middle of the 20th century and continues to the present day.

There are several drugs currently widely used in the adult population that are in multiple phase studies in pediatric populations (25, 26). Fondaparinux, a direct factor Xa inhibitor, is a once daily alternative to enoxaparin and appears to cause less osteoporosis (27). There are multiple ongoing trials on the use of the novel anticoagulant (NOAC) drugs in children, though to date, there are no approved uses in the pediatric population (28-34).

These agents (i.e., rivaroxaban, dabigatran, apixaban, and edoxaban) have already profoundly changed the management of thromboembolic disease in adults. Minor pulmonary embolisms can be treated with oral medications and discharged; hospitalization are now rarely necessary for uncomplicated deep venous thrombosis. Assuming some or all of the currently available (or future) NOACs are approved for pediatric patients, a similar shift in the management of pediatric thromboembolic disease is anticipated.

NOACs have the benefit of oral therapy and limited drug interactions and unlike warfarin, routine bloodwork is not needed. Therapeutic levels with NOACs are easily achieved in most adults and are unaffected by diet. There are, however, limitations to the new anticoagulant drugs. In addition to a lack of studies in children, these drugs are expensive and have been associated with increased risk of bleeding. While the risk of bleeding in adult patients on the novel anticoagulants appears to be lower than with warfarin, presently only the direct thrombin inhibitor, dabigatran, has an effective reversal agent; however, multiple drugs being studied for the other NOACs and the future looks encouraging for management of pediatric and adult patients with thromboembolism (28, 35).

REFERENCES

[1] Westaby S. The foundations of cardiac surgery. In: Westaby S, ed. Landmarks in cardiac surgery. Oxford: Isis Medical Media, 1997:1-47.

[2] McFadden PM, Ochsner JL. A history of the diagnosis and treatment of venous thrombosis and pulmonary embolism. Ochsner J 2002;4(1):9-13.

[3] Eini ZM, Houri S, Cohen I, Sion R, Tamir A, Sasson L, et al. Massive pulmonary emboli in children: does fiber-optic-guided embolectomy have a role? Review of the literature and report of two cases. Chest 2013;143(2):544-9.

[4] Badheka A, Bangalore Prakash P, Allareddy V. Successful use of extracorporeal membrane oxygenation in a child with obstructive shock due to massive bilateral pulmonary embolism. Perfusion 2017 Oct 1:267659117736380. doi: 10.1177/0267659117736380.

[5] Manco-Johnson MJ, Grabowski EF, Hellgreen M, Kemahli AS, Massicotte MP, Muntean W, et al. Recommendations for tPA thrombolysis in children. On behalf of the Scientific Subcommittee on Perinatal and Pediatric Thrombosis of the Scientific and Standardization Committee of the International Society of Thrombosis and Haemostasis. Thromb Haemost 2002;88(1):157-8.

[6] Collen D, Lijnen HR. The tissue-type plasminogen activator story. Arterioscler Thromb Vasc Biol 2009;29(8):1151-5.

[7] Tarango C, Manco-Johnson MJ. Pediatric thrombolysis: A practical approach. Front Pediatr 2017;5:260. doi: 10.3389/fped.2017.00260.

[8] Lungren MP, Ward TJ, Patel MN, Racadio JM, Kukreja K. Endovascular thrombolysis to salvage central venous access in children with catheter-associated upper extremity deep vein thrombosis: technique and initial results. J Thromb Thrombolysis 2015;40(3):274-9.

[9] Holzer R, Peart I, Ciotti G, Bolton-Maggs PH. Idiopathic multifocal intracardiac and pulmonary thrombosis: successful treatment with rTPA. Pediatr Cardiol 2002;23(5):548-52.

[10] Gaballah M, Shi J, Kukreja K, Raffini L, Tarango C, Keller M, et al. Endovascular thrombolysis in the management of iliofemoral thrombosis in children: A multi-institutional experience. J Vasc Interv Radiol 2016;27(4):524-30.

[11] Hamidian Jahromi A, Coulter AH, Bass P, 3rd, Zhang WW, Tan TW. Pharmacomechanical thrombectomy and catheter-directed thrombolysis of acute lower extremity deep venous thrombosis in a 9-year-old boy with inferior vena cava atresia. Vasc Med 2015;20(2):139-42.

[12] Kukreja KU, Lungren MP, Patel MN, Johnson ND, Racadio JM, Dandoy C, et al. Endovascular venous thrombolysis in children younger than 24 months. J Vasc Interv Radiol 2014;25(8):1158-64.

[13] Godown J, Dodd DA, Doyle TP, Smith AH, Janssen D, Mettler BA. Tissue plasminogen activator treatment of bilateral pulmonary emboli in a pediatric patient supported with a ventricular assist device. Pediatr Transplant 2015;19(7):E160-4.

[14] Dandoy CE, Kukreja KU, Gruppo RA, Patel MN, Tarango C. Outcomes in children with deep vein thrombosis managed with percutaneous endovascular thrombolysis. Pediatr Radiol 2015;45(5):719-26.

[15] Kukreja K, Gruppo R, Chima R, Ristagno R, Racadio J. Developing a pediatric endovascular thrombolysis program: A single-center experience. Pediatr Radiol 2013;43(8):1024-9.

[16] Qureshi AM, Petit CJ, Crystal MA, Liou A, Khan A, Justino H. Efficacy and safety of catheter-based rheolytic and aspiration thrombectomy in children. Catheter Cardiovasc Interv 2016;87(7):1273-80.

[17] Parikh S, Motarjeme A, McNamara T, Raabe R, Hagspiel K, Benenati JF, et al. Ultrasound-accelerated thrombolysis for the treatment of deep vein thrombosis: initial clinical experience. J Vasc Interv Radiol 2008;19(4):521-8.

[18] Lin PH, Annambhotla S, Bechara CF, Athamneh H, Weakley SM, Kobayashi K, et al. Comparison of percutaneous ultrasound-accelerated thrombolysis versus catheter-directed thrombolysis in patients with acute massive pulmonary embolism. Vascular 2009;17(Suppl 3):S137-47.

[19] Bavare AC, Naik SX, Lin PH, Poi MJ, Yee DL, Bronicki RA, et al. Catheter-directed thrombolysis for severe pulmonary embolism in pediatric patients. Ann Vasc Surg 2014;28(7):1794.e1-7.

[20] Morgan RW, Stinson HR, Wolfe H, Lindell RB, Topjian AA, Nadkarni VM, et al. Pediatric in-hospital cardiac arrest secondary to acute pulmonary embolism. Crit Care Med 2017 Dec 19. doi: 10.1097/CCM.0000000000002921.

[21] Knofler R, Dinger J, Kabus M, Muller D, Lauterbach I, Rupprecht E, et al. Thrombolytic therapy in children--clinical experiences with recombinant tissue-plasminogen activator. Semin Thromb Hemost 2001;27(2):169-74.

[22] Komvilaisak P, Grant R, Weitzman S, Brandao L, Blaser S, Chait P, et al. Epidural hematoma following tissue plasminogen activator (tPA) therapy for pulmonary embolism in a pediatric patient with stage IV Burkitt's lymphoma: a case report. Thromb Res 2008;121(5):709-12.

[23] Levy M, Benson LN, Burrows PE, Bentur Y, Strong DK, Smith J, et al. Tissue plasminogen activator for the treatment of thromboembolism in infants and children. J Pediatr 1991;118(3):467-72.

[24] Young G. How I treat pediatric venous thromboembolism. Blood 2017;130(12):1402-8.

[25] Kerlin BA. Current and future management of pediatric venous thromboembolism. Am J Hematol 2012;87:S68-S74.

[26] Young G. Anticoagulants in children and adolescents. Hematology Am Soc Hematol Educ Program 2015;2015:111-6.

[27] Young G, Yee DL, O'Brien SH, Khanna R, Barbour A, Nugent DJ. FondaKIDS: a prospective pharmacokinetic and safety study of fondaparinux in children between 1 and 18 years of age. Pediatr Blood Cancer 2011;57(6):1049-54.

[28] von Vajna E, Alam R, So TY. Current clinical trials on the use of direct oral anticoagulants in the pediatric population. Cardiol Ther 2016;5(1):19-41.

[29] Halton JML, Picard AC, Harper R, Huang F, Brueckmann M, Gropper S, et al. Pharmacokinetics, pharmacodynamics, safety and tolerability of dabigatran etexilate oral liquid formulation in infants with venous thromboembolism. Thromb Haemost 2017;117(11):2168-2175.

[30] Halton JML, Albisetti M, Biss B, Bomgaars L, Brueckmann M, Gropper S, et al. Phase IIa study of dabigatran etexilate in children with venous thrombosis: pharmacokinetics, safety, and tolerability. J Thromb Haemost 2017;15(11):2147-57.

[31] Goldenberg NA, Takemoto CM, Yee DL, Kittelson JM, Massicotte MP. Improving evidence on anticoagulant therapies for venous thromboembolism in children: Key challenges and opportunities. Blood 2015;126(24):2541-7.

[32] Dietrich K, Stang L, van Ryn J, Mitchell LG. Assessing the anticoagulant effect of dabigatran in children: an in vitro study. Thromb Res 2015;135(4):630-5.

[33] Bansal M, Ren CL. Anti-coagulant therapy with dabigatran for cystic fibrosis patients. Pediatric Pulmonol 2016;51(8):E29-30.

[34] Radulescu VC. Anticoagulation therapy in children. Semin Thromb Hemost 2017; 43(8):877-85.

[35] Ansell JE. Universal, class-specific and drug-specific reversal agents for the new oral anticoagulants. J Thromb Thrombolysis 2016;41(2):248-52.

In: Chronic Disease and Disability
Editors: DE Greydanus, P Anne, JD Rowlett et al.
ISBN: 978-1-53617-656-8

Chapter 12

POMPE DISEASE

Stuart Covi, MD and
Premchand Anne*, MD, MPH, MBA, FAAP, FACP, FACC
Pediatric Cardiology, Ascension St John Children's Hospital,
Detroit, Michigan, United States of America

ABSTRACT

Pompe disease is a well described, genetically inherited lysosomal storage disease due to deficiency of acid α-glucosidase, with dramatic clinical implications. Hallmarks of the disease, depending on the phenotype, can include progressive motor and respiratory decline, along with hypertrophic cardiomyopathy. Therapies including enzyme replacement have emerged as highly effective and life-altering, with improvements in both longevity and quality of life. This discussion will outline the pathophysiology, genetics, and therapies associated with Pompe disease.

INTRODUCTION

Pompe disease, also known as glycogen storage disease type II, was initially described by Dutch pathologist Joannes Cassianus Pompe (1901-1945) in 1932 in *Over idiopathische hypertrophie van het hart*, after a post-mortem autopsy was performed on a 7-month old with cardiomegaly (1). Pompe reported on the disorganized and distorted arrangement of the myocardium. Birth prevalence of Pompe disease varies by population, ranging anywhere from 1 in 146,000 to 1 in 40,000 (2-4).

Pompe disease is an inherited metabolic myopathy, induced by a deficiency or absence in the lysosomal enzyme acid α-glucosidase (previously referred to as acid maltase) (5). The deficient enzyme is responsible for cleavage of α-1,4- and α-1,6-glycosidic bonds of glycogen into glucose. The classically held view is that altered enzyme function results in lysosomal

* Correspondence: Premchand Anne, MD, Pediatric Cardiology, Ascension St John Children's Hospital, 22201 Moross, Suite 275, PB II, Detroit, MI 48236, United States. Email: Premchand.anne@ascension.org.

glycogen accumulation, swelling, and eventually rupture into the cellular cytoplasm (6). An important characteristic of Pompe disease is the involvement of cardiac and skeletal muscle, leading to hypertrophic cardiomyopathy and progressive myopathy with subsequent weakness, respectively. Later stages in the disease process consist of contractile element replacement by spilled cytoplasmic glycogen, therefore impacting function (6). Recent evidence suggests abnormal enzyme trafficking also results from autophagic buildup of cellular content, which also may play a role (7). The manifestation of enzyme deficiency can be of infantile-onset or late/adult-onset.

Genetics and Inheritance

Pompe disease has been well described as an autosomal recessive disorder, with no documented cases of affected carriers (5). Mutations of both acid α-glucosidase (GAA) alleles are required to harbor the pathogenic phenotype; interestingly, most are compound heterozygotes with two different mutations present. To date, over 500 mutations have been identified, although not all are considered pathogenic (8).

The gene for GAA is located on the chromosome 17q25.2-q25.3, a very heterogenous locus (2). More specifically, c.-32-13T>G is the most common mutation (75%) in children and adults, with a slowly progressive course of disease (5, 9). The common mutation is associated with low levels (3-20%) of normal acid α-glucosidase in sampled fibroblasts; however, the combination of the common mutation with another null mutation showed marked variability in the phenotype (age of onset and progression), thereby implicating a two-hit hypothesis (9, 10).

Secondary genetic and non-genetic factors exert a strong affect as well, with clinical course not always correlating with degree of enzyme activity. Similar levels of enzyme activity have been shown to have drastically different ages of symptoms onset (9, 11). Clinical course is extremely difficult to predict as it is closely tied to the specific nature of each mutation, which in turn affects the degree of enzyme deficiency (12). Based upon established models, signs of disease as more likely to emerge when residual enzyme activity is <30% (5).

Clinical Features

The nomenclature for Pompe's disease is "classic infantile," "childhood," and "adult" forms; however, the phenotypic distinction between childhood and adult is vague (13). Patients with the classic, or infantile, form of Pompe disease can display symptoms from the immediate postnatal period to 12 months of age. The median age of symptom onset is two months, with a median age of diagnosis at 4.7 months (14). Hypertrophic cardiomyopathy is a common finding in infantile-onset Pompe disease, yet cardiac symptoms of fluid overload and arrhythmia are less frequent (15). Symptoms most often consist of feeding difficulties, failure to thrive, respiratory infections, and hypotonia.

Physical examination findings include hypotonia, murmurs, myopathy, and hepatomegaly. At a median age of 4 months, 92% have cardiomegaly, 88% hypotonia, 78% respiratory distress, 57% feeding difficulties, and 53% failure to thrive (16). Most infantile-onset patients experience ventilator dependence or death by one year of age. The median age at initiation of ventilatory support in untreated infants is 5.9 months (range 0.1-31 months). Only 6.7% of infants are ventilator free by 18 months of age (16). The median age for death is 8.7 months (range 0.3-73 months), with a survival rate of 25.7% at 12 months and 12.3% by 18 months of age among untreated patients (16). Vertebral and femoral fractures are present in long-term survivors of infantile-onset Pompe disease (17).

Late-onset Pompe disease

In late-onset Pompe disease, clinical features can appear anywhere from infancy to late adulthood (5). Initial symptoms have been described in individuals as old as 71 years of age. Generally, this type of Pompe disease is considered slowly progressive, with a wide variety of clinical phenotypes and no criteria to define sub-types. Late-onset Pompe disease is characterized by progressive muscular involvement, respiratory insufficiency, however without cardiac involvement (18). First symptoms are often the result of muscle weakness (80%), with primary involvement of the lower limb and paraspinal muscles (18).

Respiratory failure is the most frequent cause of death (72%) (range 0.9 months-66 years) due to the dysfunction of the diaphragm, intercostal and accessory muscles (18, 19). Interestingly, respiratory and motor issues may progress at different paces so that some wheelchair bound patients have normal pulmonary function tests, while others are still ambulatory but require nocturnal ventilation (5). Other manifestations include scoliosis and lumbar hyperlordosis, and involvement of nonmuscular tissue/organs such as brain, liver, spleen, salivary glands, kidneys and blood vessels (20). Cardiac failure is a rare entity in this late-onset phenotype, occurring in only 0.4% of patients. The overall median age of death is 24.5 years of age (range 0.9-66 years) (19).

Differential diagnoses

Index of suspicion for Pompe disease, whether infantile-onset or late-onset, must be high for prompt and accurate diagnosis. Both subtypes have commonalities with muscular, respiratory, and metabolic disorders. Infantile Pompe disease has features that mimic various conditions including idiopathic hypertrophic cardiomyopathy, spinal muscular atrophy type I, mitochondrial diseases, Danon disease, and hypothyroidism amongst others (14).

Differential diagnoses for late-onset include metabolic disorders, myasthenia gravis, polymyositis, and various musculoskeletal disorders including muscular dystrophies, particularly those that involve limb girdle muscle weakness (14, 21). Approximately 7% of patients with late-onset Pompe are incorrectly diagnosed initially with either Duchenne muscular dystrophy, Becker muscular dystrophy, or spinal muscular atrophy (21).

Diagnosis

The diagnosis of Pompe disease presents a diagnostic dilemma due to its low incidence and a wide spectrum of presenting features. When taken as an aggregate, however, the phenotypic characteristics can lend to easier diagnosis. Family history can be of some utility, although only 34% of Pompe patients describe a family history of this disease (16). Currently, prenatal genetic testing is identifying mothers with single allele mutations, thereby rendering the diagnosis more likely in the presence of clinical and noninvasive test findings.

Residual activity level of the acid α-glucosidase in fibroblasts has traditionally been considered the gold standard with almost universal deficiency in those with the disease (22). Utilizing fibroblasts, the 4-methylumbelliferyl-α-D-glycopyranoside substrate-based assay can detect as little as 1-2% of residual enzyme activity level (23). Infants with Pompe have been found to have <1% residual activity, whereas children and adults have activity levels ranging from 6-22% (23).

Muscle biopsy is another traditional approach that can be used either for enzyme activity similar to fibroblasts, or histologically for direct glycogen deposition in vacuoles which can be ten-fold that of normal (14, 24). As with most muscle biopsies, the site and technique used can dramatically impact the quality of the sample.

Enzyme activity in dried bloodspots/whole blood sample using multiplexed tandem mass spectrometry has expanded newborn disease detection, and some consider it one of the most successful programs for secondary prevention of inherited disease (25-27). Pompe disease is included on the recommended uniform screening panel by the US federal advisory committee (28). Such screening offers rapid, noninvasive first tier testing and has been shown in some studies to have excellent (100%) sensitivity and specificity in infantile, and late-onset (juvenile and adult) Pompe disease (29). In addition, prenatal chorionic villi sampling at 10-12 weeks gestation is emerging as a sensitive method to quickly detect abnormal enzyme activity levels (30, 31).

While 97.6% of Pompe diagnoses are confirmed by GAA enzyme assay (16), second tier testing with molecular genetic analysis is considered essential once low GAA activity is discovered to confirm the diagnosis and predict CRIM status (32). Moreover, none of the enzymatic tests reliably discriminate between unaffected carriers and non-carriers; therefore, in such cases GAA DNA mutation analysis testing can be used for confirmatory diagnosis and genetic counseling purposes (5). Other blood serum labs including creatine kinase, AST, ALT, LDH, and urine hexose tetrasaccharide have been used as ancillary findings and can be fairly sensitive, albeit nonspecific (14).

Cardiac findings

Cardiac findings can vary drastically depending on the type of Pompe disease. In infantile-onset type, electrocardiographic (EKG) changes such as short PR interval and large QRS voltages are characteristic. Shortened PR is seen in 58%, left ventricular hypertrophy in 83-100%, and biventricular hypertrophy in 84% (15, 33, 34). Excess glycogen deposition has been proposed as the main mechanism, leading to accelerated conduction through the AV node and hypertrophy (34). Virtually all cases of infantile-onset involve left ventricular posterior wall and/or interventricular septal thickening that is progressive in nature, and in severe cases can lead to left ventricular intracavitary as well as outflow obstruction (15, 35). In stark contrast, cardiac manifestations are quite rare in late-onset type. Only 3% of those with the c.-32-13T>G genotype have mild hypertrophic cardiomyopathy and pre-excitation pattern (36).

Pulmonary testing

Pulmonary function testing can be of diagnostic use due to diaphragm weakness that occurs early in the disease process, generally before other muscle groups. This feature distinguishes Pompe from some of the other myopathies in which respiratory failure follows the loss of ambulation (37). For that reason, respiratory evaluation is critical in evaluation of Pompe disease (38). Spirometry revealing a >10% decline in forced vital capacity (FVC) from sitting to supine suggest diaphragm muscle weakness but may be missed if supine FVC is not specifically measured (37, 39).

EMG

Electromyographic findings can often (~50%) indicate myopathy with increased muscle membrane irritability activity including complex repetitive discharges (40).

Treatment

While historically outcomes were bleak, the advent of enzyme replacement therapy (ERT) has substantially improved ventilator free survival, motor function, degree of cardiomyopathy and overall survival (41, 42). ERT consists of human recombinant GAA which degrades lysosomal glycogen in cardiac and other muscle groups. Myozyme was approved by the FDA in 2006 for infantile-onset Pompe, and Lumizyme in 2010 for the late-onset type.

Cross-reactive immunological material (CRIM) status is of critical importance in determining response to enzyme therapy. CRIM positive infantile-onset children were found to have only 19% death/invasively ventilated at 27 months of age, notably better than the natural course without therapy. Unfortunately, CRIM negative infants have no residual protein expression and tend to exhibit a much poorer response to enyzme therapy. Such patients mount an immune response to rh-GAA, leading to significant clinical decline including 100% death/invasive ventilation by 27 months of age (42). In this setting, immunomodulation before commencing ERT has been successful in suppressing high antibody titers (43).

To date, there is no evidence comparing GAA therapy to placebos nor to other therapies. In addition, there is no strong clinical evidence regarding optimal dosing, although 20-40 mg/kg infusion once every two weeks is a common dose. Very often in infants, 20 mg/kg of ERT once a week is infused. One study found that higher dosing (40 mg/kg) had a higher number of infusion related adverse events than lower dosing (20 mg/kg) (44).

For late-onset Pompe disease, long term ERT has been found to improve muscle strength, activity levels, and FVC on pulmonary function testing. The largest increase has been shown in the first 2-3 years of treatment (45). Others have found similar results including improved maintenance of muscular function and quality of life scores (46).

PROGNOSTIC FACTORS

Both occurrence of symptoms and diagnosis of infantile Pompe within the first 6 months of life have been shown to significantly increase the risk of death (RR of 2.9 for symptoms and 2.1 for diagnosis) (14). In addition, patients on a high-protein diet, CPAP/BiPAP, physical or respiratory therapy at any point had a lower risk of death (14). For late-onset type, a later age of diagnosis ($\geq$ 18 years old) had a notably higher median age of death (44.9 years) in comparison to those diagnosed 0-1 years of age (6.1 years) (19). Later onset of symptoms has also been found to result in a better prognosis (19). Higher disease severity has been associated with complete absence or near-complete absence of acid α-glucosidase activity (15, 16).

CONCLUSIONS: FUTURE DIRECTIONS

Some longitudinal studies have shown that ERT results in sustained improvements in both cardiac parameters and gross motor function; however, sample sizes remain small (47-49). A phenotype of infantile survivors is emerging, however, with initial improvements followed by residual muscle weakness, or even progressive deterioration (49, 50). Due to these limitations in enzyme therapy, focus is increasingly being placed on second-generation drug therapies.

Gene therapy trials in mice models using recombinant adeno-associated virus (AAV) vectors have demonstrated the ability to restore GAA activity, improve glycogen clearance, and improve respiratory function---thereby offering a promising therapy (51, 52). Small scale early phase trials in children with ventilator dependence showed modest improvement in ventilatory function via direct intradiaphragmatic delivery of AAV gene therapy (53). Substrate reduction therapy, in which enzymes involved in glycogen synthesis are targeted, have shown a significant reduction of glycogen in skeletal muscle (54).

Fiber type conversion from fast to slow twitch muscles to eliminate autophagic buildup has been successful, however paradoxically resulted in increased lysosomal glycogen disposal in skeletal muscle (55). Suppression of autophagy in skeletal muscle to reduce lysosomal glycogen accumulation has been successful in mouse models; however, this loss of autophagy has been associated with atrophy and decreased muscle strength (18, 56). Finally, stimulation of lysosomal exocytosis via various transcription factors (TFEB, TFE3) has promise in reducing glycogen load, lysosomal size, and autophagosome processing (57, 58, 59).

Although recommended, lysosomal storage disorders are not currently mandatory in the United States on newborn screening and not all states include it on their panel. By improving the inclusion rate, Pompe disease can be detected earlier (60) and outcomes may be improved (61).

REFERENCES

[1] Van Gijn J, Gijselhart JP. Pompe and his disease. Ned Tijdschr Geneeskd 2011;155:A2878. [Dutch]

[2] Martiniuk F, Chen A, Mack A, Arvanitopoulos E, Chen Y, Rom WN, et al. Carrier frequency for glycogen storage disease type II in New York and estimates of affected individuals born with the disease. Am J Med Genet 1998;79(1):69–72.

[3] Poorthuis BJ, Wevers RA, Kleijer WJ, Groener JE, de Jong JG, van Weely S, et al. The frequency of lysosomal storage diseases in The Netherlands. Hum Genet 1999;105(1-2):151–56.

[4] Meikle PJ, Hopwood JJ, Clague AE, Carey WF. Prevalence of lysosomal storage disorders. JAMA 1999;281(3):249–54.

[5] Van der Ploeg AT, Reuser AJ. Pompe's disease. Lancet 2008; 372(9646):1342–53.

[6] Griffin JL. Infantile acid maltase deficiency. I. Muscle fiber destruction after lysosomal rupture. Virchows Arch B Cell Pathol Incl Mol Pathol 1984; 45(1):23-36.

[7] Raben N, Roberts A, Plotz PH. Role of autophagy in the pathogenesis of Pompe disease. Acta Myol 2007;26(1):45-48.

[8] Mutations in human acid alpha-glucosidase. Pompe Mutation Database. Erasmus Univeritair Medische Centrum Rotterdam. URLK: http://cluster15.erasmusmc.nl/klgn/pompe/mutations. html.

[9] Kroos MA, Pomponio RJ, Hagemans ML, Keulemans JL, Phipps M, DeRiso M, et al. Broad spectrum of Pompe disease in patients with the same c.-32-13T->G haplotype. Neurology 2007;68(2):110–15.

[10] Kroos M, Hoogeveen-Westerveld M, van der Ploeg A, Reuser AJ. The genotype-phenotype correlation in Pompe disease. Am J Med Genet C Semin Med Genet 2012;160C(1):59–68.

[11] Montalvo AL, Bembi B, Donnarumma M, Filocamo M, Parenti G, Rossi M, et al. Mutation profile of the GAA gene in 40 Italian patients with late onset glycogen storage disease type II. Hum Mutat 2006;27(10):999-1006.

[12] Hermans MM, van Leenen D, Kroos MA, Beesley CE, van der Ploeg AT, Sakuraba H, et al. Twenty-two novel mutations in the lysosomal alpha-glucosidase gene (GAA) underscore the genotype-phenotype correlation in glycogen storage disease type II. Hum Mutat 2004; 23(1):47–56.

[13] Güngör D, Reuser AJ. How to describe the clinical spectrum in Pompe disease? Am J Med Genet A 2013;161A(2):399–400.

[14] Kishnani PS, Steiner RD, Bali D, Berger K, Byrne BJ, Case LE, et al. Pompe disease diagnosis and management guideline. Genet Med 2006;8(5):267–88.

[15] van den Hout HM, Hop W, van Diggelen OP, Smeitink JA, Smit GP, Poll-The BT, et al. The natural course of infantile Pompe's disease: 20 original cases compared with 133 cases from the literature. Pediatrics 2003;112(2): 332-40.

[16] Kishnani PS, Hwu WL, Mandel H, Nicolino M, Yong F, Corzo D; Infantile- onset Pompe Disease Natural History Study Group. A retrospective, multinational, multicenter study on the natural history of infantile-onset Pompe disease. J Pediatr 2006;148(5):671–76.

[17] Van den Berg LE, Zandbergen AA, van Capelle CI, de Vries JM, Hop WC, van den Hout JM, et al. Low bone mass in Pompe disease: muscular strength as a predictor of bone mineral density. Bone 2010;47(3):643-9.

[18] Lim JA, Li L, Raben N. Pompe disease: from pathophysiology to therapy and back again. Front Aging Neurosci 2014 Jul 23;6:177. doi: 10.3389/fnagi.2014.00177.

[19] Winkel LP, Hagemans ML, van Doorn PA, Loonen MC, Hop WJ, Reuser AJ, et al. The natural course of non-classic Pompe's disease; a review of 225 published cases. J Neurol 2005; 252(8):875–84.

[20] Filosto M, Todeschini A, Cotelli MS, Vielmi V, Rinaldi F, Rota S, et al. Non-muscle involvement in late-onset glycogenosis II. Acta Myol 2013;32(2):91–4.

[21] Hagemans ML, Winkel LP, Van Doorn PA, Hop WJ, Loonen MC, Reuser AJ, et al. Clinical manifestation and natural course of late-onset Pompe's disease in 54 Dutch patients. Brain 2005;128(Pt 3):671–7.

[22] Hers HG. alpha-Glucosidase deficiency in generalized glycogen storage disease (Pompe's disease). Biochem J 1963;86(1):11–16.

[23] Reuser AJ, Koster JF, Hoogeveen A, Galjaard H. Biochemical, immunological, and cell genetic studies in glycogenosis type II. Am J Hum Genet 1978;30(2):132–43.

[24] Mehler M, DiMauro S. Residual acid maltase activity in late-onset acid maltase deficiency. Neurology 1977;27(2):178–84.

[25] Hoffmann GF, Lindner M, Loeber JG. 50 years of newborn screening. J Inherit Metab Dis 2014; 37(2):163–4.

[26] Wilcken B, Wiley V, Hammond J, Carpenter K. Screening newborns for inborn errors of metabolism by tandem mass-spectrometry. N Engl J Med 2003;348(23):2304–12.

[27] Villoria JG, Pajares S, López MR, Marin JL, Ribes A. Neonatal screening for inherited metabolic diseases in 2016. Semin Pediatr Neurol 2016;23(4):257–72.

[28] No authors listed. Newborn screening: toward a uniform screening panel and system. Genet Med 2006;8(Suppl 1):1S-252S.

[29] Umapathysivam K, Hopwood JJ, Meikle PJ. Determination of acid alpha-glucosidase activity in blood spots as a diagnostic test for Pompe disease. Clin Chem 2001;47(8):1378–83.

[30] Besançon AM, Castelnau L, Nicolesco H, Dumez Y, Poenaru L. Prenatal diagnosis of glycogenosis type II (Pompe's disease) using chorionic villi biopsy. Clin Genet 1985;27(5):479–82.

[31] Verma J, Thomas DC, Sharma S, Jhingan G, Saxena R, Kohli S, et al. Inherited metabolic disorders: prenatal diagnosis of lysosomal storage disorders. Prenat Diagn 2015;35(11):1137-47.

[32] Burton BK, Kronn DF, Hwu WL, Kishnani PS. The initial evaluation of patients after positive newborn screening: Recommended algorithms leading to a confirmed diagnosis of Pompe disease. Pediatrics 2017;140. e20160280D. doi:10.1542/peds.2016-0280D.

[33] Nihill MR, Wilson DS, Hugh-Jones K. Generalized glycogenosis type II (Pompe's disease). Arch Dis Child 1970;45(239):122–9.

[34] Gillette PC, Nihill MR, Singer DB. Electrophysiological mechanism of the short PR interval in Pompe disease. Am J Dis Child 1974;128(5):622–6.

[35] Seifert B, Snyder M, Klein A, O'Loughlin JE, Magid MS, Engle MA. Development of obstruction to ventricular outflow and impairment of inflow in glycogen storage disease of the heart: serial echocardiographic studies from birth to death at 6 months. Am Heart J 1992;123(1):239-42.

[36] Van der Beek NA, Soliman OI, van Capelle CI, Geleijnse ML, Vletter WB, Kroos MA, et al. Cardiac evaluation in children and adults with Pompe disease sharing the common c.-32-13T>G genotype rarely reveals abnormalities. J Neurol Sci 2008;275(1-2):46-50.

[37] Mellies U, Lofaso F. Pompe disease: a neuromuscular disease with respiratory muscle involvement. Respir Med 2009;103(4):477-84.

[38] Manganelli F, Ruggiero L. Clinical features of Pompe disease. Acta Myol 2013;32(2):82-84.

[39] Van der Beek NA, van Capelle CI, van der Velden-van Etten KI, Hop WC, van den Berg B, Reuser AJ, et al. Rate of progression and predictive factors for pulmonary outcome in children and adults with Pompe disease. Mol Genet Metab 2011;104(1-2):129-36.

[40] Müller-Felber W, Horvath R, Gempel K, Podskarbi T, Shin Y, Pongratz D, et al. Late onset Pompe disease: clinical and neurophysiological spectrum of 38 patients including long-term follow-up in 18 patients. Neuromuscul Disord 2007;17(9-10):698-706.

[41] Chen M, Zhang L, Quan S. Enzyme replacement therapy for infantile-onset Pompe disease. Cochrane Database Syst Rev 2017;11:CD011539. doi: 10.1002/14651858.CD011539.pub2.

[42] Kishnani PS, Goldenberg PC, DeArmey SL, Heller J, Benjamin D, Young S, et al. Cross-reactive immunologic material status affects treatment outcomes in Pompe disease infants. Mol Genet Metab 2010;99(1):26–33.

[43] Messinger YH, Mendelsohn NJ, Rhead W, Dimmock D, Hershkovitz E, Champion M, et al. Successful immune tolerance induction to enzyme replacement therapy in CRIM-negative infantile Pompe disease. Genet Med 2012;14(1):135–42.

[44] Kishnani PS, Corzo D, Nicolino M, Byrne B, Mandel H, Hwu WL, et al. Recombinant human acid [alpha]-glucosidase: Major clinical benefits in infantile-onset Pompe disease. Neurology 2007;68(2):99–109.

[45] Kuperus E, Kruijshaar ME, Wens SCA, de Vries JM, Favejee MM, van der Meijden JC, et al. Long-term benefit of enzyme replacement therapy in Pompe disease: A 5-year prospective study. Neurology 2017;89(23):2365-73.

[46] Van der Ploeg AT, Clemens PR, Corzo D, Escolar DM, Florence J, KPompe's disease. N Engl J Med 2010; 362(15):1396-406.

[47] Van Capelle CI, Poelman E, Frohn-Mulder IM, Koopman LP, van den Hout JMP, Régal L, et al. Cardiac outcome in classic infantile Pompe disease after 13 years of treatment with recombinant human acid alpha-glucosidase. Int J Cardiol 2018;269:104-10.

[48] Van der Meijden JC, Kruijshaar ME, Harlaar L, Rizopoulos D, van der Beek N, van der Ploeg AT. Long-term follow-up of 17 patients with childhood Pompe disease treated with enzyme replacement therapy. J Inherit Metab Dis 2018;41(6):1205-14. doi: 10.1007/s10545-018-0166-3.

[49] Prater SN, Banugaria SG, DeArmey SM, Botha EG, Stege EM, Case LE, et al. The emerging phenotype of long-term survivors with infantile Pompe disease. Genet Med 2012;14(9):800–10.

[50] Prater SN, Patel TT, Buckley AF, Mandel H, Vlodavski E, Banugaria SG, et al. Skeletal muscle pathology of infantile Pompe disease during long-term enzyme replacement therapy. Orphanet J Rare Dis 2013;8:90. doi: 10.1186/1750-1172-8-90.

[51] Mah C, Cresawn KO, Fraites TJ Jr, Pacak CA, Lewis MA, Zolotukhin I, et al. Sustained correction of glycogen storage disease type II using adeno-associated virus serotype 1 vectors. Gene Ther 2005;12(18):1405-9.

[52] Keeler AM, Zieger M, Todeasa SH, McCall AL, Gifford JC, Birsak S, et al. Systemic delivery of AAVB1-GAA clears glycogen and prolongs survival in a mouse model of Pompe disease. Hum Gene Ther 2019;30(1):57-68.

[53] Smith BK, Collins SW, Conlon TJ, Mah CS, Lawson LA, Martin AD, et al. Phase I/II trial of adeno-associated virus-mediated alpha-glucosidase gene therapy to the diaphragm for chronic respiratory failure in Pompe disease: initial safety and ventilatory outcomes. Hum Gene Ther 2013;24(6):630-40.

[54] Douillard-Guilloux G, Raben N, Takikita S, Batista L, Caillaud C, Richard E. Modulation of glycogen synthesis by RNA interference: towards a new therapeutic approach for glycogenosis type II. Hum Mol Genet 2008;17(24):3876–86.

[55] Takikita S, Schreiner C, Baum R, Xie T, Ralston E, Plotz PH, et al. Fiber type conversion by PGC-1α activates lysosomal and autophagosomal biogenesis in both unaffected and Pompe skeletal muscle. PLoS One 2010; 5(12):e15239. doi: 10.1371/journal.pone.0015239.

[56] Nascimbeni AC, Fanin M, Masiero E, Angelini C, Sandri M. Impaired autophagy contributes to muscle atrophy in glycogen storage disease type II patients. Autophagy 2012;8(11):1697–700.

[57] Medina DL, Fraldi A, Bouche V, Annunziata F, Mansueto G, Spamspanato C, et al. Transcriptional activation of lysosomal exocytosis promotes cellular clearance. Dev Cell 2011;21(3):421-30.

[58] Martina JA, Diab HI, Li H, Puertollano R. Novel roles for the MiTF/TFE family of transcription factors in organelle biogenesis, nutrient sensing, and energy homeostasis. Cell Mol Life Sci 2014;71(13):2483–97.

[59] Martina JA, Diab HI, Lishu L, Jeong-A L, Patange S, Raben N, et al. The nutrient-responsive transcription factor TFE3 promotes autophagy, lysosomal biogenesis and clearance of cellular debris. Sci Signal 2014;7(309):ra9. doi: 10.1126/scisignal.2004754.

[60] Chien YH, Chiang SC, Zhang XK, Keutzer J, Lee NC, Huang AC, et al. Early detection of Pompe disease by newborn screening is feasible: results from the Taiwan screening program. Pediatrics 2008;122(1):e39-45.

[61] Landau YE, Waisbren SE, Chan LM, Levy HL. Long-term outcome of expanded newborn screening at Boston Children's Hospital: benefits and challenges in defining true disease. J Inherit Metab Dis 2017;40(2):209-18.

In: Chronic Disease and Disability
Editors: DE Greydanus, P Anne, JD Rowlett et al.
ISBN: 978-1-53617-656-8

Chapter 13

SEXUAL AND REPRODUCTIVE HEALTH IN THE ADOLESCENT CARDIAC PATIENT

Maria Demma Cabral*[1*]*, MD, Nneka Holder*[2]*, MD, MPH and Sadhana Dharmapuri*[3]*, MD

[1]Department of Pediatric and Adolescent Medicine, Western Michigan University, Homer Stryker MD School of Medicine, Kalamazoo, Michigan, United States of America

[2]Department of Pediatrics, MedStar Georgetown University Hospital, Washington DC, Michigan, United States of America

[3]Division of Adolescent and Young Adult Medicine, Stroger Hospital, Chicago, Illinois, Michigan, United States of America

ABSTRACT

This discussion highlights the importance of understanding the sexual and reproductive health needs of the adolescent with cardiac disease. There are published guidelines and reports discussed in this review that provide the essential information on how to care for this special population. Like their peers, they experience physical changes and psychosocial challenges that may result in poor health outcomes, such as unintended pregnancies and sexually transmitted infections. Review of the current United States Medical Eligibility Criteria for Contraceptive Use released in 2016 is included with emphasis on women with cardiac disease and contraception.

INTRODUCTION

Advancements in scientific knowledge have led to improved medications and surgical treatments for all youth; especially adolescents and young adults at risk for complications from

* Correspondence: Maria Demma Cabral, MD, Department of Pediatric and Adolescent Medicine, Western Michigan University Homer Stryker MD School of Medicine, 1000 Oakland Drive, Kalamazoo, MI 49008, United States. Email: mariademma.cabral@med.wmich.edu.

cardiovascular disease. As the population of youth with chronic heart disease matures, they face similar challenges that their peers experience and more. Adolescents with complex congenital or acquired heart diseases require specialized care yet often receive limited sexual and reproductive health care services. Like any other chronic health conditions, this population is at risk of sexual dysfunction and fertility problems; thus, these youths will benefit greatly from early counseling on family planning and prevention of sexually transmitted infections (STIs).

PREVALENCE OF PEDIATRIC HEART DISEASE

The combined 2016-2017 National Survey of Children's Health indicated that 1.1% of children aged 0-17 years in the United States, approximately 920,000 children, currently have a heart condition (1). Cardiac conditions can be congenital or acquired. According to the U.S. Centers for Disease Control and Prevention (CDC), congenital heart disease (CHD) affects around 1 in 100 live births per year in the United States and is considered the most common type of birth defect (2). Genetic syndromes associated with extra-cardiac defects comprise 30% of CHD (3). There are no published data on the prevalence of children with acquired heart conditions (4). Common acquired heart diseases include Kawasaki disease and rheumatic heart disease. Table 1 summarizes the common genetic conditions associated with CHD and acquired heart diseases in the pediatric age group.

Research estimates from 2010 that around 1 million children and 1.4 million adults with CHD are living in the United States (5). Survival depends on heart defect severity, time of diagnosis and indicated treatment (6). Twenty-five percent of infants with CHD have these critical defects: transposition of the great arteries (TGA), hypoplastic left heart syndrome (HLHS), tetralogy of Fallot (TOF), and coarctation of the aorta (CoA). These affected infants usually require surgical interventions in the first year of life with subsequent morbidities (6). Yet 69% are expected to survive to their 18th birthday (2, 6). The prevalence of CHD is expected to increase by 5% annually due to advancements in scientific knowledge that includes medical and surgical treatments.

Table 1. Genetic conditions with CHD and acquired heart diseases in children and adolescents

Congenital heart diseases
Down syndrome
Turner syndrome
22q11.2 deletion syndrome
Williams syndrome
Noonan syndrome
Marfan syndrome
Alagille syndrome
Kabuki syndrome
Acquired heart diseases
Kawasaki disease
Rheumatic heart disease

With more individuals having asymptomatic to life-threatening heart conditions surviving into their child-bearing years, they will face similar challenges as their peers, including sexual health concerns.

Sexual and reproductive health care service provision and sexual health education

Pediatricians and family physicians, among other health care professionals (HCPs), have the opportunity to provide and support these services for everyone – with and without chronic health conditions and disabilities during health maintenance visits (7). Various medical organizations have published evidence-based guidelines and recommendations in addressing sexual as well as reproductive health care service needs in adolescence and young adulthood; these include the American Academy of Pediatrics (AAP), the American College of Obstetrics and Gynecology (ACOG), the American Academy of Family Physicians (AAFP), and other professional medical organizations in coordination with the government (8-10).

The AAP Committee on Adolescence and Committee on Psychosocial Aspects of Child and Family Health stated,

> "sexuality education is defined as teaching about human sexuality, including intimate relationships, human sexual anatomy, sexual reproduction, sexually transmitted infections, sexual activity, sexual orientation, gender identity, abstinence, contraception, and reproductive rights and responsibilities." (11)

Discussing relevant topics is important and should be developmentally appropriate; these areas include reproductive anatomy, masturbation, erections, sexual orientation as well as fantasies, orgasms and intercourse (12-14).

Compared to their healthy peers, one study of teens with CHD has shown no major differences in sexual measures such as coitarche, number of sexual partners, use of barrier protection and STIs (15). Parents and providers should not assume that an adolescent with heart disease is not interested in sexual health-related topics and will not be involved in romantic (sexual) relationships. Educating adolescents on these topics can be a powerful tool in building healthy attitudes about themselves as well as their relationships in addition to preventing potential exploitation and risky sexual practices.

Reproductive health in female adolescents and young adults with CHD

Women with CHD are eight times more likely to experience cardiovascular complications during pregnancy and have a six times greater risk of dying compared to women without CHD; thus, reproductive health counseling should start even before such a young woman is ready to start a family (16). Comprehensive reproductive health education should include information on gynecological issues that may occur during their reproductive lifetime, along with family planning needs and genetic counseling.

Women with CHD experience normal physiological changes of growth and development as experienced by their healthy peers. Depending on their cardiac defect, acyanotic or cyanotic, women with CHD can experience some abnormalities in these changes; these include delay in menarche, prolonged menstrual bleeding and/or intermenstrual bleeding. Certain CHD may require anti-coagulants, which can alter the menstrual cycle and be teratogenic (16). Provider and patient knowledge of the specific heart defect and health history can help direct a woman's decision around contraceptive choice and should be assessed when discussing these issues.

A woman's lack of knowledge about her defect and the treatment that she uses for it can impact her reproductive health choices. There has been limited research around women with CHD and their reproductive health knowledge---including contraceptive use. Most studies are of adult women's knowledge and experience with contraception and family planning counseling. In a study of women attending a collaborative family planning clinic in the United Kingdom, 35% of women had never discussed contraception with a health care provider, although 80% of these women were sexually active. Out of the women discussing contraception for the first time with the medical provider, 78% choose to start a hormonal method (17). Of those who did discuss contraception with their provider, 33% were given incorrect information. Some were told that no form of birth control was safe to use. Others were told that the birth control pill was unsafe to use, while it was safe for their particular lesion, while others were started on the combined hormonal pill when it was unsafe for them (18).

A few studies have focused on adolescents. An earlier study noted that 21% of adolescents with CHD had appropriate knowledge of what contraceptive method would be compatible with their defect, citing that only 25% of providers educated them on this information (19). A study of Dutch adolescents with CHD, found that half of the study participants knew the name of their heart defect and only 28% could describe their heart defect or locate the lesion on a diagram. Around 78% of patients knew that their heart defect was not prohibitive to sexual intercourse. Twenty percent of the adolescents understood the heritability of their condition while 14% and 35% of the female patients did not know whether intrauterine devices (IUD) and oral contraceptives, respectively, were appropriate choices for their defect. Most of the female patients had insufficient knowledge of the risks of pregnancy (20).

Another study of adolescents with CHD explored the similarities and differences between sexual activity in adolescents with CHD and their healthy peers (15). This study found that there were no differences in age of first sexual intercourse, number of partners or number of times condoms were not used in the last month (15). One study, however, reported lower rates of ever having sex with 26% of adolescents with CHD compared to 47% in the general population (21). One in four of those participants used dual effective methods and 1 in 4 used none (21).

Along with lack of knowledge about their CHD, these individuals face many barriers to accessing and maintaining healthcare; these include lack of access to subspecialty providers, lack of or increased cost of health insurance, and lack of access to quality information by providers as well as health care institutions (22). Research on contraceptive knowledge and counseling by providers for individuals with CHD is lacking. Provider knowledge of contraception in general has been shown to be variable. Although there is clear evidence that long acting reversible contraceptive (LARCs) methods are the most effective in preventing pregnancy, these methods are under-utilized in general. In women with CHD it was found that IUDs and implants were safe and effective contraceptive methods, though their use in women with CHD was low as well (22).

Fortunately, there are options that are suitable to every individual's needs and preferences. However, for some patients, certain options may have more risks than benefits. Hence, it is important to understand the general underlying heart condition and how some hormonal contraceptives may have an adverse effect. As with any unplanned birth outcome, an undesired state of pregnancy has the most damaging effects on a young person's life potential when compared to the potential side effects of hormonal contraception.

Sexual and reproductive health in adolescents and young adults with genetic syndromes associated with congenital heart diseases

For each genetic syndrome, published current clinical reports and guidelines are discussed. Table 2 provides a list of genetic conditions, the published guidelines and associated cardiac defects. Most of them mention inclusion of sexuality education as part of health care provision. It is recommended to provide the youth with easily understandable factual information on the difference between male and female body structures, physiological and psychological functioning, and appropriate sexual expression. Parents as well as guardians, in collaboration with health care providers (i.e., pediatricians, cardiologists, endocrinologists, gynecologists, others), should provide the necessary knowledge and support in acquiring personal understanding of healthy, safe relationships.

Table 2. Common genetic syndromes with published guidelines and cardiac anomalies (3)

Genetic Syndrome	Published guidelines	CHD (%)	Cardiac defects
Down syndrome	AAP clinical report: Health supervision for children with Down syndrome (2011) (23)	40-50	ASDa, VSDb, AVCDc, TOF
Turner syndrome	Clinical practice guidelines for the care of girls and women with Turner syndrome (2017) (24)	25-45	CoA, BAVd, ASe, HLHSf
22q11.2 deletion	Practical guidelines for managing patients with 22q11.2 deletion (2011) (25)	70-75	TOF, aortic arch anomalies, truncus arteriosus
Williams syndrome	Health care supervision for children with Williams syndrome (2001) (26)	75-80	Supravalvar AS, PPSg
Noonan syndrome	Noonan Syndrome: Clinical features, diagnosis, and management guidelines (2010) (27)	70-80	PSh, HCMi, ASD
Marfan syndrome	AAP Clinical Report: Health Supervision for Children with Marfan Syndrome (2013) (28)	60-80	aortic root dilation, dissection of ascending aorta

[a]atrial septal defect.
[b]ventricular septal defect.
[c]atrioventricular canal defect.
[d]bicuspic aortic valve.
[e]aortic stenosis.
[f]hypoplastic left heart syndrome.
[g]peripheral pulmonary stenosis.
[h]pulmonary stenosis.
[i]hypertropic cardiomyopathy.

Down syndrome

Down syndrome (DS) is the most common chromosomal abnormality with an estimated prevalence of 1.08 per 1,000 live births in the United Kingdom and 1.4 per 1,000 in the United States (29, 30). Forty to 50% of individuals with DS will have a CHD with almost 100% of survival the first year of life (23, 29). Cardiology follow-up in the adolescent years should be individualized based on the cardiac defect. Part of health supervision for children with DS in late childhood to adolescence is to discuss growth and development, fertility issues and pregnancy prevention.

These persons will usually follow normal trends of physical development like their peers, yet it is important for HCPs to utilize discussions that are easy to comprehend. Common topics in this regard include hygiene, menstrual management and masturbation. Individuals with DS are at increased risk for sexual abuse (23). Providing guidance on normal and healthy sexuality as well as sexual behaviors is important. One study looked at genetic counselors in providing sex education since DS is highly associated with intellectual disability; this research found that, though the opportunity was present, education offered was based on the counselor's comfort with such topics (31).

Young males were found to have diminished sex drives and can be infertile. Testicular size is typically small with corresponding reduced sperm counts and low ejaculate volumes (32). Young females with DS were found to have small, hypoplastic ovaries with delayed onset of menarche and breast development, occasionally lacking areolar glands. Half of them will never menstruate and the rest can have regular menstruation. While females can achieve pregnancy, there is a 50% risk of recurrence of the syndrome in their offspring (32). Routine gynecologic care should be offered, including discussions on fertility, contraception, and safety.

Turner syndrome

An estimated 25-50 per 100,000 females are diagnosed with Turner syndrome (TS), with 50% having a CHD, such as BAV and CoA (24). Affected phenotypic females have complete or partial absence of the second sex chromosome, with most cases not inheritable. TS is known to have hypergonadotropic hypogonadism presenting with either primary or secondary amenorrhea due to gonadal dysgenesis. A third of them, usually mosaic TS, have spontaneous thelarche and 6% will experience regular menstruation (33). Pediatric endocrinologists care for these youth early in childhood and provide assistance in growth hormone treatment as well as puberty induction (24).

Affected females have less chances of spontaneous conception as they get older and will benefit from fertility treatments. Mosaic TS women with persistent ovarian function should receive counseling on oocyte cryopreservation under the care of an expert (24). Pregnant women with TS require a team of specialists in maternal–fetal medicine and cardiology. The increased cardiovascular risk of pregnancy is related to aortic dilation with an estimated 2% risk of maternal death due to aortic dissection or rupture (24).

22q11.2 deletion syndrome

22q11.2 deletion syndrome (22q11DS) is the most common microdeletion syndrome with an estimated prevalence of 1 in 4,000 live births (25). It is the second most common cause of developmental delay and CHD following DS, with 10-15% of affected individuals having TOF (34). Patients with DiGeorge syndrome and velocardiofacial syndrome commonly will have this deletion.

There are rare instances of some individuals with 22q11DS having hypospadias, cryptorchidism, and an absent uterus (25). However, given current medical and surgical advancements, more individuals with 22q11DS have been surviving to reproductive age (35). Regardless of gender, an affected individual has a 50% likelihood of having an affected child (25). It is important to provide effective and developmentally-appropriate genetic counseling as part of health maintenance of an affected adolescent, including safe contraception given increased morbidities in pregnancy and poor birth outcomes---especially if the woman with 22q11DS has a CHD and schizophrenia (35).

Williams syndrome

An estimated 30,000 people in the United States are diagnosed with Williams syndrome (WS). Also known as Williams-Beuren syndrome, it is usually associated with multiple medical and developmental issues requiring a team of experts (36). The most common CHD identified is supravalvular AS (80%) (26). It is important to discuss sexual health-related topics especially since puberty in both girls and boys with WS has an early onset; true precocious puberty rarely occurs (26, 36). Early puberty results in stunted growth due to the early onset of menarche, with an estimated 2.9% incidence (36).

In affected males, about 15% may have cryptorchidism prompting evaluation. In the presence of a renal agenesis or malformation, it is recommended to evaluate Mullerian structures (37-38). Despite WS being an autosomal dominant inheritance, there are rare familial cases due to few affected individuals reproducing (37).

Noonan syndrome

Noonan syndrome (NS) is the second most common syndromic cause of CHD following DS, affecting up to 1 in 2,500 live births (27). Short stature and CHD are characteristic features, with pulmonary stenosis (PS) being the most common defect. Compared to the general population, delayed puberty is typical in individuals with NS; 35% of boys start puberty after 13.5 years old, and 44% of girls after 13 years old (39). This prompts referral to a pediatric endocrinologist.

Unilateral or bilateral cryptorchidism can be present in about 80% of boys with NS. Surgical orchiopexy is required and should be performed early. However, primary Sertoli cell dysfunction has been the main cause of male infertility, and not cryptorchidism (27, 40). Male adults with NS were found to have hypoestrogenism resulting in increased risk of osteopenia (41). Fertility in females with NS was shown to not be affected (41). NS can be inherited in an autosomal dominant manner with complete penetrance but variable expressivity (27).

Marfan syndrome

Marfan syndrome (MFS) is a multisystemic, autosomal dominant, hereditary connective tissue disorder with vast clinical presentations, affecting approximately 1 in 5,000 people (42). Cardiovascular defect, such as aortic dilation and valve prolapse, is the major cause of increased morbidity and mortality in affected individuals (43). Excessive growth is a characteristic feature in MFS and some prepubertal females may benefit from early high-dose estrogen therapy, although this is controversial (28). In the AAP clinical report for health supervision for children with MFS, there was no mention of sexual health-related education nor reproductive health issues; MFS, however, was mentioned as a common disorder that alters growth and puberty in males (14, 28).

Pregnancy in women with MFS is high risk and should strongly be discouraged especially if with prior history of aortic dissection. There is need for extensive education with emphasis on safe and effective contraception. Tables 3 summarizes the key recommendations for the management of patients with MFS during pregnancy, from preconception to postpartum depending on the aortic size (44). It has been reported that individuals with MFS were concerned about their personal health and recurrence risk, hence affecting their reproductive planning (45).

Table 3. Management of pregnant women with MFS (44)

Time	Recommendations
Preconception	• Assessment of maternal and fetal risks - Past medical and family history - Aortic size before conception - Prenatal diagnosis information • Evaluation of the aorta using transthoracic echocardiography (TTE) and/or CT/MRI • Initiation of beta-blockers • Elective surgery when ascending aorta > 45 mm
During pregnancy	• Serial TTE 4-12 weeks dependent on ascending aorta size - <40 mm: monthly follow-up - 40-45 mm: monthly follow-up - 45 mm: prophylactic surgery pre-pregnancy/or during pregnancy in women with rapid growth of the aorta • Continuation of beta-blockers • Conservative vs surgery based on types of aortic dissection
Delivery	• C-section when ascending aorta 40–45 and >45 mm • Vaginal delivery when diameter <40 mm
Postpartum	• Continuation of beta-blockers • Clinical aortic follow-up weekly for high risk and monthly for low risk, up to 2-6 months

Contraception and Heart Disease during Adolescence

The only contraceptive method that is assured to provide absolute protection from STIs and pregnancy is abstinence. In reality, this method is rarely chosen by many adolescents and young adults. Comprehensive information about sexual health and contraception should be offered to all adolescent patients, even those with chronic or newly diagnosed heart disease. Adolescents should be reminded that, in addition to preventing pregnancy, there is a need to prevent STIs. Surgical contraceptive options (such as tubal ligation or hysterectomy) are typically not recommended for adolescents and young adults. Barrier contraceptives (such as condoms) have demonstrated effective STI protection when used appropriately. Adolescents who are sexually active should be encouraged to use "dual method" of barrier as well as effective contraception (46).

For many healthy adolescents and young women, there are numerous contraceptive options with varying degrees of efficacy. The least effective methods of contraception with failure rates from 18 to 28%, include barrier contraceptives: male and female condoms, the contraceptive sponge, withdrawal, fertility awareness, and spermicides. Moderately effective options with reported failure rates from 6 to 12% include hormonal: injectable progesterone, combined estrogen and progesterone formulations, and barrier (diaphragm). The most effective methods with reported failure rates of 0.05-1.5% are either permanent or reversible. Permanent options are surgical (male or female sterilization).

While the most effective reversible options are LARCs or implantable devices, such as the progesterone implant, the progesterone IUD or the copper IUD (Cu-IUD). Temporary contraceptive methods include lactation and emergency contraception (46, 47). LARCs are endorsed for use in adolescents by several organizations including the AAP, the Society for Adolescent Health and Medicine (SAHM), the ACOG and the AAFP (48-51).

Utility of the 2016 United States medical eligibility criteria (US MEC) for contraceptive use in women with cardiac disease

The CDC regularly reviews certain contraceptive methods for patients with specific characteristic or medical conditions. Such medical eligibility charts are categorized based on contraceptive methods and by disease condition (52). It offers a guide for clinicians to help determine which prescribed contraceptive option may be safest and most effective for an individual patient. There is data to show that LARCs can be offered safely to most women with cardiovascular conditions (22, 53).

However, there are circumstances in which contraception is the preferred choice instead of pregnancy at any time. In these cases, it is paramount the patient understands the dangers of pregnancy and the importance of safe as well as effective contraception. The following conditions are those in which pregnancy is contraindicated:

1. Pulmonary hypertension/Eisenmenger syndrome (systemic ventricular ejection fraction <30% or systemic ventricular dysfunction with New York Heart Association (NYHA) Class III-IV) (54);
2. Severe mitral stenosis (MS), severe AS, MFS with aorta >45 mm (44);
3. Bicuspid aortic valve with aorta >50 mm, native severe coarctation (52);
4. Prior peripartum cardiomyopathy with any residual impairment of ventricular function (55).

For most adolescents and young adults with heart disease there is an option that she can choose that will be ideal for her. The risks and benefits of each contraceptive are discussed in further detail followed by Table 4 which summarizes the US MEC recommendations based on the cardiovascular conditions included.

Valvular heart disease

Valvular heart disease may be divided into complicated and uncomplicated. Common valvular defects include AS, MS, aortic regurgitation, and mitral regurgitation. Complicated valvular heart lesions are those that have coexisting atrial fibrillation, pulmonary hypertension or prior endocarditis (56). According to the US MEC, all contraceptive options can be used safely and without restriction for uncomplicated valvular heart disease (VHD). Even for combined hormonal contraceptives (CHC), the benefits of use tend to outweigh the risk of unplanned pregnancy; also, this refers to both initiation and continuation of use. Combined hormonal methods should not be recommended to patients with complicated valvular heart disease (52). Any option (excluding CHC) may be offered to patients with complicated VHD. These recommendations do not address options for an individual's status correction of complicated VHD. A case of endocarditis has been reported in a patient with TOF after insertion of an IUD (57).

Hypertension risk of prescribed contraceptives with a history of properly diagnosed hypertension depends on the severity of the disease. Risk is also determined by lack of other risk factors for hypertension. In general, the cu-IUD is an option that can be recommended regardless of severity of hypertension. Hormonal LARCs are considered generally safe; however, there is a theoretical risk when the systolic blood pressure (SBP) is > 140 mmHg or the diastolic blood pressure (DBP) is > 90 mmHg. The risk continues to increase for use of the injectable progesterone but less so for the progestin only pill (POP). This is due to some data suggesting that lower estrogen levels induced by injectable progesterone contribute to lower high-density lipoprotein (HDL) level which are associated with hypertension (52).

With respect to CHC, the risks outweigh the benefits. This is due to early studies demonstrating that users of CHC were at increased risk of stroke, acute myocardial infarction, or peripheral artery disease, compared to non-users. Combined hormonal options are not recommended when SBP is >140 mmHg or DBP is >90 mmHg. The risk of each method is the same in cases of hypertension due to underlying vascular disease. The recommendations are the same for initiation and continuation of each method (52).

Deep vein thrombosis (DVT)/ pulmonary embolism (PE)

Risk of medical complications while using hormonal contraception is based on timing, severity, family history and anticipated surgery. In the case of an active/acute DVT/PE, the risk of complication with any method is slightly elevated even with non-hormonal cu-IUD. Again, use of CHC is contraindicated in this setting. In general, the cu-IUD is the safest option for a patient who has had a history of a DVT/PE even while off of anticoagulants. Progestin-only options-- including the implant, injection and pills--- have similar safety profiles and are considered safe as well.

CHCs in the form of intravaginal ring, transdermal patch, and oral pills, are contraindicated. CHCs may be used if the risk for a recurrent DVT/PE is low; however, the risk of complication is higher than when using a progestin-only method. In the case of a DVT/PE that requires anticoagulation, CHCs are contraindicated, while the use of non-hormonal cu-IUD and progestin-only options have acceptable risk profiles. A family history of DVT/PE actually refers to a first-degree relative. With respect to family history of DVT/PE, all methods are considered safe; CHCs do have a slightly increased risk profile (52).

In terms of anticipated surgery, risk is based on the degree of post-surgical immobilization. Any method may be initiated and use may be continued if minor surgery occurs without the need for postsurgical immobilization. In general, the non-hormonal cu-IUD is considered safe, regardless of type of surgery (major vs. minor) and the degree of postsurgical immobilization. The risk of complications with hormonal options increases, especially for CHCs, when postsurgical immobilization is prolonged. CHCs are contraindicated in cases when major surgery occurs and there is prolonged post-surgical immobilization (52).

Ischemic heart disease (IHD)

The non-hormonal cu-IUD is considered the safest option for patients with current or history of ischemic heart disease (IHD). The next safest options for initiation of contraception are the progestin IUDs, implants and POPs. The risk of complications increases if a patient develops IHD while using any of these methods. There is also a higher risk for complications when using the injectable progesterone contraceptive. This risk is the same for initiation and for continued use. CHCs are contra-indicated at any time in a patient with IHD (52).

Peripartum (postpartum) cardiomyopathy

Risk of complication is based on degree of cardiac functional impairment and duration of illness. Functional impairment is defined by NYHA Functional Class. For normal or mildly impaired cardiac function (NYHA Class I): no activity restriction or NYHA Class II with mild activity restrictions ----regardless of duration of illness--- progestin-only methods (implant, injection and pills) are preferred and considered safe (54). The risk of complication increases with an IUD, either hormonal or non-hormonal. CHCs are contraindicated for patients who present within 6 months of diagnosis; the risk decreases slightly if patients present after this time frame (52).

For patients with moderate or severe cardiac functional impairment, NYHA Class III (marked activity restrictions) or NYHA Class IV (complete rest), CHCs are contraindicated (54). All other methods, including the cu-IUD and any progesterone method, carry some risk but are generally considered safe for use (52).

Obesity (body mass index or BMI > 30 kg/m^2)

In general, the non-hormonal cu-IUD as well as LARCs and POPs are considered safe and effective in patients despite BMI. The risk for potential effects on bone density has been shown in some patients who use injectable progesterone (58-66). There are also concerns about increased weight gain with use of injectable progesterone particularly in the adolescents who have a BMI >30 kg/m^2 (67). There is a slightly higher risk of complications with use of CHCs such as a higher risk of venous thromboembolic events in patients with a BMI >30 kg/m^2 who choose a CHC (52). Also, there is decreased contraceptive efficacy of the transdermal patch in patients who weigh >90 kg (68).

Multiple risk factors for atherosclerotic cardiovascular disease

This category refers to young women who have multiple risk factors for atherosclerosis, such as older age, smoking history, diabetes mellitus, hypertension, low HDL levels, high low-density lipoprotein (LDL) levels, and elevated triglyceride levels. In general, the non-hormonal cu-IUD is considered the safest option for these patients; followed by the progestin IUD, implant and POPs which all have similar risk profiles. Injectable progesterone has a slightly higher risk of further increasing the risk of complications from atherosclerosis. CHCs having the highest risk may even be contraindicated in some instances such as in a patient with several factors occurring simultaneously (52).

Table 4. Summary of US MEC recommendations for women with cardiovascular conditions (52)

Condition	Sub-condition	Cu-IUD		LNGa-IUD		Implant		DMPA		POP		CHC	
		Ib	Cc	I	C	I	C	I	C	I	C	I	C
Valvular heart disease	a. Uncomplicated	1		1		1		1		1		2	
	b. Complicated	1		1		1		1		1		4	
Hypertension	a. Adequately controlled	1		1		1		2		1		3	
	b. Elevated blood pressure levels												
	i. SBP 140-159 or DBP 90-99 mmHg	1		1		1		2		1		3	
	ii. SBP > 160 or DBP > 100 mmHg	1		2		2		3		2		4	
	c. Vascular disease	1		2		2		3		2		4	
Deep Vein Thrombosis/Pulmonary Embolism	a. History of DVT/PE, not receiving anticoagulant therapy												
	i. Higher risk for recurrent DVT/PE	1		2		2		2		2		4	
	ii. Lower risk for recurrent DVT/PE	1		2		2		2		2		3	
	b. Acute DVT/PE	2		2		2		2		2		4	
	c. DVT/PE and established anticoagulant therapy at least 3 months												
	i. Higher risk for recurrent DVT/PE	2		2		2		2		2		4	
	ii. Lower risk for recurrent DVT/PE	2		2		2		2		2		3	

Condition	Sub-condition	Cu-IUD		LNG[a]-IUD		Implant		DMPA		POP		CHC	
		I[b]	C[c]	I	C	I	C	I	C	I	C	I	C
	d. Family history (first-degree relatives)	1		1		1		1		1		2	
	e. Major surgery												
	i. With prolonged immobilization	1		2		2		2		2		4	
	ii. Without prolonged immobilization	1		1		1		1		1		2	
	f. Minor surgery without immobilization	1		1		1		1		1		1	
Ischemic heart disease	Current and history of	1		2	3	2	3	3		2	3	4	
Peripartum cardiomyopathy	a. Normal or mildly impaired cardiac function												
	i. < 6 months	2		2		1		1		1		4	
	ii. > 6 months	2		2		1		1		1		3	
	b. Moderately or severely impaired cardiac function	2		2		2		2		2		4	
Obesity	a. BMI > 30 kg/m^2	1		1		1		1		1		2	
	b. Menarche to < 18 years and BMI > 30 kg/m^2	1		1		1		2		1		2	
Multiple risk factors for atherosclerotic cardiovascular disease	older age, smoking, diabetes, hypertension, low HDL, high LDL, or high triglyceride levels	1		2		2		3		2		3/4	

[a]levonogestrel.
[b]initiation.
[c]continuation.

CONCLUSION

As a health care practitioner providing care for adolescents and young adults with cardiac disease, it is important to be aware that there are published guidelines that include provision of sexual health education. Similar to their peers, they go through significant physical and psychosocial changes and will greatly benefit from guidance of both the guardian and health care provider. For sexually active females, the US MEC is a good guide in choosing the best, safest and most effective contraceptive method in preventing unintended pregnancies (52). Empowering them with the understanding of their sexual and reproductive health needs will result in a healthy adult despite the health consequences posed by the cardiac condition that includes congenital or acquired heart diseases, post-heart transplantation or other medically complex conditions (69-74). Training in contraception is important for all those involved in the care of females with cardiovascular conditions (75).

References

[1] Child and Adolescent Health Measurement Initiative. 2016-2017 National Survey of Children's Health (NSCH) data query. Data Resource Center for Child and Adolescent Health supported by Cooperative Agreement U59MC27866 from the U.S. Department of Health and Human Services Health Resources and Services Administration's Maternal and Child Health Bureau (HRSA MCHB). 2018. URL: http://childhealthdata.org/.

[2] Congenital heart defects (CHDs): Data and Statistics. Centers for Disease and Control Prevention, 2018. URL: https://www.cdc.gov/ncbddd/heartdefects/data.html#References.

[3] Ko JM. Genetic syndromes associated with congenital heart disease. Korean Circ J 2015;45(5):357-61.

[4] Chen M, Riehle-colarusso T, Yeung LF, Smith C, Farr SL. Children with heart conditions and their special health care needs - United States, 2016. MMWR 2018;67(38):1045-9.

[5] Gilboa SM, Devine OJ, Kucik JE, Oster ME, Riehle-Colarusso T, Nembhard WN, et al. Congenital heart defects in the United States: Estimating the magnitude of the affected population in 2010. Circulation 2016;134(2):101-9.

[6] Oster ME, Lee KA, Honein MA, Riehle-Colarusso T, Shin M, Correa A. Temporal trends in survival among infants with critical congenital heart defects. Pediatrics 2013;131(5):e1502-8.

[7] Hagan J, Shaw J, eds. Bright Futures: Guidelines for Health Supervision of Infants, Children, and Adolescents. 4th ed. Elk Grove, IL: American Academy of Pediatrics; 2017.

[8] Marcell AV, Burstein GR. Sexual and reproductive health care services in the pediatric setting. Pediatrics. 2017;140(5):e20172858. doi: 10.1542/peds.2017-2858.

[9] Committee on Gynecologic Practice. Committee Opinion No 706: Sexual health. Obstet Gynecol 2017;130(1):e42-7.

[10] Adolescent health care, sexuality and contraception. American Academy of Family Physicians, 2017. URL: https://www.aafp.org/about/policies/all/adolescent-sexuality.html.

[11] Breuner CC, Mattson G. Committee on Adolescence; Committee on Psychosocial Aspects of Child and Family Health. Sexuality education for children and adolescents. Pediatrics 2016;138(2):e20161348. doi: 10.1542/peds.2016-1348.

[12] American Academy of Pediatrics. Fertility and sexual function in children with chronic health conditions, 2018. URL: https://www.healthychildren.org/English/health-issues/conditions/chronic/Pages/Reproductive-Health-in-Teens-with-Chronic-Health-Conditions.aspx.

[13] Nahata L, Quinn GP, Tishelman AC. Section on Endocrinology. Counseling in pediatric populations at risk for infertility and/or sexual function concerns. Pediatrics 2018;142(2):e20181435. doi: 10.1542/peds.2018-1435.

[14] Marcell A, Wibbelsman C, Seigel W; AAP Committee on Adolescence. Clinical report: Male adolescent sexual and reproductive health care. Pediatrics 2017;140(5): e20172858.

[15] Loomba RS, Aggarwal S, Pelech AN. Addressing sexual health in congenital heart disease: when being the same isn't the same. Congenit Heart Dis 2015;10(1):30-5.

[16] Shum KK, Gupta T, Canobbio MM, Durst J, Shah SB. Family planning and pregnancy management in adults with congenital heart disease. Prog Cardiovasc Dis 2018;61(3-4):336-46.

[17] Rogers P, Mansour D, Mattinson A, O'Sullivan JJ. A collaborative clinic between contraception and sexual health services and an adult congenital heart disease clinic. J Fam Plann Reprod Health Care 2007;33(1):17-21.

[18] Lindley KJ, Madden T, Cahill AG, Ludbrook PA, Billadello JJ. Contraceptive use and unintended pregnancy in women with congenital heart disease. Obstet Gynecol 2015;126(2):363-9.

[19] Uzark K, VonBargen-Mazza P, Messiter E. Health education needs of adolescents with congenital heart disease. J Pediatr Health Care 1989;3(4):137-43.

[20] Van Deyk K, Pelgrims E, Troost E, Goossens E, Budts W, Gewillig M, et al. Adolescents' understanding of their congenital heart disease on transfer to adult-focused care. Am J Cardiol 2010;106(12):1803-7.

[21] Fry KM, Gerhardt CA, Ash J, Zaidi A, Garg V, McBride KL, et al. Lifetime prevalence of sexual intercourse and contraception use at last sex among adolescents and young adults with congenital heart disease. J Adolesc Health 2015;56(4):396-401.

[22] Amies Oelschlager AM, Micks EA, Debiec KE, Nizamic T, Mantrala MD, Prager SW. Long acting reversible contraception in adolescents with cardiovascular conditions. J Pediatr Adolesc Gynecol 2014;27(6):353-5.

[23] Bull MJ; Committee on Genetics. Health supervison for children with Down syndrome. Pediatrics 2011;128(2):393-406.

[24] Gravholt CH, Andersen NH, Conway GS, Dekkers OM, Geffner ME, Klein KO, et al. Clinical practice guidelines for the care of girls and women with Turner syndrome: Proceedings from the 2016 Cincinnati International Turner Syndrome Meeting. Eur J Endocrinol 2017;177(3):G1-70.

[25] Bassett AS, McDonald-McGinn DM, Devriendt K, Digilio MC, Goldenberg P, Habel A, et al. Practical guidelines for managing patients with 22q11. 2 deletion syndrome. J Pediatr 2011;159(2):332-9.

[26] Committee on Genetics. American Academy of Pediatrics: Health care supervision for children With Williams Syndrome. Pediatrics 2001;107(5):1192-204.

[27] Romano AA, Allanson JE, Dahlgren J, Gelb BD, Hall B, Pierpont ME, et al. Noonan syndrome: Clinical features, diagnosis, and management guidelines. Pediatrics 2010; 126(4):746-59.

[28] Tinkle BT, Saal HM; Committee on Genetics. Health supervision for children with Marfan syndrome. Pediatrics 2013;132(4):e1059-72.

[29] Irving C, Basu A, Richmond S, Burn J, Wren C. Twenty-year trends in prevalence and survival of Down syndrome. Eur J Hum Genet 2008;16(11):1336-40.

[30] Parker SE, Mai CT, Canfield MA, Rickard R, Wang Y, Meyer RE, et al. Updated national birth prevalence estimates for selected birth defects in the United States, 2004-2006. Birth Defects Res Part A Clin Mol Teratol 2010;88(12):1008-16.

[31] Murphy C, Lincoln S, Meredith S, Cross EM, Rintell D. Sex education and intellectual disability: Practices and insight from pediatric genetic counselors. J Genet Couns 2016;25(3):552-60.

[32] Pueschel SM, Scola PS. Parents' perception of social and sexual functions in adolescents with Down's syndrome. J Ment Defic Res 1988;32(Pt 3):215-20.

[33] Pasquino AM, Passeri F, Pucarelli I, Segni M, Municchi G. Spontaneous pubertal development in Turner's syndrome. Italian Study Group for Turner's syndrome. J Clin Endocrinol Metab 1997;82(6):1810-3.

[34] Carotti A, Digilio MC, Piacentini G, Saffirio C, Di Donato RM, Marino B. Cardiac defects and results of cardiac surgery in 22q11.2 deletion syndrome. Dev Disabil Res Rev 2008;14(1):35-42.

[35] Chan C, Costain G, Ogura L, Silversides CK, Chow EW, Bassett AS. Reproductive health issues for adults with a common genomic disorder: 22q11.2 deletion syndrome. J Genet Couns 2015;24(5):810-21.

[36] Walton JR, Martens MA, Pober BR. The proceedings of the 15th professional conference on Williams Syndrome. Am J Med Genet A 2017;173(5):1159-71.

[37] Morris CA, Mervis CB, Paciorkowski AP, Abdul-Rahman O, Dugan SL, Rope AF, et al. 7q11.23 Duplication syndrome: Physical characteristics and natural history. Am J Med Genet A 2015;167A(12):2916-35.

[38] Mervis CB, Morris CA, Klein-Tasman BP, Velleman SL, Osborne LR. 7q11.23 Duplication syndrome. In: Adam MP, Ardinger HH, Pagon RA, Wallace SE, Bean LJH, Stephens K, et al, eds. GeneReviews. Seattle, WA: University of Washington, 1993-2019.

[39] Romano AA, Dana K, Bakker B, Davis DA, Hunold JJ, Jacobs J, et al. Growth response, near-adult height, and patterns of growth and puberty in patients with Noonan syndrome treated with growth hormone. J Clin Endocrinol Metab 2009;94(7):2338-44.

[40] Marcus KA, Sweep CG, van der Burgt I, Noordam C. Impaired Sertoli cell function in males diagnosed with Noonan syndrome. J Pediatr Endocrinol Metab 2008;21(11):1079-84.

[41] Roberts AE, Allanson JE, Tartaglia M, Gelb BD. Noonan syndrome. Lancet 2013;381(9863):333-42.

[42] Loeys BL, Dietz HC, Braverman AC, Callewaert BL, De Backer J, Devereux RB, et al. The revised Ghent nosology for the Marfan syndrome. J Med Genet 2010;47(7):476-85.

[43] Castellano JM, Silvay G, Castillo JG. Marfan syndrome: Clinical, surgical, and anesthetic considerations. Semin Cardiothorac Vasc Anesth 2014;18(3):260-71.

[44] Goland S, Elkayam U. Pregnancy and Marfan syndrome. Ann Cardiothorac Surg 2017; 6(6):642-53.

[45] Peters KF, Kong F, Hanslo M, Biesecker BB. Living with Marfan syndrome III. Quality of life and reproductive planning. Clin Genet 2002;62(2):110-20.
[46] World Health Organization Department of Reproductive Health and Research (WHO/RHR) and Johns Hopkins Bloomberg School of Public Health/Center for Communication Programs (CCP) Knowledge for Health Project. Family planning: A global handbook for providers (2018 Update). Baltimore, MD: CCP, 2018.
[47] Trussell J. Contraceptive failure in the United States. Contraception 2011;83(5):397-404.
[48] Ott MA, Sucato GS; Committee on Adolescence. Contraception for adolescents. Pediatrics 2014;134(4):e1244-56.
[49] Society for Adolescent Health and Medicine. Improving knowledge about, access to, and utilization of long-acting reversible contraception among adolescents and young adults. J Adolesc Health 2017;60(4):472-4.
[50] No authors listed. ACOG Committee Opinion No. 735: Adolescents and long-acting reversible contraception: Implants and intrauterine devices. Obstet Gynecol 2018; 131(5):e130-9.
[51] Klein DA, Arnold JJ, Reese ES. Provision of contraception: Key recommendations from the CDC. Am Fam Physician 2015;91(9):625-33.
[52] Curtis KM, Tepper NK, Jatlaoui TC, Berry-Bibee E, Horton LG, Zapata LB, et al. U.S. Medical Eligibility Criteria for contraceptive use, 2016. MMWR Recomm Rep 2016; 65(3):1-103.
[53] Vu Q, Micks E, McCoy E, Prager S. Efficacy and safety of long-acting reversible contraception in women with cardiovascular conditions. Am J Cardiol 2016;117(2):302-4.
[54] The Criteria Committee of the New York Heart Association. Nomenclature and Criteria for Diagnosis of Diseases of the Heart and Great Vessels. 9th ed. Ed: M Dolgin. Boston: MA: Little Brown; 1994:253-6.
[55] Lindley K, Williams D. Valvular heart disease in pregnancy. American College of Cardiology, 2018. URL:https://www.acc.org/latest-in-cardiology/articles/2018/02/12/07/29/valvular-heart-disease-in-pregnancy.
[56] Sedlak T, Bairey Merz CN, Shufelt C, Gregory KD, Hamilton MA. Contraception in patients with heart failure. Circulation 2012;126(11):1396-400.
[57] Meyerowitz EA, Prager S, Stout K, Roxby A. Endocarditis following IUD insertion in a patient with tetralogy of Fallot. BMJ Case Rep 2019 Feb 7;12(2). pii: bcr-2018-227962. doi: 10.1136/bcr-2018-227962.
[58] Lanza LL, McQuay LJ, Rothman KJ, Bone HG, Kaunitz AM, Harel Z, et al. Use of depot medroxyprogesterone acetate contraception and incidence of bone fracture. Obstet Gynecol 2013;121(3):593-600.
[59] Kaunitz AM, Darney PD, Ross D, Wolter KD, Speroff L. Subcutaneous DMPA vs. intramuscular DMPA: A 2-year randomized study of contraceptive efficacy and bone mineral density. Contraception 2009;80(1):7-17.
[60] Lara-Torre E, Edwards CP, Perlman S, Hertweck SP. Bone mineral density in adolescent females using depot medroxyprogesterone acetate. J Pediatr Adolesc Gynecol 2004; 17(1):17-21.
[61] Scholes D, LaCroix AZ, Ichikawa LE, Barlow WE, Ott SM. Injectable hormone contraception and bone density: Results from a prospective study. Epidemiology 2002; 13(5):581-7.
[62] Segall-Gutierrez P, Agarwal R, Ge M, Lopez C, Hernandez G, Stanczyk FZ. A pilot study examining short-term changes in bone mineral density among class 3 obese users of depot-medroxyprogesterone acetate. Eur J Contracept Reprod Health Care 2013;18(3):199-205.
[63] Tang OS, Tang G, Yip PS, Li B. Further evaluation on long-term depot-medroxyprogesterone acetate use and bone mineral density: a longitudinal cohort study. Contraception 2000;62(4):161-4.
[64] Wong AYK, Tang LCH, Chin RKH. Levonorgestrel-releasing intrauterine system (Mirena®) and Depot medroxyprogesterone acetate (Depo-Provera) as long-term maintenance therapy for patients with moderate and severe endometriosis: a randomised controlled trial. Aust NZ J Obstet Gynaecol 2010;50(3):273-9.
[65] Zhang MH, Zhang W, Zhang AD, Yang Y, Gai L. Effect of depot medroxyprogesterone acetate on bone mineral density in adolescent women. Chin Med J (Engl) 2013; 126(21):4043-7.

[66] Cromer BA, Lazebnik R, Rome E, Stager M, Bonny A, Ziegler J, et al. Double-blinded randomized controlled trial of estrogen supplementation in adolescent girls who receive depot medroxyprogesterone acetate for contraception. Am J Obstet Gynecol 2005; 192(1):42-7.

[67] Le YC, Rahman M, Berenson AB. Early weight gain predicting later weight gain among depot medroxyprogesterone acetate users. Obstet Gynecol 2009;114(2 Pt 1):279-84.

[68] Zieman M, Guillebaud J, Weisberg E, Shangold GA, Fisher AC, Creasy GW. Contraceptive efficacy and cycle control with the Ortho Evra™/Evra™ transdermal system: the analysis of pooled data. Fertil Steril 2002;77(2 Suppl 2):S13-8.

[69] Bonassi Machado R, Gandolpho AC, Santana N, Bocardo RC, Palandri N, Morassutti Machado R. Contraception for women with heart disease: an update. Minerva Ginecol 2017;69(3):259-68.

[70] Roos-Hesselink JW, Cornette J, Sliwa K, Pieper PG, Veldtman GR, Johnson MR. Contraception and cardiovascular disease. Eur Heart J 2015;36(27):1728-34.

[71] Carmine I. Contraception for adolescents with medically complex conditions. Curr Probl Pediatr Adolesc Health Care 2018;48(12):345-57.

[72] Abarbanell G, Tepper NK, Farr SL. Safety of contraceptive use among women with congenital heart disease: A systematic review. Congenit Heart Dis 2019;14(3):331-40.

[73] Sobhani NC, Schultz H, Kheiwa A, Killion M, Parikh NI, Harris IS, et al. Contraceptive choices in the immediate postpartum period in women with cardiac disease. Am J Cardiol 2019;123(8):1364-9.

[74] Rajapreyar IN, Sinkey RG, Joly JM, Pamboukian SV, Lenneman A, Hoopes CW, et al. Management of reproductive health after cardiac transplantation. J Matern Fetal Neonatal Med 2019 Jul 7:1-10. doi: 10.1080/14767058.2019.1636962.

[75] Brown AE, Bradbrook KE, Casey FE. A survey of adult and pediatric cardiology fellows on training received in family planning counseling. J Womens Health (Larchmt) 2019 Jan 25. doi: 10.1089/jwh.2018.7186.

In: Chronic Disease and Disability
Editors: DE Greydanus, P Anne, JD Rowlett et al.
ISBN: 978-1-53617-656-8

Chapter 14

SLEEP DISORDERS IN CHILDREN AND ADOLESCENTS

Ahsan Nazeer**, MD, Lisa Campisi, PhD, Karen Lim, MD, Durre Shahwar, MRCPsych and Nehdia Hashemi, MD

Child and Adolescent Psychiatry, Sidra Medicine, Doha, Qatar
Qatar University School of Medicine, Doha, Qatar

ABSTRACT

Sleep health issues and sleep disorders regarding pediatric persons are discussed. Research has confirmed the need for healthy sleep for all persons, including those with chronic illnesses, such as cardiovascular disorders. Normal sleep parameters for pediatric persons are defined, and developmental perspectives of sleep disorders are considered. Various sleep disorders in different pediatric ages are reviewed from infants/toddlers to adolescents. An essential approach to caring for those with chronic illnesses is to improve their sleep hygiene and screen for as well as manage overt sleep disorders that may be present.

INTRODUCTION

The benefits of restful sleep have long been established as necessary for proper brain and body development. Yet, recent estimates suggest that sleep disorders are a common occurrence in the pediatric population, affecting over 30% of children (1-3). Moreover, research suggests that sleep issues persist throughout childhood with as much as half of children who have sleep problems during the first three years of life, continuing to encounter these issues two to three years later (1-3).

The International Classification of Sleep Disorders-3 (ICSD-3) lists sixty different sleep disorders organized into seven major categories, whereas the Diagnostic and Statistical Manual of Mental Disorders-5 (DSM-5) aggregates sleep-wake disorders under ten broader categories

---

* Correspondence: Ahsan Nazeer, MD, Division Chief, Child and Adolescent Psychiatry, Sidra Medicine, C2M 224, 2nd Mezzanine, OPC, POBox 26999, Al-Luqta Street, Education City North Campus, Qatar Foundation, Doha, Qatar. Email: anazeer@sidra.org.

of disorders or disorder groups (4,5). Commonly encountered sleep disturbances in children are similar to those in adults and include insomnia, obstructive sleep apnea, parasomnia, narcolepsy, and restless legs syndrome (3-5). These disorders have an impact on children's development and affect functioning in numerous areas, including daytime attention, affect regulation, behavior, and learning.

There is now growing evidence that children with medical and psychiatric disabilities are at increased risk for sleep disorders; these include attention deficit hyperactivity disorder (ADHD), mood disorders, and autism spectrum disorder (6,7). Current literature suggests that approximately between 74%-84% of children and adolescents with psychiatric disabilities struggle with severe sleep problems (1-3, 8). Other known risk factors include medical conditions such as asthma, allergic rhinitis, epilepsy, and obesity (9-11). Commonly reported sleep symptoms include bedtime settling issues, restless sleep, shorter sleep, and frequent nocturnal awakenings in younger children as well as delayed sleep phase syndrome during adolescence (8).

Normal sleep

Ongoing research and recent clinical advances have led to improved recognition regarding the necessity of normal sleep (4, 5). We now know that sleep is an active physiological state involving higher cortical structures and that it is vital for overall brain and body development as well as behavioral and emotional control. Sleep also has an impact on executive functions that includes attention, planning, abstract thinking, working memory, and impulse control. Hence, persistently sleep disturbed children are often considered as irritable, aggressive, impulsive as well as hyperactive, and at times misdiagnosed as having ADHD. Sleep disorders in childhood also impact parental functioning, as parents often report poor sleep, fatigue, and psychological distress.

Circadian rhythms and homeostatic processes are believed to regulate the sleep-wake cycle. The circadian cycle, considered to be the body's internal clock, lasts one hour longer than the standard 24-hour day and is influenced by light, temperature, noise, bedtime routines and medications. There is a close association between circadian rhythm and body temperature. Around 4 AM, when body temperature is the lowest, individuals go into a deeper state of sleep in comparison to the morning hours when body temperature rises and sleep also becomes lighter. The rising body temperatures and light sleep are believed to be in anticipation of the greater energy demands of impending wakefulness.

The homeostatic sleep process refers to an ever-increasing drive to sleep that builds and accumulates during daytime wakefulness, eventually resulting in a period of sleep. This represents the need to sleep during nighttime hours. During sleep, an ultradian rhythm determines the timing and duration of rapid eye movement (REM) and non-rapid eye movement (NREM) sleep; these are two distinct types of sleep that alternate throughout the sleep period.

REM sleep is also called active sleep because, in this stage, the body's physiological and neurochemical processes, as well as the electroencephalographic patterns, are similar to those of the wakeful state. It is associated with irregular breathing, lower muscle tone, and increased cerebral blood flow and metabolism. Even though brain activity is highest during REM sleep, individuals appear relaxed due to the active inhibition of muscle tone from signals that originate in the pons. Consequently, when there is a disruption in these inhibitory signals, children exhibit unusual motor activity, a condition known as REM behavior disorder, a parasomnia. During REM sleep, the brain increases protein production and stimulates areas involved in learning. Infants spend almost half of their time in REM sleep, but this decline to about 25% in the childhood years.

In contrast to neuronal activation in REM sleep, NREM sleep, or quiet sleep, is characterized by physiological and behavioral inhibition. During this phase, breathing and heart rate become rhythmic, and active inhibition of muscle tone ceases. By six months of age, the differentiation of NREM sleep into four stages is complete, and sleep spindles, K- complexes as well as delta waves characterize the specific stages. Table 1 summarizes sleep patterns from birth through adolescence with corresponding proportions of REM and NREM sleep.

Table 1. Sleep patterns through adolescent years

Age	Recommended time asleep	Time spent in REM sleep
Birth (0-3 m)	16 hours	50%
Infants (3-12 m)	15 hours	25%
Toddlers (1- 3 y)	12-14 hours	25%
Preschool (3-5 y)	11-13 hours	20-25%
School-age (6-12 y)	11 hours	20%
Adolescents (12-18y)	8-9 hours	20%

A developmental perspective of sleep disorders

Table 2. DSM classification of sleep disorders

DSM-IV-TR	DSM-5
Dyssomnias:	Insomnia Disorder
Primary Insomnia	Hypersomnolence disorder
Primary Hypersomnia	Narcolepsy
Narcolepsy	
Breathing Related Sleep Disorder	*Breathing Related Sleep Disorders:*
Circadian Rhythm Sleep Disorders	Obstructive Sleep Apnea-Hypopnea
	Central Sleep Apnea
Parasomnias:	Sleep-Related Hypoventilation
Sleep Terror Disorder	
Sleepwalking Disorder	Circadian Rhythm Sleep-Wake Disorders
Nightmare Disorder	
	Parasomnias:
Medical disorders:	NREM Sleep Arousal Disorders
Substance-Induced Sleep Disorder	Nightmare Disorder
	REM Sleep Behavior Disorder
Due To General Medical Condition	
(Eliminated in DSM-5)	
	Restless legs syndrome
Due To Other Psychiatric Disorders	Substance/Medication-induced Sleep
(Eliminated in DSM-5)	dDisorder

As reported previously, sleep-wake disorders are common in the child and adolescent population, but they differ in nature and presentation across the life span (4-11). Short lived sleep disruptions, as well as transient, require different interventions than those that persist and transcend multiple developmental phases. A developmental perspective is useful for differential diagnosis, intervention, and treatment planning. Table 2 summarizes the classification of sleep disorders in the DSM-IV-TR and DSM-5 (5).

Infants/toddlers (0-3 years)

Infants spend a large portion of their early lives sleeping. Approximately 15-16 hours of 24-hour are spent sleeping in infancy. For the first three months, infants will transition from wakefulness to REM sleep. After this age, infants will begin to consolidate their sleep patterns, and transition from wakefulness into NREM sleep, with REM sleep appearing approximately 90 minutes to two hours later. Most infants awaken during the night and can self-soothe until they return to sleep. It is because of this ability to self-soothe that parents are encouraged to put infants to bed while they are still awake. Conversely, infants who are rocked or fed until asleep are more likely to seek parental comfort during nighttime awakenings. Contrary to the belief that children outgrow their sleep problems, research has indicated a more chronic course, with about 20% of children continuing to require parental soothing and rocking at three years of age (12).

Behavioral insomnia

Nighttime awakening problems are among the most common concerns for which parents seek help from a healthcare professional (4). Bedtime resistance and frequent nighttime awakening are extremely common and occur in about 20%-30% of infants. From a behavioral point of view, nighttime awakenings are linked with pre-bedtime activities, and a detailed assessment of bedtime routines as well as interactions can be helpful. Educating parents about positive routines, healthy sleeping habits and graduated extinction (e.g., waiting for progressively longer intervals before intervening, letting the infant cry for few nights) are found to be effective in clinical settings. Table 3 provides recommended parental guidelines for parents to follow to encourage good sleep hygiene.

Table 3. Recommended parental practices to promote good sleep hygiene

- Establish bedtime routines and cues
- Limit nighttime feedings to no more than first six months of life
- Place the baby in the crib while still awake to encourage self-soothing
- Use a firm mattress
- Have the baby sleep on his back
- Avoid clothes that can cause overheating at night
- Avoid co-sleeping

Sleep-related rhythmic movement disorder (RMD)

Repetitive and stereotypic movements during sleep, involving any part of the body, characterize this disorder. Parents may report having witnessed concerning behaviors, such as head banging and body rocking (1, 3). In the majority of cases, RMD is a self-limiting, normal physiological phenomenon arising in a healthy child; however, children with intellectual disabilities and other psychiatric disorders (including autism spectrum disorder and attention deficit hyperactivity disorder), also have been noted to present with this disorder (6).

The presence of these repetitive body movements should always be reported to child health care professionals, particularly if they also occur outside of the sleep period. In these more complex situations, RMD tends to persist beyond childhood and require specific treatments; these include the use of protective helmets, behavior modification, and medications such as benzodiazepines as well as atypical antipsychotics. On the other hand, reassuring parents and educating them about the benign nature of this physiological variant is sufficient in most cases.

Sleep Disordered Breathing (SDB)

Sleep-disordered breathing (SDB) is a spectrum described as a constellation of respiratory disorders that occur or get worse during sleep and has a prevalence estimated to be around 1-4% (13, 14). Infants with prematurity and complex medical problems are more likely to be diagnosed with SDB. Children with SDB have numerous effects on behavior, neurodevelopment as well as growth, and a high level of suspicion is needed to make an accurate diagnosis (15).

Preschool children (3-5 years)

By 18 months of age, children transition from two daytime naps to one, and by five years of age, 73% of children have stopped napping altogether. Preschoolers average 10-12 hours of sleep per night and commonly present with bedtime resistance and nighttime fears. Typical sleep problems during this phase include behavioral insomnia (limit testing), nighttime fears, nightmare disorders, night terrors, obstructive sleep apnea, and partial arousal parasomnia (2, 3).

Nighttime fears

Nighttime fears peak during preschool years, at which time children often refuse to go to bed. Fears of darkness, being alone, or imaginary creatures in their room are characteristic of the nighttime struggles in this age group. Some factors that lead to bedtime stalling and disturbed sleep include parental discord, child anxiety, daytime overstimulation, increased emotional arousal, and a desire to spend more time with the parents. Counseling parents about maintaining a balance between reassurance and limit setting is an essential part of the treatment.

Nightmare disorder

The nightmares of nightmare disorder occur during rapid eye movement (REM) sleep and are usually reported by children between 3 to 6 years of age (4). Typically, the nightmares occur during the middle or last third of the night and result in child awakening. During the nightmare, children have some autonomic arousal but display little body movement. They are distressed and wide-awake after the nightmare and usually have vivid recall of the event the next morning, with themes often related to being lost or abandoned. In general, nightmares are natural phenomena; however, factors that can trigger nightmares and distressing dreams include anxiety, stress, sleep deprivation, posttraumatic stress disorder (PTSD), and medications (e.g., amphetamines).

Withdrawal from REM suppressant medications (e.g., clonidine) is another cause of REM rebound and nightmares. Infrequent or medication-induced nightmares are usually self-limiting, but recurrent nightmares that cause family dysfunction require special attention. In mild cases, reassuring the parents and teaching relaxation skills to the child is adequate. In severe cases, referral to a mental health provider should be initiated.

Obstructive sleep apnea (OSA)

Obstructive sleep disorder in childhood that presents as excessive daytime somnolence usually peaks in prevalence during the preschool years (16). Children typically present with symptoms of having difficulty waking up in the morning and needing daytime naps. If the disorder remains untreated, numerous behavioral sequelae may result, including hyperactivity, inattention, aggression, learning problems, and cognitive difficulties (17). OSA causes repeated awakenings during the night, which also interferes with growth hormone secretion, which in severe cases could result in growth retardation or failure to thrive syndrome.

Snoring is found in 3% to 12% of children, and by itself, is not a sine qua non of OSA; however, as 1% to 3% of these children eventually are diagnosed with OSA, the American Academy of Pediatrics recommends that all children with habitual snoring be evaluated (16). Usual causes of sleep apnea in preschoolers include hypertrophied tonsils as well as adenoids, craniofacial abnormalities, and chronic nasal congestion. Chronic or recurrent allergies are also known risk factors for OSA due to the chronic effect of inflammation.

Similarly, childhood asthma, also characterized by airway inflammation, is associated with sleep problems that include reduced sleep time, frequent nighttime arousals, and sleep-disordered breathing (4, 9). It is thought that asthma symptoms worsen at night due to circadian fluctuations in lung functioning. Young children with asthma also show more frequent nocturnal awakenings compared to non-asthmatic children. Obesity is also increasingly thought of as a risk factor to snoring and sleep apnea in children, as it plays a role in upper airway obstruction during sleep (4, 11). As rates of childhood obesity continue to grow, increased attention to this issue and the mechanisms in which this contributes to sleep problems should be further examined.

Treatment can include tonsillectomy, adenoidectomy, and pharmacological management of nasal congestion or allergies. In surgical guidelines, some authors have also discussed surgery for sleep disorders; these include nasal, palatal, tongue, maxillomandibular, tracheal, and bariatric, surgeries (18). In unsuccessful cases and those cases for whom the severity is judged to be moderate to severe, the use of continuous positive airway pressure (CPAP) is usually successful in relieving the symptoms of OSA (19,20). In these cases, behavioral intervention and family support are thought to improve the effectiveness of the intervention, particularly in the case of younger children (19, 20).

Partial arousal parasomnia

Partial arousal parasomnias, also called disorders of arousal, include sleep terrors, sleepwalking, sleep talking, and confusional arousal (21, 22). These disorders are most common between 3 and 13 years of age but usually resolve by 10-11 years of age. Arousals usually occur within the first one to two hours of sleep and coincide with the transition from slow-wave (stage 3 and 4) sleep to REM sleep. They are sporadic, last 5 to 15 minutes, and usually occur only once per night.

During these episodes, the child may demonstrate dramatic behaviors, lack awareness of surroundings, and have only a fragmented memory of events afterward. The child also may experience intense autonomic arousal, characterized by tachypnea, tachycardia, and diaphoresis. These episodes are often difficult for parents to witness, yet parental attempts to calm and comfort the child are typically ineffective. In 60% of individuals, there is a family history of parasomnias.

When evaluating these parasomnias, medical providers need to rule out nocturnal seizures, nightmares, and post-traumatic stress disorder (PTSD). Repetitive stereotypic behaviors and odd posturing often signify an underlying seizure disorder, and polysomnography is usually indicated in these instances (10). In benign cases, parental education about the disorder is important. Getting insufficient sleep is a common trigger, and correcting this issue may be the only treatment required; other triggers, including warm showers, should be avoided as well. Although controlled studies are lacking, clozapine is the medication of choice for the treatment of these parasomnias.

Other than above, children with developmental disabilities display chronic insomnias. If behavioral therapy fails to address this problem, pharmacotherapeutic agents, including melatonin, can be considered. Other agents including clonidine, trazodone, gabapentin, and mirtazapine can also be considered. Some supplements holds promise but need further study; these include iron, vitamin D, and 5-hydroxytryptophan (23).

School-age children (6-12 years)

The school-age period is a time of decreasing parental supervision and increasing autonomy. During this phase, children need at least 10 hours of sleep per night; however, numerous daily responsibilities may conflict with this need; these include social, academic, and sports activities (19, 21, 24). The constant flow of electronic communication, from instant messaging, and Internet chat sites to cyberbullying, competes with sleep, and disrupts bedtime routines (24). Some of the common sleep problems in this age group include nighttime fears, poor sleep hygiene, parasomnias and restless leg syndrome (1-3).

Sleep hygiene

Poor sleep hygiene is one of the leading causes of sleep-onset problems and presents in about 10% of school-age children. Parental education regarding healthy sleeping habits is an important first step. Assessment of sleeping routines and the use of a daily sleep diary help with the differential diagnosis of sleep-related issues. Table 4 summarizes the basic tenets of healthy sleep hygiene.

Table 4. Sleep hygiene for children

- Maintain a regular bedtime and waking schedule seven days a week
- Establish a bedtime routine for the child
- Avoid emotional discussions thirty minutes before bedtime
- Avoid caffeinated drinks
- Avoid video games and TV thirty minutes before bed
- Consider foods high in tryptophan (warm milk and turkey)
- Consider a warm bath, comfortable clothes, family unwinding time including reading stories
- Make the bedroom dark and maintain comfortable temperature (temperatures above 75 F are uncomfortable)
- Keep bedroom for sleeping and do not associate it with timeouts or playing

Restless leg syndrome (RLS)

Restless leg syndrome (RLS) usually presents with uncomfortable sensations in the legs that get worse during the latter part of the day or after long periods of inactivity. RLS in younger children has an autosomal dominant pattern of inheritance, and there is usually a positive family history among first-degree relatives. It is present in 2% of children and has a strong association with ADHD. This condition probably is under-diagnosed in children, considering the fact the 10% of adults report an onset of symptoms before ten years of age (25).

Children usually complain of tingling and crawling sensations in their legs accompanied by an urge to move; running or walking often relieves symptoms. Low serum ferritin levels are associated with RLS in children, and those with levels below 35μg/L may benefit from iron replacement therapy (26). In severe cases, other pharmacological interventions, including clonidine or clonazepam, may be used; however, clonidine may make night terrors worse, and clonazepam can cause daytime drowsiness, due to its long half-life. Proper pharmacological counseling is thus recommended when RLS is found in children (27, 28).

Adolescents (12-18 years)

During adolescence, teenagers need between 8 and 9 hours of sleep per night, yet the majority of them sleep no more than 7 hours per night. There are numerous reasons for this sleep debt. With the emergence of puberty, teenagers experience a biological shift in the time of onset of sleep, and their bedtimes also begin to migrate to later hours; also, as they stay up later, youth may sleep in later in the morning. Besides biological factors, environmental factors contribute to chronic sleep deprivation in adolescence; these include evening social events, early school start times, work schedules, and sports activities (29-31).

Another important contributor to sleep-related behavior is the widespread use of electronic messaging and media technology. There is now growing evidence that the use of a computer or the internet, a cell phone, and other electronic technology is negatively associated with sleep patterns in adolescence. The effects are most robust in the hour before going to bed, whereby the more adolescents use technology during the pre-sleep hour, the later their bedtimes and the longer the sleep onset.

Chronic sleep deprivation leads to numerous daytime consequences, including detrimental effects on mood, behavior, and academic performance (32, 33). Moreover, chronically sleep-deprived adolescents may need to rely on stimulants or other wakefulness- promoting agents to function during the day. Cognitive behavioral therapy for insomnia (CBT-i) is effective in managing insomnia in this age group; however, further research is needed (34-36).

Delayed sleep phase syndrome (DSPS) and narcolepsy are two disorders that are common in this age group.

Delayed sleep phase syndrome (DSPS)

Delayed sleep phase syndrome (DSPS) is a circadian rhythm disorder that is present in about 5% to 10% of the adolescent population (37, 38). During adolescence, there is a change toward evening circadian preference. At the same time, the homeostatic need to sleep also lessens, leading adolescents to stay up longer. Individuals with DSPS usually present to the clinic with complaints of difficulty with early morning awakening and excessive daytime sleepiness.

In this disorder, regular sleep-wake schedules are delayed by more than two hours, and adolescents report an inability to sleep until the latter part of the night. Their efforts to get to sleep early are often unsuccessful and lead to sleep-onset insomnia; however, if they go to bed at late hours, they fall asleep quickly and have normal sleep quality. After so few hours of sleep, adolescents have difficulty waking up on time for school and are often tired as well as drowsy during the school day; this may contribute to truancy, academic difficulties, behavioral difficulties, and impaired mood.

Treatment for DSPS is complicated and requires a highly motivated adolescent. Obtaining a detailed sleep history and having the adolescent keep a sleep diary is both helpful in clarifying the differential diagnosis. Depending upon the underlying problem, phase advancement therapy and chronotherapy are two treatments that can be employed. The goal of the treatment is to align the adolescent's sleep-wake rhythm with a schedule that promotes healthy living and improves psychosocial functioning (39-41).

Narcolepsy

Narcolepsy, a lifelong condition, is a REM sleep hypersomnia characterized by irresistible attacks of daytime sleepiness, accompanied by cataplexy, hypnagogic hallucinations, and sleep paralysis (42, 43). Narcolepsy affects 1 in 2,000 individuals and has a peak onset during adolescence as well as young adulthood. Genetic factors play an important role, and 8-10% of affected individuals report having a first degree relative with a similar disorder (44, 45).

The pathophysiological mechanisms underlying narcolepsy are linked to hypocretin ligand deficiency in the brain as well as cerebrospinal fluid and to a specific human leukocyte antigen (HLA-DQB1*0602) (46, 47). The differential diagnosis includes chronic sleep deficiency, Kleine-Levin syndrome, and psychiatric disorders, including depression and ADHD. Polysomnography and multiple sleep latency testing aids in establishing the diagnosis.

Narcolepsy is a chronic condition, and treatment is usually individualized. Educating parents and teachers about this disorder helps reduce stigma and deters the misperception that the child is oppositional, lazy, or bored. Stimulant medications, including methylphenidate as well as amphetamines, and behavioral approaches are first-line treatments; behavioral approaches include scheduled daytime naps and exercise. Stimulants are wakefulness-promoting agents and are very effective in school-age children. Non-stimulant options, such as modafinil, and tricyclic antidepressants, including clomipramine, have also been used successfully (48-50).

Cardiovascular effects of sleep disorders

Numerous insomnias, especially obstructive sleep apnea, is associated with cardiopulmonary dysfunction because of its association with hypercapnia, hypoxemia, and alterations in sympathetic tone as well as pulmonary artery vasoconstriction (15, 51-53). In some children, symptoms are subtle; however, in others, sleep disorders can lead to numerous cardiopulmonary sequela, including altered arterial blood pressure regulation, changes in left ventricular function, and systemic hypertension (54-61). In severe cases, children can develop cor-pulmonale, failure to thrive, and even death.

Conclusion

Pediatric sleep disorders are common throughout childhood in those with and without chronic illnesses and an important source of parental concerns (7, 13, 17, 18, 23, 62-64). However, they are usually under diagnosed. Since children with sleep disorders often present with significant behavioral comorbidities, initial treatment usually takes place in a psychiatric clinic. Persons of all ages with chronic disease, including cardiovascular conditions (i.e., atrial fibrillation, heart failure, hypertension, others), are also at risk for abnormal sleep hygiene and overt sleep disorders with increasing research revealing links with circadian rhythm dysfunction, obstructive sleep apnea, insomnia, narcolepsy, and others (57, 60, 62). Useful strategies for providing appropriate care to children with sleep disorders include a high level of suspicion, a multidisciplinary approach using a developmental perspective to treatment and collaboration with a pediatric sleep specialist.

References

[1] Hoban TF. Sleep disorders in children. Ann NY Acad Sci 2010;1184(1):1-14.
[2] Huhdanpää H, Klenberg L, Westerinen H, Fontell T, Aronen ET. Sleep and psychiatric symptoms in young child psychiatric outpatients. Clin Child Psychol Psychiatry 2018;23(1):77-95.
[3] Kotagal S, Chopra A. Pediatric sleep-wake disorders. Neurol Clin 2012; 30(4):1193-212.
[4] Sateia MJ. International classification of sleep disorders-third edition: highlights and modifications. Chest 2014;146(5):1387-94.
[5] American Psychiatric Association. Diagnostic and statistical manual of mental disorders, 5th ed (DSM 5). Arlington, VA: American Psychiatric Publishing, 2013.
[6] Rzepecka H, McKenzie K, McClure I, Murphy S. Sleep, anxiety and challenging behaviour in children with intellectual disability and/or autism spectrum disorder. Res Dev Disabil 2011;32(6):2758-66.
[7] Deliens G, Peigneux P. Sleep–behaviour relationship in children with autism spectrum disorder: methodological pitfalls and insights from cognition and sensory processing. Dev Med Child Neurol 2019;61(12):1368-76.
[8] Hoban TF, Chervin RD. Sleep-related breathing disorders of childhood: Description and clinical picture, diagnosis, and treatment approaches. Sleep Med Clin 2007;2(3):445-62.
[9] Koinis-Mitchell D, Kopel SJ, Boergers J, Ramos K, LeBourgeois M, McQuaid EL, et al. Asthma, allergic rhinitis, and sleep problems in urban children. J Clin Sleep Med 2015;11(2):101-10.
[10] Lewandowski AS, Ward TM, Palermo TM. Sleep problems in children and adolescents with common medical conditions. Pediatr Clin North Am 2011; 58(3):699-713.

[11] Redline S, Tishler PV, Schluchter M, Aylor J, Clark K, Graham G. Risk factors for sleep-disordered breathing in children. Associations with obesity, race, and respiratory problems. Am J Respir Crit Care Med 1999;159(5 Pt 1):1527-32.

[12] Mindell JA, Kuhn B, Lewin DS, Meltzer LJ, Sadeh A; American Academy of Sleep Medicine. Behavioral treatment of bedtime problems and night wakings in infants and young children. Sleep 2006;29(10):1263-76.

[13] Mehta B, Waters K, Fitzgerald D, Badawi N. Sleep disordered breathing (SDB) in neonates and implications for its long-term impact. Paediatr Respir Rev 2019 Oct 30. pii: S1526-0542(19)30092-2. doi: 10.1016/j.prrv.2019.10.003.

[14] Bixler EO, Vgontzas AN, Lin H-M, Liao D, Calhoun S, Vela-Bueno A, et al. Sleep disordered breathing in children in a general population sample: Prevalence and risk factors. Sleep 2009;32(6):731-6.

[15] Lavergne F, Morin L, Armitstead J, Benjafield A, Richards G, Woehrle H. Atrial fibrillation and sleep-disordered breathing. J Thorac Dis 2015;7(12):E575-84.

[16] Section on Pediatric Pulmonology. Subcommittee on Obstructive Sleep Apnea Syndrome. American Academy of Pediatrics. Clinical Practice Guideline: Diagnosis and management of childhood obstructive sleep apnea syndrome. Pediatrics 2002;109(4):704-12.

[17] Krzeski A, Burghard M. Obstructive sleep disordered breathing in children – an important problem in the light of current European guidelines. Otolaryngol Pol 2018;72(5):9-16.

[18] Mandavia R, Mehta N, Veer V. Guidelines on the surgical management of sleep disorders: A systematic review. Laryngoscope 2019 May 1. doi: 10.1002/lary.28028.

[19] Beebe DW. Cognitive, behavioral, and functional consequences of inadequate sleep in children and adolescents. Pediatr Clin North Am 2011;58(3):649-65.

[20] Byars KC, Yolton K, Rausch J, Lanphear B, Beebe DW. Prevalence, patterns, and persistence of sleep problems in the first 3 years of life. Pediatrics 2012; 129(2):e276-e84.

[21] Moore M, Allison D, Rosen CL. A review of pediatric nonrespiratory sleep disorders. Chest 2006;130(4):1252-62.

[22] Stores G. Parasomnias of childhood and adolescence. Sleep Med Clin 2007; 2(3):405-17.

[23] Bruni O, Angriman M, Melegari MG, Ferri R. Pharmacotherapeutic management of sleep disorders in children with neurodevelopmental disorders. Expert Opin Pharmacother 2019;20(18):2257-71.

[24] Pieters D, De Valck E, Vandekerckhove M, Pirrera S, Wuyts J, Exadaktylos V, et al. Effects of pre-sleep media use on sleep/wake patterns and daytime functioning among adolescents: The moderating role of parental control. Behav Sleep Med 2014;12(6):427-43.

[25] Leschziner GD. Restless legs syndrome. In: Selsick H, ed. Sleep disorders in psychiatric patients. Heidelberg: Springer, 2018:175-88.

[26] Rosen GM, Morrissette S, Larson A, Stading P, Barnes TL. Does improvement of low serum ferritin improve symptoms of restless legs syndrome in a cohort of pediatric patients? J Clin Sleep Med 2019;15(8):1149-54.

[27] Trenkwalder C, Allen R, Högl B, Clemens S, Patton S, Schormair B, et al. Comorbidities, treatment, and pathophysiology in restless legs syndrome. Lancet Neurol 2018;17(11):994-1005.

[28] Winkelmann J, Allen RP, Högl B, Inoue Y, Oertel W, Salminen AV, et al. Treatment of restless legs syndrome: Evidence-based review and implications for clinical practice. Mov Disord 2018;33(7):1077-91.

[29] Crowley SJ, Wolfson AR, Tarokh L, Carskadon MA. An update on adolescent sleep: New evidence informing the perfect storm model. J Adolesc 2018;67:55-65.

[30] Galván A. The unrested adolescent brain. Child Dev Perspect 2019;13(3):141-6.

[31] Chue AE, Gunthert KC, Kim RW, Alfano CA, Ruggiero AR. The role of sleep in adolescents' daily stress recovery: Negative affect spillover and positive affect bounce-back effects. J Adolesc 2018;66:101-11.

[32] Schwarz J, Axelsson J, Gerhardsson A, Tamm S, Fischer H, Kecklund G, et al. Mood impairment is stronger in young than in older adults after sleep deprivation. J Sleep Res 2018;28:e12801.

[33] Simon SL, Diniz Behn C, Laikin A, Kaar JL, Rahat H, Cree-Green M, et al. Sleep & circadian health are associated with mood & behavior in adolescents with overweight/obesity. Behav Sleep Med 2019;20:1-10. doi: 10.1080/15402002.2019.1629444.

[34] Treece C. CBT-I for the Treatment of Insomnia. Lynchburg J Med Sci 2019; 1(4):69.
[35] van der Zweerde T, Bisdounis L, Kyle S, Lancee J, Van Straten A. Long-term effects of cognitive behavioral therapy for insomnia: a meta-analysis. Sleep Med Rev 2019;48:1-11.
[36] Schlarb AA, Bihlmaier I, Velten-Schurian K, Poets CF, Hautzinger M. Short-and long-term effects of cbt-i in groups for school-age children suffering from chronic insomnia: The Kiss-program. Behav Sleep Med 2018;16(4):380-97.
[37] Nesbitt AD. Delayed sleep-wake phase disorder. J Thorac Dis 2018;10(Suppl 1):S103-11.
[38] Snitselaar MA, Smits MG, Spijker J. ADHD symptoms in adults with delayed sleep phase disorder. Sleep Biol Rhythms 2019;17(1):11-8.
[39] Hirose M, Arakawa C, Watanabe A, Esaki Y, Kawai R, Iwata N, et al. Treatment outcome of non-24-hour sleep–wake rhythm disorder: a retrospective study of 24 consecutive cases in a sleep clinic. Fujita Med J 2018;4(3):70-6.
[40] Danielsson K, Jansson-Fröjmark M, Broman J-E, Markström A. Light therapy with scheduled rise times in young adults with delayed sleep phase disorder: therapeutic outcomes and possible predictors. Behav Sleep Med 2018;16(4):325-36.
[41] Watson LA, Phillips AJ, Hosken IT, McGlashan EM, Anderson C, Lack LC, et al. Increased sensitivity of the circadian system to light in delayed sleep–wake phase disorder. J Physiol 2018;596(24):6249-61.
[42] Mahoney CE, Cogswell A, Koralnik IJ, Scammell TE. The neurobiological basis of narcolepsy. Nat Rev Neurosci 2019;20(2):83-93.
[43] Postiglione E, Antelmi E, Pizza F, Lecendreux M, Dauvilliers Y, Plazzi G. The clinical spectrum of childhood narcolepsy. Sleep Med Rev 2018;38:70-85.
[44] Taheri S. The genetics of narcolepsy. In: Goswami M, Thorpy MJ, Pandi-Perumal SR, eds. Narcolepsy: A clinical guide. Berlin: Springer, 2016:3-10.
[45] Miyagawa T, Tokunaga K. Genetics of narcolepsy. Hum Genome Var 2019; 6(1):1-8.
[46] Ollila HM, Ravel J-M, Han F, Faraco J, Lin L, Zheng X, et al. HLA-DPB1 and HLA class I confer risk of and protection from narcolepsy. Am J Hum Genet 2015;96(1):136-46.
[47] Capittini C, De Silvestri A, Terzaghi M, Scotti V, Rebuffi C, Pasi A, et al. Correlation between HLA-DQB1* 06: 02 and narcolepsy with and without cataplexy: approving a safe and sensitive genetic test in four major ethnic groups. A systematic meta-analysis. Sleep Med 2018;52:150-7.
[48] Barateau L, Dauvilliers Y. Recent advances in treatment for narcolepsy. Ther Adv Neurol Disord 2019;12:175628641987562.
[49] Nallu S, Guerrero GY, Lewis-Croswell J, Wittine LM. Review of narcolepsy and other common sleep disorders in children. Adv Pediatr 2019;66:147-59.
[50] Pérez-Carbonell L. Treatment of excessive daytime sleepiness in patients with narcolepsy. Curr Treat Options Neurol 2019;21(11):57. doi: 10.1007/s11940-019-0595-9.
[51] Budhiraja R, Quan SF. Sleep-disordered breathing and cardiovascular health. Curr Opin Pulm Med 2005;11(6):501-6.
[52] Gianfagna F, Veronesi G, Bertù L, Cesana G, Grassi G, Stranges S, et al. Influence of sleep disturbances on age at onset and long-term incidence of major cardiovascular events: the MONICA-Brianza and PAMELA cohort studies. Sleep Med 2016;21:126-32.
[53] Oliveira CCS, Tufik S, Andersen ML. Sleep disorders impair attaining ideal cardiovascular health. Arq Bras Cardiol 2019;112(6):807-808. [Article in English, Portuguese]
[54] Drager LF, McEvoy RD, Barbe F, Lorenzi-Filho G, Redline S; INCOSACT Initiative (International Collaboration of Sleep Apnea Cardiovascular Trialists). Sleep apnea and cardiovascular disease: Lessions from recent trails and need for team science. Circulation 2017;136(19):1840-50.
[55] Farrell PC, Richards G. Recognition and treatment of sleep-disordered breathing: an important component of chronic disease management. J Transl Med 2017;15(1):114. doi: 10.1186/s12967-017-1211-y.
[56] Larsson SC, Markus HS. Genetic liability to insomnia and cardiovascular disease risk. Circulation 2019;140(9):796-8.
[57] Linz D, Baumert M, Desteghe L, Kadhim K, Vernooy K, Kalman JM, et al. Nightly sleep apnea severity in patients with atrial fibrillation: Potential applications of long-term sleep apnea monitoring. Int J Cardiol Heart Vasc 2019;24:100424

[58] Liu TZ, Xu C, Rota M, Cai H, Zhang C, Shi MJ, et al. Sleep duration and risk of all-cause mortality: A flexible, non-linear, meta-regression of 40 prospective cohort studies. Sleep Med Rev 2017;32:28-36.

[59] Nakamoto T. Sleep-disordered breathing—a real therapeutic target for hypertension, pulmonary hypertension, ischemic heart disease, and chronic heart failure? J Nippon Med Sch 2018;85(2):70-7

[60] Silvani A. Sleep disorders, nocturnal blood pressure, and cardiovascular risk: A translational perspective. Auton Neurosci 2019;218:31-42.

[61] Zinchuk A, Yaggi HK. Sleep apnea heterogeneity, phenotypes, and cardiovascular risk. Implications for trial design and precision sleep medicine. Am J Respir Crit Care Med 2019;200(4):412-3.

[62] Mediano O, Sánchez-de-la-Torre M, García-Río F. The role of sleep disorders breathing treatment as a modifiable condition for cardiovascular risk associated hypertension. Eur Heart J 2019;40(38):3207. doi: 10.1093/eurheartj/ehz602.

[63] Owens JA, Babcock D, Blumer J, Chervin R, Ferber R, Goetting M, et al. The use of pharmacotherapy in the treatment of pediatric insomnia in primary care: rational approaches. A consensus meeting summary. J Clin Sleep Med 2005;1(1):49-59.

[64] Owens JA, Rosen CL, Mindell JA, Kirchner HL. Use of pharmacotherapy for insomnia in child psychiatry practice: A national survey. Sleep Med 2010; 11(7):692-700.

In: Chronic Disease and Disability
Editors: DE Greydanus, P Anne, JD Rowlett et al.
ISBN: 978-1-53617-656-8

Chapter 15

SUDDEN CARDIAC DEATH IN THE PEDIATRIC AND ADOLESCENT POPULATION

John D Rowlett[1,*], MD, FAAP, FACP,
Wesley Arrison[2], PharmD, BCPS and Carson S Villa[3], BS
[1]Director of Pediatrics, St Joseph's/Candler Healthcare System, Savannah, Georgia, Medical College of Georgia, Augusta and Eastern Kentucky University, Richmond, United States of America
[2]Emergency Medicine, St. Joseph's/Candler Healthcare System, Savannah, Georgia, United States of America
and [3]Fourth Year Pharmacy Student, Lipscomb University, Nashville, Tennessee, United States of America

ABSTRACT

Each year nearly 7,000 children, adolescents, and young adults in the United States as well as tens of thousands worldwide die unexpectedly. Nearly 50% of these deaths occur with little or no warning. This discussion reviews the epidemiology, presentation, diagnosis, and management of sudden cardiac death (SCD). SCD is predominantly due to previously unrecognized structural abnormalities of the heart and underlying or acquired conditions that predispose persons, especially when involved in exercise, to sudden death. Topics considered include SCD presenting signs, symptoms, diagnoses, and when applicable, management of common conditions associated with SCD.

INTRODUCTION

Sudden cardiac death (SCD) in the United States and other developed countries is an uncommon but devastating event. SCD is predominantly due to previously unrecognized congenital heart abnormalities. Almost 7,000 asymptomatic children, adolescents, and young

* Corresponding Author's Email: drrowlett@gmail.com.

adults die annually in the United States from SCD. Almost half of these deaths occur with minimal or no warning signs. Causes of sudden cardiac death can vary by region of the world, ethnicities, age group, and even when looking at subpopulations within a country. In the United States, structural cardiovascular disease (e.g., hypertrophic cardiomyopathy [HCM], arrhythmogenic right ventricular cardiomyopathies [ARVC], Marfan syndrome) is responsible for about 40% of these deaths; also, many are from inherited channelopathies (i.e., Brugada and long QT syndromes, catecholaminergic polymorphic ventricular tachycardia) and commotio cordis (see Table 1).

Table 1. Major causes of sudden death in adolescents and young adults

1.	Hypertrophic cardiomyopathies
2.	Arrhythmogenic right ventricular cardiomyopathy
3.	Anomalous coronary artery
4.	Marfan syndrome
5.	Ion channelopathies (long qT, Brugada)
6.	Commotio cordis
7.	Sickle cell trait
8.	Myocarditis (not reviewed in this chapter)

Autopsies are normal in up to 40% of cases of SCD in children and adolescents (1-3). Finocchiaro and colleagues reviewed autopsies of 79 British athletes less than 18 years of age who died suddenly; 45% had structurally abnormal hearts (4). In addition to HCM and cardiomyopathies, a substantial number of athletes had anomalous coronary arteries or myocarditis as a contributing factor in their death (4). The bulk of the remaining deaths were attributed to "sudden arrhythmic death syndrome" which encompasses the channelopathies and other entities (4). The addition of post-mortem next-generation genetic testing, a "molecular autopsy," has been shown to identify formerly silent clinically relevant cardiac gene mutations in one-quarter of those SCD victims with previously unclassified causes of death (3).

In the general population, most cases of SCD occur at rest or with minimal exertion; however, in the athletes autopsied, between 60% and 80% were engaged in competitive events/training at the time of their demise (4-6). Data on Italian athletes suggests a 2.8 fold increase in SCD compared to nonathletes; researchers hypothesize exercise-induced surges in catecholamines acting on arrhythmogenic substrates (7). Additional factors, including dehydration, hyperpyrexia, and electrolyte abnormalities, are thought to contribute to the increased incidence of death during exertion (8).

There is a significant male predominance in SCD associated with exertion; the incidence of SCD in high school male athletes is nine times that of female athletes; SCD decreases to five times more likely among male collegiate athletes (compared to women) (6, 9). Data on collegiate athletes suggests that elite African-American athletes are more than twice as likely to die from SCD than white peers; the contribution of underlying hypertrophic cardiomyopathy, twice as common in the elite black athletes, is thought to be influential though other factors may be contributory (9, 10). Among division I basketball players in the United States, the incidence of SCD is 14-times that of non-athletes (9).

Etiologic topics now considered are hypertrophic cardiomyopathy (HCM), arrhythmogenic right ventricular cardiomyopathy (ARVC), anomalous coronary artery, Marfan syndrome, ion channelopathies (i.e., Brugada syndrome, Long QT syndrome), cardiovascular effects of energy drinks, commotio cordis, and sickle cell trait. Then, screening for SCD (including use of echocardiography) is considered along with the importance of emergency preparedness and legal issues in sudden cardiac death.

HYPERTROPHIC CARDIOMYOPATHY (HCM)

Hypertrophic cardiomyopathy (HCM) is the root cause of up to 35% of pediatric SCD cases and is the most common structural heart condition associated with SCD in adolescents and young adults (11). High profile athlete deaths (i.e., Hank Gathers [1990], Reggie Lewis [1993]) have received intense coverage in the United States; videos of their actual deaths are widely available on the internet. HCM is defined as a hypertrophied, asymmetric non-dilated left ventricle without underlying cardiac disease (12). HCM is definitively diagnosed by either echocardiography or cardiac magnetic resonance imaging (12).

Despite public perception of this being a common disease with a high mortality rate, the actual prevalence of the disease is low. While the true prevalence in children is not known, HCM is estimated to affect 1 in 500 young adults (13, 14). HCM is inherited as an autosomal dominant; more than 1,400 mutations in multiple genes that code for proteins of the cardiac centromere have been found. Genetic screening is helpful in family members of those with known HCM, but many cases are *de novo* mutations. In families without previous history of HCM, the most common mutations involve the β-myosin heavy chain gene on chromosome 14 q11.2-3 (15).

Symptoms of HCM range from completely asymptomatic to mildly symptomatic (exertional fatigue) to edema, shortness of breath, heart failure, irregular heart rhythms, syncope, and sudden death. Pediatric and young adult patients with HCM who do not present with sudden cardiac death may present with a positive family history or what was thought to be a benign murmur. More profound presenting symptoms short of SCD, include syncope, heart failure, and arrhythmias. Dyspnea is secondary to impaired filling of the stiffened left ventricle with concomitant elevated left ventricular and left atrial pressures with pulmonary congestion. Presentations associated with significant symptoms are associated with increased mortality (13, 14, 16). Many cases of SCD associated with HCM are in previously undiagnosed individuals.

Weissler-Snir and colleagues reviewed all HCM related SCD in persons 10-45 years of age in Ontario between 2005 and 2016 (70 million person-years) (17). Cases were classified as either definite, probably, or possibly HCM; identified were 44 definite, 3 probable, and 6 possible cases of SCD secondary to HCM (17). The majority of SCD events occurred in previously undiagnosed individuals; only 15% of these deaths were associated with vigorous activity, suggesting that exercise guidelines in some persons with HCM may be too restrictive (17).

For persons with HCM, several risk factors have been associated with increased risk of sudden cardiac death; these include extreme left ventricular hypertrophy, family history of SCD, unexplained syncope, non-sustained ventricular arrhythmias on Holter monitor, cardiac ejection fraction <50%, left apical aneurysm, and hypotensive response to exercise (16, 18). Of these, extreme left ventricular hypertrophy is the most powerful risk factor. Persons with symptomatic HCM should be considered for automatic internal cardiac defibrillator (AICD) placement. AICDs have been shown to be effective in terminating potentially fatal arrhythmias in children and adolescents with HCM.

Maron et al. reported on 224 children with HCM deemed at high risk for SCD who received AICDs for either primary (n=188) or secondary (after cardiac arrest, n=36) prevention (18). Over the 4-year study period, 19% of the defibrillators appropriately activated and terminated ventricular arrhythmias. Importantly, 3% of these patients had never previously suffered a cardiac event and were identified (and saved) based on risk factors (18). Extreme left ventricular hypertrophy was the most common risk factor in persons who had AICD termination of ventricular arrhythmias. While proven effective, AICDs use is still limited by availability and cost. Further, AICD malfunction (lead failure, inappropriate shocks) occurs in nearly 40% of patients under age 25-years (18).

Surgical septal myectomy is an "open-heart" procedure that entails removing a portion of the interventricular septum and has been shown to prolong life in infants, children, and young adults with severe outflow obstruction secondary to HCM. When performed at experienced centers, the mortality rate is less than 1% with 85% of patients having markedly improved outcomes. Complications of surgical myectomy include death, arrhythmias, infection and stroke among others (12, 19).

ARRHYTHMOGENIC RIGHT VENTRICLE CARDIOMYOPATHY (ARVC)

Arrhythmogenic right ventricular cardiomyopathy (ARVC) is an inherited, non-ischemic disorder with a reported incidence of up to 1:1,000 in the general population. It is an increasingly recognized cause of sudden death in young persons, especially athletes. Structural changes of the right ventricle (and often left) may be asymptomatic up until the sentinel event; however, signs of right heart failure (i.e., ankle swelling), syncope, and non-fatal arrhythmias are sometimes present. ARVC is inherited in different patterns including autosomal dominant and recessive; many cases are spontaneous or due to new mutations.

Pathogenesis of ARVC is unclear, though typical autopsy findings include apoptosis, fatty infiltration, fibro-fatty infiltration, and dilation of the right ventricle. Death is from ventricular tachydysrhythmias. Pre-morbid ECG in patients with ARVC may reveal non-specific T-wave inversion in leads v1-v3, right bundle branch block, and premature ventricular contractions. Echocardiography may demonstrate a hypokinetic dilated right ventricle with thinning of the wall and occasional tricuspid regurgitation. Cardiac magnetic resonance imaging (MRI) reveals fatty infiltration of the right and occasionally left ventricle as well as right ventricle free wall thinning. Transvenous biopsy of the right ventricle is highly specific but due to spotty disease, lacks sensitivity (20, 21).

In those patients with pre-morbid diagnosis of ARVC, management includes limiting sports/exertional activities and treatment with a combination of medications (i.e., beta blockers, amiodarone), catheter ablation, and implantable cardioverter-defibrillator. Patients with severe right ventricular hypokinesis may benefit from anti-coagulation to decrease risk of thromboembolic events. Heart transplantation has been successfully utilized in advanced heart failure secondary to ARVC (21-25).

ANOMALOUS CORONARY ARTERY

Coronary artery abnormalities are found in about 7% of SCD cases involving adolescents and young adults; of these, the majority are due to anomalous origin (4). The most common anomalies are the right coronary artery originating in the left sinus of Valsalva and the left coronary originating in the right sinus of Valsalva. Coronary flow, particularly during exercise, is compromised by the compression of the vessel (at the ostium) as it travels between the aorta and the pulmonary artery (8, 26).

Finocchiaro and colleagues reviewed 5,100 consecutive cases of SCD at a specialty cardiac pathology center in London and 30 cases of anomalous coronary artery origin as the culprit lesion. In eight cases, the decedent was less than 18 years of age; 50% of the deaths were associated with exercise or emotional stress (27). Based on tissue microscopy, death is felt to be more often from ischemic arrhythmias than overt infarction (27). Pre-participation screening echocardiography detected two cases of anomalous coronary artery in a cohort of more than 11,000 adolescent soccer players (28). Both underwent corrective surgery; they had successful and uneventful soccer careers (28).

MARFAN SYNDROME

Marfan syndrome is an inherited autosomal dominant collagen disorder characterized by mutations in the genes encoding for fibrillin. The estimated prevalence of Marfan syndrome is 1 in 5,000 and it accounts for about 3% of cases of SCD in young athletes. Marfan syndrome is characterized by disorders of the ocular lens (ectopia lentis [lens dislocation]), skeletal abnormalities (i.e., arm span-to-height ratio greater than 1.05, tall stature, arachnodactly, ligament laxity and hyperextensibility), and cardiac abnormalities (i.e., aortic dilation, dissection, and rupture). Accordingly, clinicians should consider the *possibility* of Marfan syndrome in taller athletes (e.g., volleyball and basketball players) (29).

Diagnosis is made by a combination of echocardiographic findings, slit-lamp examination findings, physical examination, and genetic testing. Aortic pathology is caused by cystic medial necrosis in the tunica media of the aorta. This increase in pressure may be intensified by exercise and those with Marfan syndrome should be restricted from both isotonic and isometric exercise of moderate or greater intensity. Beta blockers should be used if echocardiography demonstrates an aortic root >40mm (8, 30-32).

ION CHANNELOPATHIES

Disorders of cardiac conduction, both congenital and acquired, are responsible for most of the cases of sudden cardiac death in persons with structurally normal hearts. Brugada syndrome and long QT (congenital or acquired) may present as sudden death in otherwise healthy children and young adults.

Brugada Syndrome

First described in 1992 by two Italian cardiologists (Pedro and Josep Brugada), the Brugada syndrome is a channelopathy that is an increasingly recognized cause of sudden death (33). The true prevalence in children is not known, but it is exceedingly rare. An autosomal dominant disease with an estimated prevalence of .0005% in the general population, Brugada syndrome is defined by ECG findings (see Table 2) (34). Curiously, a third Brugada brother (Ramon), also a cardiologist, described the initial genetic mutation associated with this disease. In addition to sudden cardiac death, patients with the Brugada mutation may present with ventricular tachydysrhythmias (i.e., ventricular tachycardia, polymorphic tachycardia [TdP; Torsades de pointes---"twisting of the points"] and syncope. Provocative factors include heavy meals, alcohol consumption, cocaine, sleep, and especially in children, fever.

Table 2. ECG findings in Brugada syndrome (35)

Type 1	coved ST elevations with at least 2 mm J point elevations and gradually descending ST segment followed by a negative t-wave
Type 2	Saddle back pattern with at least 2 mm J point elevation and 1 mm ST elevation with positive or biphasic t wave
Type 3	coved or saddle-back pattern with < 2mm j4point elevation and less than 1 mm ST elevation (can occur in healthy subjects)

Prompt treatment of fever with anti-pyretics in persons with known Brugada syndrome is advised. Certain medications (i.e., flecainide, verapamil, propranolol, amitriptyline) should also be avoided (35). In addition to lifestyle advice (avoiding certain medications, alcohol, cocaine, heavy meals, limiting exercise [though this is of questionable value as some fatal events have occurred during sleep]), implantable cardiovert-defibrillator (ICD) may be beneficial. For those with persistent firing of an ICD, additional anti-arrhythmic medication (quinidine) or radiofrequency catheter ablation may be considered (36).

Long QT syndrome: Congenital and acquired

Prolongation of the QT interval, whether congenital or acquired (drug-induced), is an important cause of morbidity (seizures, syncope, ventricular dysrhythmias) and sudden cardiac death. The QT interval on an electrocardiogram (ECG) represents the time it takes for the heart to repolarize after the onset of depolarization. The interval (reported in milliseconds [ms]) is measured from the beginning of the QRS complex to the end of the T wave. Since the interval is inversely related to the heart rate, it is necessary to use the corrected QT interval (QTc) for clinical interpretation. The formula used to calculate the QTc interval is an estimate of the original QT interval if the heart rate was regulated at 60 bpm; this will eliminate any misinterpretations of the interval due to fast or slow heart rates (37).

A normal QTc value will vary based on age and gender. In general, most adult males and females are considered to have a prolonged QTc if the interval is greater than 450 ms and 470 ms, respectively. It is extremely important to take note of a prolonged QTc interval because the patient may be at risk of developing a polymorphic ventricular tachycardia (TdP) or other fatal dysrhythmias. When the QTc interval reaches a value greater than 500 ms, the patient is at a high risk for TdP, ventricular fibrillation and cardiac arrest (38).

There are some unmodifiable risk factors that could put a patient at risk for QTc prolongation. These include older age, female gender, genetic predispositions (congenital/familial long QT syndrome), structural heart disease, low left ventricular heart disease and impaired elimination due to renal or hepatic disease. In the acute setting, it is extremely important to identify and correct modifiable risk factors, including hypomagnesemia, hypokalemia and hypocalcemia (37). While correcting these electrolyte abnormalities will help reduce the risk of developing tachydysrhythmias, the risk may transiently increase in select cases of the refeeding syndrome (severe malnutrition, including patients with anorexia nervosa). Medical historians credit Hippocrates with recognizing this in his 5th century BC work "De Carnibus" (On Fleshes) in which he writes "If a person goes seven days without eating or drinking anything, in this period most die; but there are some who survive that time but still die (39)."

In persons with congenital long QT syndrome, one or more of the cardiac ion channels is altered resulting in deranged permeability that manifests as prolonged depolarization. Though it may be quiescent, congenital long QT syndrome typically presents in the second decade as syncope, seizures, or sudden cardiac death; estimated prevalence is as high as 1 in 2,000 persons (13, 40-42). Persons with known congenital long QT syndrome should be restricted from competitive sports and may benefit from beta-blocker and/or implantable defibrillators (41).

Many commonly used medications can put a patient at risk for acquired QTc prolongation (see Table 3). The online resource, *crediblemeds.org* maintains an accurate list of medications known to prolong the QTc as well as potential drug-drug interactions. Antiarrhythmic medications are frequently linked to this side effect, but not all are high risk. Sotalol and amiodarone are among the top offenders for QTc prolongation in this drug class, although the risk of developing TdP is much lower with amiodarone compared to sotalol. Also, non-cardiac medications can cause prolongation by either blocking potassium current or by enhancing the concentration of other drugs that have this affect. Many antimicrobial agents, such as macrolides, fluoroquinolones and antifungals, are associated with QTc prolongation and TdP (43, 44).

Table 3. Common drugs associated with QTc prolongation (91)

Antiarrhythmics	Antimicrobial	Psychiatric	Antidepressants	Anti-fungals	Others
Amiodarone	Azithromycin	Haloperidol	Amitriptyline	Ketoconazole	Ondansetron
Procainamide	clarithromycin	Droperidol	Imipramine	Voriconazole	Sumatriptan
Sotalol	Erythromycin	Quetiapine	Doxepin	Fluconazole	zolmitriptan
Quinidine	Levofloxacin	ziprasidone	Sertraline		Methadone
Flecanide	Ciprofloxacin	Olanzapine	Venlafaxine		Propofol
	Trimethoprim-Sulfamethoxazole				Loperamide
					Metoclopramide
					Tacrolimus

Certain antipsychotics have been associated with risk of certain death and many agents have been removed from the market or are no longer recommended in common practice. Droperidol now has a black box warning for QT prolongation and the incidence of TdP (45,

46). Schneeweiss recommends obtaining a baseline electrocardiogram before initiation of any anti-psychotic (47). Many studies have also established QTc prolongation with antiemetics, such as ondansetron; however, no current literature reports a case of TdP associated with its use (48, 49). The chance of developing prolongation is the highest within the first few days of therapy and close monitoring should be performed for patients with multiple risk factors. Most of these medications are metabolized by the liver through cytochrome isoenzymes CYP3A4, 1A2, and 2D6; this makes drug-drug interactions another risk for developing QTc prolongation (50).

Electrolytes should be monitored regularly for early intervention if there is an abnormality. If QTc prolongation occurs after a suspected medication is initiated, the medication should be promptly stopped to avoid progression into TdP. The treatment of TdP is 1- 2 grams of intravenous magnesium sulfate given over a 15-minute duration. Athletes with known or suspected channelopathies should undergo comprehensive cardiac evaluation; limited participation may be resumed--presuming appropriate precautionary measures and disease specific treatments are in place. Avoidance of all drugs which may prolong the QTc, dehydration, stimulants are mandatory. Athletes are strongly encouraged to have an emergency action plan as well as a personal external defibrillator (51).

CARDIOVASCULAR EFFECTS OF ENERGY DRINKS (EDS)

The consumption of energy drinks (ED) is now commonplace among adolescents and young adults; this includes EDs with increased concentrations of caffeine, taurine, guarana, and l-carnitine. One study estimates the global market for energy drinks in 2021 will surpass *61 billion* dollars (52). Use increases with age and about 1 in three middle- and high-school students endorse regular use of energy drinks; indeed, a survey of more than 1,500 nursing students revealed nearly 80% of them routinely consumed EDs, ranging from 1 to 30 cans weekly (52, 53). Except for caffeine, the cardiovascular effects of most of the ingredients in energy drinks have not been thoroughly studied. In general, these drinks have been shown to increase heart rate, blood pressure, and arrhythmias (including atrial fibrillation). Daily intake has been demonstrated to have an increasing effect (elevation) of blood pressure compared to occasional intake (54).

Cases of sudden cardiac death have been reported after consumption of energy drinks; however, assigning specific causation is difficult (55). The literature on this is sparse, anecdotal, and frequently industry sponsored. It is known that consumption of energy drinks is associated with short-term and sustained increases in the QTc, though the absolute as well as relative effects are highly variable, and the effects do not seem attributable to a single specific ingredient. Indeed, it is most probable that the common pathway is arrhythmogenesis, especially in those with known or unrecognized underlying predisposition to cardiac rhythm abnormalities (52, 56-58).

Water, not energy or sports drinks, should be promoted as the principle fluid for maintaining hydration (59). The risk may be compounded by various factors such as electrolyte depletion (hypokalemia, hypomagnesemia), dehydration, and increased core temperature and/or heart rate; thus, it is particularly prudent that athletes with any propensity to arrhythmia be instructed to avoid such drinks or EDs (60, 61).

Commotio cordis

Sudden impact to the chest wall, as when struck with a baseball or other object, may cause sudden cardiac death, otherwise known as "Commotio cordis" (from the Latin "agitation of the heart"). Maron reports that this has been described in the medical literature since the 1700s (62). The exact incidence of deaths secondary to commotio cordis is unknown, but it is estimated to be the second most common cause of sudden death in athletes, second only to HCM (62-64).

Since the creation of the National Commotio Cordis Registry in the United States in the 1990s, more than 200 cases have been confirmed (63, 64). Of these, more than 95% involved males, and of these, most were youth (only 9% were older than 25 years of age). Only one-fourth of these cases involved non-athletes. The most common causes were batted or thrown baseballs, lacrosse balls, hockey pucks and direct blows (football, soccer, martial arts) (62-64).

The mechanism of death is thought to be an elicited electrical impulse during the early portion of ventricular repolarization resulting in ventricular fibrillation. To date this has only been described with impacts over the cardiac silhouette; increased velocity and harder objects are more likely to be associated with commotio cordis (63-68).

The widespread availability of defibrillators at sporting events has decreased the fatality rate from commotio cordis. Though frequently fatal, those who survive such an event should undergo a comprehensive evaluation looking for underlying structural heart disease (i.e., HCM, arrhythmogenic right ventricle) or channelopathy (69). Numerous organizations are looking at the development of safer equipment, but to date chest wall protectors have not been shown to decrease the incidence of commotio cordis; many of the victims in the national registry were wearing appropriate chest wall protective equipment at the time of their demise (63).

Sickle cell trait

In 1987, Kark et al. concluded that U.S. Armed Forces recruits in basic training with sickle-cell trait (hemoglobin AS, SCT) had a substantially increased, age-dependent risk of exercise-related sudden death (70). Using published prevalence rates, they reported that recruits with hemoglobin AS were 27 times more likely to suffer unexplained sudden cardiac death than those without hemoglobin S (70). Nelson and colleagues, however, reported that SCT was not associated with a higher risk of death in a cohort of nearly 50,000 Black US soldiers, including 3564 with hemoglobin AS; however, they did find a higher risk of exertional rhabdomyolysis (71). Similarly, hemoglobin AS confers increased risk of rhabdomyolysis and in some cases, increased risk of death to athletes.

The U.S. National Collegiate Athletic Association (NCAA) began mandated SCT screening for all Division 1 athletes and has expanded it now to include all student-athletes (Divisions 1, 2, and 3) (72). Importantly, though mandatory to be screened for SCT, the NCAA does not prohibit athletes with SCT from sports participation (72). NCAA Division 1 football players with hemoglobin AS have a 37-fold increased risk of sudden cardiovascular collapse and death than other student-athletes (73).

The mechanism of collapse and death in athletes with hemoglobin AS is not precisely understood, though it appears that in some situations, progressive sickling can begin after a few minutes of high intensity exercise and "logjam" vessels, resulting in explosive rhabdomyolysis, collapse, and occasionally death. Proposed contributory factors include a combination of environmental issues (i.e., high ambient temperatures, high humidity), previous exertional rhabdomyolysis, genetic factors, dietary factors (i.e., energy drinks, caffeine) (73-76). Recognition of athletes at risk for this syndrome and tailored workouts may decrease but not eliminate this process (74-76).

Screening for SCD

There is consensus among major medical societies that athletes should have some form of preparticipation cardiac screening; there is, however, no consensus as to what this screening should entail. The American Heart Association (AHA) issued a policy statement in 1996 recommending a comprehensive personal and family history as well as physical examination but stopped short of recommending routine screening electrocardiograms (77). This approach has been demonstrated to have both a high-false positive and limited sensitivity for detecting SCD risk factors (77). In contrast, the European Society of Cardiology endorsed in 2005 the use of routine preparticipation electrocardiograms (78).

A 2019 study published by the American Heart Association suggests that the latter is a more efficacious approach. Using an enhanced (14-part) AHA evaluation with physical examination and ECG, more than 3,600 high school athletes were screened (79). The AHA and physical examination underperformed the ECG in sensitivity, specificity, and positive predictive value for identifying conditions placing athletes at risk for sudden cardiac death (79). In an editorial in the same journal, Dr. Barry Maron strongly disputes this recommendation stating that when properly applied, the AHA criteria are more effective and notes that there is no evidence that screening ECG reduces mortality for SCD (80). Dr Barry Maron is widely regarded as one of the top experts in the world on this subject; indeed, PubMed (maintained by the National Center for Biotechnology Information that is part of the US National Library of Medicine) credits this expert with more than 790 peer-reviewed articles, largely on the subject of sudden cardiac death) (62-64, 80).

One problem identified in this screening dilemma is the inter-observer variation in the interpretation of the ECG; those read by highly skilled cardiologists using different published criteria (i.e., Seattle criteria, European Society of Cardiology, International) demonstrate widely variable results; indeed, the international criteria seem to have the highest sensitivity and specificity in this regard (81). In addition to questionable efficacy, Halkin estimates that the total cost of mandatory ECG screening (and associated down-stream testing) to be more than 2 billion dollars per year at a cost of 14 million dollars per life-saved (using the Italian data for possible efficacy disputed by Maron) (82).

Landry reviewed all out-of-hospital cardiac arrests during sports participation for a five year period in Ontario and found 3 of 74 patients with SCD who could have theoretically been detected at risk for SCD with screening ECG and physical examination---noting that for each patient identified, nearly 150,000 would have to be screened (83). Of note, this cohort included patients to age 45 years of age; of the 13 events in patients ages 12-17-years, 5 were from structural lesions, 4 were thought to be primary arrhythmic, 2 were from commotio cordis, and two unknowns (83). Impressively, 8 of the 13 youth who suffered sudden cardiac arrest survived (83).

Malhotra published the results of a 20-year European study of adolescent soccer players who underwent screening history, physical examination, ECG and echocardiography (28). During the screening process, 38% of these athletes were found to have conditions predisposing to SCD and were disqualified (28). Of the remaining more than 11,000 athletes, there were 8 cases of sudden cardiac death in the following years. Upon further review, seven of these deaths were from a cardiomyopathy; five of these had completely normal screening examination. Two patient who subsequently died had been identified as having an abnormal ECG and echocardiogram (28).

Echocardiography

Echocardiography provides detailed structural and to some extent functional views of the cardiac anatomy. Echocardiograph is non-invasive and readily available in most communities in the United States; however, it is not available in some centers around the world. Limited echocardiography, in combination with comprehensive history, physical examination, and ECG has been suggested a tool for identifying athletes (and others) at risk for sudden cardiac death. Rizzo et al. screened 3,100 adolescent male soccer players and found structural cardiac lesions in 56 subjects (1.8%); none of these athletes were detected by standard screening (84). Of these, most were clinically insignificant with respect to athletic competition (i.e., bicuspid aortic valve, mild mitral valve prolapse, asymptomatic atrial septal defect); HCM was detected in two subjects (84).

Wyman screened nearly 400 asymptomatic athletes and found 5 athletes requiring more detailed evaluation by a cardiologist (85). Anderson et al. screened more than 650 adolescent athletes and found a total of 5 subjects at increased risk for sudden cardiac death; none of these were identified solely by echocardiogram (86). Importantly, multiple patients identified as having left ventricular hypertrophy on ECG were found on echocardiogram to have normal ventricles (86). Further, echocardiogram did identify otherwise undetected cardiac abnormalities NOT associated with increased short-term sudden cardiac death risk (86).

Modaff reviewed the charts of nearly 3000 athletes screened at a single university with a combination of standard preparticipation history and physical and a focused 5-minute echocardiogram (87). A total of three athletes (0.1%) were ultimately found to have abnormalities that warranted restriction of participation (1 with HCN, 1 with a dilated aorta, and 1 with large atrial septal defect; 2 of these had normal preparticipation history and physical examination) (87). In short, focused echocardiography identified 2 patients out of 2,898 with asymptomatic pathology which limited participation. Further, of more than 650 athletes with abnormal preparticipation history/physical, only 1 (0.15%) had an abnormal echocardiogram. The authors concluded that although the overall number was low, the echocardiogram can detect athletes at risk for sudden cardiac death not detected by routine testing (87). It is unclear whether these two patients would have been identified by electrocardiography, but it is probable that the patient with the large ASD would have had an bi-atrial hypertrophy.

The role of selected echocardiography to evaluate for possible Marfan syndromes in selected sports favoring increased height (i.e., volleyball, basketball) remains controversial, though the National Basketball Association now requires pre-season ECGs and stress echocardiograms in the United States (88). Harmon et al. reported that male high school basketball players had 2.5-fold increased risk of sudden cardiac death compared to male peers in other sports and nearly 15-fold increased risk of death compared to female athletes (5).

Emergency preparedness

The widespread availability of external cardiac defibrillators has contributed to increased survivability of SCD events. The interval between arrest and defibrillation is the single biggest contributor to survival. Prompt defibrillation of malignant dysrhythmias is associated with increased survival; for cases of ventricular fibrillation, the survival rate declines up to 10% for each minute defibrillation is delayed (89). Effective bystander cardiopulmonary resuscitation attenuates this decrease to 3-4 percent decline in survival per minute that defibrillation is delayed. Venue and staff preparedness are critical in improving the outcome in SCD (89).

Legal issues

In addition to content, cost, and efficacy, there are increasing legal issues involved in screening athletes and prohibiting them from competition. Applicable case law is evolving, but courts have consistently upheld the right of educational institutions (i.e., high schools, universities) to exclude athletes with high-risk cardiovascular conditions from competition; courts have supported the use of national medical association guidelines in formulating eligibility/disqualification decisions (90).

Summary

Sudden death is a reality for young persons that annually includes nearly 7000 children, adolescents and young adults in the United States as well as tens of thousands around the world. Nearly 50% of these deaths occur with little or no warning. Causes of death including sudden cardiac death can vary by region of the world, ethnicities, age group, and even when looking at subpopulations within a country (90-98). Etiologic topics reflected in this discussion include hypertrophic cardiomyopathy (HCM), arrhythmogenic right ventricular cardiomyopathy (ARVC), anomalous coronary artery, Marfan syndrome, ion channelopathies (i.e., Brugada syndrome, Long QT syndrome), potential cardiovascular effects of energy drinks, commotio cordis, and published links of sickle cell trait with SCD (2-5, 99). Also considered is the complex as well as controversial subject of SCD screening (including use of echocardiography) along with the importance of widespread availability of external cardiac defibrillators to save lives and legal issues faced by educational entities (i.e., high schools, colleges, universities) with regard to SCD (2, 100).

REFERENCES

[1] Kauferstein S, Kiehne N, Neumann T, Pitschner HF, Bratzke H. Cardiac gene defects can cause sudden cardiac death in young people. Dtsch Arztebl Int 2009;106(4):41-7.

[2] Paterick TE, Jan MF, Paterick ZR, Umland MM, Kramer C, Lake P, et al. Cardiac evaluation of collegiate student athletes: a medical and legal perspective. Am J Med 2012;125(8):742-52.

[3] Bagnall RD, Weintraub RG, Ingles J, Duflou J, Yeates L, Lam L, et al. A prospective study of sudden cardiac death among children and young adults. N Engl J Med 2016;374(25):2441-52.

[4] Finocchiaro G, Papadakis M, Robertus JL, Dhutia H, Steriotis AK, Tome M, et al. Etiology of sudden death in sports: Insights from a United Kingdom regional registry. J Am Coll Cardiol 2016;67(18):2108-15.

[5] Harmon KG, Asif IM, Maleszewski JJ, Owens DS, Prutkin JM, Salerno JC, et al. Incidence and etiology of sudden cardiac arrest and death in high school athletes in the United States. Mayo Clin Proc 2016;91(11):1493-502.

[6] Van Camp SP, Bloor CM, Mueller FO, Cantu RC, Olson HG. Nontraumatic sports death in high school and college athletes. Med Sci Sports Exerc 1995;27(5):641-7.

[7] Corrado D, Basso C, Schiavon M, Thiene G. Does sports activity enhance the risk of sudden cardiac death? J Cardiovasc Med (Hagerstown). 2006;7(4):228-33.

[8] Chandra N, Bastiaenen R, Papadakis M, Sharma S. Sudden cardiac death in young athletes: practical challenges and diagnostic dilemmas. J Am Coll Cardiol 2013;61(10):1027-40.

[9] Harmon KG, Asif IM, Klossner D, Drezner JA. Incidence of sudden cardiac death in National Collegiate Athletic Association athletes. Circulation 2011;123(15):1594-600.

[10] Harmon KG, Asif IM, Maleszewski JJ, Owens DS, Prutkin JM, Salerno JC, et al. Incidence, cause, and comparative frequency of sudden cardiac death in National Collegiate Athletic Association athletes: A decade in review. Circulation 2015;132(1):10-9.

[11] Maron BJ, Doerer JJ, Haas TS, Tierney DM, Mueller FO. Sudden deaths in young competitive athletes: analysis of 1866 deaths in the United States, 1980-2006. Circulation 2009;119(8):1085-92.

[12] Maron BJ, Maron MS. Hypertrophic cardiomyopathy. Lancet 2013;381(9862):242-55.

[13] Fant C, Cohen A. Syncope in pediatric patients: a practical approach to differential diagnosis and managment in the emergency department. Pediatr Emerg Med Pract 2017;14(4):1-28.

[14] Maskatia SA. Hypertrophic cardiomyopathy: infants, children, and adolescents. Congenit Heart Dis 2012;7(1):84-92.

[15] Maron BJ, Maron MS, Semsarian C. Genetics of hypertrophic cardiomyopathy after 20 years: clinical perspectives. J Am Coll Cardiol 2012;60(8):705-15.

[16] Maron BJ. Clinical course and management of hypertrophic cardiomyopathy. N Engl J Med 2018;379(20):1977.

[17] Weissler-Snir A, Allan K, Cunningham K, Connelly KA, Lee DS, Spears DA, et al. Hypertrophic cardiomyopathy-related sudden cardiac death in young people in Ontario. Circulation 2019;140(21):1706-1716.

[18] Maron BJ, Spirito P, Ackerman MJ, Casey SA, Semsarian C, Estes NA, 3rd, et al. Prevention of sudden cardiac death with implantable cardioverter-defibrillators in children and adolescents with hypertrophic cardiomyopathy. J Am Coll Cardiol 2013;61(14):1527-35.

[19] Behr ER, McKenna WJ. Hypertrophic cardiomyopathy. Curr Treat Options Cardiovasc Med 2002;4(6):443-53.

[20] Asimaki A, Tandri H, Huang H, Halushka MK, Gautam S, Basso C, et al. A new diagnostic test for arrhythmogenic right ventricular cardiomyopathy. N Engl J Med 2009;360(11):1075-84.

[21] Basso C, Corrado D, Marcus FI, Nava A, Thiene G. Arrhythmogenic right ventricular cardiomyopathy. Lancet 2009;373(9671):1289-300.

[22] Fontaine G, Tonet J, Gallais Y, Lascault G, Hidden-Lucet F, Aouate P, et al. Ventricular tachycardia catheter ablation in arrhythmogenic right ventricular dysplasia: a 16-year experience. Curr Cardiol Rep 2000;2(6):498-506.

[23] Corrado D, Basso C, Thiene G, McKenna WJ, Davies MJ, Fontaliran F, et al. Spectrum of clinicopathologic manifestations of arrhythmogenic right ventricular cardiomyopathy/dysplasia: a multicenter study. J Am Coll Cardiol 1997;30(6):1512-20.

[24] Corrado D, Leoni L, Link MS, Della Bella P, Gaita F, Curnis A, et al. Implantable cardioverter-defibrillator therapy for prevention of sudden death in patients with arrhythmogenic right ventricular cardiomyopathy/dysplasia. Circulation 2003;108(25):3084-91.

[25] Corrado D, Calkins H, Link MS, Leoni L, Favale S, Bevilacqua M, et al. Prophylactic implantable defibrillator in patients with arrhythmogenic right ventricular cardiomyopathy/dysplasia and no prior ventricular fibrillation or sustained ventricular tachycardia. Circulation 2010;122(12):1144-52.

[26] Basso C, Maron BJ, Corrado D, Thiene G. Clinical profile of congenital coronary artery anomalies with origin from the wrong aortic sinus leading to sudden death in young competitive athletes. J Am Coll Cardiol 2000;35(6):1493-501.

[27] Finocchiaro G, Behr ER, Tanzarella G, Papadakis M, Malhotra A, Dhutia H, et al. Anomalous coronary artery origin and sudden cardiac death: Clinical and pathological insights from a National Pathology Registry. JACC Clin Electrophysiol 2019;5(4):516-22.

[28] Malhotra A, Dhutia H, Finocchiaro G, Gati S, Beasley I, Clift P, et al. Outcomes of cardiac screening in adolescent soccer players. N Engl J Med 2018;379(6):524-34.

[29] McClain LG. The tall athlete and Marfan syndrome. Need for clinical differentiation. J Adolesc Health 1989;10(6):564-6.

[30] Yetman AT, Bornemeier RA, McCrindle BW. Long-term outcome in patients with Marfan syndrome: is aortic dissection the only cause of sudden death? J Am Coll Cardiol 2003;41(2):329-32.

[31] Maron BJ, Zipes DP. Introduction: eligibility recommendations for competitive athletes with cardiovascular abnormalities-general considerations. J Am Coll Cardiol 2005;45(8):1318-21.

[32] Maron BJ, Ackerman MJ, Nishimura RA, Pyeritz RE, Towbin JA, Udelson JE. Task Force 4: HCM and other cardiomyopathies, mitral valve prolapse, myocarditis, and Marfan syndrome. J Am Coll Cardiol 2005;45(8):1340-5.

[33] Brugada P, Brugada J. Right bundle branch block, persistent ST segment elevation and sudden cardiac death: a distinct clinical and electrocardiographic syndrome. A multicenter report. J Am Coll Cardiol 1992;20(6):1391-6.

[34] Probst V, Denjoy I, Meregalli PG, Amirault JC, Sacher F, Mansourati J, et al. Clinical aspects and prognosis of Brugada syndrome in children. Circulation 2007;115(15):2042-8.

[35] Postema PG, Wolpert C, Amin AS, Probst V, Borggrefe M, Roden DM, et al. Drugs and Brugada syndrome patients: review of the literature, recommendations, and an up-to-date website (www.brugadadrugs.org). Heart Rhythm 2009;6(9):1335-41.

[36] Kautzner J, Peichl P. Catheter ablation to prevent sudden cardiac death. Int J Cardiol 2017;237:29-33.

[37] Al-Khatib SM, LaPointe NM, Kramer JM, Califf RM. What clinicians should know about the QT interval. JAMA 2003;289(16):2120-7.

[38] Roden DM. Drug-induced prolongation of the QT interval. N Engl J Med 2004;350(10):1013-22.

[39] Wikipedia. Refeeding syndrome, 2019 URL: https://en.wikipedia.org/w/index.php?title=Refeeding_syndrome&oldid=921216264.

[40] Levine E, Rosero SZ, Budzikowski AS, Moss AJ, Zareba W, Daubert JP. Congenital long QT syndrome: considerations for primary care physicians. Cleve Clin J Med 2008;75(8):591-600.

[41] Roden DM. Clinical practice. Long-QT syndrome. N Engl J Med 2008;358(2):169-76.

[42] Devinsky O. Sudden, unexpected death in epilepsy. N Engl J Med 2011;365(19):1801-11.

[43] Yap YG, Camm AJ. Drug induced QT prolongation and torsades de pointes. Heart 2003;89(11):1363-72.

[44] Ray WA, Murray KT, Hall K, Arbogast PG, Stein CM. Azithromycin and the risk of cardiovascular death. N Engl J Med 2012;366(20):1881-90.

[45] Taylor DM. Antipsychotics and QT prolongation. Acta Psychiatr Scand 2003;107(2):85-95.

[46] Ray WA, Chung CP, Murray KT, Hall K, Stein CM. Atypical antipsychotic drugs and the risk of sudden cardiac death. N Engl J Med 2009;360(3):225-35.

[47] Schneeweiss S, Avorn J. Antipsychotic agents and sudden cardiac death--how should we manage the risk? N Engl J Med 2009;360(3):294-6.

[48] Moffett PM, Cartwright L, Grossart EA, O'Keefe D, Kang CS. Intravenous ondansetron and the QT interval in adult emergency department patients: An observational study. Acad Emerg Med 2016;23(1):102-5.

[49] Li K, Vo K, Lee BK, Addo N, Coralic Z. Effect of a single dose of i.v. ondansetron on QTc interval in emergency department patients. Am J Health Syst Pharm 2018;75(5):276-82.

[50] Bauman J. The role of phamacokinetics, drug interactions, and pharmacogentics in the acquired long qt syndrome. Eur Heart J Suppl 2001; 3(Suppl K):k93-k100. doi. 10.1016/S1520-765X(01)90012-4.

[51] Ackerman MJ, Zipes DP, Kovacs RJ, Maron BJ. Eligibility and disqualification recommendations for competitive athletes with cardiovascular abnormalities: Task Force 10: The Cardiac Channelopathies: A Scientific Statement From the American Heart Association and American College of Cardiology. J Am Coll Cardiol 2015;66(21):2424-8.

[52] Shah SA, Szeto AH, Farewell R, Shek A, Fan D, Quach KN, et al. Impact of high-volume energy drink consumption on electrocardiographic and blood pressure parameters: A randomized trial. J Am Heart Assoc 2019;8(11):e011318.

[53] Kim IK, Kim KM. Energy drink consumption patterns and associated factors among nursing students: a descriptive survey study. J Addict Nurs 2015;26(1):24-31.

[54] Steinke L, Lanfear DE, Dhanapal V, Kalus JS. Effect of "energy drink" consumption on hemodynamic and electrocardiographic parameters in healthy young adults. Ann Pharmacother 2009;43(4):596-602.

[55] Enriquez A, Frankel DS. Arrhythmogenic effects of energy drinks. J Cardiovasc Electrophysiol 2017;28(6):711-7.

[56] Wassef B, Kohansieh M, Makaryus AN. Effects of energy drinks on the cardiovascular system. World J Cardiol 2017;9(11):796-806.

[57] Ehlers A, Marakis G, Lampen A, Hirsch-Ernst KI. Risk assessment of energy drinks with focus on cardiovascular parameters and energy drink consumption in Europe. Food Chem Toxicol 2019;130:109-21.

[58] Basrai M, Schweinlin A, Menzel J, Mielke H, Weikert C, Dusemund B, et al. Energy drinks induce acute cardiovascular and metabolic changes pointing to potential risks for young adults: A randomized controlled trial. J Nutr 2019;149(3):441-50.

[59] Committee on Nutrition and the Council on Sports Medicine and Fitness. Sports drinks and energy drinks for children and adolescents: are they appropriate? Pediatrics 2011;127(6):1182-9.

[60] Clauson KA, Shields KM, McQueen CE, Persad N. Safety issues associated with commercially available energy drinks. J Am Pharm Assoc 2008;48(3):e55-63; quiz e4-7.

[61] Woosley RL. Arrhythmogenic foods - A growing medical problem. Trends Cardiovasc Med 2019 Aug 24. pii: S1050-1738(19)30116-1. doi: 10.1016/j.tcm.2019.08.007.

[62] Maron BJ, Doerer JJ, Haas TS, Estes NA, 3rd, Link MS. Historical observation on commotio cordis. Heart Rhythm 2006;3(5):605-6.

[63] Maron BJ, Estes NA, 3rd. Commotio cordis. N Engl J Med 2010;362(10):917-27.

[64] Maron BJ, Doerer JJ, Haas TS, Estes NA, Hodges JS, Link MS. Commotio cordis and the epidemiology of sudden death in competitive lacrosse. Pediatrics 2009;124(3):966-71.

[65] Link MS, Wang PJ, Pandian NG, Bharati S, Udelson JE, Lee MY, et al. An experimental model of sudden death due to low-energy chest-wall impact (commotio cordis). N Engl J Med 1998; 338(25):1805-11.

[66] Link MS, Maron BJ. Sudden cardiac death caused by innocent chest wall blows. Ital Heart J 2005; 6(4):281-3.

[67] Link MS. Commotio cordis: ventricular fibrillation triggered by chest impact-induced abnormalities in repolarization. Circ Arrhythm Electrophysiol 2012;5(2):425-32.

[68] Madias C. Commotio cordi. In: UptoDate. Waltham, MA: UpToDate 2019. URL: https://www.uptodate.com/contents/commotio-cordis.

[69] Link MS, Estes NA, 3rd, Maron BJ. Eligibility and disqualification recommendations for competitive athletes with cardiovascular abnormalities: Task Force 13: Commotio Cordis: A Scientific Statement From the American Heart Association and American College of Cardiology. Circulation 2015;132(22):e339-42.

[70] Kark JA, Posey DM, Schumacher HR, Ruehle CJ. Sickle-cell trait as a risk factor for sudden death in physical training. N Engl J Med 1987;317(13):781-7.

[71] Nelson DA, Deuster PA, Carter R, 3rd, Hill OT, Wolcott VL, Kurina LM. Sickle cell trait, rhabdomyolysis, and mortality among U.S. army soldiers. N Engl J Med 2016;375(5):435-42.

[72] Maron BJ, Harris KM, Thompson PD, Eichner ER, Steinberg MH. Eligibility and disqualification recommendations for competitive athletes with cardiovascular abnormalities: Task Force 14: Sickle cell trait: A Scientific Statement From the American Heart Association and American College of Cardiology. J Am Coll Cardiol 2015;66(21):2444-6.

[73] Harmon KG, Drezner JA, Klossner D, Asif IM. Sickle cell trait associated with a RR of death of 37 times in National Collegiate Athletic Association football athletes: a database with 2 million athlete-years as the denominator. Br J Sports Med 2012;46(5):325-30.

[74] Quattrone RD, Eichner ER, Beutler A, Adams WB, O'Connor FG. Exercise collapse associated with sickle cell trait (ECAST): case report and literature review. Curr Sports Med Rep 2015;14(2):110-6.

[75] Harris KM, Haas TS, Eichner ER, Maron BJ. Sickle cell trait associated with sudden death in competitive athletes. Am J Cardiol 2012;110(8):1185-8.

[76] Eichner ER. Sickle cell trait in sports. Curr Sports Med Rep 2010;9(6):347-51.

[77] Fudge J, Harmon KG, Owens DS, Prutkin JM, Salerno JC, Asif IM, et al. Cardiovascular screening in adolescents and young adults: a prospective study comparing the Pre-participation Physical Evaluation Monograph 4th Edition and ECG. Br J Sports Med 2014;48(15):1172-8.

[78] Corrado D, Pelliccia A, Bjornstad HH, Vanhees L, Biffi A, Borjesson M, et al. Cardiovascular pre-participation screening of young competitive athletes for prevention of sudden death: proposal for a common European protocol. Consensus Statement of the Study Group of Sport Cardiology of the Working Group of Cardiac Rehabilitation and Exercise Physiology and the Working Group of Myocardial and Pericardial Diseases of the European Society of Cardiology. Eur Heart J 2005; 26(5):516-24.

[79] Williams EA, Pelto HF, Toresdahl BG, Prutkin JM, Owens DS, Salerno JC, et al. Performance of the American Heart Association (AHA) 14-Point evaluation versus electrocardiography for the cardiovascular screening of high school athletes: A prospective study. J Am Heart Assoc 2019;8(14):e012235.

[80] Maron BJ, Thompson PD, Maron MS. There is no reason to adopt ECG s and abandon American Heart Association/American College of Cardiology history and physical screening for detection of cardiovascular disease in the young. J Am Heart Assoc 2019;8(14):e013007.

[81] Malhotra A, Dhutia H, Yeo TJ, Finocchiaro G, Gati S, Bulleros P, et al. Accuracy of the 2017 international recommendations for clinicians who interpret adolescent athletes' ECGs: a cohort study of 11 168 British white and black soccer players. Br J Sports Med 2019 Jul 5. pii: bjsports-2017-098528. doi: 10.1136/bjsports-2017-098528.

[82] Halkin A, Steinvil A, Rosso R, Adler A, Rozovski U, Viskin S. Preventing sudden death of athletes with electrocardiographic screening: what is the absolute benefit and how much will it cost? J Am Coll Cardiol 2012;60(22):2271-6.

[83] Landry CH, Allan KS, Connelly KA, Cunningham K, Morrison LJ, Dorian P. Sudden cardiac arrest during participation in competitive sports. N Engl J Med 2017;377(20):1943-53.

[84] Rizzo M, Spataro A, Cecchetelli C, Quaranta F, Livrieri S, Sperandii F, et al. Structural cardiac disease diagnosed by echocardiography in asymptomatic young male soccer players: implications for pre-participation screening. Br J Sports Med 2012;46(5):371-3.

[85] Wyman RA, Chiu RY, Rahko PS. The 5-minute screening echocardiogram for athletes. J Am Soc Echocardiogr 2008;21(7):786-8.

[86] Anderson JB, Grenier M, Edwards NM, Madsen NL, Czosek RJ, Spar DS, et al. Usefulness of combined history, physical examination, electrocardiogram, and limited echocardiogram in screening adolescent athletes for risk for sudden cardiac death. Am J Cardiol 2014;114(11):1763-7.

[87] Modaff DS, Hegde SM, Wyman RA, Rahko PS. Usefulness of focused screening echocardiography for collegiate athletes. Am J Cardiol 2019;123(1):169-74.

[88] Waase MP, Mutharasan RK, Whang W, DiTullio MR, DiFiori JP, Callahan L, et al. Electrocardiographic findings in National Basketball Association athletes. JAMA Cardiol 2018;3 (1):69-74.

[89] Drezner JA, Courson RW, Roberts WO, Mosesso VN, Jr., Link MS, Maron BJ. Inter-association task force recommendations on emergency preparedness and management of sudden cardiac arrest in high school and college athletic programs: a consensus statement. Clin J Sport Med 2007;17(2):87-103.

[90] Murray CJ, Lopez AD, Mortality by cause for eight regions of the world: Global Burden of Disease Study. Lancet 1997;349(9061):1269-76.

[91] He PX, Wu L, Jiang J. Etiology, prevention and treatment of sudden cardiac death in youth. Zhonghua Xin Xue Guan Bing Za Zhi 2018;46(8):665-7. [Article in Chinese]

[92] Corrado D, Zorzi A, Vanoli E, Gronda E. Current challenges in sudden cardiac death prevention. Heart Fail Rev 2019 Jul 26. doi: 10.1007/s10741-019-09830-0.

[93] Offerhaus JA, Bezzina CR, Wilde AAM. Epidemiology of inherited arrhythmias. Nat Rev Cardiol 2019 Oct 3. doi: 10.1038/s41569-019-0266-2.

[94] Chin A. Sudden cardiac death in Africa. Cardiovasc J Afr 2014;25(4):151-2.

[95] Bonny A, Tibazarwa K, Mbouh S, Wa J, Fonga R, Saka C, et al. Epidemiology of sudden cardiac death in Cameroon: the first population-based cohort survey in sub-Suharan Africa. Int J Epidemiol 2017;46(4):1230-8.

[96] Mathers CD, Boerma T, Ma Fat D. Global and regional causes of death. Br Med Bull 2009;92:7-32.

[97] GBD 2016 Causes of Death Collaborators. Global, regional, and national age-sex specific mortality for 264 cause of death, 1980-2016: a systematic analysis for the Global Burden of Disease Study 2016. Lancet 2017;390(10100):1151-1210.

[98] Vora A, Burkule N, Contractor A, Bhargava K. Prevention of sudden cardiac death in athletes, sportspersons and marathoners in India. Indian Heart J 2018;70(1):137-45.

[99] Paterick TE, Paterick TJ, Fletcher GF, Maron BJ. Medical and legal issues in the cardiovascular evaluation of competitive athletes. JAMA 2005;294(23):3011-8.

[100] Marzuillo P, Benettoni A, Germani C, Ferrara G, D'Agata B, Barbi E. Acquired long QT syndrome: a focus for the general pediatrician. Pediatric Emerg Care 2014;30(4):257-61.

SECTION 2: CHRONIC DISEASE, PALLIATIVE CARE AND DEATH

In: Chronic Disease and Disability
Editors: DE Greydanus, P Anne, JD Rowlett et al.
ISBN: 978-1-53617-656-8

Chapter 16

MENTAL HEALTH AND CHRONIC DISEASE: ISSUES IN CARDIOVASCULAR DISEASE

Nelli El-Ghazal, PhD, Christina Helen Vlahos, PhD, Muhammad Waqar Azeem, MD and Ahsan Nazeer*, MD
Child and Adolescent Psychiatry, Department of Psychiatry,
Sidra Medicine, and Weil Cornell Medical School, Doha, Qatar

ABSTRACT

This discussion reflects on mental health issues in pediatric persons with cardiovascular disorders. Research notes that chronic diseases, including cardiovascular illness, may lead to the development of mental health conditions, which have a negative social and academic impact on the lives of pediatric persons. Though more research is needed, clinicians need to be aware of these issues so that they can intervene in a timely manner to improve the quality of life of these patients and families.

INTRODUCTION

Cardiovascular disease (CVD) in children, whether occurring congenitally, as a result of viral infections or acquired later in childhood, brings with it a slew of medical and non-medical concerns (1). Advancements in the medical field, particularly in the areas of diagnosis and treatment of heart conditions in children, has resulted in 90% of children surviving into adolescence and adulthood. During the last decade, concerns are gaining attention regarding these children's development, exercise, quality of life (QoL), psychosocial functioning, and cognitive development (2, 3). Children with CVD have been identified as having more cognitive, developmental, psychological, and behavioral concerns than their same-age peers. However, in many cases, the presence of the disease in and of itself is not necessarily related

* Correspondence: Ahsan Nazeer, MD, Division Chief-Child and Adolescent Psychiatry, Sidra Medicine, C2M 224, 2nd Mezzanine, OPC, PO Box 26999, Al Luqta Street, Education City North Campus, Qatar Foundation, Doha, Qatar. Email: anazeer@sidra.org.

to other non-medical complications; indeed, it is more so the interaction of the disease with treatment, environmental, and demographic variables that is related to these deficits (3).

Of all the types of CVD in children, congenital heart defects (CHD) are the most common physical disability and occurs in approximately 1% of live births. Of those born with CHD, about 25% will require medical intervention such as surgery to survive, adding another risk factor to their overall quality of life (4). The majority of the available research on the developmental and psychological impact of heart disease, is mostly in the context of CHD, as opposed to general cardiovascular disease (5).

Quality of Life

As CHD patients are living longer, it is imperative to recognize the quality of life in the context of overall life expectancy as a measure of the success of their treatment (6). Quality of life is a subjective experience that accounts for overall life satisfaction while integrating emotional, physical, and social wellbeing. Given that the manifestation and severity of CHD can vary, the restrictions and adjustments to everyday life that CHD patients will have to make, per their disease, will also vary. These restrictions may affect one or multiple aspects, including the social, environmental, or physical domains of the patient's life (7).

In general, there is no consensus on whether CHD significantly impairs the quality of life of patients as compared to their healthy peers. This inconsistency is due to the complex nature of both CHD and the quality of life as observable and measurable factors. Fortunately, the mere presence of a CHD, in and of itself, does not seem to be enough of a predictor of impairment in quality of life. Instead, it is the personal and medical experiences along the CHD treatment path that are more likely to contribute to the patient's perceptions of their quality of life.

In studies of adult patients, researchers have found that the quality of life in CHD patients is proportionate, if not better, than in healthy controls (8). However, no similar pattern has arisen in children with CHD. One possible reason may be the variation in perspectives of families whose children have CHDs, with more positive attitudes being directly related to a positive quality of life outcomes. Along with the above, the quality and intensity of medical treatment and parents' satisfaction with care may also be tied to varying reports of quality of life.

A sense of the low quality of life in patients is linked to cardiac instability, increased disease severity, impaired motor functioning, and decreased autonomy (9, 10). Furthermore, increased medical and surgical interventions are also related to a lower quality of life ratings. For example, operative procedures create a significant interruption to life, including the day-to- day activities and experiences that would otherwise be identified as 'typical' for children. It is, therefore, not surprising that the above children have a more negative outlook on their overall functioning and quality of life (11).

Furthermore, postoperative complications, length of hospital stay, and need for ongoing medication use are also linked to lower quality of life reporting. There are conflicting reports on whether the duration and number of certain medical procedures (e.g., the duration of circulatory arrest or cardiopulmonary), have an impact on the quality of life. Further research is needed to address the above question (12, 13).

Regardless of whether CHD patients undergo surgery or not, parents of children with CHD may lower their expectations of and underestimate their child's physical ability. Such increased limitations on children's behavior and experiences, with or without surgery, are generally related to lower quality of life. This issue is particularly pertinent when children are withheld from desirable activities in which their peers engage.

Another concern is also the loss of known health and psychological benefits of exercise, as well as the reduced access to social interactions. Despite the drawbacks of increased limitations, authors understand that at times caution about daily functioning may be warranted for complicated patients. This is why it is essential that the decisions about the extent of physical activity should only be taken on a case-by-case basis and only after extensive consultation with the patients' cardiologists.

In one study, physical functioning scores on Pediatric Quality of Life Inventory (PedsQoL), as reported by parents and children, were lower for children with severe cardiovascular disease than in children with less severe disease (5). Physical symptoms were much more consistently rated by patients and their parents, particularly with increased CHD severity. However, non-physical symptoms were different. Parent ratings of physical appearance, treatment anxiety, and communication of their children were related to disease severity, whereas patients' self-report ratings were not associated with disease severity (5).

The degree of disease severity is also a risk factor for the poor quality of life ratings, not only due to the limitations imposed on the child but also because of the physical discomfort experienced as well as the amount of medical intervention necessary. Another notable disease characteristic is whether the amount of oxygen in the body is lowered as the result of the CHD (cyanotic), as it is generally related to lower quality of life than when the oxygen amount is not impacted.

Another essential factor to consider is the impact of CHD on school attendance, which is particularly salient with increased CHD severity and medical interventions. Poor school attendance also raises a concern regarding patients' acquisition of knowledge and availability for learning, which is then linked to lower ratings of quality of life. However, the academic experience is more than just the academic and learning components of the school; it also encompasses the children's social integration as well as functioning.

Time away from the school because of medical necessity also means time away from opportunities to develop social skills and relationships. Because of the above, CHD students miss out on a fundamental shared experience with other children. Though the lack of social support is a risk factor in the QoL ratings, the presence of it is a protective factor and increases the reported quality of life. It is, therefore, essential that social opportunities should be intentionally sought out and tailored to the patient's limitations.

Demographic risk factors have also been examined concerning the QoL. Some studies have reported a positive relationship between patient age and quality of life, which may be linked to the patients' ability to understand as well as manage the disease more independently. Although some self-report ratings indicated a positive relationship between age and quality of life, parent ratings have indicated the opposite, i.e., age and quality of life are negatively related. This is another area in which a clear understanding has not yet developed, and further studies are needed.

Higher intelligence quotient (IQ) was also related to higher levels of quality of life, potentially for the same reason that underlies the relationship with older age. There are inconsistent findings concerning the relationship between gender and quality of life, but data indicate that males tend to do better in this regard. Although the reason for this relationship is unclear, it may be beneficial to examine behavioral and physical activity limitations placed on CHD patients through a gender norm lens to determine whether lower limitations are present for male patients, which would inadvertently be related to a higher quality of life ratings.

Family factors have also been found to be related to patient quality of life. Parental unemployment and inter-familial conflicts because of the overall level of family stress are related to lower quality of life ratings. Family socioeconomic status has been examined, but results are inconsistent with regard to its relation to the quality of life. It is important to note that the parents more often report quality of life impairments than by the child. In particular, parents who have children with developmental, language, or cognitive delays; tend to report more psychological problems (11, 14, 15). This trend may be because children do not have a point of comparison or may not have the cognitive skills to understand the extent of their deficits. However, these findings may also be overestimated if the parents are overprotective of their child.

EMOTIONAL AND BEHAVIORAL DIFFICULTIES

Chronic illness has generally been established as a factor related to emotional or psychological distress; this finding is consistent for patients with CHD. These children are at a higher risk for emotional, behavioral, and psychological difficulties than the general population (16). Compared to the general population where one in five adults has a psychiatric disorder, one in three CHD patients are noted to have a psychiatric disorder (5, 14-17).

Some data indicate that the prevalence of lifetime psychopathology in the CHD population is 18.7%, with double the rates in females than in males. These psychological difficulties are typically classified within the broader categories of behavior that are *internalizing* (i.e., withdrawal, anxiety, depression, dysphoria, etc.) and *externalizing* (i.e., defiance, impulsivity, hyperactivity, disruptiveness, aggression, and antisocial features) (7, 11). It is important to note that even if patients present with externalizing behaviors, they are generally more at risk for major depression, bipolar disorder, and substance abuse in the future (2). In another study, feeling angry was the most frequent emotional problem noted by both parents and children with CHD (5). One (12.5%) in eight children among the study sample, also reported worrying about the future, while the most common cognitive problems reported by parents and patients were related to memory and attention (5).

There have also been connections made between CHD and attention-deficit/hyperactivity disorder, internalizing problems, limitations in socialization, and low self-esteem (3). As the children grow into adolescence, peer acceptance, and participation in activities with peers become increasingly important. Fear of the unexpected nature of CHD and the possibility of a sudden cardiac event may also contribute to a level of stress in these patients. These differences between CHD patients and their healthy peers have been established in multiple countries including the United States, Canada, China, Norway, and Germany; such results indicate that irrespective of cultural differences, these difficulties seem to be prevalent in the population of patients with CHD (3, 6, 7).

Surgery has also been identified as a potential risk factor with regard to patient psychological/behavioral functioning and development (3, 11). Except for patients with transposition of the great arteries (TGA), children who have undergone other surgical repairs have more psychological difficulties; this difference in the outcome maybe because of the better postoperative prognosis, or because of the low incidence of genetic disorders in TGA group (11, 16). Most of the psychological complications postoperatively tend to be, attentional, social, and somatic. One study indicated that 5 to 10-year-olds who had undergone surgery as newborns were rated as "clinically significant" on inattention and hyperactivity at a rate of 3-4 times the general population (16, 18).

Some findings indicate that older age at the time of surgery may also be a risk factor. The number of surgical procedures and the duration of the hospital stay were also a predictor for externalizing problems. The relationship between CHD and the development of internalizing, externalizing, attention, and social difficulties may be associated with the level of intensity of the treatment (i.e., the more intense the treatment, the greater the behavioral problems) (11). Despite the positive relationship between treatment severity and psychological and behavioral difficulties, there is an inconsistency in the available data on whether a relationship exists between disease severity and the level of psychological as well as cognitive functioning.

Some specific treatments or conditions may also be related to greater psychological or behavioral difficulties. For example, there are some indications that deep hypothermic circulatory arrest (DHCA) seems to be linked to long term behavioral and emotional issues; however, this association should be taken with caution because of the limitations in the research methodology. Prolonged hypoxia is also noted to be a risk factor in the development of psychological difficulties in TGA patients; however, like many other findings, this is also not consistent across studies.

Another factor that has been identified to impair psychological functioning is premature birth. In one study, parents of 3.5 year-olds who met this criterion reported more internalizing problems than parents of the control group (16). Low birth weight and less than 36-week gestation are added risk factors to a number of surgeries and deep hypothermic circulatory arrest in predicting the future internalizing problems.

Demographic factors have also been found to be related to psychological and behavioral functioning. Some studies have found that older adolescents have had more difficulty adjusting, but this has not been a consistent finding. Patients aged 12 to 17 years have been reported to be more withdrawn while older patients (19-26 years) were reportedly more anxious, had more difficulty with attention, and had more externalizing problems. Conversely, younger children have reported fewer externalizing and internalizing behaviors than controls.

Based on parent reports in one study, children aged 5 to 7 years showed no differences from their same age peers, whereas those 13-18 show psychological functioning significantly below their peers. Therefore, it appears that age may be more related to psychological problems than is the presence or severity of CHD. This is consistent with other chronic illnesses and maybe because adolescents have greater exposure to risk factors throughout their lifetime than do younger children. Additionally, the hormonal and brain changes that occur in adolescence may trigger the expression of genetic vulnerabilities in conjunction with stressful experiences related to CHD.

It is important to note the numerous variables that affect the results of available studies. First, there are noted to be inconsistencies on parents, teachers, and self-report measures of psychological as well as behavioral difficulties. When rating CHD patient's functioning, parents tend to report fewer symptoms than their children, and teachers report less deviant behaviors than parents. The difference between parent and self-report may be due to the potentially unobservable nature of internalizing behaviors also, as parents have more insight into their child's functioning than teachers; hence, the discrepancy in ratings.

Second, the Child Behavior Checklist (CBCL), which is an instrument to access psychological functioning, and is commonly used in studies accessing QoL, consists of an internalizing scale that includes physical symptom items. Since these children already have a physical condition, that scale may not be an accurate reflection of their internalizing feelings, as they may endorse specific items based on actual physical symptoms, whereas the item may measure a somatic complaint in a healthy child.

Finally, some family factors may be linked to behavioral difficulties; these include early parental distress, maternal fear, poor parental behavior management skills, high maternal worry about their children, and maternal psychological symptoms. Because parental well-being is related to psychological adjustment of CHD patients, an integrated family approach to care and wellness is imperative.

Cognitive and Academic Impact

Another area that has received an increased focus is the cognitive and academic functioning of CHD patients (6, 14, 15). Because this area is still emerging, the research remains inconsistent with regards to identifying a clear or consistent relationship between CHD and cognitive functioning. One salient point to note is that the majority of cognitive testing in study samples is conducted in persons with ages of four and eighteen. As the reliability and validity of cognitive testing are low in younger children, therefore the research findings need to be interpreted in this context.

Unlike difficulties with emotional functioning or quality of life, the presence of CHD has been identified, in and of itself, as a predictor of developmental delays; this is especially true when complications occur at birth (19). The presence of CHD is often accompanied by other symptoms such as trouble breathing, fatigue, dizziness, low weight, frequent respiratory infections, arrhythmias, and cyanosis. Depending on the degree of these symptoms, children with CHD can experience physical and motor constraints that directly impact their cognitive and emotional development. Children with CHD have been noted to have a distinct neuropsychiatric profile, including deficits in executive control and cognitive performance, inattention, difficulties with social interaction, and impairment in the pragmatic language (20).

Delays in cognitive development and psychosocial functioning are more likely to become evident as children grow and develop language skills. By school age, children with critical congenital heart disease (CCHD) have lower scores on intelligence and achievement subsets of psychological batteries, display impairments in fine and gross motor function, and have a higher likelihood of learning disabilities (21).

There are also cultural and environmental factors that come into play, such as living conditions, quality and quantity of medical care, perinatal risks, family as well as social interactions, and housing conditions that affect the functioning (22). The following factors have not been noted to be related to delays: age and education of the parents, number of children per family, care before and after delivery, breastfeeding, mother’s health, and use of controlled medication or substances; however, future studies should continue to investigate these factors further.

In children with CCHD, neurocognitive development may be affected by hypoxic-ischemic injury to brian during brain development, and impairments in progression as well as the rate of early brain maturation (23, 24). The severity of the CHD also has an impact on the overall cognitive functioning of patients. Specifically, more severe patients exhibit both lower verbal and performance IQ than same-age peers. There were also differences in cognitive ability based on the type of CHD present. Those with an atrial septal defect and ventricular septal defect had higher overall, verbal, and performance *intelligence quotient* (IQ) than the normative sample; on the other hand, those with hypoplastic left heart syndrome (HLHS) and TGA had lower IQs than the normative sample, especially in the area of perceptual reasoning ability.

Specific to treatment procedures for CHD patients, a relationship in the literature is emerging between deep hypothermic circulatory arrest and cognitive score. Some have found a relationship between the length of time of arrest and IQ; however, others have found IQ to be impacted not by the cooling itself, but by the length of the cooling period, with shorter cooling periods being linked to lower IQ (25, 26). Some studies have shown that even when children with CHD have a similar IQ to their healthy peers, they continue to demonstrate deficits in visual-spatial and visual-motor skills, as well as speech-language impairments and executive functioning (27).

There are also reports of inattention and hyperactivity in the complex CHD population in schools. In parent's reports, the most common school and cognitive concerns were related to memory and attention; however, these individuals also have impairment in behavioral regulation, lower working memory, and problems with organizational as well as planning skills (28-30). In some samples, the rate of students with attention and executive functioning concerns was three to four times as high as the general population (15). Cyanotic patients were more likely to exhibit more concerns with poor attention and executive functioning skills than acyanotic patients. Although the exact prevalence of ADHD as a diagnosis in this population cannot be conclusively stated, it is a significant risk factor to consider in the management of these children.

Research has also noted larger than normal numbers of CHD patients receiving remedial services as compared to the same-age peers in school (15). In general, parents note more academic difficulties in their children than do teachers. However, teachers may have a higher threshold for behavior and academic difficulties because they may also be comparing the cardiac patient to other children who are in a special education classroom, where there is a high prevalence of behavioral and developmental issues. In contrast, parents may be comparing their children to typically developing same-age peers. Therefore, the consistent and systematic identification of patients with CHD's need for support is imperative so as to improve their school functioning and, in turn, their social functioning; such is consequently linked to psychological adjustment and quality of life.

Quality of Life in Pediatric Heart Transplant Patients

Cardiac transplant is a life-saving surgery, and in addition to the preservation of life, the majority of recipients do not have any limitations on physical activity. However, the need for a transplant is difficult to understand for anyone, and while growing up, cardiac transplant patients struggle with a slew of psychosocial problems. For adolescents who are developing the ability to build peer relationships, to think in new ways and explore new thoughts, the idea of a major surgery triggers fears, worries, concerns about body image, and the overall quality of life.

The children who have more psychosocial difficulties before the procedure continue to have numerous hospitalizations after the procedure (31). A significant number of patients (33%), have behavioral problems, 25% have emotional difficulties, 20-24% have psychological distress, and others have academic and school-related difficulties (32, 33). Other studies have identified concerns regarding the inability to keep up with peers and being teased. In a small study sample, more than 40% of the transplant recipients reported being teased and bullied because of their surgery scars and medication side effects, including hirsutism (34). Few studies have noted feelings of resentment, anger, difficulty talking to others regarding their fears and feelings, and worries about transplant rejection and life expectancy (17, 18, 35-37). Current research has not found any correlation between the psychological-psychosocial functioning as well as age and time since transplant and socioeconomic status (18); however, psychosocial functioning was noted to be significantly correlated with family and school functioning in multiple studies (17, 38).

PARENTAL MENTAL HEALTH

As noted above, the survival of the children with CHD has improved considerably during the last decade; however, about 25% of the children with CHD have CCHD and require two or more surgeries in the first year of life with varied outcomes (39). These children undergo numerous hospitalizations, multiple surgeries, and are at increased risk of medical complications, all of which poses a significant emotional and physical burden to the parents (40-43). These risks are further exacerbated, mainly when the medical procedures occur during the immediate postpartum period, in which mothers already are at risk of the development of postpartum depression. Studies have noted an exponential increase in postpartum depression among mothers of children who spend time in the Intensive Care Unit (ICU) after birth (44). It is also well noted that impairment in maternal mental health leads to the dysfunctional parent-child relationship and results in long term emotional, behavioral, and cognitive problems in children (45-47).

Different studies have evaluated the long-term psychological functioning of the parents of children with CHD and CCHD and have focused on general distress, stress, trauma, and depression and anxiety symptoms. Studies that specifically focused on trauma symptoms noted symptoms of acute stress disorder (ASD) and post-traumatic stress disorder (PTSD) among both parents. In a study of infants who underwent surgery before three months of age, 35% of the mothers and 18% of the fathers reported symptoms of ASD, one month after discharge (48). In another study, 25% of the parents met the criteria for PTSD one-month post-surgery, while 12% still met PTSD criteria six months after surgery (49).

Studies have also focused on the symptoms of depression and anxiety in parents. Research has noted an increased prevalence of depression among mothers of children undergoing two or more cardiac procedures (50). Symptoms of depression and anxiety were present within four weeks of cardiac procedures and were also associated with impaired bonding and lower level of maternal attachment with their infants (51). Surprisingly, in some cases, symptoms of mood and anxiety persisted as long as five years post-surgery (52). There is a considerable level of heterogeneity among the studies defining and measuring the global level of stress, distress, and overall quality of life of parents. However, most of the studies have noted elevated levels of stress/distress before surgery and improvement in the mood by two months post-surgery (53). In summary, parents of children with CCHD are at increased risk of mental health problems, with 80% experiencing symptoms of trauma, about 50% reporting mood, and anxiety problems, and 30-80% experiencing psychological distress (54).

Psychopharmacological considerations in children with CHD/CVD

A variety of psychotropics are associated with cardiac side effects, including cardiac arrhythmias and sudden cardiac death. Different medications have different propensity to affect the heart. Antipsychotic medications that are used for the management of behavioral problems in children with autism and intellectual disability, along with psychosis and treatment of mood disorder, warrants particular attention in this regard. In the literature, the most common cardiovascular adverse effects of typical and atypical antipsychotics in children were orthostatic hypotension, tachycardia, QTc interval prolongation, and arrhythmias. There are also reports of electrocardiographic (ECG) changes, myocarditis, and cerebrovascular events that further questions the cardiovascular safety of these medications in children and adolescents (55-58). In one study, the use of antipsychotics was associated with cardiomegaly, heart disease not otherwise specified (NOS), tachycardia, and arrhythmia NOS (59). In the same study, youth receiving typical (first generation, conventional) antipsychotics, multiple antipsychotics, and individuals with congenital heart defects, were at increased risk of developing cardiovascular-related events. Children with pre-existing cardiac conditions are particularly at risk of the development of these side effects; however, these risks need to be considered in the context of symptomatic relief that these medications can bring to debilitating mental health symptoms.

Hypotension, syncope and rhythm disturbances

Orthostatic hypotension (decrease in systolic BP > 20mm/Hg) is the most common side effect of antipsychotic medications and is reported to occur in more than 70% of the individuals. Low potency antipsychotics, including chlorpromazine and thioridazine, are more likely to cause postural hypotension than atypical antipsychotics. Among atypical antipsychotics, clozapine is associated with the most significant hypotension and benign sustained tachycardia (an average increase in the cardiac rate of 10-15 beats per minute). This effect is mediated via antagonism on the alpha one adrenergic receptor. Syncope is another side effect that is prevalent in individuals treated with clozapine (6%) as a comparison to the ones treated with risperidone (0.2%) and quetiapine (1%). Oral and intramuscular olanzapine is also associated with clinically significant bradycardia in 7.5% of the patients (58).

QTc prolongation and cardiac conduction delays

QTc prolongation is of particular importance while treating a patient with pre-existing cardiac conditions, who already have prolonged or abnormal cardiac repolarization. Prolonged QTc leads to torsade de pointes with symptoms of palpitations, syncope, and at times fibrillation and sudden cardiac death. There is no direct correlation of degree of QTc prolongation and the development of torsades; however, the risk appears to increase with QTc prolongation of 500ms significantly. Several psychotropics are associated with QTc prolongation, including haloperidol, ziprasidone, citalopram, methadone, and lithium (list not exhaustive). Other than electrophysiological changes and direct effects on cardiac adrenoreceptors (antagonism), it is speculated that psychotropics treatment may have predisposed or exacerbated metabolic changes and ultimately leading to cardiovascular events.

Stimulants and sudden cardiac death

Children with CHD suffer from impairment in numerous psychosocial domains, including impairment in cognition, speech as well as language difficulties, learning disabilities, inattention, impulsivity, and impairment in executive functioning (15, 20, 60). Higher prevalence of ADHD with elevated scores in inattention and hyperactivity at times warrant the use of stimulants for adequate behavioral control and to improve academic functioning (61, 62). Stimulant medications cause a slight increase in heart rate and blood pressure, and their cardiovascular safety has been hotly debated in the literature (63).

A recent study from South Korea found an increase in the risk of arrhythmias among children and adolescents who were prescribed methylphenidate for ADHD. The risk was substantially higher (three-fold increase) in individuals with pre-existing heart disease, and the highest risk was observed during the initial three days of the start of the treatment. A higher risk of hypertension was also noticed from day four to seven (64). This study is at odds with the United States' studies of private and Medicaid insurances as those studies have not found elevated cardiac side effects among individuals with or without pre-existing heart disease who were started on methylphenidate (65-67). The average rate of sudden cardiac death in children with CHD ranges from 1/454 to 1/7157 cases, and the results of the above study suggest that children with CHD are at three times more risk of suffering from sudden cardiac death than their peers (68).

CONCLUSION

Current research regarding the psychological, behavioral, and developmental impact of CHD on children provides important information to guide management and care that they receive (1-3, 5, 17). However, the current body of literature on this topic presents its limitations, which hinders the clinician's ability to integrate the findings and draw a meaningful conclusion for a variety of CHD patients. One limitation is that few studies, if any, have examined the psychological or cognitive effects longitudinally, which makes it difficult to plan the allocation of resources and to document the benefits of early interventions. Another one is the rapidly developing treatments in this area, which creates much variability in the patients' cohort to generalize the research results.

Future research should investigate more narrow-band psychological and cognitive functions as opposed to broader internalizing or externalizing behaviors, as well as verbal or performance IQ. Including a psychologist as part of the patient's medical team could also offer a more proactive approach to treatment and interventions for psychological and cognitive deficits. There is little research on the impact of treatment and psychological interventions; therefore, research should also investigate the effectiveness of those interventions.

Finally, as about 20% of the adolescents with CHD struggle with some form of mental illness (i.e., developmental disorders, anxiety disorder, impulse control disorders, and mood disorder), it is imperative to screen individuals for these disorders. It is best to embed mental health professionals in CHD clinics, and if this is not possible, an early referral needs to be made to the appropriate child and adolescent mental health service. It is also essential to further examine the impact of a child's cardiovascular disease on families. With a better understanding of the impact on family dynamics, employment, and overall stress, appropriate advocacy and clinical services can be established to improve the overall wellbeing of the child and the family.

REFERENCES

[1] Areias ME, Pinto CI, Vieira PF, Teixeira F, Coelho R, Freitas I, et al. Long term psychosocial outcomes of congenital heart disease (CHD) in adolescents and young adults. Transl Pediatr 2013;2(3):90-8.

[2] Lane DA, Millane TA, Lip GYH. Psychological interventions for depression in adolescent and adult congenital heart disease. Cochrane Database Syst Rev 2013;10: CD004372.

[3] Latal B, Helfricht S, Fischer JE, Bauersfeld U, Landolt MA. Psychological adjustment and quality of life in children and adolescents following open-heart surgery for congenital heart disease: a systematic review. BMC Pediatr 2009;9(1):6. doi: 10.1186/1471-2431-9-6.

[4] Bernier PL, Stefanescu A, Samoukovic G, Tchervenkov CI. The challenge of congenital heart disease worldwide: epidemiologic and demographic facts. Semin Thorac Cardiovasc Surg Pediatr Card Surg Annu 2010;13(1):26-34.

[5] Uzark K, Jones K, Slusher J, Limbers CA, Burwinkle TM, Varni JW. Quality of life in children with heart disease as perceived by children and parents. Pediatrics 2008; 121(5):e1060-e7.

[6] Karsdorp PA, Everaerd W, Kindt M, Mulder BJM. Psychological and cognitive functioning in children and adolescents with congenital heart disease: A meta-analysis. J Pediatr Psychol 2006;32(5):527-41.

[7] Johnson B. Behaviour problems in children with congenital heart disease. BMH Med J 2015;2(1):14-9.

[8] Moons P, Van Deyk K, De Bleser L, Marquet K, Raes E, De Geest S, et al. Quality of life and health status in adults with congenital heart disease: a direct comparison with healthy counterparts. Eur J Cardiovasc Prev Rehabil 2006;13(3):407-13.

[9] Marino BS, Shera D, Wernovsky G, Tomlinson RS, Aguirre A, Gallagher M, et al. The development of the pediatric cardiac quality of life inventory: a quality of life measure for children and adolescents with heart disease. Qual Life Res 2008;17(4): 613-26.

[10] Marino BS, Tomlinson RS, Wernovsky G, Drotar D, Newburger JW, Mahony L, et al. Validation of the pediatric cardiac quality of life inventory. Pediatrics 2010; 126(3):498-508.

[11] Utens E. Prediction of behavioural and emotional problems in children and adolescents with operated congenital heart disease. Eur Heart J 1998;19(5):801-7.

[12] Landolt MA, Valsangiacomo Buechel ER, Latal B. Health-related quality of life in children and adolescents after open-heart surgery. J Pediatr 2008;152(3):349-55.

[13] O'Connor AM, Wray J, Tomlinson RS, Cassedy A, Jacobs JP, Jenkins KJ, et al. Impact of surgical complexity on health-related quality of life in congenital heart disease surgical survivors. J Am Heart Assoc 2016;5(7). pii: e001234. doi: 10.1161/JAHA.114.001234.

[14] Mari MA, Cascudo MM, Alchieri JC. Congenital heart disease and impacts on child development. Braz J Cardiovasc Surg 2016;31(1):31-7.
[15] Shillingford AJ, Glanzman MM, Ittenbach RF, Clancy RR, Gaynor JW, Wernovsky G. Inattention, hyperactivity, and school performance in a population of school-age children with complex congenital heart disease. Pediatrics 2008;121(4):e759-e67.
[16] Brosig CL, Whitstone BN, Frommelt MA, Frisbee SJ, Leuthner SR. Psychological distress in parents of children with severe congenital heart disease: the impact of prenatal versus postnatal diagnosis. J Perinatol 2007;27(11):687-92.
[17] Uzark KC, Sauer SN, Lawrence KS, Miller J, Addonizio L, Crowley DC. The psychosocial impact of pediatric heart transplantation. J Heart Lung Transplant 1992;11(6):1160-7.
[18] Brosig C, Hintermeyer M, Zlotocha J, Behrens D, Mao J. An exploratory study of the cognitive, academic, and behavioral functioning of pediatric cardiothoracic transplant recipients. Prog Transplant 2006;16(1):38-45.
[19] Mussatto KA, Hoffmann RG, Hoffman GM, Tweddell JS, Bear L, Cao Y, et al. Risk and prevalence of developmental delay in young children with congenital heart disease. Pediatrics 2014;133(3):e570-e7.
[20] Wernovsky G. Current insights regarding neurological and developmental abnormalities in children and young adults with complex congenital cardiac disease. Cardiol Young 2006;16(Suppl 1):92-104.
[21] Bellinger DC, Wypij D, Rivkin MJ, DeMaso DR, Robertson RL, Dunbar-Masterson C, et al. Adolescents with d-transposition of the great arteries corrected with the arterial switch procedure. Circulation 2011;124(12):1361-9.
[22] Newburger JW, Sleeper LA, Bellinger DC, Goldberg CS, Tabbutt S, Lu M, et al. Early developmental outcome in children with hypoplastic left heart syndrome and related anomalies. Circulation 2012;125(17):2081-91.
[23] Limperopoulos C, Tworetzky W, McElhinney DB, Newburger JW, Brown DW, Robertson RL, et al. Brain volume and metabolism in fetuses with congenital heart disease. Circulation 2010;121(1):26-33.
[24] von Rhein M, Buchmann A, Hagman n C, Huber R, Klaver P, Knirsch W, et al. Brain volumes predict neurodevelopment in adolescents after surgery for congenital heart disease. Brain 2013;137(1):268-76.
[25] Fuller S, Rajagopalan R, Jarvik GP, Gerdes M, Bernbaum J, Wernovsky G, et al. Deep hypothermic circulatory arrest does not impair neurodevelopmental outcome in school-age children after infant cardiac surgery. Ann Thorac Surg 2010;90(6):1985-95.
[26] Snookes SH, Gunn JK, Eldridge BJ, Donath SM, Hunt RW, Galea MP, et al. A systematic review of motor and cognitive outcomes after early surgery for congenital heart disease. Pediatrics 2010;125(4):e818-e27.
[27] Bellinger DC. Are children with congenital cardiac malformations at increased risk of deficits in social cognition? Cardiol Young 2008;18(1):3-9.
[28] Calderon J, Bellinger DC. Executive function deficits in congenital heart disease: why is intervention important? Cardiol Young 2015;25(7):1238-46.
[29] Cassidy AR, White MT, DeMaso DR, Newburger JW, Bellinger DC. Executive function in children and adolescents with critical cyanotic congenital heart disease. J Int Neuropsychol Soc 2015;21(1):34-49.
[30] Marelli A, Miller SP, Marino BS, Jefferson AL, Newburger JW. Brain in congenital heart disease across the lifespan. Circulation 2016;133(20):1951-62.
[31] DeMaso DR, Douglas Kelley S, Bastardi H, O'Brien P, Blume ED. The longitudinal impact of psychological functioning, medical severity, and family functioning in pediatric heart transplantation. J Heart Lung Transplant 2004;23(4):473-80.
[32] Todaro JF. Cognitive and psychological outcomes in pediatric heart transplantation. J Pediatr Psychol 2000;25(8):567-76.
[33] Wray J, Radley-Smith R. Longitudinal assessment of psychological functioning in children after heart or heart–lung transplantation. J Heart Lung Transplant 2006; 25(3):345-52.
[34] Green A, McSweeney J, Ainley K, Bryant J. In my shoes: Children's quality of life after heart transplantation. Prog Transplant 2007;17(3):199-208.
[35] Green A, Meaux J, Huett A, Ainley K. "It Has its Ups and Downs": Adolescents' quality of life after heart transplantation. ProgTransplant 2011;21(2):115-20.

[36] Mintzer LL. Traumatic stress symptoms in adolescent organ transplant recipients. Pediatrics 2005;115(6):1640-4.
[37] Wray J, Radley-Smith R. Depression in pediatric patients before and 1 year after heart or heart-lung transplantation. J Heart Lung Transplant 2004;23(9):1103-10.
[38] Hirshfeld AB, Kahle AL, Clark BJ, Bridges ND. Parent-reported health status after pediatric thoracic organ transplant. J Heart Lung Transplant 2004;23(9):1111-8.
[39] Centers for Disease Control and Prevention (CDC). Critical congenital heart defects, 2019. URL: https://www.cdc.gov/ncbddd/heartdefects/cchd-facts.html.
[40] Connor JA, Kline NE, Mott S, Harris SK, Jenkins KJ. The meaning of cost for families of children with congenital heart disease. J Pediatr Health Care 2010;24(5):318-25.
[41] Hopkins J, Marcus M, Campbell SB. Postpartum depression: A critical review. Psychol Bull 1984;95(3):498-515.
[42] Ross LE, McLean LM. Anxiety disorders during pregnancy and the postpartum period. J Clin Psychiatry 2006;67(8):1285-98.
[43] Vesga-López O, Blanco C, Keyes K, Olfson M, Grant BF, Hasin DS. Psychiatric disorders in pregnant and postpartum women in the United States. Arch Gen Psychiatry 2008;65(7):805-15.
[44] Lefkowitz DS, Baxt C, Evans JR. Prevalence and correlates of posttraumatic stress and postpartum depression in parents of infants in the neonatal intensive care unit (NICU). J Clin Psychol Med Settings 2010;17(3):230-7.
[45] Lyons-Ruth K, Wolfe R, Lyubchik A. Depression and the parenting of young children: Making the case for early preventive mental health services. Harv Rev Psychiatry 2000;8(3):148-53.
[46] McPeak KE, Sandrock D, Spector ND, Pattishall AE. Important determinants of newborn health. Curr Opin Pediatr 2015;27(1);138-144.
[47] Mirhosseini H, Moosavipoor SA, Nazari MA, Dehghan A, Mirhosseini S, Bidaki R, et al. Cognitive behavioral development in children following maternal postpartum depression: A review article. Electron Physician 2015;7(8):1673-9.
[48] Franich-Ray C, Bright MA, Anderson V, Northam E, Cochrane A, Menahem S, et al. Trauma reactions in mothers and fathers after their infant's cardiac surgery. J Pediatr Psychol 2013;38(5):494-505.
[49] Helfricht S, Latal B, Fischer JE, Tomaske M, Landolt MA. Surgery-related posttraumatic stress disorder in parents of children undergoing cardiopulmonary bypass surgery: A prospective cohort study. Pediatr Crit Care Med 2008;9(2):217-23.
[50] Hearps SJ, McCarthy MC, Muscara F, Hearps SJC, Burke K, Jones B, et al. Psychosocial risk in families of infants undergoing surgery for a serious congenital heart disease. Cardiol Young 2013;24(4):632-9.
[51] Jordan B, Franich-Ray C, Albert N, Anderson V, Northam E, Cochrane A, et al. Early mother-infant relationships after cardiac surgery in infancy. Arch Dis Child 2014; 99(7):641-5.
[52] Guan G, Liu H, Wang Y, Han B, Jin Y. Behavioural and emotional outcomes in school-aged children after surgery or transcatheter closure treatment for ventricular septal defect. Cardiol Young 2013;24(5):910-7.
[53] Wray J, Sensky T. Psychological functioning in parents of children undergoing elective cardiac surgery. Cardiol Young 2004;14(2):131-9.
[54] Woolf-King SE, Anger A, Arnold EA, Weiss SJ, Teitel D. Mental health among parents of children with critical congenital heart defects: A systematic review. J Am Heart Assoc 2017;6(2). pii: e004862. doi: 10.1161/JAHA.116.004862.
[55] Cheng-Shannon J, McGough JJ, Pataki C, McCracken JT. Second-generation antipsychotic medications in children and adolescents. J Child Adolesc Psychopharmacol 2004;14(3):372-94.
[56] Correll CU, Penzner JB, Parikh UH, Mughal T, Javed T, Carbon M, et al. Recognizing and monitoring adverse events of second-generation antipsychotics in children and adolescents. Child Adolesc Psychiatr Clin N Am 2006;15(1):177-206.
[57] McIntyre RS, Konarski JZ. Tolerability profiles of atypical antipsychotics in the treatment of bipolar disorder. J Clin Psychiatry 2005;66(Suppl 3):28-36.
[58] Wagstaff AJ, Easton J, Scott LJ. Intramuscular olanzapine. CNS Drugs 2005;19(2):147-64.
[59] McIntyre RS, Jerrell JM. Metabolic and cardiovascular adverse events associated with antipsychotic treatment in children and adolescents. Arch Pediatr Adolesc Med 2008;162(10):929-34.

[60] Hansen E, Poole TA, Nguyen V, Lerner M, Wigal T, Shannon K, et al. Prevalence of ADHD symptoms in patients with congenital heart disease. Pediatr Int 2012;54(6): 838-43.
[61] Marino BS, Lipkin PH, Newburger JW, Peacock G, Gerdes M, Gaynor JW, et al. Neurodevelopmental outcomes in children with congenital heart disease: Evaluation and management. Circulation 2012;126(9):1143-72.
[62] Sistino JJ, Atz AM, Simpson KN, Ellis C, Ikonomidis JS, Bradley SM. The prevalence of attention-deficit/hyperactivity disorder following neonatal aortic arch repair. Cardiol Young 2014;25(4):663-9.
[63] Martinez-Raga J, Knecht C, Szerman N, Martinez MI. Risk of serious cardiovascular problems with medications for zttention-deficit hyperactivity disorder. CNS Drugs 2012;27(1):15-30.
[64] Shin JY, Roughead EE, Park B-J, Pratt NL. Cardiovascular safety of methylphenidate among children and young people with attention-deficit/hyperactivity disorder (ADHD): nationwide self controlled case series study. BMJ 2016;353:i2550.
[65] Cooper WO, Habel LA, Sox CM, Chan KA, Arbogast PG, Cheetham TC, et al. ADHD drugs and serious cardiovascular events in children and young adults. N Engl J Med 2011;365(20):1896-904.
[66] Schelleman H, Bilker WB, Strom BL, Kimmel SE, Newcomb C, Guevara JP, et al. Cardiovascular events and death in children exposed and unexposed to ADHD agents. Pediatrics 2011;127(6):1102-10.
[67] Winterstein AG, Gerhard T, Kubilis P, Saidi A, Linden S, Crystal S, et al. Cardiovascular safety of central nervous system stimulants in children and adolescents: population based cohort study. BMJ 2012;345:e4627. doi: 10.1136/bmj.e4627.
[68] Jackson JW. The cardiovascular safety of methylphenidate. BMJ 2016;353:i2874.

In: Chronic Disease and Disability
Editors: DE Greydanus, P Anne, JD Rowlett et al.
ISBN: 978-1-53617-656-8

Chapter 17

PSYCHOSOCIAL ADAPTATION TO CHRONIC ILLNESS AND DISABILITY (CID) FOR CHILDREN AND ADOLESCENTS: A GLOBAL PERSPECTIVE

Roger W Apple*[*], *PhD
Division of Developmental and Behavioral Pediatrics,
Department of Pediatric and Adolescent Medicine, Western Michigan University,
Homer Stryker MD School of Medicine, Kalamazoo, Michigan, United States of America

ABSTRACT

The purpose of this chapter is to provide a general overview of psychosocial adaptation to chronic illness and disability (CID) as it pertains to children and adolescents. Providing a global perspective of how children and adolescents adapt psychosocially to CID will aid medical and mental health providers in conceptualizing how these factors impact their patients and ultimately designing and implementing effective treatment. The importance of psychosocial factors relating to adaptation of CID for children and adolescents cannot be stressed enough as physicians are often the first provider these patients visit; additionally many patients with CID may not understand the significance of psychosocial factors and not seek out mental health services without the encouragement from the medical team. The necessity of multidisciplinary teams is stressed due to the fact that CID impacts the whole person (physiologically, psychologically, psychosocially, and environmentally) and teams need to include professionals who can adequately address all of these factors. Definition, overarching concepts, coping strategies, assessment, and interventions will be discussed.

INTRODUCTION

Psychosocial adaptation to chronic illness and disability (CID) is a complex phenomenon to understand for patients, medical and mental health care providers, and an even more complex phenomenon when children and adolescents are the patients (1). The purpose of this chapter is

[*] Corresponding Author's Email: Roger.apple@med.wmich.edu.

to provide a global perspective of some of the most common psychosocial characteristics present in children and adolescents as they adapt to chronic illness and disability as well as discuss definition, overarching concepts, assessment, and treatment and interventions. This is very important in primary care as physicians are usually in contact with children with chronic illness and disability long before they are possibly referred to a psychologist (2).

Chronic Illness and disability impact the whole person (physiologically, psychologically, psychosocially, and environmentally). Medical teams need to be able to treat all of the various parts as a whole (not individually) to be most effective and lead to improved outcomes (3). This also means that health care centers should provide multidisciplinary treatment (medical, psychology, social work, etc.) in the same location through the collaboration of multidisciplinary teams. This approach will likely improve outcomes as opposed to referring patients to outside resources to treat the individual components. In fact, some suggest that the term *medical team* be replaced with a new term (i.e., care team, treatment team, multidisciplinary team) that signifies the necessary multidisciplinary team which is needed to fully respond to children and adolescents with CID. This transformation in primary care is critically important because there is often a psychological component to children and adolescents struggling with CID (4).

SEARCH METHODS

Several databases were searched including PubMed, PsychInfo, PsychArticles, as well as Google Scholar to identify the most salient literature. Literature was sought out for counseling children and adolescents with chronic illness, counseling techniques for children with CID; however, these search criteria yielded only general information regarding how physicians might counsel their patients which is very different than counseling techniques that are used by psychologists. Further searches were conducted and the term *psychosocial adaptation* yielded the most salient information regarding the psychological functioning of children and adolescents diagnosed with CID. With this information treatment teams will be better able to adapt treatment interventions to meet the specific needs of children and adolescentss diagnosed with CID. Specific information was sought out for definition of psychosocial adaptation, overarching concepts of psychosocial adaptation, coping strategies, assessment, and interventions.

FINDINGS

This chapter provides a global perspective on psychosocial adaptation to CID for children and adolescents. Focusing on global psychosocial characteristics of children and adolescents diagnosed with various chronic illnesses and disabilities was done intentionally to look at the common characteristics in the attempt to provide a resource to physicians and mental health providers, in general, to respond appropriately to a variety of psychosocial factors that occur in most chronic illnesses.

While there is ample literature regarding psychosocial adaptation in general; the information found using the search term *psychosocial adaptation* can be used to fill a void in the literature specific to helping mental health providers design evidenced based interventions for children and adolescents with CID. In fact, rehabilitation literature has an abundant amount of information regarding psychosocial adaptation.

DEFINITION

At first glance it would appear quite simple to define *psychosocial adaptation*; however, when considering several definitions it became apparent that it is not so simple in part because *psychosocial adaptation* is more of a concept rather than a term. Additionally, this chapter is not merely defining *psychosocial adaptation*; it is defining *psychosocial adaptation* in relation to children and adolescents diagnosed with CID. Because of this the term *adaptation* will be defined generally followed by *psychosocial adaptation* defined more specifically, and lastly a list of common CID seen in children and adolescents to help give context to the definition.

Adaptation

Adaptation, in general, refers to the "individual's personal and highly individual response to disability- or illness-related disruptions across a wide range of life domains. These disruptions may be experienced, for example, in interpersonal relationships, in interaction with the physical environment, and as changes in psychological or emotional health and function" (5).

Psychosocial adaptation

Even though there continues to be some variation in definition across the literature a general consensus describes psychosocial adaptation as "…responding to the functional, psychological, and social changes that occur with the onset and experience of living with a disability, chronic illness, or associated treatments" (5, 6). Others have described a definition that seems to focus more on healthy adaptation indicating that it is a process where a person moves from a negative reaction to a positive state of well-being (6). This last process could also be referred to as a process of acceptance.

Lastly, when defining psychosocial adaptation to CID the unique developmental characteristics of children and adolescents must be taken into consideration. For example, age of diagnosis is very important in a child's or adolescent's ability to comprehend a complex diagnosis of CID. For very young children, less than five years of age, may not yet understand the concept of death and certainly not the full ramifications of CID. When the age of onset is during adolescence the impact can potentially be much more amplified due to increased ability to understand such concepts and can often lead to increased feelings of depression.

Common chronic illnesses and disabilities

While reviewing the definitions of CID it became clear that conditions considered to be a chronic illness or disability varied depending on the study, article, or topic being covered. The following CID were identified during the literature search for this chapter (7–9) (see Table 1). There are many other conditions that can be considered as a chronic illness or disability such as heart conditions, mobility issues, as well as vision and hearing problems. Having such a vast array of CID is part of the problem in terms of a clear definition and response from the treatment team.

Table 1. Chronic illness and disabilities (7-9)

Spinal cord injuries	other allergies
Traumatic brain injuries	allergic skin conditions
Multiple Sclerosis	other skin conditions
Diabetes	Migraine
Cancer	Diabetes
Pain	End Stage Renal Disease
Heart problems	Ulcerative colitis
Traumatic and physical injuries	Spina bifida
Asthma	Cystic Fibrosis
allergic rhinitis	Crohn's Disease

Psychosocial Adaptation to Chronic Illness: Overarching Concepts

The psychosocial factors that impact children's and adolescents' adaptation to chronic illness and disability have such a significant impact on their functioning that these factors must be considered in order to be able to provide the best medical treatment and for the patient to be able to accept and implement treatment recommendations. This section will focus on describing the overarching psychosocial concepts impacting adaptation to CID from a global perspective. This will provide a general foundation of information that can help treatment teams with an overarching understanding of psychosocial adaptation to CID for children and adolescents.

Psychosocial adaptation in the literature

To help understand psychosocial adaptation to CID the literature often categorizes the topic into various stages, domains, concepts, or constructs (6, 7, 10). However, there is little consistency across the literature regarding global categorization with each individual study or paper categorizing psychosocial adaptation to CID differently. One approach from a qualitative study looking at psychosocial adaptation for patients undergoing long-term hemodialysis identified these four stages: slipping into, restricted to a renal world, and stuck in an endless process (10). In another paper written to facilitate counselors' understanding of psychosocial adaptation of CID three domains were identified: basic concepts, psychosocial responses (chronic illness triggered responses), and coping strategies (6).

Positive constructs

The field of positive psychology has worked to identify factors related to successful adaptation, six constructs were identified for successful and healthy adaption to CID (7) which include: optimism, hope, resilience, benefit-finding, meaning-making, and post-traumatic growth. These six constructs could help the medical team have a positive impact on successful adaptation. Specific positive factors that have been associated with improved psychosocial adaptation include hope and optimism and/or a positive outlook (1). Benefit finding has been associated as both a coping strategy early on in CID and as an outcome measure as it helps patients identify positive outcomes of CID and helps them cope at the beginning. Meaning-making is when people make sense of the global meanings and the meanings associated with the specific event – i.e., onset of CID. Posttraumatic growth refers to the growth that can be experienced after the initial shock of the diagnosis of CID. Posttraumatic growth can be seen as a coping mechanism to cognitively process the trauma and improve psychological functioning. It was found that these 6 constructs were associated with greater psychosocial adaptation. The benefit of these six constructs(7) is that they are all healthy coping mechanisms and could be used to design interventions for individuals who do not innately have high levels of these constructs. The following Table 2 lists several positive outcomes associated with health psychosocial adaptation to CID (7).

Table 2. Positive outcomes (7)

Positive self-worth
Life satisfaction
Global psychological adjustment
Physical independence
Improved social and familial roles
Reintegration into occupation roles
Positive reframing
Problem focused coping
Acceptance
Ability to maintain a stable equilibrium
Lower symptoms of PTSD, anxiety, depression
Higher levels of self-efficacy and positive affectivity
Self-efficacy
Self-esteem
Optimism
Hope
Acceptance of disability
Mastery
Internal locus of control

However, when negative adaptation occurs there is often a lack of focus on the emotional and psychosocial wellbeing of the patient and a perceived lack of understanding by the medical team from the patients' viewpoint (1). This evidences the huge need for increased understanding on behalf of the treatment teams regarding the psychosocial factors of adaptation to CID.

Additional positive factors that impact successful adaptation include: constructive internal dialogue, positive thinking, and hope for the future (11). Attention is drawn to the fact that various factors can function as protective factors and/or risk factors depending on the unique psychosocial characteristics of each adolescent. This is crucial for treatment teams to understand so as to not misinterpret their patient's experience of any identified factors as always a protective factor and/or always a risk factor.

The concept of symbolic interactionism from Grounded Theory indicates that behavior is determined by adaptation to the environment making healthy adaptation even more critical (10). The following table lists several mechanisms often associated with coping in children and adolescents diagnosed with CID.

Table 3. Coping mechanisms (6, 7, 10)

Disengagement
Engagement
Optimism
Hope
Resilience
Benefit-finding
Meaning-making
Post-traumatic growth
Positive outlook
Constructive internal dialogue Positive thinking
Hope for the future

Child and adolescent developmental considerations

Chronic illness and disability can often be embarrassing leaving many children and adolescents feeling neglected, isolated, or forgotten about. Other children can also often be cruel and tease children about their illness causing increased anxiety, depression, and low self-esteem. In school settings some teachers and staff may not fully understand CID and as a result may not be as supportive as possible of a child's needs, such as frequently needing to use the rest room to avoid accidents. Problems with social life are also common for children and adolescents with CID and can be so problematic that they find the hospital more comforting and do not necessarily want to leave. Another factor facing children and adolescents is that their parents often put pressure on them to be grateful to the medical team for which they may have a strained and difficult relationship (4).

Children and adolescents are at an increased risk of psychosocial adaptation problems than those without CID and will often experience: "...lower self-image, poorer body image, problems with psychological well-being, behavior problems, and social adjustment" (8). A higher risk of psychosocial problems has been found in children and adolescents with conditions with an uncertain prognosis, an "invisible condition", and chronic pain. Other risk factors include: "...male gender, low self-esteem, poor psychological health, poor school achievement, and lower sociable temperament" (8). Research is inconsistent whether or not CID in childhood or adolescence has a negative impact on adult functioning.

Emotional impact of CID

Children and adolescents adapting to CID almost always experience an emotional and/or psychosomatic component which necessitates the integration of psychologists into the medical team (4). Integration of psychologists is essential because families are often caught off guard when referred to a psychologist or are skeptical of the presence of psychologists on the medical team if they are not fully integrated. Families tend to be much more accepting when they can meet the psychologist as part of the medical team and at regular medical appointments as opposed to going to a different location for mental health care. The following Table 4 lists common emotional effects on children and adolescents adapting to CID (4).

Table 4. Emotional effects on children with CID (4)

- Lower educational achievement
- Less anxious in the face of illness compared to normal peers
- Denial may be a helpful coping mechanism for children
- Children with CI are often in a regressed state which makes it even more difficult for them to understand information about their illness
  - Adult explanation are too complicated even for adolescents
- More emphasis should be paid to educating parents rather than children/adolescents
- Huge capacity for misinterpretation compared to adults
- Belief they acquired illness due to doing something wrong or bad
- Providing scientific explanations of what is going on often will not help alleviate a child's anxiety; rather, always try and elicit the child's perception of what is causing the illness
- Capacity to adjust is often quite dependent on emotional functioning of parents
- If children are unable to express emotion well there could be an exacerbation of physical symptoms – psychosomatic

Protective/risk factors

For successful psychosocial adaptation adolescents must learn to manage the developmental tasks all adolescents must face while at the same time manage their chronic illness (11). Positive protective factors include constructive internal dialogue, positive thinking, and hope for the future. Attention is drawn to how the same factors can function as protective factors and/or risk factors depending on the unique psychosocial characteristics of each adolescent. Unfortunately, most interventions are medical and do not focus specifically on psychosocial factors. Categories of risk and protective factors include: religiosity/faith, daily routine and time, emotions, hospitalization, health and body; and family, friends, support structure and socialization. The following (see Table 5) are two lists with specific positive factors and specific risk factors impacting successful adaptation to chronic illness (11).

Table 5. Protective and risk factors (11)

Protective Factors	Risk Factors
• Faith/belief in non-tangible resources • Adapting daily routines to fit medical procedures • Positive internal dialogue/positive thinking • Creative adjustment to challenges • Laughter/humor • Acceptance/acknowledgement • Responsibility/self-discipline • Positive attitude • Self-care and emotional awareness • Positive actions such as sports / encouraging words • Good communication between doctor/patient and that treatment protocols are understood by the patient • Hospitalization (many aspects) – emotional support, opportunity to talk about religious beliefs, having visitors, crafts, rest time "creative adjustment". • Support of families – help adolescent understand the need for treatment • Friends • Expanded support system beyond medical team – life coaches	• Why me? • Medical procedures that are time consuming and uncomfortable • Not restful idleness • Missing out on social activities, school • Feeling isolated – will try to hide illness • Lack of peer acceptance – leads to lower levels of self-worth for adolescents • Loss/regret • Bereavement – death of friends with CF • Mood swings/negative emotions • Hospitalization (many aspects) • Feelings of powerlessness • Invasive procedures • Struggling to breathe, tiredness, poor sleep • Feeling like a different person • Stress • Worry about the future • Illness impacts whole life

Family

The literature provides an abundance of support linking family and CID seen in children and adolescents (12–17). The role of family is often mentioned in discussions regarding CID for children and adolescents; however, the literature also agrees that much more research needs to be done on the topic (15, 17). The term *family* in relation to CID is considered in many different ways. Family can be looked at in terms of caregiver reaction to their child's illness in terms of both negative and positive outcomes (12, 16). *Family* can be considered in terms of how CID impact the entire family unit in regards to several factors including financial, embarrassment, changing social roles of parent and child, impact on siblings, and problems impacting the extended family (13). Family is also considered in terms of psychosocial interventions and the importance of choosing to include or not include family in those interventions (14, 18). The focus on this section of the chapter is overarching concepts related to CID; however, the importance of family in relation to CID for children and adolescents is stressed.

Team integration

The importance of comprehensive integrated care cannot be ignored when treating CID. Integrated care programs will lead to the most effective care and improved outcomes (3). In regard to psychosocial adaptation integrated care is critically important because more mental health problems are seen in primary care than in any other health care setting. Management of chronic illness is almost always accompanied by a wide array of psychosocial factors that need to be addressed as part of a comprehensive team approach that focuses on treating the whole person as opposed to the individual parts. The development of integrative behavioral health models into medical teams in treating chronic illness will help to put the patient at the center of their health care. Children and adolescents with CID place strong value on emotional support from the medical team so much so that they indicate it helps with overall medical outcomes (3).

Understanding that CID impacts the whole person helps justify the importance of meeting psychosocial needs as part of the method to improve treatment outcomes. The idea that one system manage medical care and another manage mental health and behavioral health contradicts integrated care models. Such a design that separates treatment actually implies separating mind from body and will increase the overall costs of health care (3).

If psychosocial issues are not addressed they can be a barrier to treatment (1). Integrated teams should address the following psychosocial factors: "... patients culture, belief system, values, socioeconomic status, family conditions, religion, psychosocial status, and well-being" (3). Access to mental health providers at medical appointments can help patients with psychosocial adjustment and health care behaviors; without integrated mental health providers many children and adolescents with CID would not access mental health services.

ASSESSMENT OF PSYCHOSOCIAL ADAPTATION

Livneh and Antonak (6) wrote a wonderful paper to help mental health professionals understand psychosocial adaptation to CID. Within this article assessment of CID was discussed from a global perspective as opposed to illness specific assessment. The authors identified the following six measures:

Table 6. Global measures of psychosocial adaptation to CID (6)

Millon Behavior Health Inventory (MHBI)
Psychosocial Adjustment to Illness Scale (PAIS)
Acceptance of Disability Scale (AD)
Sickness Impact Profile (SIP)
Reactions to Impairment and Disability Inventory (RIDI)
Handicap Problems Inventory

Others have also suggested using more focused psychological assessments (9). This could help providers better understand individual patient characteristics and develop patient and/or illness specific interventions. The following assessments were described:

However, Livneh and Antonak (6) suggested counselors and therapists be cautious using traditional psychological assessments that have not been developed and normed for patients with CID. This is because sometimes the physical symptoms of CID can be similar to mental health symptoms. For example, fatigue is often associated with depression as well as many chronic illnesses, and using assessment tools that do not take into account the symptoms of the physical illness may over-identify mental health symptoms. Of most concern is that mental health staff be knowledgeable about co-morbid psychological conditions and be able differentiate symptoms (9).

Table 7. Specific psychological assessments (9)

Behavior Assessment System for Children – Second Edition (BASC-2)*
Children's Depression Inventory (CDI)*
Posttraumatic Stress Reaction Index (PSRI)
Pediatric Quality of Life Inventory (PEDS-QL)

When to conduct psychosocial adaptation assessment

There is some variability regarding when to use psychosocial assessments. Often treatment teams will administer assessments for all new patients and then yearly thereafter or whenever it appears as though there could be a need for assessment. Team integration also plays a large role in assessment. If the treatment team includes a psychologist or social worker that person can often do the necessary assessments and make decisions on when it is appropriate to refer out to a psychologist for more comprehensive evaluation. If there is not a mental health provider on the team nurses, nurse practitioners, physician's assistants, and even the medical doctors can often administer the assessments. It is even possible to train graduate level psychology students to help with simple assessment screening with the proper supervision.

PSYCHOSOCIAL TREATMENT AND INTERVENTION

Providing effective treatment to children and adolescents struggling with CID can be challenging. In fact, providing effective treatment to children and adolescents struggling with treatment adherence alone can be very difficult and yield mixed results (9). Adding in the often multiple and complex psychosocial factors that impact overall adaptation to CID can make effective psychosocial treatment extremely difficult. The focus on psychosocial treatment and intervention in this chapter was intentional as it can be a common mistake to focus treatment on only the medical problems or lack of improved medical outcomes (11). A good example is focusing on the treatment regimen for children and adolescents diagnosed with diabetes. In this case focusing on the treatment regimen alone is likely not the best target of intervention, but rather to focus on the often multiple and complex psychosocial factors impacting the treatment regimen such as affective characteristics, acceptance, personal uniqueness, peer group acceptance, acceptance of treatment by family and school, and treatment integration (1). The following Table 8 lists several interventions and strategies for treating the psychosocial aspect of CID (4, 9, 20).

Just as multiple psychosocial factors impact CID multiple treatment interventions are typically necessary (9). For example, the child with diabetes struggling with treatment adherence might benefit best from a combination of treatments and interventions such as an initial assessment with parents, behavior contracting, motivational interviewing, and objective feedback. Often children and adolescents may accept counseling to help navigate through a crisis but will soon stop after the immediate problems are resolved. However, many children with CID will adamantly deny any emotional problems related to their illness or that the illness is impacted by emotional functioning (4). Livneh and Antonak (6) suggested global interventions which often include 4 steps: 1) exploring the meaning of CI, 2) provide relevant medical information, 3) providing supportive family/group experiences, and 4) teaching adaptive coping skills. However, more treatments and intervention strategies validated for children and adolescents are needed.

Table 8. Interventions and strategies for children and adolescent with CID (4, 9, 20)

- initial assessment with parent and child
- assessment of psychological adjustment
- Individual counseling
- Family and Marital work
- Family Systems
- Parent and staff groups
- Adolescent groups
- Cognitive Behavioral Therapy
- Behavior Therapy
- psycho-dynamic therapies
- behavior management
- behavior contracting
- behavior plans
- behavioral adherence promotion
- reinforcement
- motivational interviewing
- supportive therapies
- objective feedback about adherence
- psychoeducation
- relaxation, biofeedback, or self-hypnosis
- respiratory muscle biofeedback
- music therapy
- dance and movement therapy
- tele-medicine

CONCLUSION

Psychosocial adaptation to chronic illness and disability for children and adolescents is a complex phenomenon that impacts the whole person and presents a myriad of factors that must be addressed by a multidisciplinary team including but not limited to: medical professionals (physicians, nurses, nurse practitioners, physician assistants), allied health professionals (occupational therapists, physical therapists, dieticians), and mental health professionals (psychologists, social workers, counselors). In supporting the medical home philosophy it would be ideal for multidisciplinary teams to collaboratively provide all services in one location. Such a holistic approach would better meet the complex needs of children and adolescents diagnosed with CID and likely lead to improved medical and psychosocial outcomes.

One significant factor impacting a global discussion of CID are the vast number of illnesses and disabilities that qualify as CID that are often quite different in presentation with the only commonality being the *chronicity* of the illness or disability. This chapter did provide a global overview of CID which is very important when beginning to work with children and adolescents with CID. The literature regarding CID provides little consistency about the process of psychosocial adaptation to CID for children and adolescents. There are some processes defined by individual authors or studies devoted to specific CID but few global processes are described. Some of the most encouraging information comes from the field of positive psychology that has identified many factors which contribute to successful psychosocial adaptation. However, more scholarship and research remains to be done regarding the psychosocial adaptation of specific CID for children and adolescents.

Fortunately, there are multiple assessment and intervention strategies for children and adolescents diagnosed with CID. Now, the task remains for the integration of professions to create the necessary multidisciplinary teams that can created unified intervention approaches that meet the specific and complex needs of children and adolescents adapting to chronic illnesses and disabilities.

REFERENCES

[1] Apple RW. Adolescents' experience of the factors influencing their diabetes treatment regimen - ProQuest 2009. URL: http://search.proquest.com/docview/89200242.

[2] Goldberg ID, Regier DA, McInerny TK, Pless IB, Roghmann KJ. The role of the pediatrician in the delivery of mental health services to children. Pediatrics 1979;63:898–909.

[3] Jortberg BT, Miller BF, Gabbay RA, Sparling K, Dickinson WP. Patient-centered medical home: how it affects psychosocial outcomes for diabetes. Curr Diab Rep 2012;12(6):721–8.

[4] Bruce T. Emotional sequelae of chronic inflammatory bowel disease in children and adolescents. Clin Gastroenterol 1986;15(1):89–104.

[5] Bishop M. Quality of life and psychosocial adaptation to chronic illness and disability: Preliminary analysis of a conceptual and theoretical synthesis. Rehabil Couns Bull 2005;48(4):219–31.

[6] Livneh H, Antonak RF. Psychosocial adaptation to chronic illness and disability: A primer for counselors. J Couns Dev 2005;83(1):12–20.

[7] Martz E, Livneh H. Psychosocial adaptation to disability within the context of positive psychology: Findings from the literature. J Occup Rehabil 2016;26(1):4-12.

[8] Huurre TM, Aro HM. Long-term psychosocial effects of persistent chronic illness. A follow-up study of Finnish adolescents aged 16 to 32 years. Eur Child Adolesc Psychiatry 2002;11(2):85–91.

[9] Cortina S, Somers M, Rohan JM, Drotar D. Clinical effectiveness of comprehensive psychological intervention for nonadherence to medical treatment: A case series. J Pediatr Psychol 2013;38(6):649–63.

[10] Lin C-C, Han C-Y, Pan I-J. A qualitative approach of psychosocial adaptation process in patients undergoing long-term hemodialysis. Asian Nurs Res (Korean Soc Nurs Sci) 2015;9(1):35–41.

[11] Hugo CJ, van der Merwe M. South African adolescents with cystic fibrosis: A qualitative exploration of their bio-psychosocial fields. J Child Adolesc Ment Health 2014;26(3):177–91.

[12] Nabors L a, Kichler JC, Brassell A, Thakkar S, Bartz J, Pangallo J, et al. Factors related to caregiver state anxiety and coping with a child's chronic illness. Fam Syst Health 2013;31(2): 171–80.

[13] Satterwhite BB. Impact of chronic illness on child and family: an overview based on five surveys with implications for management. Int J Rehabil Res 1978;1(1):7–17.

[14] Martire LM. The relative efficacy of involving family in psychosocial interventions for chronic illness: Are there added benefits to patients and family members? Fam Syst Health 2005;23(3):312–28.

[15] Berge JM, Patterson JM. Cystic fibrosis and the family: A review and critique of the literature. Fam Syst Health 2004;22(1):74–100.

[16] Cohen MS. Families coping with childhood chronic illness: A research review. Fam Syst Health 1999;17(2):149–64.

[17] White K, Kolman ML, Wexler P, Polin G, Winter RJ. Unstable diabetes and unstable families: a psychosocial evaluation of diabetic children with recurrent ketoacidosis. Pediatrics 1984;73(6):749–55.

[18] Scharff L, Langan N, Rotter N, Scott-Sutherland J, Schenck C, Tayor N, et al. Psychological, behavioral, and family characteristics of pediatric patients with chronic pain: A 1-year retrospective study and cluster analysis. Clin J Pain 2005;21(5):432–8.

[19] Millon® Behavioral Medicine Diagnostic. URL: http://www.pearsonclinical.com/psychology/products/100000231/millon-behavioral-medicine-diagnostic-mbmd.html.

[20] Goldbeck L, Fidika A, Herle M, Quittner AL. Psychological interventions for individuals with cystic fibrosis and their families. Cochrane Database Syst Rev 2014;6:CD003148.

In: Chronic Disease and Disability
Editors: DE Greydanus, P Anne, JD Rowlett et al.
ISBN: 978-1-53617-656-8

Chapter 18

PHYSICIAN USE OF BRIEF COUNSELING MODELS IN A PEDIATRIC OUTPATIENT SETTING

Roger W Apple**, PhD and Katie White, MA

Division of Developmental and Behavioral Pediatrics,
Department of Pediatric and Adolescent Medicine, Western Michigan University,
Homer Stryker MD School of Medicine, Kalamazoo, Michigan, United States of America

ABSTRACT

Brief counseling models can be used as brief counseling and intervention strategies by physicians in the outpatient setting for patients struggling with psychosocial stressors, engaging in risky behaviors, engaging in behaviors that negatively affect their health, or patients who simply are ambivalent or unaware of their need for change. These brief counseling models offer physician's an efficient and structured approach to behavior change that will add little, if any, time to appointments. Several models will be discussed including: BATHE, The Five A's, FRAMES, Motivational Interviewing, Stages of Change (transtheoretical model), Solution Focused Therapy, and Problem Solving Therapy. Additionally, this chapter devotes a discussion to the importance of the physician – patient relationship in regards implementing brief counseling models. Lastly, an overall discussion of these models in a pediatric outpatient setting is provided as well as limitations and implications for improvement.

INTRODUCTION

This chapter was written to highlight the need and importance of physicians using brief counseling models in the pediatric outpatient setting. As pediatricians are often the first stop, and sometimes only stop, for children and adolescents with mental health concerns knowledge and ability to implement brief counseling models is essential. In addition to providing brief

* Correspondence: Roger W Apple, PhD, Division of Developmental and Behavioral Pediatrics, Department of Pediatric and Adolescent Medicine, Western Michigan University, Homer Stryker MD School of Medicine, Kalamazoo, Michigan, United States. Email: Roger.apple@med.wmich.edu.

counseling for psychosocial issues, these models can also be used as a guide for structured conversations with patients regarding their psychosocial concern, medical concern, health risk behavior, or substance use problem. However, the use of brief counseling models specific to the pediatric outpatient setting is not prevalent in the literature and it is the intent that this chapter will begin to help fill that gap.

There are several different approaches to brief counseling models that can be chosen based on patient needs. The Five A's and Frames models are typically used for treating excessive smoking and drinking for patients ready for change; the Stages of Change and Motivational Interviewing models are used for improving health risk behavior for patients less ready for change; and Problem Solving, Solution Focused, and BATHE models are typically used for mental health and psychosocial issues (1). In setting the stage for a discussion of these models this chapter will first provide information regarding definition of brief counseling models, the role of the physician-patient relationship in implementation, considerations of use in pediatric outpatient settings, and a brief overview of each model.

DATABASE SEARCH

Several databases were searched including PubMed, PsychInfo, PsychArticles, as well as Google Scholar to identify the most salient literature. Searching for literature was difficult due to a variety of terminology used to described what this chapter is calling *Brief Counseling Models*. Other terms used include behavior change models, behavior readiness models, counseling, and cross-cultural communication models. In all, seven models were identified that can provide physicians with a structured framework in which to effectively communicate with their patients regarding psychosocial and substance use problems.

FINDINGS

This chapter provides an overview of seven brief counseling models that are rarely presented together in the literature. Presenting a variety of models in one chapter will provide physicians with an abundance of options to choose from in order to best help them respond to their patients' needs. Brief descriptions of each model are offered as well as tables which provide suggestions for implementation. In addition, this chapter fills a void in the literature as it presents these models for use in the pediatric outpatient setting. Lastly, this chapter stresses the importance of the physician-patient relationship in the application of these models. All too often various interventions are discussed only in regards to the technical components of the interventions; this chapter stresses the importance of the physician-patient relationship in the effective delivery of brief counseling models. Without a healthy physician-patient relationship the likelihood of successful implementation will significantly decrease.

DEFINITION

Brief counseling models are suggested as a useful tool for an outpatient office setting because they are "time limited, their focus is on current concerns rather than on the past" (2) "they adopt an active role and encourages the client to become actively engaged in the change process" (2). The brief counseling models outlined below are brief interventions that can be used by physicians to assist their interaction with patients who may be struggling with a psychosocial stressor, engaging in risky behavior, participating in behaviors that negatively affect their health, or patients who simply are ambivalent or unaware of their need for change. In training physicians the medical model generally puts the physician as the expert when giving the patient advice or information regarding ways to change (3). The physician reviews medical data, interprets how a patient's behavior is impacting their health and then the physician gives a persuasive message on how and why to change which gives the patient two options; to either accept it or resist it (3). This can make it difficult for the patient to collaborate with their physician and as a result may become ambivalent or non-compliant with their want to change.

Brief counseling models "offer an efficient means of targeting behavioral, developmental, and social problems" and are patient-centered (4). This allows the patient to be directly involved in their want and need for change. It puts them in charge of their life and allows the physician to be there as an educator who helps the patient develop a plan; it allows them to provide encouragement to the patient and develop a collaborative rapport which can increase a successful outcome. Using brief counseling models have "been shown to improve pediatric health outcomes ranging from adherence to functional status" (4).

The models discussed are useful in sparking conversation and initiating awareness. This is the first step in creating change. Many factors go into whether or not behavior changes will occur and center on the motivation and desire of the patient. These tools can help a physician begin a conversation in a manner that is focused on the needs of the patient and what they are willing to do at that particular moment in the hopes that it will eventually elicit change.

ROLE OF THE PHYSICIAN-PATIENT RELATIONSHIP

The role of the physician – patient relationship is crucial for effective care in any medical setting. Nobile et al. (5) reports that the physician-patient relationship is one of the most complex interpersonal relationships in society because it revolves around a number of important issues; physical health and emotional well-being which can become complicated because the knowledge and perspective of the patient and physician are often different. These perspectives are becoming more profound and altered because of the advancement in technology and medicine (5). The method in which a physician communicates with their patient can become the way to obtain a constructive relationship or an ineffective one. Because of this, communication is one of the most complex tools a physician must learn.

Communication becomes even more complicated when physicians practice in a pediatric outpatient setting because this setting elicits a number of multifaceted issues that adult settings do not. D. Purvis (6) illustrated this by stating that pediatric physicians must learn how to not only communicate with a population that varies in emotional development and cognitive abilities due to age but also with a population that ranges from patients being; infants that are unaware because of their age, uniformed children and invincible teenagers, who are either unable to verbalize their wants and needs or are intimidated because of the setting and participants. In addition to a complicated patient population pediatric medicine requires the participation of the child's parents or caregivers. This creates a triad of interaction which requires the physician to not only be a leader but also a follower (6). The way in which a physician communicates with both the child and parents can impact the success of further interactions and adherence to treatment plans (5).

Physicians in this setting also encounter a variety of presenting complaints that often go beyond the scope of medicine. These problems can range from parental complaints regarding behavior, developmental issues, concerns about academics, and reports of mood disorders and substance use. It is also suggested that the more somatic complaints a patient presents with the more likely they are suffering from a psychological disorder rather than from a medical problem (7). These complaints result in physicians providing nearly 50% of mental health services in the United States (8). Pediatric primary care physicians are therefore the first to encounter these problems and become the first in line to provide therapy to assist their patients. Physicians in this role often report problems related to time constraints and ineffective training and expertise as the most significant barriers they encounter when trying to help their patients and families in need of brief counseling (5, 8).

In addition to learning skills such as active listening, empathy, including patient decision making, and providing care that is patient centered (6), learning interventions like brief counseling models can also assist physicians in effectively helping their patients. Since the physician is often the first line of defense when it comes to combating mental health issues, skills like having the ability to listen to the patient, provide support, legitimizing their concerns, elicit and reflect feelings, showing respect and establishing a healing relationship, are effective communication skills that will build a strong trustful rapport (7) which will then become critically important when implementing behavior change models.

CONSIDERATIONS IN A PEDIATRIC SETTING

Several considerations arise in determining the practicality of the described brief counseling models with the pediatric population. A primary concern is the vast variation in cognitive abilities in pediatric patients generally ranging in age from 0 to 18 years. In pediatric settings a physician may wonder if questions should be directed toward the patient and/or the parent; this is not clear in the models we have described. We are suggesting that when asking questions pertaining to the models described that rephrasing the questions to meet the child's or adolescents' level of understanding may be necessary. Also, when interacting with younger pediatric patients (up to age 9 or 10 years) the parent may be the one that responds to a majority of the questions with the child and/or adolescent gradually increasing their role in responding to questions as age and cognitive ability develop.

Children of all ages can experience a variety of mental health concerns and screening for them is just as important as it is with adults. It is estimated that 1 in 5 children/adolescents in the United States suffer from some type of mental health issue and if left untreated can be harmful for their development (9).

Pediatric patients often have mental health concerns such as delayed development, social problems, behavior concerns, and affective concerns, that when identified and treated early, can help prevent the developing of more significant symptoms and disorders.

In addition, utilizing these brief counseling models in a pediatric outpatient setting can also help identify mental health concerns of caregivers that may be directly impacting the child's or adolescent's functioning. If a caregiver is suffering from a mood disorder, substance abuse problem, or is struggling with parental responsibilities, these areas can be recognized and appropriate services can be recommended. Caregiver functioning is critical to the mental health functioning of children and adolescents and it is an area that should not be overlooked.

These brief counseling models are meant to open the lines of communication between the patient and the physician and assist them in uncovering possible psychosocial concerns that may be influencing the patients' medical concerns (7). Once a physician identifies an area of concern they can continue treatment in an outpatient setting or refer the patient to a psychologist for further evaluation if needed. Using these simple models can help the physician create a trusting relationship with their patients. As a result of using these models pediatricians can help shape how a patient responds to the health care system.

If children and adolescents feel they are "being respected, listened to, and understood...can set the stage for a child's future performance" (6) and shape their life-long attitude toward their physician and response to interventions and recommendations.

BRIEF COUNSELING MODELS

All of the brief counseling models discussed below have been deemed beneficial in primary care settings, but their usefulness is not as well documented in pediatric outpatient settings. This chapter helps fill that void in the literature by providing suggestions on how to incorporate these models in pediatric outpatient settings, however, further research is needed to determine effectiveness within this population.

It will likely be best not to use the following models with only the child for a variety of reasons; lack of understanding, the child likely having little control over environmental factors, and dependence on parental support. When using these techniques when communicating with both the parent and child will likely promote the best outcome. It is important to remember that physicians are often the first professionals to meet with children and adolescents struggling with psychosocial concerns and these models provide tools to begin a conversation of effective communication and potential change.

Health risk behavior models

Endorsed by the American Academy of Pediatrics, the 5 A technique uses an evidenced based sequence that was developed as a tool to help patients change risky behavior such as smoking and alcohol use and for increasing healthy behaviors like eating and exercising (8, 10, 11). The 5 A's is a single model that is based on the principles of cognitive behavioral therapy and can be used to address all of the listed health risk behaviors; alcohol and tobacco use, unhealthy eating and shortage of physical activity, which are behaviors that have become the leading cause of disease, death and loss of functioning in the United States (11, 12). It is a tool that is used to gage a patient's risk, their current behaviors, and their readiness to change (13). This model also allows the physician to; give advice about change, provides collaboration between the physician and patient to set goals, encourages the physician to help the client address hurdles they may come in contact with during this change, and this model suggests the physician schedule follow up appointments to track progress (13). Research has shown that this model increases a patients motivation (13) and is a technique that is more effective than the physician just making recommendations alone (8) which in turn likely increases the odds of a patient being successful in obtaining their goals. Table 1 was created and modified to show how the 5 A's can be used in a pediatric setting (8, 10, 12).

Table 1. Five A's

FIVE A's	Implementation	Physicians Interventions
Ask	Begin by *asking* the patient or the caregiver about potential risky behavior that may have been identified during the course of the appointment. This is to help the physician identify the behavior and to determine if the patient/caregiver identifies this as problematic. For instance in a pediatric setting a pediatrician maybe concerned about a child's unhealthy weight and determine this as a health risk behavior	The physician can use communication, results from written assessments, or data from physiologic risk factors like body mass index to identify risky behavior
Advise	Once the pediatrician along with the patient/caregiver have singled out a potential risky behavior the physician can *advise* them of risks if the behavior continues and benefits if they cease the risky behavior Keeping in mind the importance of communication with a patient and caregiver this advice should be specific to the patient's symptoms, and patient's and caregiver's values and concerns and should be brief in delivery.	The physician can provide evidence to support the advice they are giving by showing specific data of the consequences or benefits of either continuing or ceasing the behavior. This can help support the physician's advice
Assess	During this step a physician should ask questions that helps them *assess* how motivated the patient/caregiver is to change the risky behavior and to determine a reasonable time line to begin. This step should be done in a collaborative way	If a patient is motivated you can set a specific time frame to begin. If they are not motivated to change you can help the patient/caregiver determine a time frame when they may be more interested in change.
Assist	During this stage the physician can *assist* the patient/caregiver in developing a goal-setting plan, which again should be collaborative in nature. The physician and patient/caregiver should identify barriers, talk about overcoming those barriers, and the physician should provide support and encouragement for the patient/caregiver as they begin working toward the set goals.	The physician can help the patient/caregiver remember the goals by providing written documentation of the plan. The physician may want to provide additional resources who may have more expertise for the specific need that was identified
Arrange	The physician should *arrange* follow up appointments or communication via phone to keep in contact with the patients/caregivers to determine their adherence to the set goal plan	In addition to the physician keeping in contact with the patient/caregiver the physician would benefit from having an open line of communication with any other professional involved in the action plan

* Table modified for a pediatric setting.

FRAMES

This model is used to help change a patient's health risk behavior and non-adherence with chronic disease treatment plans (1). This model focuses on the premise that it is the patient's responsibility to want and make changes (1). The physician's role is to offer strategies that may help the patient and assist the patient by collaboration in tailoring what works best for them (1, 8). Table 2 shows suggestions of how to use the FRAMES method in a pediatric setting (1, 8).

Table 2. FRAMES

Component	Purpose	Considerations in Pediatrics
Feedback about personal risk	Provide objective feedback about health risk behavior such as problems with treatment adherence.	Feedback will need to match the patient's developmental ability to understand. Many children and even adolescents will not understand complex explanations about their health risk behavior.
Responsibility of Patient	Responsibility – FRAMES works to empower the patient to view themselves as the one who has the control over the condition or problem.	During this stage patients and family will often both be responsible for treatment. If sole responsibility is put on the child rather than the family, failure is likely.
Advice to change	Depending on the patient's willingness to change physician can offer advice for behavior change.	Again, information will need to be tailored to ability to understand.
Menu of strategies	Offer a wide range of options – a "menu" for behavior change strategies.	Collaborating with the child and family is important as well as offering strategies offered by the child.
Empathetic style	Use of empathy is highly encouraged in this model providing the patient with a sense of understanding on behalf of the physician.	Often younger children and adolescents may not fully understand their condition or treatment. The physician using empathy to convey that the illness and treatment to the child may be confusing and not make sense will likely help the child trust the physician.
Promote Self efficacy	Support and encourage self-efficacy and the patient's ability to change.	As mentioned above, the entire family's ability to change will need to be supported.

* Table modified for a pediatric setting.

Psychosocial models

The BATHE model can help a physician screen for anxiety, depression and situational disorders (7) which may account for physical complaints that a patient originally sought services for in an outpatient setting (14). It is a tool that was specifically developed for physicians in a primary care setting by a psychologist and a family physician (1). This technique is popular with physicians because it allows them to build rapport easily with their patients, it is simple to understand and its implementation is fast, usually completed within five to seven minutes (15, 16). Studies regarding this method have shown positive results for patient satisfaction because they felt their physician was sympathetic and concerned about their problems (14, 17). The BATHE method suggests that the questions be asked in a uniform and systematic manner. Table 3 was created and adapted to show how the physician can implement the BATHE model in a pediatric setting (1, 7, 8, 15, 16).

Table 3. BATHE

Component	Implementation	Example for pediatric setting
Background	Begin with a simple direct question to get background regarding the concern and to determine the heart of the problem that the patient/caregiver has.	"It sounds like your main concern is about your child's behavior at school."
Affect	The physician should pose a question to ask how the patient/caregiver feels about their concern.	"How does this make you feel when he has outbursts at school?"
Troubles	The physician should ask a question to narrow down the most troubling thing. It is important to remember that what the physician thinks is the most troublesome issue may not be what the patient/caregiver perceives as most troublesome.	"What troubles you most about your child's behavior?"
Handling	The physician asks a question that helps them find out how the patient/caregiver is handling the situation, what the patients/caregivers internal resources are and provides direction for intervention	The physician may find out that the parent is teaching the child to defend themselves with aggressive behavior. You can reflect back to them that this suggestion may be a contributing factor to their child getting into trouble at school.
Empathy	The physician asks an empathetic question with the intention to build rapport and trust between the patient and physician.	"I know you only want to teach your child to protect themselves when you are not there and this situation must be very difficult for you."

* Table modified for a pediatric setting.

Problem Solving Therapy

Table 4. Problem Solving Therapy

Component	Description	Implementation in a Pediatric Setting
Problem Definition	Conduct a thorough clinical interview and define the problem with behavioral evidence.	The younger the patient the more involved the family will need to be in the clinical interview to help clarify the problem as accurately as possible. As the child's age increases they can have an increasing role in providing information during this stage.
Generating alternative solutions	Use brainstorming in collaboration with the patient and/or family to generate possible alternative solutions to the problem.	As in Problem Definition the family will need to be involved depending on the age of the patient. Also, when working in a pediatric setting consultation with and obtaining the school perspective is often necessary. It is also important to remember that ideas generated by children are often not what an adult would suggest but should be considered fully to build a collaborative relationship.
Decision Making	Discuss with the patient and family the benefits and/or consequences of generated solutions.	Helping children narrow down solutions may take longer than with an adult population. Offering children options which include adult and child generated solutions and giving them the ability to choose is recommended.
Solution verification and implementation	Review generated solutions with the patient and family and collaboratively develop a plan.	Work with the child and/or family to develop and implement the plan. Involving the caregivers and school may also be beneficial.

* Table modified for a pediatric setting.

Problem Solving Therapy is a brief counseling model that is a specific approach but also a term in a general way to indicate strategies which can be used to solve a variety of problems and concerns (8, 18–20). The model begins by having the physician use questions to identify a specific problem, collaboration with the patient and/or family to generate solutions, make decisions, followed by reviewing solutions and implementation. Problem Solving Therapy can be used to treat a variety of pediatric conditions including anxiety and depression (19), obesity (18), and psychosocial factors associated with pediatric oncology (20). Table 4 helps to explain how this model can be implemented in a pediatric setting (8, 18–20).

Solution Focused Therapy

This model focuses on how to solve a patient's problem rather than focusing on the problem itself and makes the patient the expert and the physician a collaborator (2). It helps the patient increase their desired behavior or obtain their desired goal (21). It is a technique that helps a patient imagine how and what they would like to have different about their life and then explores ways to make that happen (22). Table 5 provides insight into how the solution focused model works in a pediatric setting (2, 22).

Table 5. Solution Focused Therapy

Type	Question	Interventions	Examples in a pediatric setting
Miracle Question	Suppose when you go to sleep tonight, a miracle happens and your problem is solved. When you wake up in the morning, how will you know that a miracle has occurred? What will be different?	After obtaining a specific change that a patient would like to make help them explore solutions to make this happen	A parent or child may respond that their miracle would be to no longer argue every day with one another
Exception Question	Can you think of a time in the past week when you did not have the problem? Or the problem was not as troublesome?	Help the patient identify and recognize that the problem may not occur all the time and help identify what made that particular time better	A child and parent may state that last week when they were driving to a store they were able to have a conversation that did not lead to an argument
Scaling Question	On a scale from 1 to 10, how did you feel last week? On a scale from 1 to 10, how motivated are you?	Help them recognize their role in the ability to make change which can be determinant on motivation	This question can help understand how motivated each party is to work on the issue or whether this identified problem is a chronic problem over a longer period of time or if there is a more identifiable problem (like arguing over curfew as the specific problem rather than communication as a whole.)

* Table modified for a pediatric setting.

Motivation and commitment models

Unlike the previous models, motivational interviewing has preliminarily been supported as a useful technique in the pediatric setting because of its impressive results when used in the adult population in the treatment of behavior change (3, 23). Motivational interviewing is a "goal-directed, client-centered counseling approach to help patients increase intrinsic motivation and strengthen commitment for change through the exploration and resolution of ambivalence" (3). The goal of motivational interviewing is enhancing the connection between the patient and the physician into a more collaborative relationship allowing the patient to remain autonomous in creating their plan to change. Motivational interviewing uses specific techniques; open ended questions that require a detailed response, affirmations that express empathy and understating, reflections of feeling and reflective listening (2). Motivational interviewing can also be used for treatment adherence concerns in chronic illnesses such as cystic fibrosis (24). Table 6 describes how motivational interviewing can be implemented in a pediatric setting (3, 8, 23, 24):

Table 6. Motivational Interviewing

Component	Examples in a Pediatric Setting
Agenda Setting	Ask the child for permission to discuss their illness, condition, or behavior. Asking permission helps establish acceptance of the problem, willingness to participate in treatment, and a collaborative relationship.
Exploration	Explore the patient's readiness for change. During this stage it will also be important to assess the caregiver's readiness for change and ability to follow through with recommendations.
Providing Information	After the agenda is set and problem explored the physician can now provide information specific to the condition as well as to the treatment. Providing education and support before this stage could be detrimental because the provider has not yet illustrated that they understand the problem.
Summarizing	Summarize the patient and family's perspective acknowledging what has worked, what has not, and what they are willing to do to move forward. This will also encourage the patient and family to further clarify their perspective if necessary.
Generating options & Contracting	Review information from steps above and generate options allowing the patient and family to choose a plan that works best for them. At this stage the physician will encourage the patient and family to follow recommendations and to return and a subsequent visit to review.

*Table modified for a pediatric setting.

Stages of Change (transtheoretical model)

This model was developed as a way to help clinicians and patients understand that change occurs in a series of stages. It does not suggest that change is linear but often will occur by cycling through the stages several times (2). Understanding this can help a physician determine what intervention to start with depending on what stage a patient may be in. Utilizing this model begins with the physician initiating awareness and then using this awareness to increase motivation until the patient is ready for action (8). Motivation has been deemed the most important factor for movement in this spectrum (25). In a pediatric setting determining a parent's motivation to change is critical in helping a pediatric patient and can be influenced by a parents; willingness and readiness to change, the severity of the child's problem and level of worry a parent has about the child's problem (25). Promoting and building self-efficacy is a key component in the ability to move through the stages of change with evidence that individuals in higher stages have more self-confidence (26, 27). This model stresses that relapse is a very possible outcome and encourages a physician to understand this and to "accept the patient in whatever stage they are in, while concurrently supporting progress toward healthier behavioral changes." (3) (pg. 418). Table 7 was created and adapted to show how the physician can implement the stages of model in a pediatric setting (2, 8, 26, 27).

Table 7. Stages of Change

Stage	Implementation	Examples in a pediatric setting
Pre-contemplation	During this stage a patient has little awareness into any problem or need for change and has no intention to change their behavior.	"You (the patient) or your son's (caregiver) body mass index is well over the 90th%" Have you ever tried diet modifications to help him lose weight?" "What happened when you did try this?" In this stage a patient or caregiver may not see the harmful effects of having a b.m.i this high or they may have tried diets in the past that were unsuccessful.
Contemplation	A patient is aware that they need to change and plans to in the next 6 months but may still be ambivalent and not have a specific plan.	"What would be the advantages/disadvantages or concerns to trying a diet modification or exercise routine?"
Preparation	The patient plans to take action in the immediate future (within a month) and a realistic plan.	"What date do you want to start this diet/exercise routine?" Also discuss possible problems and specific plans to begin the change.
Action	The patient takes concrete steps to change the behavior.	"How has your exercise/diet routine been going?" Ask questions regarding any changes in the plan, setbacks, unexpected events, and how they overcame it to continue on their journey.
Maintenance	The patient has maintained a change for at least six months and is taking steps to prevent relapse.	Explaining to the patient/caregiver that relapses are common and providing praise and support for not giving up can be empowering

* Table modified for a pediatric setting.

Conclusion

The need for physicians' use of brief counseling models in the pediatric outpatient setting is critical to best meet the needs of their patients as the physician is often the first, and sometimes only, treating professional that children and adolescents visit when struggling with health risk behaviors and psychosocial problems. Brief counseling models offer a time-limited and structured approach that physicians can use to facilitate such conversations, develop collaborative relationships, and make the patient the center of treatment. In applying these models in a pediatric setting it is important to note that physicians may need to modify the model to meet the needs of pediatric patients such as including parents in conversations and asking questions that children and adolescents are able to understand. It will also be important to take in to consideration the impact of parental functioning on the functioning of the child or adolescent. Brief counseling models offer some mental health intervention in a medical setting for children and adolescents and can help prepare outpatient settings for the growing surge of integrated behavioral health models.

REFERENCES

[1] Searight HR. Efficient counseling techniques for the primary care physician. Prim Care 2007;34(3):551–70,vi – vii.

[2] Clinical Psychology. In: Psychology EPPP Preparation. Ventura, CA: Association for Advanced Training In The Behavioral Sciences, 2014:16–9.

[3] Suarez M, Mullins S. Motivational interviewing and pediatric health behavior interventions. J Dev Behav Pediatr 2008;29(5):417–28.

[4] Erickson SJ, Gerstle M, Feldstein SW. Brief interventions and motivational interviewing with children, adolescents, and their parents in pediatric health care settings: A review. Arch Pediatr Adolesc Med 2005;159(12):1173–80.

[5] Nobile C, Drotar D. Research on the quality of parent-provider communication in pediatric care: implications and recommendations. J Dev Behav Pediatr 2003;24(4):279–90.

[6] Purvis J. The challenge of communicating with pediatric patients. Rosemont, IL: American Academy Orthopaedic Surgeons, 2009.

[7] Lieberman JA, Stuart MR. The BATHE method: Incorporating counseling and psychotherapy into the everyday management of patients. Prim Care Companion J Clin Psychiatry 1999;1(2):35–8.

[8] Searight HR. Realistic approaches to counseling in the office setting. Am Fam Physician 2009;79(4):277–84.

[9] Kataoka SH, Zhang L, Wells KB. Unmet need for mental health care among US children: Variation by ethnicity and insurance status. Am J Psychiatry 2002;159(9):1548–55.

[10] van Dillen SME, Noordman J, van Dulmen S, Hiddink GJ. Quality of weight-loss counseling by Dutch practice nurses in primary care: an observational study. Eur J Clin Nutr 2015;69(1):73–8.

[11] Pbert L, Druker S, DiFranza JR, Gorak D, Reed G, Magner R, et al. Effectiveness of a school nurse-delivered smoking-cessation intervention for adolescents. Pediatrics 2011;128(5):926–36.

[12] Goldstein MG, Whitlock EP, DePue J. Multiple behavioral risk factor interventions in primary care. Summary of research evidence. Am J Prev Med 2004;27(2 Suppl):61–79.

[13] Jay M, Gillespie CC, Schlair S, Sherman S, Kalet AL. Physicians' use of the 5As in counseling obese patients: is the quality of counseling associated with patients' motivation and intention to lose weight? BMC Health Serv Res 2010;10(1):159.

[14] Leiblum SR, Schnall E, Seehuus M, DeMaria A. To BATHE or not to BATHE: patient satisfaction with visits to their family physician. Fam Med 2008;40(6):407–11.

[15] Lieberman JA III. Depression: A common illness uncommonly diagnosed. Psychiatr Ann 2002;32(9):522-6.

[16] Poon VH. Short counseling techniques for busy family doctors. Can Fam Physician 1997;43:705–8, 711–3.

[17] Kim JH, Park YN, Park EW, Cheong YS, Choi EY. Effects of BATHE interview protocol on patient satisfaction. Korean J Fam Med 2012;33(6):366–71.

[18] Resnicow K, Davis R, Rollnick S. Motivational interviewing for pediatric obesity: Conceptual issues and evidence review. J Am Diet Assoc 2006;106(12):2024–33.

[19] Weersing VR, Gonzalez A, Campo JV, Lucas AN. Brief Behavioral Therapy for Pediatric Anxiety and Depression: Piloting an integrated treatment approach. Cogn Behav Pract 2008;15(2):126–39.

[20] Kazak AE, Rourke MT, Alderfer MA, Pai A, Reilly AF, Meadows AT. Evidence-based assessment, intervention and psychosocial care in pediatric oncology: a blueprint for comprehensive services across treatment. J Pediatr Psychol 2007;32(9):1099–110.

[21] Bannink FP. Solution-Focused Brief Therapy. J Contemp Psychother 2007;37(2):87–94.

[22] Gingerich W, Eisengart S. SFBT: A review of the outcome research. Family Process 2004. doi.org/10.1111/j.1545-5300.2000.39408.x.

[23] Erickson SJ, Gerstle M, Feldstein SW. Brief interventions and motivational interviewing with children, adolescents, and their parents in pediatric health care settings: A review. Arch Pediatr Adolesc Med 2005;159(12):1173–80.

[24] Duff AJA, Latchford GJ. Motivational interviewing for adherence problems in cystic fibrosis. Pediatr Pulmonol 2010;45(3):211–20.

[25] Godoy L, Carter AS. Identifying and addressing mental health risks and problems in primary care pediatric settings: a model to promote developmental and cultural competence. Am J Orthopsychiatry 2013;83(1):73–88.

[26] Naar-King S, Wright K, Parsons JT, Frey M, Templin T, Ondersma S. Transtheoretical Model and substance use in HIV-positive youth. AIDS Care 2006;18(7):839–45.

[27] Tung W-C, Gillett PA, Pattillo RE. Applying the Transtheoretical Model to physical activity in family caregivers in Taiwan. Public Health Nurs 2005;22(4):299–310.

In: Chronic Disease and Disability
Editors: DE Greydanus, P Anne, JD Rowlett et al.
ISBN: 978-1-53617-656-8

Chapter 19

PEDIATRIC PALLIATIVE CARE IN CONGENITAL HEART DISEASE: A CASE-BASED APPROACH IN INFANTS AND CHILDREN

Natalie Kontos*[1]*, DO and
Premchand Anne*[1,2,*]*, MD, MPH, MBA, FAAP, FACP, FACC
[1]Pediatrics and [2]Pediatric Cardiology, Ascension St John Children's Hospital, Detroit, Michigan, United States of America

ABSTRACT

The purpose of this review is to discuss pediatric palliative care in the infant, toddler and young child population of critical congenital heart disease patients. It addresses how the parents, siblings and patients are affected. It will emphasize the importance of a cohesive approach to the patient and their family as a unit and how each separate piece of the puzzle needs to be addressed for providing optimal care to these critically ill patients.

INTRODUCTION

Congenital heart disease (CHD) affects about 1% of births every year in the United States, with about 25% of them having critical CHD (CCHD) (1). The leading cause of death in infants in 2016 was congenital anomalies; congenital anomalies also accounted for the second and third most common causes of death in children ages 1-4 years and 5-9 years, respectively (2). Of babies born with CCHD, about 75% are expected to survive to one year of age and 69% are expected to survive to 18 years (1). These statistics demonstrate how many children affected by congenital heart disease are potential candidates for palliative care intervention.

Each infant/child with their family unit and their medical condition is unique. Pediatric cardiac patients are among some of the most unique; they are not "little adults" with heart

* Correspondence: Premchand Anne, MD, Pediatric Cardiology, Ascension St John Children's Hospital, 22201 Moross, Suite 275, PB II, Detroit, MI 48236, United States. Email: Premchand.anne@ascension.org.

problems. Their heart defects, repairs and symptom management are very different from heart diseases afflicting adults. The statistics on CCHD can only give broad strokes of information. They cannot account for all the variants that are seen in this specific population. At least 15% of CHD is associated with an underlying genetic condition (1). This association between congenital cardiac disease and genetic abnormalities increases the likelihood that palliative care will benefit these patients and their families.

This discussion focuses on three cases: d-transposition of the great arteries (d-TGA), tetralogy of Fallot, and hypoplastic left heart syndrome (HLHS) to illustrate diverse ways in which pediatric palliative care (PPC) teams can impact children and their families. D-TGA affects approximately 1 in 3,300, while Tetralogy of Fallot affects 1 in every 2,518 babies and HLHS affects 1 in 4,344 babies (3-5). There are more than ten critical congenital heart conditions (CCHD). Although all three conditions (d-TGA, Tetralogy and HLHS) can be diagnosed prenatally, they are often not diagnosed until after birth (3-5). When PPC service is consulted shortly after diagnosis, the service can help the parents navigate the long medical road ahead of them and their child.

Pediatric palliative care has a goal of improving the quality of life while the disease process progresses (6). All PPC teams hope to achieve coordination of care and facilitation of informed decision-making by patients, families and health care professionals (7). The American Academy of Pediatrics (AAP) policy statement states that core commitments should include the following: 1) shared decision making allowing engagement of the patient and their support system; 2) providing care for all ages and during all stages of illness; and 3) focusing on general education about pediatric palliative care and pediatric hospice care and, if possible, an early consultation of these services (8).

The American Academy of Pediatrics (AAP) has acknowledged the importance of pediatric palliative care for all pediatric patients. The National Hospice and Palliative Care Organization (NHPCO) published a list of features from the palliative care philosophy that include care and services that are coordinated by an interdisciplinary team (a partnership between patients, families, palliative care providers and non-palliative health care providers), provision of services available to accompany, or act independently of curative or life-prolonging care, support of the patient and their family during the process of death and dying including bereavement (9).

Both AAP and the NHPCO recognize the importance of palliative care intervention for the patient and their family unit. In 2007, the NHPCO completed a survey on pediatric services to member-providers. Overall, 78% of responding hospices stated they serve pediatric patients, and 36.6% have a formal pediatric program (9). These numbers will continue to increase over the coming years. This discussion can serve as a tool to help clinicians when faced with difficult congenital heart disease scenarios. While the number of pediatric programs are small in comparison to the adult palliative care programs, the services provided by Pediatric Palliative Care (PPC) and Pediatric Hospice Care (PHC) are immeasurable to the patients and their families (9). One consideration, that must be kept in mind, is that many parents may initially find it difficult to accept the help from the PPC team. This is because the outcome is often unknown. Therefore, early and often consultation with a PPC team is highly recommended (7).

PARENTAL GRIEF

The goal of Pediatric Palliative Care and Pediatric Hospice Care (PPC-PHC) is to help the family and the child manage the disease and in extreme cases, be “prepared” for death. Experiencing grief is an important component in this process. There are no experts in showing families how they should grieve; however, the PPC-PHC can guide families in the process. The following are some well-established goals (10):

1) Maintain connection with the family and their child until death;
2) Facilitate communication;
3) Help the family develop memories that they can cherish long after the death;
4) Help parents negotiate the medical system;
5) Provide respite care;
6) Help parents with the concept of “appropriate death”;
7) Help parents talk about choices for the funeral or memorial service in advance, if they choose.

Consultation should occur early in patients with CCHD (6). The PPC-PHC teams can work to help the family with realistic expectations along with symptom management. PPC-PHC teams can also provide bereavement care before, during, and after the death of a child (8). PPC-PHC providers should work closely with the family to ensure that they feel supported during their child’s illness. This support can range from concerns about financial problems, and ensuring access to mental health services, spiritual support, and bereavement support (8). The PPC-PHC team can communicate with the patient and their families and set short-, intermediate-, and long-term goals. This should be done often and at any time requested by the family.

The process of parental grief is very complicated. The parents of children with CCHD must work through many separate phases of grief. With the advances in medicine and early diagnosis, most parents of children with CCHD experience grief after initial diagnosis during the gestational period, then again after birth and after each procedure. For the parents whose children die just after diagnosis, the process of grief is very different than parents whose children survive for days and months to many years.

Table 1. Common phases of parental grief (12)

Shock	A numb feeling sometimes so profound that parents can feel empty
Denial	A feeling that the situation did not happen; waiting for the child to appear again
Replay	Trying to change the outcome of the situation; centered on “what ifs”
Yearning	Begging/Praying for “just 5 more minutes”
Confusion	The inability to process daily activities because the parent is so overcome with their emotions
Guilt	Wondering if there was something the parent did/did not do to cause the diagnosis/outcome
Powerlessness	Feeling of not being in control either in the death of their child or sometimes other aspects of their life surrounding their child’s death
Anger	Comes in many forms. Anger that others get to move on (see their children go to school/graduate), Anger that they as the parent could not control the outcome
Loss of hope(s)	A feeling that acknowledges the loss of milestones for a child (not graduating, getting married, etc)

Regardless of when their child dies, all parents experience the typical stages of grief. These five stages, initially recorded in the Kübler-Ross model, include Denial, Anger, Bargaining, Depression and Acceptance (11). Parental grief is often more complicated than these five stages alone; parents will often go back and forth between stages and experience various forms/phases of grief (see Table 1) (12). Also, many parents go through a version of these stages at diagnosis as well as at the death of their child. Parents can also experience grief many years after their child's death and it can sometimes occur spontaneously.

Case of a Child Diagnosed Prenatally with HLHS

Mr. and Mrs. Smith present for their 20-week fetal anatomy scan. This is their second successful pregnancy and they have a healthy 8-year-old daughter. During the ultrasound, the fetal cardiac anatomy is found to be abnormal. The maternal-fetal medicine (MFM) physician reviews the images and is concerned about hypoplastic left heart syndrome (HLHS). She schedules Mrs. Smith for a fetal echocardiogram the following day.

At this point, Mr. and Mrs. Smith are aware that their baby may have a heart defect, with some information given by the MFM physician regarding the anatomy. They are not told about the potential extent of the defect and the implications of the defect. They spend the next 24 hours in shock and denial about the potential diagnosis. As most parents do, they go home and search on the internet about hypoplastic left heart syndrome. Mrs. Smith is now feeling guilty; did she do something to cause this defect? Mr. Smith is feeling powerless; how can he help his wife and unborn child through this possible diagnosis. At this point, Mr. and Mrs. Smith are dealing with the uncertainty of the diagnosis. They know that in 24 hours they could be told that their unborn child has a significant cardiac defect.

On the morning of the fetal echocardiogram, Mr. Smith seems distant. Mrs. Smith tries to remain optimistic that "it won't be that bad." During their appointment, it is confirmed that their unborn child has HLHS. Mr. Smith is in shock and keeps repeating "this can't be happening." Mrs. Smith is still trying to remain optimistic. She wants to discuss the potential treatments and ways to "fix" her child. The pediatric cardiologist sets a meeting with a pediatric cardiothoracic surgeon and Pediatric Palliative Care for the following week.

At the meeting with the cardiothoracic surgeon, there is discussion of potential surgical interventions to palliate the baby's heart. It is at this point, that the palliative care physician asks the parents what they want for their child. At first, Mr. and Mrs. Smith are confused by her question. Of course, they want their child to live a long happy life. The palliative care physician explains that the three surgeries that are typically utilized to correct the heart come with risks. She explains that these risks include increased risk for infection, stroke, and complications with anesthesia, including death. She tries to help the parents understand that even if the surgical correction goes 100% as planned, their child will continue to need medical follow-up with possibility of future surgical interventions. She asks the parents how much the parents are willing to go through or have their child endure. This is a lot for the parents to consider during their first meeting. It is likely a topic that will need to be revisited many times prior to the baby's birth.

Discussions with this family need to focus on the perinatal period along with the long-term care of the child. Genetic testing is something that the PPC team may discuss with this family.

It is thought that environmental and genetic factors are the main causes of CHD (13). While the overall development of CHD is not well understood, heritable genetic factors may play a larger role than once thought (13). There should be discussions about the future quality of life of their child and their family (14).

Considering today's medical advancements, it seems to most physicians, that parents would want everything done for a child. This, however, is a dangerous assumption. While most parents would want everything done, not every parent is prepared to care for a medically fragile child. It is important that the potential future outcomes are discussed with families as early as possible. This will help decrease the potential for abuse/neglect in the future along with help for the parents to psychologically and emotionally prepare for the life ahead for them and their child.

It is also very possible that the pregnant mother and father dyad may opt for termination of pregnancy. While the termination of a pregnancy is a difficult topic, it is one that must be considered. As clinicians, it is important to set aside our personal beliefs and discuss all options with our patients. It is also imperative to remain as unbiased and objective as possible (6). Termination of the pregnancy may be "the only option" for a family despite many of available options. In this instance, Mr. and Mrs. Smith have a very healthy and energetic child at home. After speaking with the palliative care team, they understand that it may be difficult to continue their current lifestyle, without any adaptations, and care for a medically fragile child. The importance of these discussions cannot be underestimated. When a woman becomes pregnant, she does not expect a bad outcome. Being pregnant with a child with CCHD is life changing and may not be how some families envision their final family picture. The PPC team helps with goal setting, medical decision making and bereavement support throughout the entire life and death of a child.

SIBLING GRIEF

Siblings of children with CCHD experience grief in a different manner than the parents of the affected child. Being the sibling of a child with CCHD or any life limiting illness can be difficult depending on the degree of parental attention and care provided to and needed by the sibling with CCHD. The siblings may often feel forgotten or not included in the life of their ill sibling. Many may want/prefer, if old enough, to be included in the discussions about their sibling's illness (14). Just as their parents crave control over their child's condition, their siblings also feel the need to be in control; this lack of control can manifest in a number of reactions (see Table 2) (15). The siblings need to be reassured of their place in the family. Sometimes the parents will have to utilize respite care services, so they can attend the school play or after school activities with their healthy children.

Respite care services are provided so that the primary caregiver, in many families the mother, can have relief from the stress associated with caring for an ill child. Respite care can help improve family stability and the relationship of the parents with their other children and family members. Recent studies show that a sibling's grief process is influenced by the grief of their parents, level of family cohesion and their immediate caregiving environment (16). Open and honest discussions have been found to help siblings cope with death. This may need to be altered depending on the age/understanding of the child.

Many siblings of children with CCHD, like those of children with cancer, often "pause" their grief (16). These children need to have their feelings and emotions addressed to be sure that they adjust to their new life without their sibling (17). Most children, especially when young, have difficulty expressing their feelings. Siblings need to be able to express their emotions, no matter how distressing they are to their parents (17). PPC-PHC is important in setting goals for the patient, but they can also help set goals for the siblings. PPC-PHC team can facilitate support groups for siblings of CCHD patients. This allows these children an opportunity to speak openly with other children in similar circumstances. PPC-PHC service can further provide guidance on how to grieve as a family instead of in isolation (14).

Table 2. Common sibling reactions to grief (15)

Fear	Concern that they might die; uncertainty of future for themselves/family; can manifest as nightmares, withdrawn behavior, acting out
Regression	Acting younger than their age to get attention
Overachieving	Some children try to become the "golden child" to compensate for feeling helpless
Displays of power	Acting out/misbehaving to get attention
Guilt	Differs depending on the age of the child; may feel responsible to the illness or the death
Anger	Can be directed at their sibling or parents
Sorrow	Feeling that can indicate that they are acknowledging the situation; meeting with other sorrowful children can be helpful.

CASE OF CHILD DIAGNOSED WITH TETRALOGY OF FALLOT

Mari is a 12-month-old female with history of Tetralogy of Fallot. She has two older siblings, Amber, who is 4 years old and Ben, who is 12 years old. Mari had her first repair in infancy and has done well clinically. She had been doing well medically until her recent follow up with cardiology at 12 months of age. Her echocardiogram showed that the right ventricle to pulmonary artery conduit that was placed during the repair has a large aneurysm. Her cardiothoracic surgeon feels that it would be best for this to be repaired prior to the complete repair of her heart. Shortly after the procedure, Mari suffers a stroke. She is hospitalized much longer than initially planned. During this time, Mari's parents are at the hospital daily. They were at Amber's dance recital prior to Mari suffering her stroke and subsequently missed Ben's science fair.Amber does not understand why her parents are always at the hospital. She is worried that she caused her sister to get sick again. She tells her mom that "Mari is sick because I didn't dance good."

Amber would benefit from the intervention of the palliative care service to help her understand the situation at her age level. She is unable to comprehend that Mari was sick before going into the hospital, because she looked well. On the other hand, Ben knows that Mari is very sick and tells his parents that it is "okay" that they missed his science fair. However, Ben has been "acting out" since the science fair and getting into fights with his classmates. It is common for siblings, especially adolescent-aged, to "act out" during these circumstances (18). Mari has been followed by many subspecialists since her birth. For the parents and her siblings, PPC has been a place of solace and comfort. They have seen Mari daily since her stroke and every few months prior to her procedure. They have spoken with the parents to try to help them manage Ben's outbursts and Amber's trouble understanding the tense medical situation.

Pediatric Palliative Care has helped with arranging respite services. This has helped Mari's parents spend more one-on-one time with their two other children. It has allowed them to attend more activities despite Mari's medical fragility. Mari's parents are grateful for the respite services but struggle with the guilt of leaving Mari in the hospital "all alone." When the family meets with Pediatric Palliative Care, Amber and Ben are included.; it can be helpful to include the other children, so they can have a sense of control. Amber knows that Mari loves bubbles and asks to blow bubbles for her sister. Ben knows that Mari loves when he sings to her. He asks if he can make a recording of him singing to play for Mari when he is not there. These gestures, seem very small to people outside of this families' situation, but are very helpful in helping Mari's siblings feel connected to her treatment and welfare.

PATIENT GRIEF

The life of a child with CCHD is very different from an average child. These children visit their pediatricians and pediatric cardiologists many more times a year than their healthy counterparts. They are usually well acquainted with several types of hospital procedures and protocols. Even at an early age, these children will have been through more examinations and procedures than most adults do in their entire life. It is important that all children with CCHD understand, based on their age, the trajectory of their illness and potential outcomes, including death. This is going to look very different in a 1-year-old compared to an older child (see Table 3) (19). PPC clinicians are educated to identify the best way to approach these topics with the children. With the focus of this discussion on infants and young children, we will not discuss the complexity of care for older children and adolescents.

Table 3. Understanding death by age (19)

	Toddler, 1-2 year of age	**Preschool, 2-6 year of age**
Cognitive Stage	Egocentric, magical, concrete, little concept of body integrity	Lacking ability to think abstractly
Developmental task	To initiate autonomy	To develop a sense of initiative
Impact of illness	Loss of independence; interferes with development of self-control	Loss of certain accomplishments
Major fears	Separation; loss of control	Loss of control, bodily injury, being left alone, the dark, unknown
Concept of death	Death recognized as immobility; viewed as reversible, temporary	Death recognized as immobility; viewed as reversible; begins to develop mature concept of death
Emotional Care	Provide stability, security, calm environment	Provide stability, security; facilitate preparation, communication, supportive care
Spiritual Care	Reassure that it is not the child's fault/punishment; encourage/facilitate use of spiritual support	Demonstrate love, trust, caring Reassure that it is not the child's fault; encourage/facilitate use of spiritual support

As children grow more aware of their illness, it is important to include them in the decision making. It can be difficult as a clinician to know the "right amount" of information to share with a young patient. PPC-PHC team members can offer considerable guidance in this regard (14). It is not uncommon that a child will want to protect their parents from their emotions. They may want to "be brave, like dad says." This will make it important that that child has a "safe adult" with whom to communicate about their emotions (14). This "safe adult" can be anyone with whom the child can communicate their concerns openly and honestly. In addition, the PPC-PHC team can provide the patient with notebooks/journals and even tape recorders to note their questions or concerns. Allowing an open conversation about the child's illness can help not only the patient cope with their illness, but also their family. Children with CCHD can be exposed to support groups for children with similar conditions and partake in camps as well as groups with shared interests. This helps alleviate the loneliness that is often felt and allow them to feel more comfortable asking questions about their condition (14).

CASE OF CHILD WITH D-TGA

Nathan is a 6-year-old male with a history of dextro-transposition of the great arteries (d-TGA). Nathan had his Arterial Switch Operation when he was three weeks old and has done well with his follow up visits. His parents had been supported by their institutions PPC team since he was diagnosed prenatally. At his 4-year-old checkup, his parents and pediatrician are very happy with Nathan's development. At his cardiology follow up, he was found to have an area of myocardial ischemia. He was sent for a cardiac catheterization which showed coronary obstruction. After the procedure, Nathan's parents sat down for a meeting with his cardiologist, cardiothoracic surgeon, and the PPC team. During the meeting, it was decided that surgical intervention would be the best option to optimize Nathan's heart function. With some help from the PPC-PHC team, Nathan was included at this meeting. The team explained the problem with his heart, in terms that Nathan could understand. After the meeting, Nathan and his parents were given time to process all the information they were given.

Nathan decided to draw a picture about how he was feeling. This was something he had done many times in the past. Art therapy has been shown to help children express their emotions, especially when they are unable to verbalize them (14). Nathan's family has used art therapy throughout his life to help communicate about his condition and associated emotions.

Another available resource is spiritual guidance. Many families, while not religious, are spiritual. It is important that this spirituality is acknowledged and utilized to help the child and the family cope with the diagnosis. Consultation with a hospital chaplain can be very helpful (14). Nathan's family priest has been present at the hospital before each significant procedure. He has prayed over Nathan and with his family during the procedures. This has helped Nathan feel safe and protected, along with offering spiritual support for his parents. Nathan and his parents are aware that this surgery is necessary for Nathan to continue to grow and develop.

One of Nathan's best friends, Michael, has the same heart defect. Their parents met when they were both hospitalized after their Arterial Switch Operations. Michael had done well until he too had coronary obstruction on his most recent cardiac catheterization. He had his surgical repair done just last month; however, Michael did not do well after the surgery. He suffered a stroke and now has trouble talking. Nathan tells his mother that he "hopes that doesn't happen to him." His mother finds it hard to comfort him, due to her own unease about the procedure. She contacts her priest and the PPC team. They bring Nathan and his parents into a room to discuss his feelings about the surgery and the outcome of Michael's surgery. While the PPC team cannot guarantee that Nathan will have a good outcome, they do their best to ease his concerns. Nathan and his parents go to the hospital on the day of his surgery knowing that they have the support of their priest and their PPC team.

BARRIERS TO PPC SERVICES

There are many barriers that may be met with the introduction of PPC. First, the public misconception that palliative care is the same as hospice care. There are no limitations to when palliative care can be initiated, although it is best utilized when initiated early in the disease process (20). Hospice care is specifically designated for those patients whose death is imminent, usually in the following 6 months (21).

A second barrier is the course of illness in pediatric patients is somewhat unpredictable. Children born with CCHD are almost always a candidate for some type of palliation. Since most children are candidates for palliation, most clinicians find it difficult to explore end-of-life discussions (20). The thought of a child dying when palliation is available is difficult. It is for this reason that PPC is so important. Palliative care can support the family, the patient and the medical staff caring for the child.

A third barrier is the lack of trained PPC physicians. Hospice and Palliative Medicine have only been recognized as a specialty since 2006 (8). Due to the relative "newness" of the field, many physicians are unaware of the capabilities of a board-certified Hospice and Palliative Medicine physician. It is important that medical students and residents are exposed to Hospice and Palliative Medicine during their training. This will hopefully allow them to feel more comfortable having end-of-life discussions with families or with consulting PPC early in the disease process. The care that is provided by a PPC physician is aimed at relief of suffering, improvement in quality of life, facilitation of informed decision-making and assistance in care coordination (8). PPC physicians can be integral member of the care team for a child with CCHD.

The care for a child with CCHD is difficult. It is a difficult course for the patient, the family, and the medical team. PPC-PHC can help ease the burden for all three. In the end, PPC-PHC along with the family strive for a good life and a good death, when the time comes (22).

CONCLUSION

Pediatric Palliative Care is a well-known service available to children and adults in the Oncology world. Children with CCHD have a long and difficult medical course that would benefit greatly from PPC. PPC can help parents focus on allowing their child to live the most complete life possible regardless of their diagnosis. All available literature about pediatric palliative care shows that early intervention is most effective for the welfare of the child (23). Early intervention can allow the PPC team to establish a connection with the family before the disease takes its toll on the patient, sibling and parental levels. Early introduction to the PPC team establishes a bond between the family and the PPC team that will hopefully carry them throughout the life of their child – allowing easier advanced care planning, goal setting, assurance of continuity of care and emotional support (23).

PPC physicians receive special training in symptom management as well as difficult discussions with family members. Currently, there is research that supports PPC services in the care of an ill child; however, in the CCHD population, the research is lacking (23). This discussion highlights some of the benefits of PPC in the CCHD population and encourage the use of PPC in this population.

> "The question is not how to get cured, but how to live."
> Joseph Conrad (1857-1924)

REFERENCES

[1] CDC. Congenital heart defects: Data and statistics. URL: https://www.cdc.gov/ncbddd/heartdefects/data.html.

[2] CDC. 10 leading causes of death by age group, United States – 2016. URL: https://www.cdc.gov/injury/wisqars/LeadingCauses.html.

[3] CDC. Congenital heart defects: Facts about dextro-transposition of the great arteries. URL: https://www.cdc.gov/ncbddd/heartdefects/d-tga.html.

[4] CDC. Congenital heart defects: Facts about tetralogy of Fallot. URL: https://www.cdc.gov/ncbddd/heartdefects/tetralogyoffallot.html.

[5] CDC. Congenital heart defects: Facts about hypoplastic left heart syndrome. URL: https://www.cdc.gov/ncbddd/heartdefects/hlhs.html.

[6] Rychik J. What does palliative care mean in prenatal diagnosis of congenital heart disease? World J Pediatr Congenit Heart Surg 2013;4(1):80-4.

[7] Hoell Jl, Warfsmann J, Gagnon G, Trocan L, Balzer S, Oommen PT, et al. Palliative care for children with a yet undiagnosed syndrome. Eur J Pediatr 2017; 176(10):1319-27.

[8] Section on Hospice and Palliative Medicine and Committee on Hospital Care. Pediatric palliative care and hospice care commitments, guidelines and recommendations. Pediatrics 2013;132(5);966-72

[9] Friebert, S. Williams, C. NHPCO's facts and figures: Pediatric palliative and hospice care in America, 2015 edition. URL: https://www.nhpco.org/sites/default/files/public/quality/Pediatric_Facts-Figures.pdf.

[10] Carter BS, Levetown M, Friebert SE. Palliative care for infants, children, and adolescents: A practical handbook, 2nd ed. Baltimore, MA: Johns Hopkins University Press, 2011:285-7.

[11] Kübler-Ross E. On death and dying. Abingdon, UK: Routledge, 1969.

[12] Grieving the death of a child. URL: https://healgrief.org/grieving-the-death-of-a-child/.

[13] Cai M, Huang H, Su L, Lin N, Wu X, Xie X, et al. Fetal congenital heart disease: Associated anomalies, identification of genetic anomalies by single-nucleotide polymorphism array analysis, and postnatal outcome. Medicine (Baltimore) 2018; 97(50):e13617. doi: 10.1097/MD.0000000000013617.

[14] Carter BS, Levetown M, Friebert SE. Palliative care for infants, children, and adolescents: A practical handbook, 2nd ed. Baltimore, MA: Johns Hopkins University Press, 2011;209-23.

[15] Helping children cope and deal with grief. URL: https://healgrief.org/helping-children-cope-deal-with-grief/.

[16] Carter BS, Levetown M, Friebert SE. Palliative care for infants, children, and adolescents: A practical handbook, 2nd ed. Baltimore, MD: Johns Hopkins University Press, 2011:284-85.

[17] Warnick AL. Supporting youth grieving the dying or death of a sibling or parent: Considerations for parents, professionals, and communities. Curr Opin Support Palliat Care 2015;9(1):58-63.

[18] Chin WL, Jaaniste T, Trethewie S. The role of resilience in the sibling experience of pediatric palliative care: What is the theory and evidence? Children (Basel) 2018;5(7). pii. 97. doi:10.3390/children5070097.

[19] Walsh T, Caraceni A, Fainsinger R, Foley K, Glare P, Gohi C, Lloyd-Williams M, Olarte J, Radbruch L. Palliative medicine, 1st Ed. Philadelphia, PA: Saunders, 2009:1085-7.

[20] Bertaud S, Lloyd DF, Laddie J, Razavi R. The importance of early involvement of paediatric palliative care for patients with severe congenital heart disease. Arch Dis Child 2016;101(10):984-7.

[21] Ranallo L. Improving the quality of end-of-life care in pediatric oncology patients through the early implementation of palliative care. J Pediatr Oncol Nurs 2017;34(6):374-80.

[22] Pierucci R, Kirby R, Leuthner S. End-of-life care for neonates and infants: The experience and effects of a palliative care consultation service. Pediatrics 2001; 108(3):653-60.

[23] May R, Thompson J. The role of pediatric palliative care in complex congenital heart disease: three illustrative cases. J Palliat Med 2017;20(11):1300-03.

In: Chronic Disease and Disability
Editors: DE Greydanus, P Anne, JD Rowlett et al.
ISBN: 978-1-53617-656-8

Chapter 20

CHRONIC DISEASE AND THE DYING ADOLESCENT

Donald E Greydanus*, MD, DrHC(Athens)
Department of Pediatric and Adolescent Medicine, Western Michigan University Homer Stryker MD School of Medicine, Kalamazoo, Michigan, United States of America

ABSTRACT

Death is a reality for children and adolescents as over 53,000 children and 3,000 adolescents succumb annually to one or more chronic illnesses. Death of these precious patients may occur in the hospital, often the neonatal or pediatric intensive care units. No one is prepared for such tragic events—neither the patient, nor the family, nor hospital staff. This article considers complex issues related to the hospitalized dying adolescent and offers recommendations for the staff as hospital individuals often struggle with providing the youth a peaceful, dignified, and painless death.

Do not stand at my grave and weep
I am not there. I do not sleep.
I am a thousand winds that blow
I am the diamond glints on snow
I am the sunlight on ripened grain
I am the gentle autumn rain
When you awake in the morning's hush
I am the soft uplifting rush
Of quiet birds in circling flight
I am the soft star that shines at night
Do not stand at my grave and cry
I am not there.....I did not die.

Anonymous, Dedicated to Adele Dellenbaugh Hofmann, MD (1926-2001)

* Correspondence: Donald E Greydanus, MD, DrHC(Athens), Professor of Pediatrics and Founding Chair, Department of Pediatric and Adolescent Medicine, Western Michigan University, Homer Stryker MD School of Medicine, 1000 Oakland Drive D48G, Kalamazoo, MI 49008-1284, United States. Email: Donald.Greydanus@med.wmich.edu.

INTRODUCTION

Approximately 53,000 children and 3,000 adolescents die each year in the United States as a consequence of chronic illness (1, 2). Youth can die from acute causes as well. Over 14,000 youth die each year from unintentional injuries (mostly motor vehicle accidents), approximately 5,000 from homicide, and 4,000 from suicides (3).

Death is perhaps the most difficult aspect of human existence for all to face. Humans tend to ignore and/or deny the inevitability of their own mortality. As life ebbs away from youth despite the best that health care professionals (HCPs) can do, HCPs must confront the uncomfortable reality of their patient's mortality and share uncomfortable emotions with the teenager and family---including grief, helplessness, loss, anger, and others (4). It is a most bitter and poignant concept that a youth is dying at a point when many decades of living should be ahead.

The literature on theories and methods for conceptualizing issues related to death and dying is controversial. One of the most well-known theorists and advocates for addressing the needs of the dying is working with individuals who are dying is Elizabeth Kübler-Ross. She proposed and employed the concept that the dying experience emotions in distinct stages (5, 6). Recent empirical research contends that Kübler-Ross' theories on death and dying are controversial. These experts offer that not all dying patients go through "stages of death and dying." Their research concludes that individuals who are dying are more resilient than previously thought. The researchers do offer that these results are dependent on the dying person receiving several types of supports: a) palliative care, b) strong family support c) are involved in their treatment decisions, and d) have good communications with their specialists and HCPs regarding their care (7).

The current authors acknowledge the growing body of literature challenging the concept of "stages of death and dying;" however, we have found the Kübler-Ross framework to be clinically useful and effective in our respective clinical work. Therefore, we will focus this discussion on adolescents dying from chronic illness and the complex factors this poses for the youth, family, and hospital staff including health care professionals (HCPs) (4) We choose to direct that focus from the Kübler-Ross framework (5, 6).

EFFECTS OF DYING ON ADOLESCENT DEVELOPMENT

Typical psychosocial development may be slowed or accelerated because of the impact of a youth's impending death. This process impedes all cognitive, social, and emotional growth because the youth's resources are redirected towards day-to-day survival (8-10) (see Table 1). These youth may experience fear about dying and not understand why this is happening to them.

As the adolescent develops s/he becomes more adult-like in appearance and in thought processes. As maturity proceeds most youth develop a Piagetian Formal Operational Thinking Stage in which adult thinking skills arise even though adult experience in life has not (3). Thus, the maturing youth may have a concept of death similar to that of the adult and like most adults, has difficulty accepting his/her own immediate mortality. The dying process occurs at a time when most youth are developing a) enthusiasm for life, b) uncompromised idealism, c) are at a developmental stage where they are beginning to experiment, and d) may be engaging in potentially high risk behavior. The final stages of chronic illness force the dying teenager to see the reality, totality, and the finality of his/her death.

Table 1. Stages of adolescent development: Cognitive and psychosocial (8-10)

Early Adolescence (10 – 14 year of Age) • Cognitive Growth results in major changes in mental abilities thought processes, thinking skills and problem solving skills, better judgment, initial abstract thought • Preoccupation with rapidly changing events with onset of puberty • Better ability to adopt another person's spatial perspective • A clear sense of their own body image worry over perceived abnormalities • Clear sense of social standing with peer • Establishment and maintenance of same-sex friendships • The process of emancipation begins
Middle Adolescence (14 – 18 year of Age) • Major changes in cognitive abilities, altruism, developing theories about life and ability to have a rich fantasy life (especially sexual fantasies) • Independence/ symbolic move away from parents/ home environment • Identification with non-parental adult role models • Experimentation with sex/sexuality, substance use or abuse • Strong reliance on peers setting personal rules • Compares their physical characteristics with peers • Able to independently weigh consequences of decisions before taking action; understand consequences of risk-taking behaviors, but peer pressure may override caution • Beginning to development of a positive self-image and increased confidence as he or she consistently experiences success
Late Adolescence (18 – 21+ years of age) • Issues of emancipation from parents are essentially resolved • Finalization of secure, acceptable body image and gender role • Establishment of adult (mutual respect and gratification) versus narcissistic sexual relationships; prefers intimacy versus isolation • Acquisition of adult lifestyle, vocational skills • More complex cognitive abilities: Abstract thinking, Altruism, Empathy skills, Personal values, future oriented • Capable of establishing and maintaining stable, mutually caring and satisfying interpersonal (including sexual) relationships • Uses own judgment for setting personal rules. Less influenced by peers • More actively participating is sexual experimentation

The struggle with understanding such a reality can be extremely difficult for someone who should be at the beginning of life, nearing the initiation of adulthood with its promise of emancipation from childhood and parents as well as the emergence of true independence in the exploration of life. How stressful to be so close to living without parental control and devastating to lose such control within sight of the universal adolescent quest for autonomy! The adolescent who is dying from chronic illness often spends considerable time in the hospital milieu, particularly in the intensive care unit as the illness worsens (11). Such loss of autonomy and destruction of one's idealized vision of life as an adult can be overwhelming to this young patient.

Negative reactions can result in combative or complaining behavior that may include provocative acting out. Other youth can become depressed and withdraw from his/her environment. which may involve the teenager developing increased feelings of resentment and anger over loss of control with reduced self-esteem.

This youth can be the greatest mourner of his/her fate as physical and sexual integrity deteriorates within view of adult life (4). This can intensify his/her search for beliefs, ethics, values, spirituality, and the potential for an afterlife. This patient may be in varying stages of grief as noted by the brilliant and now classic work of Kübler-Ross: Denial, anger, bargaining, depression, and acceptance (5, 6).

ISSUES WITH ADOLESCENT CONSENT, ACCENT, OR REFUSAL OF TREATMENT

Care for the adolescent has been complicated by the concepts of consent and confidentiality (3, 12-14). Though not yet a legal adult and not of a child status, the teenager often exists in a unique status with some legal rights. Youth in this part of the 21st century can be treated by HCPs in the United States without parents' permission for certain conditions and issues such as emergency care, sexually transmitted diseases, substance use, contraception, evaluation of pregnancy, and others.

Such care is granted to youth without parental knowledge if the clinician feels this is in the best interest of the youth (3). The concept of the Mature Minor Doctrine has developed which, though not a legal concept per se, states that youth can be treated as adults (i.e., without parental permission) under certain circumstances, such as one who is living alone unassisted (i.e., "on the streets"), is a parent, is in the military, is of a certain age (often 16 years or older), and others (3, 12-14).

However, the dying youth in the hospital does not usually meet the criteria for the Mature Minor Doctrine and usually has parents intimately involved in each step of the diagnosis and management of the youth's chronic illness. The precise rights of this hospitalized and dying teenager become obscured and perhaps forgotten in the mix of hovering parents and a wide variety of hospital personnel. Some youth may not want any rights apart from their parents. One recent study of youth dying from cancer noted that all the involved adolescents, when asked what they requested, stated they wanted what the family felt was best for their treatment (15).

This sets the stage for some potentially difficult problems. Can this relatively "young" patient form wishes for care independent from the wishes of his or her parents? Should this patient even be told when death seems the mostly likely outcome? What if the parents do not want their "child" to know such a grim prognosis? Does the teenager have to consent or even assent to treatments approved of by the parents? Does this patient have to provide consent for potentially mutilating surgery, such as limb amputation? Does the adolescent have the right to refuse treatment at some point in the management process from diagnosis to death (16, 17)?

Typically when rights of the parents' conflict with rights of the youth, HCPs often choose to side with the parents whose insurance may be paying the HCPs for their time as well as covering the overall hospital bill. The HCPs and the hospital may decide to suspend the full privilege of confidentiality in the teen patient-doctor relationship and make it a 100% parent-doctor relationship that involves the patient when the parent-doctor relationship chooses. Such an approach, however, may lead to anger on the part of this grieving youth who may choose to act out. They may express their disagreement by becoming verbally or physically angry and may even refuse treatment options. Indeed, the needs of this patient may seem complex and overwhelming to parents and hospital staff (18). For example, can the parents and staff affirm decisions made by the dying youth about life and death---especially if these decision are in conflict with that of parents and/or treating attendings (19)?

PARENTAL ISSUES

The parents whose youth is dying are going through their own Kübler-Ross stages of grief that may not be in sync with where their "child-adolescent" is struggling. Parents become involved in a complex array of feelings often not understood by the teenager, hospital staff, nor even themselves. Families of the 21st century are estranged from the idealized view of families in the mid-twentieth century of America with frequent divorce and single parent households.

Parents must deal with causal guilt and wonder if they caused this illness through their own genetic structure, failure for early diagnosis, and/or lack of financial resources for the "best care." Parents are typically nurturers and mourn when their best efforts at nurturing fail. Parents despair at the loss of a beloved family member who is perceived as an extension of themselves. They are forced to deal with the loss of parental hopes of immortality through the life of their child. Anger may arise from their reality that their own precious child is one of the few to die. They question why not many others? Parents may be reluctant to discuss death with their child who typically suspects but can be confused by the parental response of denial or avoidance of impending death (20).

Parents may become confused and angry over the potentially negative reaction of their teenager who does not accept that normal issues of emancipation are suspended and becomes distressed over being forced to give up dreams of independence for the reality of being sent back to a dependent relationship with parents. Parents may become depressed and/or angry as their child intensifies feelings of alienation with the result of increasing confrontational behavior (4).

Though impending death makes the teenager ever more dependent on parents, his or her negative behavior can make the entire situation more stressful and perplexing for grieving parents. Parents may have had emancipation-based conflicts with their youth before chronic illness intervened and this new forced dependency can be overwhelming for all family members. If there is lack of trust with the health care team, more stress is added. Parents may be unable to sustain the loss of a loved child and not be able to continue with their lives in a healthy manner after the death of their offspring (20).

ISSUES FOR HEALTH CARE PROFESSIONALS AND HOSPITAL STAFF

Caring for a dying youth raises multiple complex issues with HCPs and hospital staff as well. Some HCPs choose the field of medicine to some extent because of the power and authority this field can convey as well as an often unconscious need of HCPs to care for themselves (i.e., an inherent dependency gratification mechanism) (4). Both of these concepts can be threatened by having a young patient become so sick that HCPs cannot save them. Some HCPs have an unconscious need to control their own fears of death by preventing death in others under their care. The dying teenager exposes this need in a threatening manner.

Some choose medicine as an expression of one's "ideal" self. These concepts are limited by having a child or teenager die despite the HCP's best efforts. Complicating these issues is the fact that the adolescent patient is relatively close in age to many of the hospital staff and young clinicians or to family members of older providers or staff.

The patient and family may place pseudo-mythical powers in hospital staff and such confidence can be eroded by the dying patient. The calm, strong, and empathetic HCP may lose some of these positive attributes and not be able to provide constant hope as well as support to the patient and family. The hospital personnel are human and vulnerable; thus, when caring for such a difficult situation, some may develop feelings of object loss, guilt, frustration, and depression from their "failure" to heal one's patients.

Some HCPs may react by limiting their visits to patient or family to few situations and "only when necessary." HCPs may react by intellectualization as a coping mechanism; they place mental distance between their emotions and the issues involved with a specific patient. Such detachment may lead to the teen patient feeling isolated with thoughts of personal devaluation and despair. At a time when it is needed the most, the teen and/or family may be deprived of emotional support from hospital staff.

Anxieties are raised in the hospital staff and challenge how staff deal with stress in dealing with the implications of mortality; indeed, these issues are subtle and yet complex and may lead staff to either using negative mechanisms of coping (i.e., withdrawal from the dying patient) or more action-oriented mechanisms (i.e., increased communication and support of the patient and family). Staff who feel helpless or frustrated may develop inner anger leading to more inner guilt. This same cycle can be seen in the patient and/or family. More avoidance of the patient can occur or some react by offering "false" hope in seeking atonement from the patient or family for failure to "save" the young patient.

Some HCPs or staff can become over-protective, over-productive with orders (i.e., tests or treatments), and even over-heroic with ordering of essentially "useless" procedures. The staff can become irritable and difficult for others to deal with leading to more negative feelings. Staff may find it very challenging as the patient they have known for a while deteriorates. The HCP may experience emotions which lead to depression and sadness; this can happen to all HCPs and staff, who are involved in the care of this patient. It is a complex task for HCPs and hospital staff to acknowledge and accept such feelings while limiting negative effects as the patient continues on an inevitable course of death (4). The hospital staff must join the patient and family in controlling these difficult emotions.

IMPENDING DEATH OF THE TEEN PATIENT

As death becomes eminent the time of anticipatory grief and mourning can become overwhelming for the patient, family, and hospital staff. The patient may remain in the hospital or be transferred to hospice care. If s/he remains in the hospital, the most involved staff should remain actively involved with the patient and family---can sit by the bed, hold the patient's or family member's hand, and allow silence as needed. The presence of the staff remains important to contribute to a peaceful, painless, and dignified death. The family should be reassured that "all was done that was possible" and that mourning is normal. The importance of spirituality and religious beliefs of the family should always be respected (21, 22). Staff should be provided with opportunities to mourn and resolve overwhelming feelings as well (23).

The teen and/or family have the right to refuse pointless (i.e., non-life extending or non-curative) procedures and the youth has a right to full control of pain right to the end of his/her life (24-27). Principles of palliation have been developed over the past few decades and are very helpful for the patient, family, and regular hospital staff (28-32). The family should receive all necessary information to help them and their teenager make informed decisions about management options. Certainly attention to known physiologic principles of dying should be provided (33, 34).

Pre-planning or advanced plans of caring are very helpful for this complex situation (35). On-going communication with family members is important and staff should not withdraw from the patient or family (36). It is critical that family members be allowed to fully mourn under the ubiquitous umbrella of feeling that they remain the loving family, have done all they could do, and can allow the inevitability of death to occur in a dignified manner consistent with their spiritual or religious beliefs (36-38). The treating physicians and hospital staff should not become an obstacle to allowing the teenager to die a dignified, painless, and peaceful death (4, 39).

A very difficult situation arises if parents refuse to allow their child to know the reality of a terminal prognosis. This creates a singular dilemma for this vulnerable patient and the staff. Though this teenager is a minor and parent-dependent, s/he is not a child and is assuming more self-responsibility. In general it is best for the HCP to work with these parents to allow them to understand that it is in the best interests of their "teen-child" to know the truth and allow full disclosure of his/her fears and worries. A strong rapport with the family is most helpful in this regard. However, the HCP and hospital staff should prepare for potential negative reactions on the part of the family and/or patient that includes depression, guilt, and even rage.

MANAGEMENT CONCEPTS FOR THE HOSPITAL STAFF

There may be a denial of the overall diagnosis and sometimes the teen or family feel the hospital stay is "only for a few tests." However, there is usually considerable anxiety and ambivalence in such situations that is found just below the surface of denial or seeming calm.

Staff should avoid negative feelings that can lead to guilt feelings, thoughts of rejection by the patient, or overdoing investigative/therapeutic procedures/tests to assuage staff frustration. Patients who develop extreme depression or acting-act behavior should receive expert psychological or psychiatric evaluation.

Conflicts can arise when a teenager is on a downward course in a teaching hospital where staff and parents may resent the ongoing education while the patient is dying. This can become an intricate and yet common dilemma. Young residents may develop anxieties about someone not much younger than themselves who is dying. Teaching should continue but attending HCPs should understand potential conflicts and remain vigilant to potentially negative feelings on the part of the residents, staff, and/or family.

All staff also need training and support to recognize signs of emotional difficulty in adolescents, their families, and peers. These signals can easily be missed or misunderstood by parents, or staff who may react by using similar mechanisms as avoidance or counter-hostility. Problem-solving staff conferences are useful to pinpoint negative behaviors, identify underlying etiologic factors, and develop strategy for improvement of these behaviors. Those most involved in care plans can visit the patient frequently and seek to understand what is occurring. Remind team members that this is not the time for the hospital milieu to isolate and abandon this vulnerable patient and family just because improvement and cure are not possible anymore.

The treatment team has to develop a written philosophy of care, expectations, and creed that the patient and his or her family are the focus of all efforts. In helping the dying teen and his/her family during this difficult process, it is helpful for the staff to appreciate the K?bler-Ross stages of grieving as noted earlier and that these stages can be found in the youth, family, and even the various members of the hospital staff. Anyone can be fixed at a particular stage and even develop a retrograde motion in which they resort to an earlier stage (4). It is helpful for the staff to hold regular meetings with each other to review each person's feelings and agree to develop a unified plan in working with the youth and family. Gaining the confidence and cooperation of the patient and family is needed and staff must avoid a three-way battle for control of the management plan (21-39) (see table 2).

Table 2. Effectively treating the dying adolescent (21-39)

- Meet with patient and family at the beginning of care
    - Explain your philosophy of care
        - Full Disclosure
            - Honest and open communication with patient and family
            - Direct, straightforward answers geared to the adolescent's cognitive developmental level
        - Involvement of patient in decision making process
            - Encourage and facilitate patient involvement and leadership in treatment decisions
        - Intent for patient to have palliative care
        - Educate parents about the stages of development and how they relate to the dying adolescent's needs
        - Acknowledgement of potential emotions and grieving process the patient, family and staff may experience
        - Discuss how combative, complaining, and resistive behavior will be managed. Explain never punitive to patient or family, but supportive and understanding of needs of patient and family
- Provide the family and patient with a written copy of your philosophy of care.
- Have every member of family sign off that you have reviewed this philosophy with them

Appreciation of adolescent consent and assent concepts is important as well as encouraging optimal functioning on the youth's part when this is possible. The hospital staff should seek to engage this maturing teen as an active partner in treatment options while minimizing youth dependence and functional impairments to the extent possible. The direct purpose is to promote normal adolescence that is realistic to promote independence, self-care, and mobility. Realistic measures to promote socialization, ongoing education, and compensatory activities are needed. Hope for improvement should be offered when circumstances warrant while effective as well as prompt pain relief is always an essential part of the overall management plan. If the youth is in a true dying state, concerns of addiction to pain medications should be avoided.

Frank and open inter-staff meetings are essential to allow the development of these overall goals. A healthy exchange of ideals and feelings is essential for all staff members involved in the care of this patient and family. A closely coordinated team is ideal for this emotional and difficult situation. Problem-solving conferences are critical and can be held as often as necessary—weekly or even daily. For example, it is important to recognize who will identify various important parts of the management plan to the patient and family in addition to when and where this will occur. Sometimes the patient and/or family will choose who(m) this should be such as a nurse or clinician specialist who sees them on a regular basis and with whom trust has been established.

Allow ventilation of staff feelings and review of how both the patient and family are doing. Confusion or disagreement over management goals and implementation should be cleared up and unified. Confusion with regard to overall prognosis should be avoided. The team conference can review a management plan to deal with the totality of the patient's and family's needs. Failure to share issues with critical staff members leads to isolation of some staff from management issues, causes blurred roles, and can lead to inappropriate responses or conflicting messages given to the teen and family.

Team leaders and nurse managers must remember that in most situations, the patient's primary care clinician will not be involved in the hospitalized care of this patient (40). Having HCPs who are not thoroughly cognizant of this patient and family can be challenging to the overall management plan, especially for clinicians who are around sporadically during a "shift-work" employment program. One manner to address this problem is to post the philosophy, treatment plan, and agreements in the patient's chart. Another technique is to ask the dying adolescent and his or her parents to a) sign a release of information for the PCP and his or her practice b) with the intent of keeping that person or group updated on the patient's care plan. Once this is obtained, as events and care plan change, the PCP (and practice) should be informed.

CONCLUSION

Caring for a dying child or adolescent is an emotional roller coaster for the patient, family, health care professionals and the hospital staff. The role of clinicians in this arena has been debated for decades and this includes helping the dying person maintain one's dignity and comfort (41-43). Though some die at home, others will die or spend much of their dying state in the hospital milieu, often the pediatric intensive care unit for adolescents (44). These issues involve children and youth around the world (45, 46). Some focus on the cost of dying while others focus on ethical issues that are involved (47, 48). The need for training in this arena is currently acklowedged (49).

What we know in the 21st century is that these patients deserve the human right of a dignified, tranquil, pain-free passing. They deserve health care professionals and hospital or hospice staff who are dedicated to their care and are willing to provide a unified message of care and professionalism under the most trying of circumstances.

It is most useful to have an understanding of how the Kübler-Ross stages of grief can affect all who are involved. Issues of thanatophobia by all concerned should be understood as well as concepts of brain injury induced by illness and the dying process (51-53). Frequent meetings are recommended for members of the hospital staff to identify barriers and obstacles that involve the patient, the family, and/or staff.

It is not recommended that health care professionals or staff isolate this precious and vulnerable patient simply because the patient is perceived as a "failure"—i.e., beyond the control of those feeling they are omniscient, fee-for-profit, work shift-based health care providers. We should reassure the parents that they remained loving parents of their cherished child even to death and allow this child or adolescent to remain captain of his or her fate right to the end of life (54, 55).

> Beyond this place of wrath and tears
> Looms but the horror of the shade,
> And yet the menace of the years
> Finds, and shall find, me unafraid.
>
> It matters not how strait the gate,
> How charged with punishments the scroll,
> I am the master of my fate:
> I am the captain of my soul
>
> (William Ernest Henley, 1849-1903, Invictus)

REFERENCES

[1] Sarwar SR, Mangewala V, Baron R. Helping the angels: a review of understanding and helping dying children. Innov Clin Neurosci 2013;10(3):31-4.
[2] Freyer DR. Care of the dying adolescent: Special considerations. Pediatrics 2004;113(2):381-8.
[3] Greydanus DE. Overview on adolescence. In: Greydanus DE, Patel DR, Omar HA, Feucht C, Merrick J, eds. Adolescent medicine: Pharmacotherapeutics in general, medical, and sexual health. Berlin: De Gruyter, 2012:9-31.
[4] Hofmann AD, Becker RD, Gabriel HP. The hospitalized adolescent. A guide to Managing the ill and injured. New York: Free Press, 1976.
[5] Kübler-Ross E. On death and dying. Abingdon, UK: Routledge, 1969.
[6] Kübler-Ross E. On grief and grieving: Finding the meaning of grief through the five stages of loss. New York: Simon Schuster, 2005.
[7] Konigsberg RD. New ways to think about grief: As the nation mourns those killed in Tucson, a new look at the science of loss shows we're more resilient than we thought. TIME 2011 Jan 29.
[8] Erickson EH. Identity, youth and crisis, New York: WW Norton, 1968.
[9] Piaget J. Intellectual evaluation from adolescence to adulthood. Hum Dev 1972;15:1-12.
[10] King A. Adolescence. In: Lewis M, ed. Child and adolescent psychiatry. A comprehensive textbook, 3rd ed. Philadelphia, PA: Lippincott Williams Wilkins, 2002:332-42.
[11] Polikoff LA, McCabe ME. End-of-life care in the pediatric ICU. Curr Opin Pediatr 2013;25(3):285-9.
[12] Sigman GS, O'Connor C. Exploration of physicians of the mature minor doctrine. J Pediatr 1991;119:520-5.
[13] Lyren A, Silber TJ. Consent, confidentiality in the care of adolescents. In: Greydanus DE, Patel DR, Pratt HD, eds. Essential adolescent medicine. New York: McGraw-Hill, 2006:29-42.
[14] McDonnell WM. Adolescent health care. In: Donn SM, eds. Medicallegal issues in pediatrics. Elk Grove Village: IL: American Academy of Pediatrics, 2012:131-30.
[15] Lyon ME, Jacobs S, Briggs L, Cheng YI, Wang J. Family-centered advance care planning for teens with cancer. JAMA Pediatr 2013; 167(5):460-7.

[16] Traugott I, Alpers A. In their own hands: adolescents' refusal of medical treatment. Arch Pediatr Adolesc Med 1997;151:922-7.

[17] Moreno J, Schonberg K. Case four: saying "no" to treatment in terminal illness. In: Blustein J, Levine C, Dubler N, eds. The adolescent alone: Decision making in health care in the United States. Cambridge, UK: Cambridge University Press, 1999:205-11.

[18] Easson WM. The seriously ill or dying adolescent: special needs and challenges. Postgrad Med 1995;78:183-4,187-9.

[19] Weir RF, Peters C. Affirming the decisions adolescents make about life and death. Hastings Cent Rep 1997;27:29-40.

[20] Nuss SL. Redefining parenthood: surviving the death of a child. Cancer Nurs 2014;37(1):E51-60.

[21] Kraus IVV. Do they play Bach in heaven? Am J Hosp Palliat Care 2013 Jul 26.

[22] Wiener L, McConnell DG, Latella L, Ludi E. Cultural and religious considerations in pediatric palliative care. Palliat Support Care 2013; 11(1):47-67.

[23] Cook KA, Mott S, Lawrence P, Jablonki J, Grady MR, Norton D, et al. Coping while caring for the dying child: nurses' experiences in an acute care setting. J Pediatr Nurs 2012;27(4):e11-21.

[24] Leikin S. A proposal concerning decisions to forgo life-sustaining treatment for young people. J Pediatr 1989;115:17-22.

[25] Freyer DR. Children with cancer: special considerations in the discontinuation of life-ustaining treatment. Med Pediatr Oncol 1992;20:136-42.

[26] Doyle L, Henning P. Stopping treatment for end-stage-renal failure: the rights of children and adolescents. J Pediatr Nephrol 1994;8:768-91.

[27] Robinson WM, Ravilly S, Berde C, Wohl ME. End-of-life care in cystic fibrosis. Pediatrics 1997;100:205-9.

[28] Committee on Bioethics and Committee on Hospital Care. American Academy of Pediatrics. Palliative care for children. Pediatrics 2000;106(2):351-7.

[29] Freyer DR, Kuperberg A, Sterken DJ, Pastyrnak SL, Hudson DR, Richards T. Multi-disciplinary care of the dying adolescent. Child Adolesc Psychiatr North Am 2006;15(3):693-715.

[30] Flavelle SC. Experience of an adolescent living with and dying of cancer. Arch Pediatr Adolesc Med 2011;165(1):28-32.

[31] Van der Geest IM, Darlington AS, Streng IC, Michiels EM, Peiters R, van den Heuvel- Elbring MM. Parents' experiences of pediatric palliative care and the impact on long-term parental grief. J Pain Symptom Manage 2013 Oct 9. Pii. S0885-3924 (13)00471-5. doi: 10.1016/jpainsymman.2013.07.007.

[32] Waldman E, Wolfe J. Palliative care for children with cancer. Nat Rev Clin Oncol 2013;10(2):100-7.

[33] Bricker LA, Kinzbrunner BM, Kavanaugh KJ, Greydanus DE. Nutrients and fluids at the end of life: physiologic and ethical guideposts over uncertain terrain. Int J Disabil Human Dev 2012;11:123-35.

[34] Tisdale MJ. Mechanisms of cancer cachexia. Physiol Rev 2009;89: 381-5.

[35] Walter JK, Rosenberg AR, Feudtner C. Tackling taboo topics: How to have effective advanced care planning decisions with adolescents and young adults with cancer. JAMA Pediatr 2013;167(8):693-95.

[36] Youngblut JM, Brooten D. Perinatal and pediatric issues in palliative and end-of-life care from the 2011 Summit on the Science of Compassion. Nurs Outlook 2012;60(6):343-50.

[37] McGraw SA, Truog RD, Solomon MZ, Cohen-Bearak A, Sellers DE, Meyer EC. "I was able to still be her mom"—parenting at end of life in the pediatric intensive care unit. Pediatr Crit Care Med 2012;13(6): e350-6.

[38] Savulescu J. Just dying: the futility of futility. J Med Ethics 2013;39(9):583-4.

[39] MacDonald F. Care of the dying adolescent. Can Fam Physician 1979;25:1090-1.

[40] Goldstein R, Rimer KP. Parents' views of their child's end-of-life care: subanalysis of primary care involvement. J Palliat Med 2013;16(2):198-202.

[41] Fraenkel M. Medical attendance during terminal illness. Am J Public Health Nations Health 1948;38(7):970-6.

[42] 42 Sahu S, Nag DA, Swain A, Samaddar DP. Biochemical changes in the injuried brain. World J Biol Chem 2017;8(1):21-31.

[43] Albert RH. End-of-life care: managing common symptoms. Am Fam Physician 2017;95(6):356-361.

[44] Baralatei FT, Ackermann RJ. Care of patients at the end of life: management of non-pain symptoms. FP Essent 2016;447:18-24.

[45] Carey EC, Dose AM, Humeniuk KM, Kuan YC, Hicks AD, Ottenberg AL, et al. The experience of hospital death. Am J Hosp Palliat Care 2017 Jan 1:1049909116689547. doi: 10.1177/1049909116689547.

[46] Snaman JM, Kaye EC, Lu JJ, Sykes A, Baker JN. Palliative care involvement is associated with less intensive end-of-life care in adolescents and young adult oncology patients. J Palliat Med 2017 Jan 18. doi: 10.1089/jpm.2016.0451.

[47] Chong LA, Khalid F, Khoo TB, Teh SH, Kuan GL, Aina Mariana AM, ete al. Clinical spectrum of children receiving palliative care in Malaysian hospitals. Med J Malaysia 2017;72(1):32-36.

[48] Trachtenberg AJ, Manns B. Cost analysis of medical assistance in dying in Canada. CMAJ 2017;189(3):E101-E105. doi: 10.1503/cmaj.160650.

[49] van Nistelrooij I, Visse M, Spekkink A, de Lange J. How shared is decision-making? A care-ethical view of role of partner and family. J Med Ethics Mar 29. pii: medethics-2016-103791. doi: 10.1136/medethics-2016-103791.

[50] Miranda SP. Learning to drive—early exposure to end-of-life conversations in medical training. N Engl J Med 2017;376(5):413-415.

[51] Eskola K, Bergstraesser E, Zimmermann K, Cignacco E. Maintaining family life balance while facing a child's imminent death—a mixed methods study. J Adv Nur 2017 Mar 22. doi: 10.1111/jan.13304.

[52] McConnell T, Porter S. The experience of providing end of life care at a children's hospice: A qualitative study. BMC Palliat Care 2017;16(1):15. doi: 10.1186/s12904-017-0189-9.

[53] Clark K. Care at the very end-of-life:dying cancer patients and their chosen family's needs. Cancers (Basel) 2017;9(2):11. pii: E11. doi: 10.3390/cancers9020011.

[54] Lee MK, Yun YH. Family functioning predicts end-of-life care quality in patients with cancer: Multicenter prospective cohort study. Cancer Nurs 2017 Apr 20. doi: 10.1097/NCC.0000000000000495.

[55] Blanke C, LeBlanc M, Heshman D, Ellis L, Meyskens F. Characterizing 18 years of the Death with Dignity act in Oregon. JAMA Oncol 2017 Apr 6. doi: 10.1001/jamaoncol.2017.0243.

[56] Hartogh GD. Suffering and dying well: On the proper aim of palliative care. Med Health Care Philos 2017 Apr 3. doi: 10.1007/s11019-017-9764-3.

SECTION 3: ACKNOWLEDGMENTS

In: Chronic Disease and Disability
Editors: DE Greydanus, P Anne, JD Rowlett et al.
ISBN: 978-1-53617-656-8

Chapter 21

ABOUT THE EDITORS

Donald E Greydanus, MD, DrHC(Athens), FAAP, FIAP (HON) is Professor and Founding Chair of the Department of Pediatric and Adolescent Medicine, as well as Pediatrics Program Director at the Western Michigan University Homer Stryker MD School of Medicine (WMED), Kalamazoo, Michigan, USA. He is also Clinical Professor of Pediatrics and Human Development at Michigan State University College of Human Medicine (Grand Rapids & East Lansing, Michigan, USA). He is a 2017 Mayo Clinic Distinguished Alumnus (Rochester, Minnesota, USA). Received the 1995 American Academy of Pediatrics' Adele D. Hofmann Award for "Distinguished Contributions in Adolescent Health", the 2000 Mayo Clinic Pediatrics Honored Alumnus Award for "National Contributions to the field of Pediatrics," and the 2003 William B Weil, Jr., MD Endowed Distinguished Pediatric Faculty Award from Michigan State University College of Medicine for "National and international recognition as well as exemplary scholarship in pediatrics." Received the 2004 Charles R Drew School of Medicine (Los Angeles, CA) Stellar Award for contributions to pediatric resident education and awarded an honorary membership in the Indian Academy of Pediatrics—an honor granted to only a few pediatricians outside of India. Was the 2007-2010 Visiting Professor of Pediatrics at Athens University, Athens, Greece and received the Michigan State University College of Human Medicine Outstanding Community Faculty Award in 2008. In 2010 he received the title of Doctor Honoris Causa from the University of Athens (Greece) as a "distinguished scientist who through outstanding work has bestowed praise and credit on the field of adolescent medicine (Ephebiatrics)." In 2010 he received the Outstanding Achievement in Adolescent Medicine Award from the Society for Adolescent Medicine "as a leading force in the field of adolescent medicine and health." In 2014 he was selected by the American Medical Association as AMA nominee for the ACGME Pediatrics Residency Review Committee (RRC) in Chicago, Illinois, USA. Past Chair of the National Conference and Exhibition Planning Group (Committee on Scientific Meetings) of the American Academy of Pediatrics and member of the Pediatric Academic Societies' (SPR/PAS) Planning Committee (1998 to Present). In 2011 elected to The Alpha Omega Alpha Honor Society (Faculty member) at Michigan State University College of Human Medicine, East Lansing, Michigan. Former member of the Appeals Committee for the Pediatrics' Residency Review Committee (RRC) of the Accreditation Council for Graduate Medical Education (Chicago, IL) in both adolescent medicine and general pediatrics. Numerous publications in adolescent health and lectureships in many countries on adolescent health. Email: donald.greydanus@med.wmich.edu

Premchand Anne, MD, MPH, MBA, FAAP, FACP, FACC is a Clinical Assistant Professor in the Department of Pediatrics at Wayne State University of School of Medicine, Detroit, Michigan, USA and Clinical Associate Professor in the Department of Pediatrics at Michigan State University College of Osteopathic Medicine, East Lansing, Michigan, USA. He is the director of the Division of Pediatric Cardiology and pediatric residency program director at Ascension St. John Children's Hospital, Detroit, Michigan, USA. His clinical practice involves care of pediatric patients with congenital and acquired cardiovascular disorders, adult patients with congenital heart disease, and pediatric and adult patients with dyslipidemias. Dr Anne participates in multidisciplinary pediatric and adult clinics. Dr Anne graduated from Wayne State University School of Medicine with a Doctor of Medicine in 2002. He completed a combined internal medicine/pediatrics residency at the Detroit Medical Center, Detroit, Michigan in 2006 and completed a pediatric cardiology fellowship at Children's Hospital of Michigan in 2009. Thereafter, he joined Ascension St John Children's Hospital as faculty in the Department of Pediatrics and later as faulty in the Department of Internal Medicine at Ascension St John Hospital. During medical school, Dr. Anne was able to complete a Masters in Public Health from University of Michigan School of Public Health, Ann Arbor, Michigan in 2002. He also completed a Masters in Business Administration at Walsh College of Business and Accountancy, Troy, Michigan in 2015. Dr. Anne has served as a consultant to the Pediatric Advisory Committee and currently serves as a member of the Pediatric Advisory Committee for the Office of Pediatric Therapeutics at the United States Food and Drug Administration. Email: Premchand.anne@ascension.org.

John D Rowlett, MD, FAAP, FACP, is a Professor of Pediatrics at the Medical College of Georgia (Augusta) and Eastern Kentucky University (Richmond). Dr Rowlett was born in Richmond, Kentucky where he attended Model Laboratory School before matriculating to Eastern Kentucky University. He attended the University of Kentucky College Of Medicine and completed a combined residency in Internal Medicine and Pediatrics at what is now the Homer Stryker College of Medicine at Western Michigan University in Kalamazoo, Michigan. Upon completion of his residency, Dr Rowlett served as Chief Resident in Internal Medicine and then completed a fellowship in Adolescent Medicine under Dr. Donald Greydanus (also at Western Michigan University). During his chief residency and fellowship, Dr Rowlett served as an attending in the pediatric critical care unit at Bronson Methodist Hospital. Upon completion of his fellowship, Dr Rowlett accepted a position at the Children's Hospital at Memorial Medical Center in Savannah, Georgia where he established the division of adolescent medicine in addition to serving as an attending in the general pediatric and internal medicine clinics, the pediatric emergency room, and the pediatric critical care unit. While at Memorial Dr Rowlett served on local, regional, state, and national committees focusing on adolescents and injury prevention. In 2000, Dr Rowlett accepted a position with Georgia Emergency Associates and has been the director of pediatric emergency medicine for the past 15 years. In this capacity, Dr Rowlett oversees pediatric emergency care for three hospitals with a combined annual census of nearly 200,000 visits. In 2017, Dr Rowlett established the inpatient pediatric hospital medicine service at St Joseph's/Candler. Dr Rowlett has published extensively in the fields of emergency medicine, injury prevention, general pediatrics, adolescent medicine, and medical essays. He and his wife Sharon have three children. Dr Rowlett has played competitive tennis for nearly 50 years and continues to do so in his spare time. Email: drrowlett@gmail.com

Joav Merrick, MD, MMedSci, DMSc, born and educated in Denmark is professor of pediatrics, child health and human development, Division of Pediatrics, Hadassah Hebrew University Medical Center, Mt Scopus Campus, Jerusalem, Israel and Kentucky Children's Hospital, University of Kentucky, Lexington, Kentucky United States and professor of public health at the Center for Healthy Development, School of Public Health, Georgia State University, Atlanta, United States, the former medical director of the Health Services, Division for Intellectual and Developmental Disabilities, Ministry of Social Affairs and Social Services, Jerusalem, the founder and director of the National Institute of Child Health and Human Development in Israel. Numerous publications in the field of pediatrics, child health and human development, rehabilitation, intellectual disability, disability, health, welfare, abuse, advocacy, quality of life and prevention. Received the Peter Sabroe Child Award for outstanding work on behalf of Danish Children in 1985 and the International LEGO-Prize ("The Children's Nobel Prize") for an extraordinary contribution towards improvement in child welfare and well-being in 1987. In 2017 appointed a Kentucky Colonel by the Commonwealth of Kentucky, the highest honor the governor can bestow to a person. Email: jmerrick@zahav.net.il

In: Chronic Disease and Disability
Editors: DE Greydanus, P Anne, JD Rowlett et al.
ISBN: 978-1-53617-656-8

Chapter 22

About the Department of Pediatric and Adolescent Medicine, Western Michigan University Homer Stryker MD School of Medicine (WMed), Kalamazoo, Michigan, United States

Mission and service

The Western Michigan University Homer Stryker MD School of Medicine was started in 2012 and its first class of medical students began in 2014. The Department of Pediatric and Adolescent Medicine has a pediatric residency program which is accredited by the Accreditation Council for Graduate Medical Education (ACGME) in Chicago, Illinois, USA and the current residency program in Pediatrics started in 1990.

The WMed Department of Pediatric and Adolescent Medicine has a commitment to a comprehensive approach to the health and development of the child, adolescent, and the family. The Department has a blend of academic general pediatricians and pediatric specialists. Our academic pediatric practice provides a broad spectrum of general well and sick child care (birth through 21 years) including immunizations, monitoring general physical and emotional growth, motor skill development, sports medicine (including participation evaluations and evaluation of common sports injuries), child abuse evaluations, and psychosocial or behavioral assessment. WMed Pediatrics believes in immunizations as a protection against preventative disease processes. WMed is recognized as a Patient-Centered Medical Home (PCMH) model of care delivery. A PCMH is a way to deliver coordinated and comprehensive primary care to our infants, children, adolescents and young adults. It is a partnership between individuals and families within a health care setting, which allows for a more efficient use of resources and time to improve the quality of outcomes for all involved through care provided by a continuity care team.

Research activities

The Department has a variety of research projects in adolescent medicine, neurobehavioral pediatrics, adolescent gynecology, pediatric diabetes mellitus, asthma, and cystic fibrosis. The WMed Department of Pediatric and Adolescent Medicine has published a number of medical textbooks: Essential adolescent medicine (McGraw-Hill Medical Publishers), The pediatric diagnostic examination (McGraw-Hill), Pediatric and adolescent psychopharmacology (Cambridge University Press), Behavioral pediatrics, through 4th Edition, Nova Science, New York, Pediatric practice: Sports medicine (McGraw-Hill), Handbook of clinical pediatrics (Singapore: World Scientific), Neurodevelopmental disabilities: Clinical care for children and young adults (Dordrecht: Springer), Adolescent medicine: Pharmacotherapeutics in medical disorders (Berlin/Boston: De Gruyter), Adolescent medicine: Pharmacotherapeutics in general, mental, and sexual health (Berlin/Boston: De Gruyter), Pediatric psychodermatology (Berlin/Boston: De Gruyter), Substance abuse in adolescents and young adults: A manual for pediatric and primary care clinicians (Berlin/Boston: De Gruyter), and tropical pediatrics (New York: Nova); Second edition in press.

The Department has edited a number of journal issues published by Elsevier Publishers covering pulmonology (State of the Art Reviews: Adolescent Medicine—AM:STARS), genetic disorders in adolescents (AM:STARS), neurologic/neurodevelopmental disorders (AM:STARS), behavioral pediatrics (Pediatric Clinics of North America), pediatric psychopharmacology in the 21st century (Pediatric Clinic of North America), nephrologic disorders in adolescents (AM:STARS), college health (Pediatric Clinics of North America), adolescent medicine (Primary Care: Clinics in Office Practice), behavioral pediatrics in children and adolescents (Primary Care: Clinics in Office Practice), adolescents and sports (Pediatric Clinics of North America), and developmental disabilities (Pediatric Clinics of North America). The Department has also edited a journal issue on musculoskeletal disorders in children and adolescents for the American Academy of Pediatrics' AM:STARs; in April of 2013 a Subspecialty Update issue was published in AM:STARs.

The department has developed academic ties with a variety of international medical centers and organizations, including the Queen Elizabeth Hospital in Hong Kong, Indian Academy of Pediatrics (New Delhi, India), the University of Athens Children's Hospital (First and Second Departments of Paediatrics) in Athens, Greece and the National Institute of Child Health and Human Development in Jerusalem, Israel.

Contact

Professor and Chair, Dilip R Patel, MD
and Professor and Founding Chair Donald E Greydanus, MD
Department of Pediatric and Adolescent Medicine
Western Michigan University Homer Stryker MD School of Medicine
1000 Oakland Drive, D48G, Kalamazoo, MI 49008-1284, United States of America
E-mail: Donald.greydanus@med.wmich.edu and dilip.Patel@med.wmich.edu
Website: http://www.med.wmich.edu

In: Chronic Disease and Disability
Editors: DE Greydanus, P Anne, JD Rowlett et al.
ISBN: 978-1-53617-656-8

Chapter 23

About the Department of Pediatrics, Ascension St John Children's Hospital, Detroit, Michigan, United States

Mission and service

The Ascension St John Children's Hospital (ASJCH) is a hospital within a hospital. The Department of Pediatrics has a pediatric residency program that has been accredited by the Accreditation Council of Graduate Medical Education (ACGME), Chicago, Illinois, USA. The pediatric residency program has been in existence since 1973.

The mission of ASJCH's Department of Pediatrics incorporates attention to the comprehensive care of all pediatric patients (birth through 21 years), with particular attention to the poor and vulnerable children, through the designation of a Patient-Centered Medical Home (PCMH). The Department of Pediatrics is composed of general pediatricians and subspecialists, who provide a broad range of expertise to address the concerns of the pediatric patients. The faculty within the Department of Pediatrics is also tasked with training pediatric residents into competent pediatricians first and foremost, and to be successful general pediatricians or prepare them for pediatric subspecialty training. The pediatric faculty has clinical appointments and are affiliated with Wayne State University School of Medicine, Michigan State University College of Osteopathic Medicine, Central Michigan University College of Medicine, and St. George's University School of Medicine.

Research activities

The faculty in the Department of Pediatrics is involved in quality-improvement and research projects, very often with a pediatric resident as the principal investigator. The Department is involved in studies focused on various topics including echocardiogram yields, aortopathies, juvenile-onset diabetes mellitus and endocrinopathies, dyslipidemia screening and management, Crohn's and ulcerative colitis, celiac disease, and neonatal outcomes. The faculty has published a number of journal articles and book chapters pertaining to pediatric care.

Contact

Department Chair Muthayipalayam Thirumoorthi, MD
Department of Pediatrics
Ascension St John Children's Hospital
22151 Moross Road, Suite 222, PB II, Detroit, MI 48236, United States of America
E-mail: Muthayipalayam.Thirumoorthi@ascension.org
Website: https://healthcare.ascension.org/Locations/Michigan/MIDET/Detroit-Ascension-St-John-Childrens-Hospital-at-22201-Moross-Rd

In: Chronic Disease and Disability
Editors: DE Greydanus, P Anne, JD Rowlett et al.
ISBN: 978-1-53617-656-8

Chapter 24

About the National Institute of Child Health and Human Development in Israel

The National Institute of Child Health and Human Development (NICHD) in Israel was established in 1998 as a virtual institute under the auspices of the Medical Director, Ministry of Social Affairs and Social Services in order to function as the research arm for the Office of the Medical Director. In 1998 the National Council for Child Health and Pediatrics, Ministry of Health and in 1999 the Director General and Deputy Director General of the Ministry of Health endorsed the establishment of the NICHD.

Mission

The mission of a National Institute for Child Health and Human Development in Israel is to provide an academic focal point for the scholarly interdisciplinary study of child life, health, public health, welfare, disability, rehabilitation, intellectual disability and related aspects of human development. This mission includes research, teaching, clinical work, information and public service activities in the field of child health and human development.

Service and academic activities

Over the years many activities became focused in the south of Israel due to collaboration with various professionals at the Faculty of Health Sciences (FOHS) at the Ben Gurion University of the Negev (BGU). Since 2000 an affiliation with the Zusman Child Development Center at the Pediatric Division of Soroka University Medical Center has resulted in collaboration around the establishment of the Down Syndrome Clinic at that center. In 2002 a full course on “Disability” was established at the Recanati School for Allied Professions in the Community, FOHS, BGU and in 2005 collaboration was started with the Primary Care Unit of the faculty and disability became part of the master of public health course on “Children and society”. In the academic year 2005-2006 a one semester course on “Aging with disability” was started as part of the master of science program in gerontology in our collaboration with the Center for Multidisciplinary Research in Aging. In 2010 collaborations with the Division of Pediatrics,

Hadassah Hebrew University Medical Center, Jerusalem, Israel around the National Down Syndrome Center and teaching students and residents about intellectual and developmental disabilities as part of their training at this campus.

Research activities

The affiliated staff have over the years published work from projects and research activities in this national and international collaboration. In the year 2000 the International Journal of Adolescent Medicine and Health and in 2005 the International Journal on Disability and Human Development of De Gruyter Publishing House (Berlin and New York) were affiliated with the National Institute of Child Health and Human Development. From 2008 also the International Journal of Child Health and Human Development (Nova Science, New York), the International Journal of Child and Adolescent Health (Nova Science) and the Journal of Pain Management (Nova Science) affiliated and from 2009 the International Public Health Journal (Nova Science) and Journal of Alternative Medicine Research (Nova Science). All peer-reviewed international journals.

National collaborations

Nationally the NICHD works in collaboration with the Faculty of Health Sciences, Ben Gurion University of the Negev; Department of Physical Therapy, Sackler School of Medicine, Tel Aviv University; Autism Center, Assaf HaRofeh Medical Center; National Rett and PKU Centers at Chaim Sheba Medical Center, Tel HaShomer; Department of Physiotherapy, Haifa University; Department of Education, Bar Ilan University, Ramat Gan, Faculty of Social Sciences and Health Sciences; College of Judea and Samaria in Ariel and in 2011 affiliation with Center for Pediatric Chronic Diseases and National Center for Down Syndrome, Department of Pediatrics, Hadassah Hebrew University Medical Center, Mount Scopus Campus, Jerusalem.

International collaborations

Internationally with the Department of Disability and Human Development, College of Applied Health Sciences, University of Illinois at Chicago; Strong Center for Developmental Disabilities, Golisano Children's Hospital at Strong, University of Rochester School of Medicine and Dentistry, New York; Centre on Intellectual Disabilities, University of Albany, New York; Centre for Chronic Disease Prevention and Control, Health Canada, Ottawa; Chandler Medical Center and Children's Hospital, Kentucky Children's Hospital, Section of Adolescent Medicine, University of Kentucky, Lexington; Chronic Disease Prevention and Control Research Center, Baylor College of Medicine, Houston, Texas; Division of Neuroscience, Department of Psychiatry, Columbia University, New York; Institute for the Study of Disadvantage and Disability, Atlanta; Center for Autism and Related Disorders, Department Psychiatry, Children's Hospital Boston, Boston; Department of Pediatric and Adolescent Medicine, Western Michigan University Homer Stryker MD School of Medicine,

Kalamazoo, Michigan, United States; Department of Paediatrics, Child Health and Adolescent Medicine, Children's Hospital at Westmead, Westmead, Australia; International Centre for the Study of Occupational and Mental Health, Düsseldorf, Germany; Centre for Advanced Studies in Nursing, Department of General Practice and Primary Care, University of Aberdeen, Aberdeen, United Kingdom; Quality of Life Research Center, Copenhagen, Denmark; Nordic School of Public Health, Gottenburg, Sweden, Scandinavian Institute of Quality of Working Life, Oslo, Norway; The Department of Applied Social Sciences (APSS) of The Hong Kong Polytechnic University Hong Kong.

Targets

Our focus is on research, international collaborations, clinical work, teaching and policy in health, disability and human development and to establish the NICHD as a permanent institute in Israel.

Contact

Professor Joav Merrick, MD, MMedSci, DMSc
National Institute of Child Health and Human Development, Jerusalem, Israel.
Email: jmerrick@zahav.net.il

SECTION 4: INDEX

INDEX OF NAMES

K

L

M

N

O

P

R

S

T

W

INDEX OF TERMS

#

A

B

C

D

E

F

G

H

I

K

L

M

N

O

P

Q

R

S

T

U

V

W

X

Y

Z